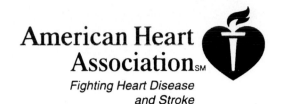

American Heart
Association℠

*Fighting Heart Disease
and Stroke*

Monograph Series

INVASIVE CARDIOLOGY

*Current Diagnostic
and Therapeutic Issues*

Previously published:

Cardiovascular Applications of Magnetic Resonance
Edited by Gerald M. Pohost, MD

Cardiovascular Reponse to Exercise
Edited by Gerald F. Fletcher, MD

Congestive Heart Failure: Current Clinical Issues
Edited by Gemma T. Kennedy, RN, PhD,
and Michael H. Crawford, MD

Atrial Arrhythmias: State of the Art
Edited by John P. DiMarco, MD, PhD
and Eric N. Prystowsky, MD

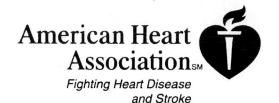

American Heart
Association℠
*Fighting Heart Disease
and Stroke*

Monograph Series

INVASIVE CARDIOLOGY

Current Diagnostic and Therapeutic Issues

Edited by

George W. Vetrovec, MD

*Professor of Medicine,
Associate Chairman of Medicine,
Medical College of Virginia,
Richmond, Virginia*

and

Blase A. Carabello, MD

*Professor of Medicine,
Cardiology Division and the Gazes Cardiac Research Institute,
Medical University of South Carolina and the
Ralph II. Johnson Department of Veterans Affairs,
Charleston, South Carolina*

FUTURA

Futura Publishing
Company, Inc.
Armonk, NY

Library of Congress Cataloging-in-Publication Data
Invasive cardiology : current diagnostic and therapeutic issues /
    edited by George W. Vetrovec and Blase A. Carabello.
        p.   cm. — (American Heart Association monograph series)
    Includes bibliographical references and index.
    ISBN 0-87993-608-8
    1. Heart—Diseases—Treatment.   2. Heart—Diseases—Diag-
nosis.   I. Vetrovec, George W.,   1943–   II. Carabello, Blase A.
III. American Heart Association.   IV. Series.
    [DNLM: 1. Cardiovascular Diseases—diagnosis—congresses.
2. Cardiovascular Diseases—therapy—congresses.   3. Cardiology—methods—congresses.   WG 120 I62 1995]
RC683.8.I63   1995
6174′1059—dc20
DNLM/DLC
for Library of Congress   94-44643
                                                                                    CIP

Published by
Futura Publishing Company
135 Bedford Road
Armonk, New York 10504

LC #: 94-44643
ISBN #: 0-87993-608-8

Preface

The advent of modern cardiology is associated with a number technological advances, particularly involving invasive diagnostic and therapeutic techniques. Early invasive techniques were pioneered by Werner Forssmann and Andre Cournaud for right heart catheterization. The development of selective coronary angiography by Mason Sones and Melvin Judkins represented another major breakthrough. The composite of these pioneering activities led to improved anatomic, hemodynamic, and physiologic understanding of normal and diseased cardiac states. These foundations led to the recognition that invasive cardiac strategies were feasible and important for diagnostic, and potentially, for therapeutic applications.

In 1977, encouraged by the early revascularization experiments of Dotter and Judkins, Dr. Andreas Gruentzig performed the first coronary balloon angioplasty. The subsequent evolution of nonsurgical revascularization has been dramatic, with the development of multiple technologies for lesion modification. The practicing cardiology community has applied these techniques widely with a resulting explosion of invasive procedures, yielding significant clinical benefits. While the early success and excitement of these technologies has stimulated further development, evaluation of appropriate applications of these techniques continues.

Despite all of the knowledge, experience, research, and clinical activities, many questions remain. For example, restenosis is a major unsolved issue. Likewise, the pathophysiology of many of these technologies remains incompletely answered, which may provide even better understanding of vascular ischemic and myocardial function. Thus, the "science" associated with the new technologies potentially extends beyond the recognized clinical utility, providing an important background of knowledge for future investigations and new therapies.

The development of this text is the work of members of the Cardiac Catheterization Committee of the American Heart Association Council of Clinical Cardiology. These experts in the field guided the editors in selecting pertinent topics and respected authorities to highlight the current state of the art of invasive cardiology. The authors have made every attempt to broadly assess issues in invasive cardiology, while at the same time striving to assemble experts to discuss the known status of various techniques

v

and devices. This text provides an excellent "snapshot" of one moment in time regarding the current state of interventional cardiology. The ensuing chapters document much of our current knowledge of invasive cardiology. While many questions remain, this information provides a sound basis for ongoing education and investigation to further refine the role of invasive cardiological techniques.

The editors of this text would like to thank all of those who contributed their time and expertise to this significant endeavor.

George W. Vetrovec, MD
Blase Carabello, MD

Contributors

Robert J. Applegate, MD Bowman Gray School of Medicine, Wake Forest University, Winston-Salem, NC

Thomas M. Bashore, MD Director of Cardiac Catheterization, Duke University Medical Center, Durham, NC

Lee N. Benson, MD Division of Cardiology, The University of Toronto School of Medicine, The Hospital for Sick Children, Toronto, Ontario, Canada

Gregory Braden, MD Bowman Gray School of Medicine, Wake Forest University, Winston-Salem, NC

Jeffrey A. Brinker, MD Division of Cardiology, Johns Hopkins University Hospital, Baltimore, MD

Robert M. Califf, MD Associate Professor of Medicine, Division of Cardiology, Department of Medicine, Duke University Medical Center, Durham, NC

Blase Carabello, MD Professor of Medicine, Cardiology Division and the Gazes Cardiac Research Institute, Medical University of South Carolina and the Ralph H. Johnson Department of Veterans Affairs, Charleston, SC

Michael J. Cowley, MD Professor of Medicine, Division of Cardiology, Medical College of Virginia, Richmond, VA

Alain Cribier, MD Centre Hospitalier et Universitaire de Rouen, Hôpital Charles Nicolle, Rouen, France

David C. Cumberland, MD Professor of Interventional Cardiology, Dept of Clinical Sciences, University of Sheffield in Sheffield, England and Consultant Cardiovascular Radiologist, Northern General Hospital Trust, Sheffield, England

Jack T. Cusma, PhD, Duke University Medical Center, Durham, NC

Ezra Deutsch, MD Assistant Professor of Medicine and Director, Cardiac Catheterization Laboratory, Temple University School of Medicine, Philadelphia, PA

John S. Douglas, Jr, MD Associate Professor of Medicine, Emory University School of Medicine and Co-Director, Cardiovascular Laboratory, Emory University Hospital, Atlanta, GA

vii

Michael C. Fishbein, MD Professor of Pathology, UCLA and Associate Pathologist, Cedars-Sinai Medical Center, Dept of Pathology & Laboratory Medicine, Los Angeles, CA

Donald F. Fortin, MD Assistant Professor of Medicine and Director of Data Management, Duke University Medical Center, Durham, NC

Mark Freed, MD William Beaumont Hospital, Royal Oak, MI

Sheldon Goldberg, MD Director, Division of Cardiology, Thomas Jefferson University Hospital, Philadelphia, PA

Thomas B. Graboys, MD Director, Lown Cardiovascular Center and Associate Clinical Professor of Medicine, Harvard Medical School, Brookline, MA

Julian Gunn, MD Cardiology Fellow, Northern General Hospital Trust, Department of Cardiology, Sheffield, England

Robert A. Harrington, MD Division of Cardiology, Duke University Medical Center, Durham, NC

John W. Hirshfeld, Jr, MD Director, Cardiac Catheterization Laboratory and Professor of Medicine, University of Pennsylvania School of Medicine, Philadelphia, PA

David R. Holmes, Jr, MD Professor of Medicine, Mayo Clinic Foundation, Rochester, NY

Jeffrey M. Isner, MD Chief of Cardiovascular Research, St. Elizabeth's Hospital of Boston, Boston, MA

Alice K. Jacobs, MD Associate Professor of Medicine, Boston University School of Medicine, and Director, Cardiac Catheterization Laboratory, Section of Cardiology, Boston University Medical Center Hospital, Boston, MA

Marianne Kearney, BS St. Elizabeth's Medical Center, Boston, MA

Morton J. Kern, MD Director, J.G. Mudd Cardiac Catheterization Laboratory, St. Louis University Hospital, St. Louis, MO

Spencer B. King, III, MD Director, Interventional Cardiology, Emory University Hospital, Atlanta, GA

Lloyd W. Klein, MD Rush-Presbyterian-St. Luke's Medical Center, Chicago, IL

Michael A. Kutcher, MD Associate Professor of Medicine and Director, Intervention Cardiology, Bowman Gray School of Medicine, Wake Forest University, Winston-Salem, NC

Larry A. Latson, MD Cleveland Clinic Foundation, Cleveland, OH

Mark A. Lawson, MD Division of Cardiovascular Disease, University of Alabama at Birmingham, Birmingham, AL

Guy Leclerc, MD Notre Dame Hospital, Cardiology Division, Montreal, Quebec, Canada

Brice Letac, MD Professeur à la Faculté de Médecine, Centre Hospitalier et Universitaire de Rouen, Hôpital Charles Nicolle, Rouen, France

William C. Little, MD Professor of Medicine and Chief of Section on Cardiology, Bowman Gray School of Medicine, Wake Forest University, Winston-Salem, NC

Frank Litvack, MD Cedars-Sinai Medical Center and Associate Professor of Medicine, UCLA School of Medicine, Los Angeles, CA

Andrew I. MacIsaac, MBBS, FRACP Center for Research in Cardiovascular Intervention, Stanford University Medical Center, Stanford, CA

Kenneth G. Morris, MD Chief of Cardiology, VA Medical Center and Assistant Clinical Professor, Duke University Medical Center, Durham, NC

Sigrid Nikol, MD Med Klinik, Klinikum Grosshadern, Munich, Germany

Robert A. O'Rourke, MD Division of Cardiology, Department of Medicine, University of Texas Health Science Center at San Antonio, San Antonio, TX

Igor F. Palacios, MD Director of Interventional Cardiology, Cardiac Catheterization Laboratories, Massachusetts General Hospital and Associate Professor of Medicine, Harvard Medical School, Boston, MA

Harry R. Phillips, III, MD Associate Professor of Medicine, Duke University Medical Center, Durham, NC

J. Geoffrey Pickering, MD, PhD University Hospital, London, Ontario, Canada

Gerald M. Pohost, MD Director, Division of Cardiovascular Disease, University of Alabama, Birmingham, AL

Eric R. Powers, MD Division of Cardiology, University of Virginia, Charlottesville, VA

Stephen R. Ramee, MD Ochsner Clinic, New Orleans, LA

Geoffrey A. Rose, MD Cardiac Ultrasound Laboratory, Massachusetts General Hospital, Boston, MA

Robert D. Safian, MD Director, Interventional Cardiology, William Beaumont Hospital, Royal Oak, MI

Robert S. Schwartz, MD Assistant Professor of Medicine, Division of Cardiovascular Diseases and Internal Medicine, Mayo Clinic and Foundation, Rochester, MN

Robert J. Siegel, MD Division of Cardiology, Cedars-Sinai Medical Center, Los Angeles, CA

Robert D. Simari, MD Assistant Professor of Medicine, Mayo Clinic, Rochester, MN

Gustavo A. Solis, MD Bowman Gray School of Medicine, Wake Forest University, Winston-Salem, NC

George Sopko, MD, MPH Division of Heart and Vascular Diseases, National Heart Lung & Blood Institutes, National Institutes of Health, Bethesda, MD

Kumar Sridhar, MD Thomas Jefferson University Hospital, Philadelphia, PA

Sanjay S. Srivatsa, MD Cardiology Fellow, Mayo Clinic, Rochester, MN

Richard S. Stack, MD Associate Professor of Medicine, Duke University Medical Center, Durham, NC

Wolfgang Steffen, MD Allgemeines Krankenhaus, Dept of Cardiology, Vienna, Austria

Carl L. Tommaso, MD Associate Professor of Medicine, School of Medicine, Northwestern University, Chicago, IL

George W. Vetrovec, MD Professor of Medicine, Associate Chairman of Medicine, Medical College of Virginia, Richmond, VA

Lawrence Weir, PhD St. Elizabeth's Medical Center, Boston, MA

Arthur E. Weyman, MD Chief, Cardiac Unit, Massachusetts General Hospital, Boston, MA

Christopher J. White, MD Director of Invasive Cardiology, Health Care International, Clydebank, Scotland

Patrick L. Whitlow, MD, FACC Director, Interventional Cardiology, Department of Cardiology, The Cleveland Clinic Foundation, Cleveland, OH

Contents

Chapter 1

Angiographic Contrast Agents:
Current Issues

Jeffrey A. Brinker, MD

Traditionally, contrast enhanced x-ray imaging of the chambers of the heart, coronary arteries, and great vessels has formed the diagnostic basis on which many prognostic and therapeutic decisions were made. With the introduction of less invasive imaging techniques, such as ultrasound, radionuclide, and magnetic resonance imaging, the need for many angiographic procedures has diminished. However, direct introduction of contrast material into the coronary arteries remains the gold standard for the delineation of coronary anatomy. No other currently available technique can portray the entire circulatory system with a similar degree of detail. While it is true that what we see is a mere anatomical "shadowgram" incapable of definitively describing the vessel lumen and wall, the angiogram would appear to supply sufficient anatomical information for clinical practice. The newer techniques of intravascular ultrasound and angioscopy can provide remarkable images that may complement but not supplant angiography. These techniques add considerable expense, are more invasive, are limited by physical constraints, and require angiographic control for proper placement. While they increase our understanding of the pathophysiology of ischemic disease and the mechanisms of coronary intervention, these techniques have not yet been shown to have the clinical applicability to justify routine use. Perhaps the greatest challenge to angiography will come from magnetic resonance imaging, the feasibility of which has recently been demonstrated.[1] Magnetic resonance imaging combines the benefits of being noninvasive as well as freedom from the toxicity of radiation. A number of constraints still apply to its use; however, the potential of this technique, which might include analysis of ventricular function as well as determination of coronary and cardiac blood flow, is intriguing.

From Vetrovec GW, Carabello BA, (eds.) *Invasive Cardiology: Current Diagnostic and Therapeutic Issues.* Armonk, NY: Futura Publishing Company, Inc.: © 1996.

Enthusiasm for coronary revascularization, both surgical and catheter based, has resulted in the rapid growth of selective coronary angiography. This technique is widely used in hospitals and nontraditional settings where it has been shown to be relatively safe and effective. Currently, some 1.4 million such procedures are performed annually in the United States; about three quarters of these are performed for diagnostic purposes while the remainder support the performance of a variety of coronary interventions. Until recently cardiologists have given little thought to the contrast media used to perform these procedures. These agents were thought to be relatively benign and because they cleared from the circulation rapidly they were not really considered drugs. The available "dyes" were inexpensive, differed little from each other, and were not heavily marketed by their manufacturers. While side effects such as hypotension and bradycardia were common, these side effects were usually transient and required little, if any, treatment. The potential for severe anaphylactoid reaction was recognized but this was uncommon, thought to be a true allergic reaction, and considered to be more a peculiarity of the patient than of the contrast media.

In the mid-1980s, alternatives to high osmolal ionic contrast became widely available in the United States. These new lower osmolal media (LOM) were soon shown to cause less hemodynamic and electrophysiologic perturbation than the traditional high osmolal ionic (HOM) agents.[2] The former were also better tolerated by patients causing less discomfort, fewer "allergic" manifestations, and less nausea and vomiting. These agents appeared ideal except for their cost, which was about 15 times more than HOM. While radiologists recognized the superiority of the nonionic media, cost limited their use.[3] This was not the case in the cardiac catheterization laboratory, however, where conversion to the nonionics was nearly universal.

Controversy continues as to the relative merits of the different contrast media. This debate has been fueled by the marketing claims of pharmaceutical companies producing LOM—the profits from which contribute greatly to their revenues. No less important, however, has been the advocacy by physicians to one or another of these products. Conflicting reports about almost every aspect of angiographic contrast have appeared in the literature. Much of this has been directed at the cardiology community, which historically has been almost oblivious to the differences between available contrast agents, not only because of the increasing angiographic volume but also because of the higher overall cost of the procedures. This higher overall cost minimizes the proportion of cost that is due to contrast. This chapter provides a perspective from which to interpret the available information.

Evolution of Contrast Agents

Within a year after the demonstration of x-ray imaging by Roentgen in 1895, experiments were conducted using radiopaque agents injected into cadaveric blood vessels. Heuser is credited with performance of the first in vivo human angiogram in 1919; he used potassium iodide to opacify the veins of an upper extremity. Subsequently many other agents, such as lipoidal, strontium bromide, thorium, and sodium iodide were used, and each found to have significant toxicity. Uroselectan, an organic iodide, was developed in 1929 for intravenous urography and found to be better tolerated than its predecessors. While a variety of similar compounds was subsequently synthesized (Iopax, Neo-Iopax, Skiodan, Diodrast, Urokon) none proved to have the success that accompanied the introduction in the 1950s of the fully substituted triiodinated benzoates.

These agents (diatrizoate, iothalamate, and metrizoate) are ionic monomers in which the organic anion is associated with a sodium or methyglucamine cation (Figure 1). In solution they yield two osmotically active particles for every three iodine atoms and are called ratio 1.5 contrast media. They have an osmolality four to six times that of plasma. While these HOM became the agents of choice for angiography and are still widely used for this purpose,

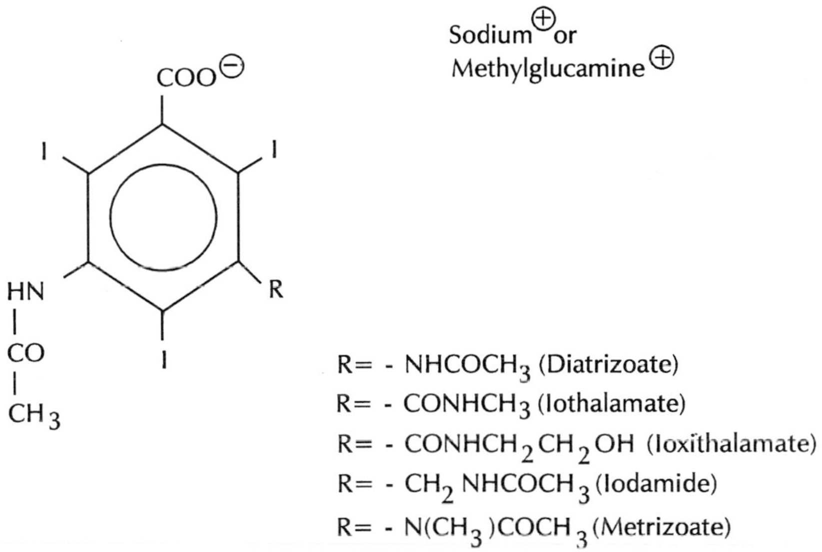
Sodium⊕ or
Methylglucamine⊕
COO⊖
I
I
HN
CO
CH3
I
R
R= - NHCOCH3 (Diatrizoate)
R= - CONHCH3 (Iothalamate)
R= - CONHCH2CH2OH (Ioxithalamate)
R= - CH2 NHCOCH3 (Iodamide)
R= - N(CH3)COCH3 (Metrizoate)

FIGURE 1. *Structure of traditional high osmolal contrast (ratio 1.5) used for cardiac angiography and consisting of triiodinated benzene anion and mixture of sodium and methylglucamine cations. The specific compound is defined by the side chain at R.*

their ionic nature and high osmolality resulted in significant toxicity. They caused pain when used for peripheral arteriography, were neurotoxic, and were associated with a variety of cardiotoxic phenomena (decreased contractility, bradyarrhythmia, and tachyarrhythmia). While some of the toxicity of HOM may be due to the specific anions and cations comprising these compounds, osmotoxicity has been considered the primary cause.

In an effort to reduce osmolality, Almen hypothesized that one could transform the ionic monomer into a nonionic monomer. This would produce a ratio 3 compound (three iodine atoms for each osmotically active particle) with essentially half the osmolality. Metrizamide was the first nonionic agent to become available, and it was rapidly adopted for myelography. Although it was shown to be useful for peripheral angiography, metrizamide never became popular with cardiologists because it was not stable in solution and had to be reconstituted from a powder prior to use. In the mid-1980s, however, two other nonionic agents (iohexol and iopamidol) that were stable in solution became available in the United States. Osmolality may also be reduced by the creation of an ionic dimer consisting of two osmotically active particles for every six iodine atoms. Such an agent, ioxaglate, was approved at the same time as the nonionic agents (Figure 2).

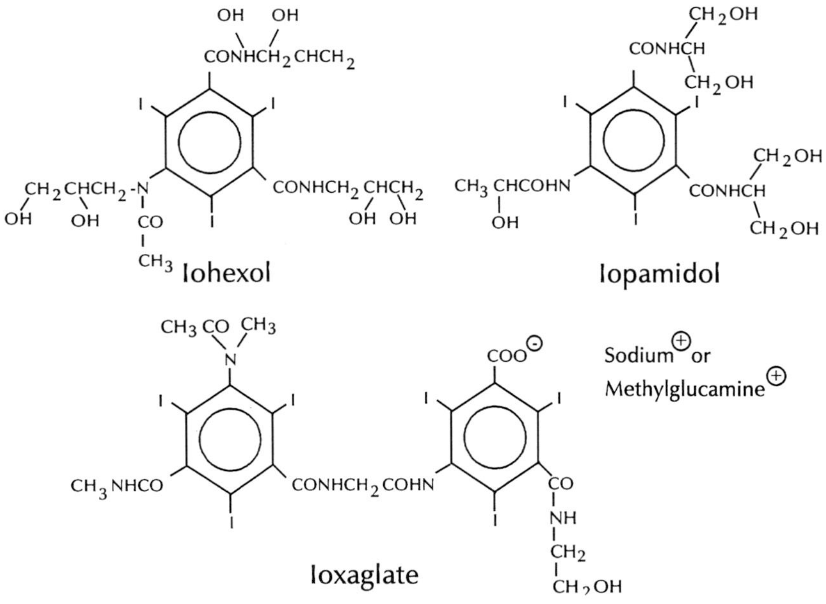

FIGURE 2. *Structures of typical ratio 3 compounds: nonionic monomers iohexol and iopamidol; ionic dimer ioxaglate.*

It should be emphasized that while the ratio 3 agents have been called low osmolal (and they are compared with the HOM), they still have about twice the osmolality of plasma. Recently, nonionic dimers were produced (Figure 3) that are ratio 6 compounds (six iodine atoms for each osmotically active particle) and may be isoosmolal or even hyposmolal to plasma. Preliminary studies using iotrolan and iodixanol in coronary angiography are under way.

The Ideal Contrast Agent

Angiographic contrast materials differ with respect to osmolality, ionicity, iodine content, additives, and viscosity (Table 1). These characteristics may influence the safety and efficacy of the agent. Cost is another differentiating factor (although there is surprisingly little variation among the expensive LOM). Based on current information, hypothetically, the ideal contrast agent would have the properties listed in Table 2. Other characteristics such as anticoagulant properties, sodium content, a prolonged intravascular presence, and the ability to adhere to the endolumi-

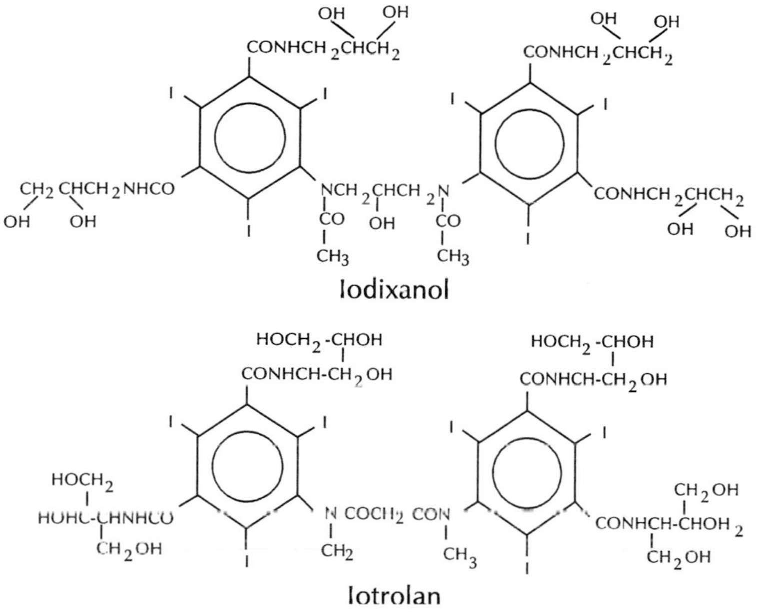

FIGURE 3. *Structures of the ratio 6 nonionic dimers iodixanol and iotrolan.*

TABLE 1

Contrast Media

Brand Name	Compound	Osmolality mOsm/kg H$_2$O	Viscosity (CP) Rm Temp	37°F	Iodine mg/ml	LD$_{50}$ Sodium+ (mEq/L)	Mouse (g iodine/kg)	Additives
Hypaque	Sodium-meglumine diatrizoate	1,690	13.3	9.0	370	160	5.3–8.0	Calcium disodium EDTA
Renografin-76	Sodium-meglumine diatrizoate	1,940	10.0	8.4	370	190	5.3–8.0	Sodium citrate, disodium EDTA
Hexabrix	Sodium-meglumine ioxaglate	600	15.7	7.5	320	150	11.2	Calcium disodium EDTA
Omnipaque	Iohexol	844	20.4	10.4	350	5	24.2	Tromethamine calcium disodium EDTA
Isovue	Iopamidol	796	20.7	9.4	370	2	21.8	Tromethamine calcium disodium EDTA
Optiray	Ioversol	702	9.9	5.8	320	2	17	Tromethamine calcium disodium EDTA
Visipaque	Iodixanol	290	26	11.8	320	19	>21	Tromethamine calcium disodium EDTA + 0.15 mEq.L Ca$^+$

EDTA = diaminetetraacetic acid; I = iodine; LD$_{50}$ = lethal dose in 50% of injected animals; Rm Temp = room temperature.

TABLE 2

Properties of an Ideal Contrast Agent

Efficacy

>   Optimal iodine concentration (370 mg/mL)
>   Low viscosity at room temperature

Safety

>   Isosmolality
>   Nonionic
>   Noncalcium binding
>   Inert additives for stabilization
>   Rapid elimination

nal surface might be useful for specific applications for which "designer" contrasts may be developed. The ideal contrast medium for cardiac angiography does not yet exist. The available agents all have the potential to provoke significant untoward reaction, and they vary in the degree to which they are tolerated by patients.

Efficacy

The sole purpose of a contrast material is to opacify the intravascular space through which it travels. Any other action might be considered a side effect, although under specific circumstances some of these side effects may be desirable. The degree of opacification afforded by a contrast is a function of its iodine content. The traditional HOM used for coronary angiography have an iodine content of 370 mg/mL. The LOM, however, are limited in their maximum iodine concentration by increasing viscosity. There seems to be little difference in the degree of coronary opacification achieved clinically with contrasts having iodine concentrations of 320 to 370 mg/mL[4], although it has been suggested that in pediatric cardiac angiography, superior imaging is obtained with a medium containing 370 mg of iodine per milliliter compared with one having 320 mg of iodine per milliliter.[5]

Under some conditions (eg, need for high flow rates through small lumen catheters or around coaxial systems) differences in viscosity may be clinically detectable. Viscosity of all contrast agents may be reduced by warming prior to administration. It has also been suggested that hemodynamic and electrophysiologic perturbation accompanying coronary angiography may be reduced if contrast is delivered at body temperature.[6] This effect is independent of a reduction in viscosity, however, and may be extended to electrolyte solutions. Because of increased viscosity (and price), nonionic agents should not be used for balloon inflation.

Safety

Given the lack of difference in the ability of various contrasts to provide clinically acceptable angiograms (assuming an iodine concentration of 320 to 370 mg/mL), safety and patient tolerance become the major basis for comparison. Much of our knowledge of contrast toxicity comes from large registries in which the majority of patients received intravenous contrast. While the incidence of any "reaction" is relatively high (5% to 10%), most are classified as mild, requiring little or no treatment. There is, however, the potential for serious complication with death occurring in approximately 1 of 40,000 contrast examinations resulting in about 500 deaths each year in the United States.[7,8] Most of the life-threatening contrast reactions are allergy-like and believed by many to result from the liberation of vasoactive peptides and amines in predisposed individuals. The activation of these agents is presumably related to hyperosmolality of the contrast rather than a true antigen-antibody reaction.[9,10] It has been suggested that the incidence of such reaction is less in patients receiving intra-arterial contrast than in those having intravenous administration.[11] The reason for this may be the dilution of contrast prior to reaching the lungs when given by the former route.

If hyperosmolality of contrast is an important etiologic factor for severe reaction, the LOM should be beneficial. Three large prospective studies[12–14] enrolling hundreds of thousands of patients have convincingly demonstrated that the incidence of mild, moderate, and severe reactions are reduced in patients receiving LOM compared with HOM. The type of contrast predicted the type of reaction whether the patient was considered at high risk or not; low-risk patients given HOM had a higher incidence of untoward events than high-risk patients given LOM. Although LOM has been shown to reduce the incidence of severe reactions, in many studies there is no convincing evidence that the risk of death is altered. Death has accompanied the use of LOM[15] although direct attribution to contrast is not clear. Pretreatment with steroids at least 12 hours prior to contrast administration decreases the incidence of side effects associated with intravenous HOM.[16] It is not clear whether this strategy is as effective as the use of a nonionic contrast agent; it is less practical but more cost effective.

Significant adverse events are more frequently encountered with selective coronary angiography than with intravenous contrast administration. However, attribution of a specific event to contrast may not be obvious because of the invasive nature of the procedure and the underlying heart disease. In registries,[17] classification of contrast-related complications may be restricted to allergy-like phenomenon while cardiac arrhythmia, pulmonary edema, acute infarction, and death may, in fact, be contrast-mediated. The spectrum of contrast-related adverse events associated with coronary angiography is depicted in Table 3. While transient slowing of heart rate and a drop in blood pressure is an almost universal observation when HOM is injected into the coronary artery, it is usually not considered a complication unless specific treatment is necessary. However, in patients with decompensated cardiac function, significant valve disease, or severe coronary obstruction a fall in blood pressure may initiate a cycle of ischemia leading to further hypotension and sustained underperfu-

---

TABLE 3

Adverse Reactions Related to Intracoronary Contrast Medium

Allergic

    Hives
    Pruritus
    Rash
    Bronchospasm
    Anaphylactoid reaction

Discomfort

    Pain/heat
    Nausea/vomiting
    Flushing

Cardiotoxic

    Hypotension
    Increased ventricular diastolic pressure
    Bradyarrhythmia (sinus and/or AV block)
    Tachyarrhythmia (ventricular tachycardia/fibrillation)

Renal Toxicity

    Decreased renal function

sion of the myocardium. In our experience this has been the leading cause of refractory hypotension and death from diagnostic angiography with HOM. In our experience one half of all significant complications accompanying cardiac angiography with HOM are contrast related (Table 4).[18]

While there appears to be relatively little difference in toxicity among the HOM compounds, some formulations contain additives (eg, sodium citrate) that intensely bind with calcium. These formulations have been shown to be associated with a higher incidence of cardiac arrhythmia and hypotension[19-21] than similar HOM without these additives. The calcium binding agents have no benefit associated with them, and contrast agents containing them probably should no longer be used. Unfortunately one of the latter, Renografin-76, is often used as a comparator to LOM in randomized controlled trials. Because of this the advantages of LOM may be magnified.[22]

Both ionic and nonionic LOM have consistently been shown to be associated with fewer untoward events than HOM when used for cardiac angiography. It should be noted that most randomized studies exclude high-risk patients such as those with a history of contrast reaction, hemodynamic instability (severe heart failure or hypotension), unstable angina, acute myocardial infarction, renal failure, and those patients in whom catheter intervention is anticipated. Barrett et al[23] characterized 12% of their diagnostic catheterization patients as being at too great a risk to receive HOM. Of those moderate- and low-risk patients who were randomized, adverse reactions requiring treatment were three times more common in patients receiving HOM (29% versus 9%). Severe or prolonged events including ventricular fibrillation, prolonged hy-

---

TABLE 4

Complications of Cardiac Catheterization Associated With HOM: The Johns Hopkins Hospital 1980–1981

Procedures	1,144
Severe complications (%)	33 (2.8)
Contrast Related (%)	17 (1.7)
Hypotension–death	3
Prolonged hypotension	3
Ventricular arrhythmia	7
Renal failure	4*

*One patient also had cholesterol embolization and later died.

potension, and cardiac arrest were more frequently encountered in the HOM group (2.9% versus 0.8%). Hill et al[24] found an almost identical difference in the incidence of severe cardiac adverse reactions in stable patients receiving Renografin-76 compared with iohexol. Steinberg et al[25] studied a similar group of patients and found that those receiving HOM had a threefold incidence of total adverse reaction, however, there was no difference in severe reactions between the two groups. An important difference between the Barrett and Hill studies compared with that of Steinberg was the use of HOM containing calcium binders in the former, but not in the latter.

Ionic Versus Nonionic LOM

Differences between nonionic ratio 3 compounds have not been clinically demonstrable in spite of manufacturer claims concerning such characteristics as iodine content, viscosity, hydrophilia, etc. However, differences between the nonionic agents and ioxaglate do appear, the ionic LOM. Gertz et al[26] found a higher incidence of adverse reactions, nausea, vomiting, and allergy-like phenomena (eg, bronchospasm and urticaria) among patients receiving the ionic dimer for cardiac angiography compared with a nonionic. There is evidence that ioxaglate should not be administered along with the vasodilating agents tolazoline or papaverine because of chemical incompatibility.[27]

There have been suggested benefits associated with ionic agents compared with nonionic agents. These include a reduced incidence of ventricular fibrillation and a lessened potential for a thromboembolic phenomenon. Evidence for a reduction in ventricular fibrillation comes primarily from animal studies using prolonged contrast infusion through an impacted coronary catheter.[28,29] This model suggests that the presence of sodium, even when added to nonionic media, protects against ventricular fibrillation. Using another animal model in which programmed ventricular electrical stimuli are delivered during bolus intracoronary injection of contrast agent, nonionic agent appear to be less arrhythmogenic than either HOM or ionic LOM.[30] While both of these models appear to be relevant to the clinical situation, studies have failed to demonstrate a difference in the occurrence of significant arrhythmia between the nonionics and ioxaglate. There have however been conflicting reports based on surrogate indices of malignant ventricular arrhythmia.[31,32]

Contrast and Coagulation

The risk of thromboembolism during coronary angiography has been recognized from the earliest experiences with this technique.[33] Clots that collected on guide wires or at the site of vascular access may be stripped off by the catheter tip as it advances to the coronary ostium and then embolized with contrast injection. Injury to the aorta or coronary orifice may result in platelet aggregation with subsequent embolization. If the catheter dislodges a clot adhering to the left atrium (after transseptal catheterization), aorta, or left ventricle thromboembolism may also result. Shortly after the nonionic contrast agent was introduced in the United States, reports associating these agents with coronary thromboembolic phenomenon surfaced.[34] Because the controversy surrounding this issue has not been completely settled, it is important to examine the existing information.

All contrast materials may be considered anticoagulant in that when they are mixed with blood, they retard clot formation to a greater degree than saline. As might be expected the nonionics, which produce the least overall physiologic perturbation, minimally effect the coagulation system and therefore are the least anticoagulant. It has been suggested[35] that, unlike ionic contrast, the nonionics do not inhibit the generation of thrombin. Thus, while nonionics inhibit fibrin polymerization, contact with blood in a syringe may establish a procoagulant milieu. The clinical relevance of these observations has been questioned and preliminary studies fail to show a difference between ionic and nonionics with regard to platelet activation and thrombin generation.[36–38] A prospective study evaluating 8,517 patients undergoing diagnostic angiography with nonionic agents concluded that the incidence of thrombotic events (0.18%) was no different than that encountered with ionic contrast whether or not the patients received systemic anticoagulation and/or antiplatelet therapy.[39]

The relation between contrast material and clot in patients undergoing coronary intervention is more controversial. Acute coronary occlusion related at least in part to thrombus formation may complicate 5% to 8% of coronary interventions. This is more likely to occur in the presence of a preexisting clot, eg, unstable angina and myocardial infarction. This complication is also related to the degree of antiplatelet and anticoagulant therapy achieved during the procedure. The stimulus for coronary thrombus formation is intense after disruption of the intima by any of the interventional techniques, and aggressive anticoagulation is necessary. Hwang et al[40] found that in the presence of systemic anticoagulation the relative differences in the intrinsic anticoagulant properties of contrast medium are unimportant. Others, however, suggest that the additional anticoagulant effect of ionic agents is beneficial.[41]

A number of studies comparing ionic and nonionic contrast use during interventional procedures have been reported. Lembo et al[42] noted that the incidence of malignant ventricular arrhythmias was greater with Renografin-76 than with a nonionic. There was no difference in the rates of death, myocardial infarction, or the need for bypass surgery in this relatively large (913 patients) randomized group. Gasperetti et al[43] reported a higher incidence of postangioplasty thrombus in patients receiving a nonionic agent. This was most marked in those with unstable angina. No difference in clinical events accompanied the angiographic findings. Esplugas et al[44] demonstrated a greater incidence of thrombus angiographically and on the guide wires of patients receiving nonionic contrast during angioplasty. There was, however, no evidence that this was of clinical significance. Piessens et al[45] found a higher incidence of in-laboratory thrombotic events in patients randomized to nonionic contrast. However, there was no difference between the contrasts when all thrombotic events (in and out of the catheterization laboratory) were considered. There was also no difference between contrasts when the total of "hard" end points (infarction, bypass surgery, and death) were compared. Royer et al[46] claimed an incidence of acute coronary occlusion in 15% of patients receiving a nonionic agent compared with 6% of those in whom ioxagalate was used. Patency could be reestablished in only half of the former but all of the latter. The incidence of procedural and postprocedural ischemic complications after percutaneous transluminal angioplasty in patients with acute ischemic syndromes appears to be less when ioxaglate than when a nonionic agent was used.[47]

While the angiographic incidence of thrombus appears to be increased in patients receiving nonionic agents as part of an interventional procedure, the clinical sequelae of this do not appear to be significant. Indeed, since their introduction, the use of nonionic contrast agents has increased such that it is now used in the majority of interventional procedures performed in the United States. This has been accompanied by a decrease in significant complications despite a more complicated and higher risk case mix. Reasons for the discrepancy between the apparent increase in thrombi detected angiographically and clinical outcome are not obvious but may include the following: the postinterventional filling defects noted are not thrombi, but represent some other phenomenon such as red cell aggregates that are easily disrupted; the thrombi seen are easily dealt with by redilatation or prolonged heparin therapy; the angiographic demonstration of periprocedural thrombus is not in itself predictive of clinical outcome; or an inadequate number of patients has been enrolled in controlled trials to detect an excess of clinical events.

The exact relation between nonionic contrast and coronary thromboembolic events remains to be clarified by a properly controlled randomized trial. The FDA has mandated labeling changes for all contrast media recognizing the potential for clots to form consequent to prolonged contact with blood. This labeling also specifies that nonionic media inhibit coagulation to a lesser degree than ionic media. The angiographer should avoid prolonged contact between blood and contrast agent in catheters and syringes. Attention should be given to wiping guide wires clean and to the proper flushing of catheters. Plastic syringes are preferred over glass for the retardation of thrombus formation.[48] With good procedural technique there does not appear to be a need to anticoagulate patients undergoing diagnostic angiography via the percutaneous femoral approach regardless of the contrast used. There is no evidence to support the routine addition of heparin to contrast prior to administration.

The interventionalist should ensure an adequate degree of heparin anticoagulation that must be confirmed by ACT (> 300–350 seconds) repeated at intervals of about 45 minutes. Patients coming to the laboratory on intravenous heparin require the same amount of procedural heparin as those not already receiving this drug.[49] Antiplatelet therapy is mandatory and the risk of coronary occlusion may be related to the duration of aspirin treatment.[50] New antiplatelet and anticoagulant drugs may further decrease the risk of coronary occlusion. There does not at the present time appear to be sufficient evidence to support the claim that ionic LOM offers any advantage of clinical significance over the nonionic agent.

Contrast and the Kidney

Impairment of renal function after contrast exposure occurs in about 1.4% of patients with normal baseline function and in up to 90% of those with preexisting renal insufficiency and diabetes.[51] The mechanism of contrast associated nephropathy is unclear but may be related to inhibition of prostaglandin-induced vasodilatation of the efferent arterioles resulting in an increase in renal vascular resistance.[52] A variety of risk factors for contrast associated nephropathy have been identified (Table 5) of which preexisting renal disease appears the most predictive. Studies of contrast associated nephropathy have been complicated by lack of a standard definition. While initial reports found no differences in nephrotoxicity between LOM and HOM[53,54] more recent studies[55-57] suggest a modest benefit of the former, although the clinical importance of this remains questionable. While it may be reasonable to use LOM in patients with existent renal insufficiency, especially those in whom the use of a high volume of contrast is anticipated, attention to adequate hydration should be the angiographer's primary defense against contrast associated nephropathy. The possibility that postangiography renal dysfunction might be the result of cholesterol embolization rather than contrast toxicity should considered. The former is more likely to occur in elderly hypertensive patients with advanced diffuse atherosclerosis. Cutaneous manifestations, elevated blood pressure and sedimentation rate, and eosinophilia may be present.[58]

Ratio 6 Nonionics

Clinical studies with iodixanol suggest that this agent may be better tolerated than ratio 3 nonionic agents. Less renal excretion of alkaline phosphatase and N-acetylgluscosamidase accompanies the use of iodixanol, suggesting reduced nephrotoxic potential.[59] In a study of low- and moderate-risk patients, there appeared to be no significant hemodynamic or electrophysiologic difference between iodixanol and iohexol, which is surprising considering the difference in osmolality.[60] Further study in high-risk patients may determine whether the ratio 6 agents have a better safety profile than the nonionic monomers.

TABLE 5

Risk Factors for Contrast Associated Nephropathy

Preexisting renal insufficiency
Diabetes mellitus
Low cardiac output
Inadequate periprocedural hydration
Multiple myeloma
Total dose of contrast

Cost Effectiveness of Contrast Agents

While LOM has been demonstrated to be better tolerated than HOM for coronary angiography, the cost effectiveness of these agents continues to be debated. The predominance of adverse reactions associated with HOM are cardiac related, considered minor, and relatively easily treated.[23-25,61] No controlled study has demonstrated a reduction in death rate or significant morbidity (myocardial infarction, stroke, or renal failure necessitating prolonged hospitalization) with LOM and the low risk associated with iodine perse remains.[62] Although the cost of the LOM is decreasing (currently about $0.85 per milliliter) it is still about 10 to 20 times that of the HOM. This cost differential is greater in the United States than in some other countries because of the somewhat higher price of the LOM here but also because of the very low domestic price of HOM ($0.04 to $0.10 per milliliter). It has been estimated that the cost of contrast alone for a facility performing 2,500 coronary angiographic procedures with HOM would increase from $21,000 to $540,000 if total conversion to LOM occurred.[22] In the present cost-sensitive environment, the universal use of LOM has been questioned.[63] Studies of cost effectiveness have demonstrated that only a portion of the differential in cost between HOM and LOM is recouped by a reduction in expenditures used to treat contrast reactions.[64] Cost effectiveness would be increased if the use of LOM were limited to those patients thought to be at increased risk for complications.[24,25]

Based on observations that the LOM cause less physiologic perturbation it is believed that these agents would be most beneficial to patients at highest risk. Unfortunately there is a paucity of controlled studies focusing on high-risk patients to confirm this (mm) and currently most practitioners would think it unethical to randomize truly high-risk patients to HOM. While it is possible to construct guidelines for the use of LOM (Table 6), this approach has practical limitations: some determinants of risk (such as extent of coronary disease) may not be known prior to angiographic study; physicians may tend to treat selected patients with LOM regardless of their risk stratification because of the improved tolerance of the latter, thus establishing a double standard for "VIPs"; failure to recognize a risk factor resulting in administration of HOM could result in litigation should a complication occur.[65,66]

Surveys to determine the usage of contrast materials in the

TABLE 6

Guidelines for the Use of LOM

Indicated

Hemodynamic instability
Congestive heart failure
Severe pulmonary hypertension
Severe coronary artery disease
Severe valvular disease
Previous contrast reaction
Dysproteinemia
Hemoglobinopathy
Electrophysiologic instability
Acute ischemic syndromes

Probably Indicated

Asthma
Other allergy
Extreme patient apprehension
Painful angiography (internal mammary, peripheral artery)
Coronary/other cardiac interventional procedure
Renal compromise (?)
Anticipated need for large volume of contrast
Age >60 years

United States suggest that the majority of diagnostic and interventional cardiac procedures use LOM (Figure 4). Most facilities using LOM do so in essentially all patients, due to the lack of risk stratification. The nonionics are the most frequently used of the LOM (70% to 80%) while ioxaglate is selected in a relatively small proportion of patients, primarily those undergoing interventional procedures. There has been little change in the use of LOM over the last few years despite pressure to cut costs. The reasons for this are not clear, but probably relate to the degree of comfort associated with use of these agents enjoyed by both patients and their physicians. Hospitals appear surprisingly accepting of the cost differential possibly because of concerns over litigation and possibly because they must compete for physicians and patients who prefer the LOM.

Often overlooked strategies to decrease the hospital's expenditures for LOM include: joining with other institutions for volume bargaining with vendors; minimizing contrast waste by analyzing physician practice; and consideration of multidosing systems. Currently several companies have designed systems for contrast deliv-

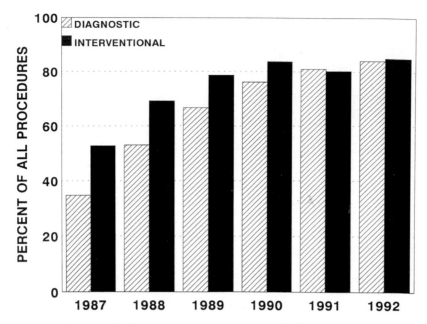

FIGURE 4. *Bar graph illustrating the percentage of all interventional (solid) and diagnostic (hashed) cardiac procedures performed with low osmolal contrast. (Source: industry marketing data).*

ery that provide for conservation of contrast. While these reservoir devices have yet to be approved by the FDA for multiple dosing of contrast, they are being used as such by some institutions. Their approval accompanied by the pharmaceutical companies' cooperation in packaging contrast could result in a considerable cost savings.

Summary

The cardiac angiographer must be aware of the differences between available contrasts in order to choose the best one for the particular patient. Many prefer the nonionics because they appear to offer the maximum protection against adverse reactions allowing the procedure to go as smoothly as possible. There is an opinion that one has the ability to use as much contrast as necessary to complete the procedure (we have used as much as 1000 cm³ in complicated interventional cases). There is the additional sense of security in knowing that the best possible contrast is being used. The better tolerance of LOM is of special importance in those pro-

cedures in which discomfort or a cough may produce motion artifacts. Procedures performed in free-standing or mobile facilities
may also benefit from the use of LOM. If cost was not an issue the
LOM would probably be used universally, and of these, the nonionic agents appear to offer the most benefit. High-risk patients
should receive LOM regardless of cost concerns. Traditional HOM
formulated with calcium binding agents should not be used for
coronary angiography. While the extent to which the nonionic
agents may predispose to thromboembolic events when used in interventional procedures is not clear, the clinical significance of this
does not appear great. Ioxaglate seems to fall between the traditional HOM and the nonionics in terms of patient tolerance. It is associated with more anticoagulant activity than the nonionics and
may be preferred by some for interventional procedures. Use of
ionic contrast does not diminish the requirement for meticulous
angiographic technique nor does it reduce the need for aggressive
anticoagulant and antiplatelet therapy for interventional procedures. The role of the ratio 6 nonionic agent remains to be established. They would appear to be the best tolerated of all contrast
material, yet the degree of additional benefit seems relatively small
considering the reduction in osmolality.

The ideal contrast does not yet exist, and so development continues. While the variety of available agents provides the physician
with choice, it also places on the physician a responsibility to
choose wisely.

References

1. Manning WJ, Li W, Edelman RR. A preliminary report comparing
   magnetic resonance coronary angiography with conventional angiogaraphy. *N Engl J Med*. 1993;328:828–832.
2. Ciuffo AA, Fuchs RM, Guzman PA, et al. Benefits of nonionic contrast
   in coronary arteriography: preliminary results of a randomized double-blind trial comparing iopamidol with renografin-76. *Invest Radiol*.
   1984;19(suppl):S197–S202.
3. Steinberg EP, Anderson GF, Powe NR, et al. Use of low-osmolality contrast media in a price-sensitive environment. *AJR*. 1988;151:271–274.
4. Kern MJ, Roth RA, Aguirre FV, et al. Effect of viscosity and iodine concentration of nonionic radiographic contrast media on coronary arteriography in patients. *Am Heart J*. 1992;123:160–165.
5. Saito H, Kimura K, Takamiya M, et al. Comparison of ionic and nonionic low-osmolar contrast media in coronary arteriography: a
   crossover study in children. *Invest Radiol*. 1988;12:910–913.
6. Jacobsen EA, Mortensen E, Refsum H, et al. The effect of the temperature of contrast media on cardiac electrophysiology and hemodynamics
   during coronary arteriography. *Invest Radiol*. 1992;27:942–946.

7. VanSonnenberg E, Neff CC, Pfister RC. Life-threatening hypotensive reactions to contrast media administration: comparison of pharmacologic and fluid therapy. *Radiology.* 1987;162:15–19.
8. Liberman P, Siegle RL, Taylor WW Jr. Anaphylactoid reactions to iodinated contrast material. *J Allergy Clin Immunol.* 1978;62:174–180.
9. Lasser EC. A coherent biochemical basis for increased reactivity to contrast material in allergic patients: a novel concept. *AJR.* 1987;149: 1281–1285.
10. Findlay SR, Dvorak AM, Kagey-Sobotka A, et al. Hyperosmolar triggering of histamine release from human basophils. *J Clin Invest.* 1981; 67:1604–1613.
11. Shehadi WH, Toniolo G. Adverse reactions to contrast material. *Radiology.* 1982;137:299–302.
12. Katayama H, Yamaguchi K, Kozuka T, et al. Adverse reactions to ionic and nonionic contrast media: a report from the Japanese Committee on the Safety of Contrast Media. *Radiology.* 1990;175:621–628.
13. Palmer FJ. The R.A.C.R. survey of intravenous contrast media reactions: a preliminary report. *Australas Radiology.* 1988;32:8–11.
14. Wolf GL, Arenson RL, Cross AP. A prospective trial of ionic vs. nonionic contrast agents in routine clinical practice: a comparison of adverse effects. *Am J Radiol.* 1989;152:939–944.
15. Curry NS, Schabel SI, Reiheld CT, et al. Fatal reactions to intravenous nonionic contrast material. *Radiology.* 1991;178:361–362.
16. Lasser EC, Berry CC, Talner LB, et al. Pretreatment with corticosteroids to alleviate reactions to intravenous contrast material. *N Engl J Med.* 1987;317:845–849.
17. Johnson LW, Lozner EC, Johnson S. Coronary arteriography 1984–87: a report of the registry of the society for cardiac angiography and interventions; I. results and complications. *Cathet Cardiovasc Diagn.* 1989;17:5–10.
18. Brinker JA. Selection of a contrast agent in the cardiac catheterization laboratory. *Am J Cardiol.* 1990;66:26F–33F.
19. Murdock DK, Johnson SA, Loeb HS, et al. Ventricular fibrillation during coronary angiography: reduced incidence in man with contrast media lacking calcium binding additives. *Cathet Cardiovasc Diagn.* 1985;11:153–159.
20. Murdock DK, Walsh J, Euler DE, et al. Inotropic effects of ionic contrast media: the role of calcium binding additives. *Cathet Cardiovasc Diagn.* 1984;10:455–463.
21. Matthai WH, Groh WC, Kurnik PB. Calcium binding contrast media should not be used in cardiac angiography—comparison between calcium binding and non-calcium binding formulation. *Circulation.* 1993;88(suppl I):I-352. Abstract.
22. Hirshfeld J. Low-osmolality contrast agents—who needs them? *N Engl J Med.* 1992;326:482–484.
23. Barrett BJ, Parfrey PS, Vavasour HM, et al. A comparison of nonionic, low-osmolality radiocontrast agents with ionic, high-osmolality agents during cardiac catheterization. *N Engl J Med.* 1992;326:431–436.
24. Hill JA, Winniford M, Cohen MB, et al. Multicenter trial of ionic versus nonionic contrast media for cardiac angiography. *Am J Cardiol.* 1993;72:770–775.
25. Steinberg EP, Moore RD, Powe NR, et al. Safety and cost effectiveness of high-osmolality as compared with low-osmolality contrast material

in patients undergoing cardiac angiography. *N Engl J Med*. 1992;326: 425–430.

26. Gertz EW, Wisneski JA, Miller R, et al. Adverse reactions of low osmolality contrast media during cardiac angiography: a prospective randomized multicenter study. *J Am Coll Cardiol*. 1992;19:899–906.

27. Zagoria RJ, D'Souza VJ, Baker AL. Recommended precautions when using low-osmolality or nonionic contrast agents with vasodilators. *Invest Radiol*. 1987;22:513–514.

28. Morris TW. The importance of sodium concentration on the incidence of fibrillation during coronary arteriography in dogs. *Invest Radiol*. 1988;23(suppl 1):S137.

29. Morris TW. Ventricular fibrillation during right coronary arteriography with ioxaglate, iohexol and iopamidol in dogs. *Radiology*. 1988;23: 205–208.

30. Piao ZE, Murdock DK, Hwang MH, et al. Contrast media-induced ventricular fibrillation: a comparison of hypaque-76, hexabrix, and omnipaque. *Invest Radiol*. 1988;23:466–470.

31. Piscione F, Focaccio A, Santinelli V, et al. Are ioxaglate and iopamidol equally safe and well tolerated in cardiac angiography? A randomized, double-blind clinical study. *Am Heart J*. 1990;120:1130–1136.

32. Vik-Mo H, Folling M, Barth P, et al. Influence of low osmolality contrast media on electrophysiology and hemodynamics in coronary angiogaraphy: differences between an ionic (ioxaglate) and a nonionic (iohexol) agent. *Cathet Cardiovasc Diagn*. 1990;21:221–226.

33. Adams DF. How safe is the coronary angiogram? *Cardiovasc Intervent Radiol*. 1982;5:168–173.

34. Grollman JH, Liu DK, Astone RA, et al. Thromboembolic complications in coronary angiography associated with the use of nonionic contrast medium. *Cathet Cardiovasc Diagn*. 1988;14:159–164.

35. Fareed J, Walenga JM, Saravia GE, et al. Thrombogenic potential of nonionic contrast media? *Radiology*. 1990;174:321–325.

36. Wiesel M-L, Zupan M, Wolff F, et al. Potential thrombogenicity of angiographic contrast agents. *Thromb Res*. 1991;64:291–294.

37. Arora R, Khandelwal M, Gopal A. In vivo effects of nonionic and ionic contrast media on beta-thromboglobulin and fibrinopeptide levels. *J Am Coll Cardiol*. 1991;17:1533–1536.

38. Hill JA, Grabowski EF. Relationship of anticoagulation and radiographic contrast agents to thrombosis during coronary angiography and angioplasty: are there real concerns? *Cathet Cardiovasc Diagn*. 1992;25:200–208.

39. Davidson CJ, Mark DB, Pieper KS, et al. Thrombotic and cardiovascular complications related to nonionic contrast media during cardiac catheterization: analysis of 8,517 patients. *Am J Cardiol*. 1990;65:1481–1484.

40. Hwang MH, Piao ZE, Murdock DK, et al. Risk of thromboembolism during diagnostic and interventional cardiac procedures with nonionic contrast media. *Radiology*. 1990;174:453–457.

41. Grines CL, Diaz C, Mickelson J. Acute thrombosis in a canine model of arterial injury: effect of ionic versus nonionic contrast media. *Circulation*. 1989;80(suppl II):II-411. Abstract.

42. Lembo NJ, King SB, Roubin GS, et al. Effects of nonionic versus ionic contrast media on complications of percutaneous transluminal coronary angioplasty. *Am J Cardiol*. 1991;67:1046–1050.

43. Gasperetti CM, Feldman MD, Burwell LR, et al. Influence of contrast media on thrombus formation during coronary angioplasty. *J Am Coll Cardiol.* 1991;18:443–450.
44. Esplugas E, Cequier A, Jara F, et al. Risk of thrombosis during coronary angioplasty with low osmolality contrast media. *Am J Cardiol.* 1991;68:1020–1024.
45. Piessens JH, Stammen F, Vrolix MC, et al. Effects of an ionic versus a nonionic low osmolar contrast agent on the thrombotic complications of coronary angioplasty. *Cath Cardiovasc Diagn.* 1993;28:99–105.
46. Royer T, Berrocal D, Rosenblatt E, et al. Acute thrombosis in coronary angioplasty: effect of ionic versus nonionic contrast media. *Eur Heart J.* 1990;11:363. Abstract.
47. Grines CL, Zidar F, Jones D, et al. A randomized trial of ionic vs nonioinc contrast in myocardial infarction or unstable angina patients undergoing coronary angioplasty (PTCA). *Circulation.* 1993;88(suppl I): I-352. Abstract.
48. Grabowski EF. A hematologist's view of contrast media, clotting in angiography syringes and thrombosis during coronary angiography. *Am J Cardiol.* 1990;66:22F–25F.
49. Blumenthal RS, Wolff MR, Resar JR, et al. Preprocedural anticoagulation does not reduce angioplasty heparin requirements. *Am Heart J.* 1993;125:1221.
50. Barnathan ES, Schwartz JS, Taylor L, et al. Aspirin and dipyridamole in the prevention of acute coronary thrombosis complicating coronary angioplasty. *Circulation.* 1987;76:125–134.
51. Berkseth RO, Kjellstrand CM. Radiologic contrast-induced nephropathy. *Med Clin North Am.* 1984;68:351–370.
52. Porter GA. Experimental contrast-associated nephropathy and its clinical implications. *Am J Cardiol.* 1990;66:18F–22F.
53. Parfrey PS, Griffiths SM, Barrett BJ, et al. Contrast material-induced renal failure in patients with diabetes mellitus, renal insufficiency, or both: a prospective controlled study. *N Engl J Med.* 1989;320:143–149.
54. Schwab SJ, Hlatky MA, Pieper KS, et al. Contrast nephrotoxicity: a randomized controlled trial of a nonionic and an ionic radiographic contrast agent. *N Engl J Med.* 1989;320:149–153.
55. Katholi RE, Taylor GJ, Woods WT, et al. Nephrotoxicity of nonionic low-osmolality versus ionic high-osmolality contrast media: a prospective double-blind randomized comparison in human beings. *Radiology.* 1993;186:183–187.
56. Moore RD, Steinberg EP, Powe NR, et al. Nephrotoxicity of high-osmolality versus low-osmolality contrast media: randomized clinical trial. *Radiology.* 1992;182:649–655.
57. Taliercio CP, Vlietstra RE, Ilstrup DM, et al. A randomized comparison of the nephrotoxicity of iopamidol and diatrizoate in high risk patients undergoing cardiac angiography. *J Am Coll Cardiol.* 1991;17: 384–390.
58. Rosman HS, Davis TP, Reddy D, et al. Cholesterol embolization: clinical findings and implications. *J Am Coll Cardiol.* 1990;15:1296–1299.
59. Klow NE, Levorstad K, Berg KJ, et al. Iodixanol in cardioangiography in patients with coronary artery disease: tolerability, cardiac and renal effects. *Acta Radiol.* 1993;34:72–77.
60. Hill JA, Cohen MB, Kou WH, et al. Iodixanol, a new isosmotic non-

ionic contrast agent, compared to iohexol in cardiac angiography. *Am J Cardiol.* In press.

61. Hlatky MA, Morris KG, Pieper KS, et al. Randomized comparison of the cost and effectiveness of Iopamidol and Diatrizoate as contrast agents for cardiac angiography. *J Am Coll Cardiol.* 1990;16:871–877.

62. Martin FIR, Tress BW, Colman PG, et al. Iodine-induced hyperthyroidism due to nonionic contrast radiography in the elderly. *Am J Med.* 1993;95:78–82.

63. Lange RA, Hillis LD. Nonionic contrast media: is it for everyone undergoing cardiovascular angiography? *Coronary Artery Dis.* 1992;3:345–346. Editorial.

64. Powe NR, Davidoff AJ, Moore RD, et al. Net costs from three perspectives of using low versus high osmolality contrast medium in diagnostic angiocardiography. *J Am Coll Cardiol.* 1993;21:1701–1709.

65. Feldman RL, Jalowiec DA, Hill JA, et al. Contrast media-related complications during cardiac catheterization using hexabrix or renografin in high-risk patients. *Am J Cardiol.* 1988;61:1334–1337.

66. Eisner JM, Casey BJ. Malpractice, informed consent, and the use of low-osmolality contrast media. *Conn Med.* 1988;52:87–91.

Chapter 2

Configuring the Cardiac Catheterization Laboratory for the 1990s

Thomas M. Bashore, MD,
Jack T. Cusma, PhD, Donald F. Fortin, MD,
and Kenneth G. Morris, MD

Historical Issues

Like many advances in medicine, invasive cardiology was accidentally discovered. In 1929, a German urologist, Werner Forssmann, inserted a ureteral catheter into his own left antecubital fossa for the purpose of proving that medications could be delivered closer to the heart.[1] After Forssmann inserted the catheter, he walked from the operating room to the x-ray suite to obtain a roentgenogram. In effect, that x-ray suite was the first cardiac catheterization laboratory. Catheterization of the left heart initially required great courage on the part of patient and physician. Successful direct left ventricular puncture,[2] suprasternal puncture,[3] posterior thoracic puncture,[4] and even transbronchial techniques[5] were reported. A radiologist named Radner[6] is generally given credit for the first coronary angiogram, which was obtained in 1945 by direct puncture of the manubrium with a cannula. Radner injected 20 to 30 mL of thorium (an early radiographic contrast) through a needle into the ascending aorta and the faint hint of the coronary arteries in humans was visualized for the first time (Figure 1). Eventually, Sones, who was working in Cleveland, reported selective coronary angiography[7] and the secrets of the coronary arteries were about to be revealed.

In order to view these secrets, however, advances in x-ray

From Vetrovec GW, Carabello BA, (eds.) *Invasive Cardiology: Current Diagnostic and Therapeutic Issues.* Armonk, NY: Futura Publishing Company, Inc.: © 1996.

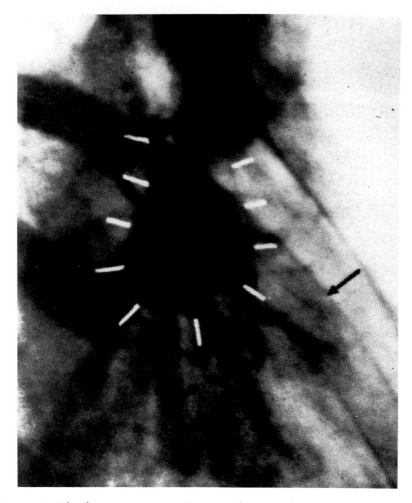

FIGURE 1. *The first coronary angiogram. The manubrium is punctured by the needle, and Radner in 1945 is given credit for the first visualization of coronary arteries by radiographic techniques. (Reproduced with permission from Reference 6.)*

imaging and radiographic contrast agents were required. Because of cardiac motion, it was immediately obvious that a continuous sequence of x-rays would be necessary. One method described by the late Jim Warren (personal communication) used a 2×4 piece of wood with cassettes mounted on it. The film cassettes were then manually pulled to capture the heart at sequential intervals. Early film changers were built using either individual cassettes or a continuous roll of film. Advances finally led to the use of 16-mm movie film and then to 35-mm film. All of these hardware advances paralleled the development of the image intensifier and the video camera. The modern cardiac catheterization laboratory is now able to produce high-quality image generation with an acceptable exchange medium that can be used universally. Therefore, are further developments necessary?

There are many advantages to moving away from a cine-film-based system to computerized imaging. The image quality attained using digital images now approaches that of cine film and has the advantage that it can undergo postprocessing. This allows for image enhancement, cine-loop reviewing, freeze-frame or road mapping capabilities, and immediate playback. By having data in a digital archival device, the data can be accessed from remote sites and the enormous problem of cine-film storage (and loss) can be dramatically reduced. All this can be achieved at a cost less than cine-film.

Because digital data are inherently transportable, the data can be moved within a facility and between facilities once appropriate networks—many currently under construction—are completed. Digital imaging is inherently flicker-free and can also reduce the standard framing rates used (to 15 frames per second for coronary arteries and probably 20 frames per second for ventriculography). This reduces x-ray exposure and wear-and-tear on x-ray systems. Imaging and nonimaging data (such as the catheterization report itself) can also be stored together for the first time.

In the future, just as vinyl records have become obsolete, virtually all film-based radiographic methods will become footnotes to history. The configuration of the cardiac catheterization laboratory is beginning to reflect this revolution. By the end of the 1990s, the advantages of a filmless environment will be obvious, and we all will wonder how we lived without it. We are at the end of an era, and although the transition may be awkward at times, the reasons for achieving the filmless laboratory and its promise of networking images is clear.

Biplane Versus Single Plane Equipment

When considering the purchase of cardiac catheterization x-ray systems, it is necessary to determine whether biplane equipment is necessary. A recent ACC/AHA Task Force[8] noted that biplane systems have several advantages over single plane systems, especially in pediatrics; however, routine use of biplane systems for coronary angiography has diminished greatly, particularly as cost has become a major issue.

Coronary interventional techniques have emphasized the need for excellent real-time fluoroscopic images, especially in an era of tiny, barely radiopaque devices. The increased exposure to x-rays that accompanies long procedures has increased awareness of the need to minimize exposure as well. A sample survey from the Society of Cardiac Angiography and Interventions from 1990[9] reported that in existing procedural rooms, approximately 33% were biplane, 33% had digital acquisition equipment installed, and about 45% had some offline digital angiographic system.

The added cost of a digital imaging system approximates that of adding a lateral x-ray system. In the adult cardiology catheterization suite, a single plane system with digital angiographic capabilities is now the more popular choice. This has been reflected in the marketplace, where industry estimates show that in 1992, only about 15% of cardiac catheterization laboratories sold in this country were biplane, whereas from 75% to 95% of new laboratories had some digital angiographic capability installed. In fact, some sources have suggested that up to 50% of catheterization laboratories sold in Europe, and approximately 30% of laboratories sold by some vendors in the United States in the last year were without cine-film capability. Add-on digital angiographic equipment that augments the x-ray display capabilities similar to built-in systems can now be purchased at a substantial reduction in cost and are not even included in the figures given. Therefore, it would appear that the adult cardiology community has chosen digital over biplane angiography when purchases are being considered.

A Brief Tutorial on How Images are Made

To better appreciate how these changes are reflected in the construction of the modern catheterization laboratory, a brief review of how images are made may be useful. Figure 2 simplistically summarizes the fundamentals of a cineangiographic laboratory. The basic x-ray system includes the generator, the x-ray tube, collimators and grids, the image intensifier, automatic exposure control, high-quality optics, the cine camera, and the video system. A variety of gantries and tables are available as well. Cine-film requires processing and then viewing on a cine-film projector.

The x-ray generator output is altered either by changing the number of electrons (mA) or the voltage (kVp) across the x-ray tube. Secondary switching or grid controlled switching is used to

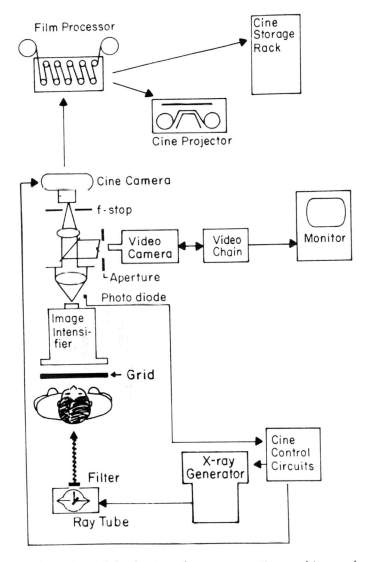

FIGURE 2. *Overview of the basics of x-ray generation and image formation in the cineangiographic laboratory. See text for details. (Reproduced with permission from Reference 10.)*

turn the output on and off in coordination with cine camera function. A high-milliampere circuit feeds electrons to the x-ray tube cathode or filament, which subsequently becomes heated. Electrons then escape by a process called thermionic emission, generally at temperatures in excess of 2200°C. A high voltage potential set up across the x-ray tube (about 60,000 V) causes these "boiled off" electrons to slam into a tungsten anode and release x-rays in the process. Although this is an incredibly inefficient system (with most of the energy being converted to heat and only 1% to x-rays), it is practical.

Considerable heat in the x-ray tube is generated in the process. The anode is rotated rapidly (10,000 rpm) in an effort to dissipate this heat. Because of x-ray divergence, the anode is also angled 8°–10° to minimize the size of the wave front of x-rays leaving the tube. This latter width, known as the focal spot, greatly influences the image resolution. A larger focal spot (0.6 or 0.8 mm) is used for long source-to-image distances and a smaller focal spot (0.3 mm) is used for short distances or in pediatrics. The x-rays diverge immediately and collimators or filters are also used to reduce this spread and "noise" in the system.

The x-rays then penetrate the patient and the table. Terrific scattering occurs, and the lower energy x-rays are absorbed, leaving the high-energy component (a process known as beam hardening). After attenuation in the patient, the x-rays must then pass through a grid that decreases the number of scattered x-rays reaching the face of the image intensifier, improving the contrast, but increasing the demand on the tube. On the face of the image intensifier is an input phosphor that produces light photons when struck by these x-rays. In close contact with the input phosphor is a photoemissive photocathode. When light from the input phosphor strikes this photocathode, electrons are emitted. Electrons that originated in the generator are once again electrons in the image intensifier.

In the image intensifier these electrons are accelerated toward the smaller output phosphor. This results in a much brighter image on the output screen than was on the input screen. Usually the input phosphor in cardiac catheterization laboratories is 9 inches across. When less of the input screen is used to capture the image, the image on the output screen will appear magnified. Typically, image intensifiers are formatted for 9/6/4.5- or 9/7/5-inch modes. Because the total x-ray exposure is a function of the total number of electrons reaching the output phosphor, a much higher number of x-rays must be generated to produce an adequate image when a smaller input phosphor field is used.

The output phosphor emits light photons when struck by the electrons. The image can be viewed by the human eye directly on the output phosphor. From this point, the image is handled by a light distributor system. Automatic exposure controls using a photodiode feed information back to the generator to control energy output and adjust exposure appropriately. An aperture varies focal length depending on the image intensifier mode. The light is then split between the cine camera and television fluoroscopy system. Typically, 85% of the light goes to the cine camera during cine filming and 15% to the fluoro camera. Currently exposure controls favor the cine requirements. The video chain feeds the image to a monitor and to a videotape recorder of some kind, where archival and playback are available.

The cine-film with its latent image is then developed by a film processor, much like any 35-mm film, and viewed on a cine-film projector. To prevent flicker, the projector shutter is run at twice the speed of the film, thus showing each frame twice. Since flicker becomes obvious at about 50 frames per second under normal conditions, flicker becomes a problem if the original film is shot at < 25 frames per second.

Current cardiac angiographic systems use a video pickup tube to provide an electronic video image from the image intensifier. The face of this tube has a layer of tiny light-sensitive globules stacked in horizontal lines (525 or 1,050 lines). Inside the tube an electron beam scans these globules, and a video signal is produced each time a dot is discharged. The pattern of light that strikes the television camera face is reflected in the resulting video signal. Each globule on the pickup tube has its corresponding dot on the television monitor. The video signal activates an electron gun in the television monitor that discharges the corresponding globule on the television screen. The television screen is scanned horizontally in a fashion similar to the television camera. Because a television monitor can display only 30 frames per second, each frame is separated into two fields, one reflecting even and one reflecting odd lines (interlaced mode). Sixty fields per second are thus normally seen by the viewer.

The entire cineangiographic system has undergone many improvements. Image intensifier modifications have steadily reduced the number of x-rays needed to generate quality images. X-ray tubes now have much higher heat capacity, an important issue during prolonged procedures. These tubes also have a steeper cooling curve to reduce delays between cine runs. Larger anodes help with heat efficiency as well. The generators have greater output, and both the image intensifiers and the television cameras have made major advances. Pincushion distortion due to the curvature at the edges of the image intensifier has been markedly reduced. Use of scan converters has eliminated flicker in the playback of images on the monitor. Fluoroscopic images have improved by pulsing the x-rays during fluoroscopy, reducing motion artifact. Attention to details of each portion of the x-ray system has resulted in the high-resolution, excellent contrast images produced by the catheterization laboratory x-ray systems in use today.

Configuration of the Cardiac Catheterization Laboratory in a Cine-less Environment

While 35-mm cineangiography remains the standard, film presents many limitations that have become more evident with the advent of interventional cardiac catheterization procedures. The ability to immediately use the images to guide therapy in the angioplasty suite, the potential for reduction in x-ray exposure and its consequences on equipment and personnel, and the advantages of having images that are transportable are all features of digital angiography. As image quality has substantially improved, acceptance of the resultant digital images has grown greatly in the cardiology community. Conversion to an "all-digital" laboratory allows for elimination of the cine camera, the film processor, the cine projector, and bulky storage of cans of films.

Figure 3 represents a generic system in operation wherein a digital angiographic device is simply added to the basic cineangiographic x-ray equipment. In this scenario, the exposure remains geared to cine-film, and the digital system adjusts to it. Because most laboratories are currently designed for both cine and digital-angiographic capabilities, this is the most common laboratory design currently being sold. Figure 4 depicts the incorporation of an integrated digital angiographic system that assumes control over exposure as well. As cine film is eliminated, this design will undoubtedly become more prevalent.[10] Note that the cine-film storage, cine projector, film processor, and cine camera have all been eliminated. Within the integrated system is the capacity to send data to an archival media for long-term storage. The laboratory then truly becomes the "all-digital" catheterization laboratory.

Current cardiac angiography systems digitize the video signal by converting it to a numerical digit using an analog-to-digital converter. The conversion of these video data can also be performed using a single computer chip, a charge-coupled device (CCD), thereby eliminating the video pickup tube. This has revolutionized the home video camera market. Recently such a camera has been introduced for the catheterization laboratory. An example of how this configuration might appear is shown in Figure 5.

Formation of a digital image is accomplished by scanning, sampling, and quantization. Each frame of the study is divided into

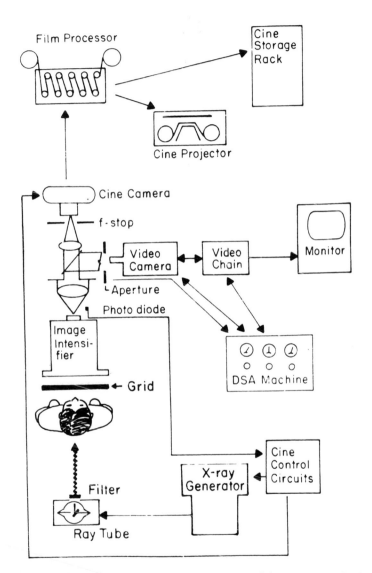

FIGURE 3. *The cineangiographic catheterization laboratory with digital angiographic capabilities. The digital angiographic device (DSA machine) attached to the video chain is added to the basic x-ray system. The system remains dedicated to cine film, but digital angiography features are available. (Reproduced with permission from Reference 10.)*

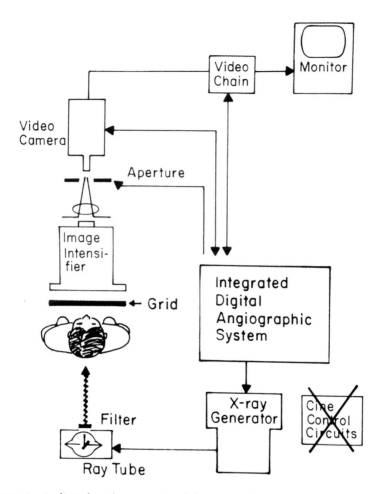

FIGURE 4. *A digital catheterization laboratory. In this scenario, the digital system controls the generator, video camera, and optics. The cine camera, cine projector, film processor, and cine storage problem are eliminated. (Reproduced with permission from Reference 10.)*

a series of squares or rectangles called picture elements or pixels. Typical pixel arrays are 512×512 or 1024×1024. The size of the pixels partially defines the system resolution. The brightness of the image within each pixel is represented by sampling the intensity and converting it to a gray scale number (quantization). How many gray scales are represented is a function of the number of binary digits (bits) assigned to each pixel. The total number of gray scales is an exponential function: $2^{(\# \text{ bits})}$. Typically, 8 bits are assigned per pixel (providing for 256 gray levels).

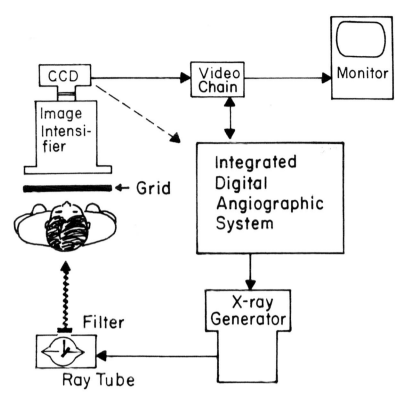

FIGURE 5. *All-digital catheterization laboratory with elimination of the video pickup camera in favor of a CCD camera and direct digitization of the image. (Reproduced with permission from Reference 10.)*

A digital image thus converts the original analog video image from the television camera to an array of numbers that can be read by a computer and stored on such media as magnetic or optical disks or tape. The image can also be filtered to reduce noise and improve contrast at the discretion of the physician. Digital systems allow for scan conversion or displaying the horizontal lines on the television monitor in sequence (noninterlaced) resulting in flicker-free images. Digital images can be immediately displayed after acquisition, and a run can repeatedly be visualized in a cine loop format. Freeze-frame, road mapping, and zooming are readily accomplished. Because of the flicker-free nature of these digital images, display at 15 frames per second is generally acceptable clinically. Table 1 summarizes some of the major clinical comparisons between cine film and digital imaging systems.

TABLE 1

Catheterization Laboratories for the 1990s:
Cine film Versus Digital Imaging

	Cinefilm	Digital
Image quality	Excellent	Excellent
Development delay	Yes	No
Image manipulation	No	Yes
X-ray exposure	Significant	Less than cine
Electronically transportable	No	Yes
Accepted interchange medium	Yes	No
Storage problem	Yes	Yes

The Archival and Interchange Media Problem

The two major disadvantages of digital imaging are the lack of an acceptable standard for exchange of the images among various laboratories and the inability to provide long-term archival of the digitized data at low cost. These disadvantages are not minor concerns, since it is estimated that about 30% of all cardiac catheterization laboratories do not have in-house cardiothoracic surgery. Patients studied in these settings who need interventional procedures or surgery obviously must be transferred to a center where these services are available. Some means must be made available to view the data. While super VHS videotape is available and is used most frequently as the final archival medium, the limited quality provided by super VHS generally makes it an unsuitable substitute. An alternative clearly is needed.

The alternative to cine-film must be able to handle an enormous amount of computer information. If 8 bits define a byte, then each image that is 512×512×8 bits deep contains 256,000 bytes of data. Each second of image data requires storage of 7.5 million bytes (7.5 megabytes). Given that the average diagnostic catheterization results in 100–120 seconds of cine film, a complete catheterization study requires that 900 million to 1 billion bytes (1 gigabyte) of data be stored. Increasing the matrix size to 1024×1024 results in a fourfold increase in these storage requirements, and, although there are no data to show that there is an improvement in quantitative or diagnostic accuracy using this greater matrix density,[11] there is clearly a trend to push toward these higher resolution images. The point is that a great deal of information must be stored and readily available.

Over the years, disk technology has improved to the point at which real-time storage of this kind of data is now possible. Unfortunately the size of these real-time disks remains limited. This results in patient studies quickly becoming overwritten. The average diagnostic study (including the ventriculogram) produces from 1300–1500 images. Even using real-time disks in parallel the maximum storage of these devices is around 12,000 images without compression (up to 48,000 with a data compression factor of 4). A better long-term alternative is clearly needed given these limitations.

A variety of replacement media for such long-term image storage has been proposed, including digital optical disks, streamer tape, magneto-optic disks, 8-mm DAT tape, and real-time digital video cassettes (DD2 or D3). Many media are being evaluated, but no clear archival media has yet to be accepted. A recent review of the current options has been published by Reiber.[12]

The requirements for an acceptable archival storage media include image quality that is at least as good as cine-film, an adequate capacity for storage of an entire patient's study, real-time acquisition and retrieval, small size, an adequate shelf-life (at least 10 years), compatibility among laboratories, and general case of use. At this time the FDA has also stated that the data cannot be compressed to save space because of the danger of data loss.

There are two major options being considered: storage of the data on a unit record (such as a digital tape or disk) or storage in a mass storage device (such as a jukebox with either multiple tapes or disks arrays). An ideal system would likely offer both. For networking, a singular mass storage device that would allow multiple inputs to the data has the clear advantage. This provides a capability that current cine-film (or any unit record storage) lacks—access to the image data by multiple people or at multiple sites. Whatever archival devices emerge as practical must also be compatible with the interchange medium to be passed among different catheterization laboratories. Because it has generally been felt that data needs to be stored for up to 10 years, a busy cardiac catheterization laboratory might need a mass storage device that holds up to 30,000 gigabytes of data.

Simon[13] recently reviewed the status of some of the digital archiving systems currently available or under development and this analysis is shown in Table 2. As shown in this table, no system totally fulfills all the archival needs at a reasonable cost. Many active sites are now investigating these devices; hopefully, the archival issue will be resolved in the next few years. In an era of cost containment, it cannot be overstated that this solution must not be more expensive than current cine film (which costs anywhere from $70.00 to $100.00 per patient to produce).

TABLE 2

Catheterization Laboratories for the 1990s: Digital Archive Systems

	Optical Disk	8-mm Exabyte	3400 Laser Tape	DD2
Capacity (GB)	6	5	50	165
Cost/MB ($)	5.8	7	0.5	0.001
Transfer rate (MB/sec)	0.6	0.5	5	15
Access time (sec)	0.4	45	15	206
Single unit cost ($)	N/A	10	N/A	40
Medium life (Yrs)	20	2	20	5

Data from Simon, R: *Advances in Quantitative Coronary Arteriography*, 1993; 113.

The replacement of cine film also requires that an appropriate interchange medium exist. This means that a standard format and a standard physical media must be agreed upon by industry and the cardiology community for this to take place. In a cooperative venture, the American College of Cardiology, the American College of Radiology, and the National Electrical Manufacturers Association have been working to promote a common interchange standard for all radiographic images. This standard is known as Digital Imaging and Communications in Medicine (DICOM), and currently version 3.0 has been released. This cooperative effort will, hopefully, allow any radiographic format (ie, echocardiography, computed tomography, magnetic resonance imaging, etc.) to be converted to a common standard that is compatible with any viewing device. As of this report, no final decision had been reached regarding the media to be promoted, but rewritable CD-ROM or magneto-optic disk options appear to be the most favored.

Once a solution for the archival issues and the interchange media are resolved, there is little reason to continue to pursue systems using film-based technology. The catheterization laboratory for the 1990s will evolve into a cineless environment with all of the ensuing advantages.

Networking and Telecommunications

One of the advantages that has only recently been explored is the networking of these images. Networking has the potential capability of distributing image information to any device (workstation, printer, display device, etc) capable of receiving and interpreting the information for display purposes. As an example, catheterization reports can be enabled with selected still images or actual digital video. The potential uses for this technology are only limited by the imagination of the developers. This increases incentives to vendors and clinicians to work together to solve the archival and interchange format difficulties. Cusma et al[14] has recently summarized the requirements for networking being developed in one institution. Figure 6 displays a prototype system.

Display workstations capable of retrieving and displaying the large volume of raw digital information available along conventional networks are not yet available. As a result of the inability to transmit and receive the digital information in a synchronous fashion over conventional Ethernet networks alternative technologies are being embraced. The ongoing development and implementation of new technologies such as FDDI (100 megabits/sec), ISDN (1.5 megabits/sec), and the higher capacity ATM (100 megabytes/sec) may provide the necessary broad communications pipelines required for the transmission of these data. At the present time the

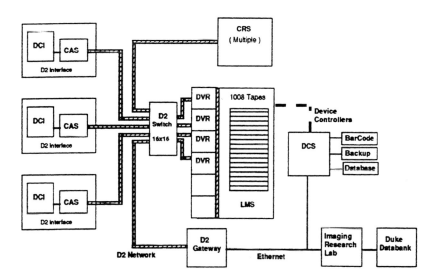

FIGURE 6. *Prototypical example of a networking environment. Built around a central core archival device (in this case a digital tape mass storage device (LMS: library management system). Input from cardiac catheterization laboratories (DCI [digital cardiac imaging] and CAS [cardiac acquisition station]) feeds through a D2 switch to the archival device. The library is controlled by the device controller station (DCS). Display functions are provided by any cardiac review station (CRS). The data can be sent to or received from a database via a LAN gateway. (Reproduced with permission from Reference 14.)*

introduction of these technologies into the medical workplace is still relatively new.

Once the conversion from a cine-film to a digital acquisition environment occurs, the potential capability of distributing such information to any device (workstation, printer, display device, etc.) capable of receiving and interpreting the information will expand our abilities to communicate enormously.

Development of such systems must be user-friendly. Vendors contemplating development of these must include the clinicians' input in their development plans if they are to be successful. An elaborate acquisition and retrieval system must rival the ease of use of the traditional cine-film projector for the timid and computer phobic physicians to abandon their older technology.

The opportunities to combine demographic and other descriptive information with image data is obvious. Networking allows for multiple users to access the same studies by use of local downloading of the information to workstations. Windowing allows simultaneous display of images at the same time that results (ie, the computer-generated coronary angiographic report) are displayed (Figure 7). Database formation should allow display of only portions of the angiogram; for instance, display of a PTCA lesion run

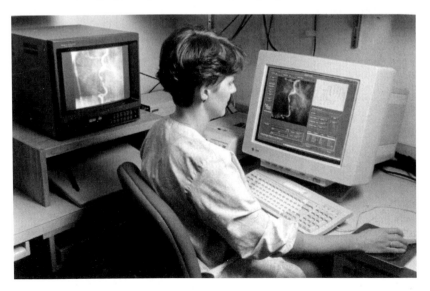

FIGURE 7. *Prototypical workstation environment. Using graphical interfaces, simultaneous display of digital images with graphical report information can be achieved, which provides an opportunity for application of analytic software (such as shown here) or simply a display of results (such as a graphical coronary tree) while viewing images.*

without the need to load cine film and find the particular run each time. In this way, for instance, patients with multiple studies could be viewed rapidly by calling up only the particular runs of interest and displaying them in sequence.

Conversion to an all-digital system also greatly facilitates use of quantitative coronary angiography with its inherent advantages over visual estimates of disease severity. In addition, it opens the way for telecommunication between physicians and hospitals to provide important consultative functions. This may become particularly important as regulation of health care becomes a reality and the need for ready access to data becomes a larger issue.

The opportunities are exciting. The time has come to abandon cine film. In configuring the cardiac catheterization laboratory for the 1990s, these trends will become more evident.

References

1. Forssmann W. The catheterization of the right side of the heart. *Klin Wochenschr*. 1929;8:2085–2087.
2. Ponsdomenach ER, Beato-Nunez V. Heart puncture in man for Diodrast visualization of the ventricular chambers and great arteries. I. Its experimental and anatomorphysiological bases and technique. *Am Heart J*. 1951;41:643–650.
3. Hansen AT, Hansen RF, Sundoe E, et al. Percutaneous diagnostic puncture of the heart and great vessels. *Acta Med Scand*. 1960;169:273–282.
4. Bjork VO, Balmstrom G, Uggla LG. Left ventricular pressures in man. *Ann Surg*. 1953;138:718–725.
5. Facquet JM, Lemoire JM, Alhomme P, et al. La measure de la pression auriculare gauche par vole transbronchique. *Arch Mal Coeur*. 1952;45:741–745.
6. Radner S. An attempt at roentgenologic visualization of coronary blood vessels in man. *Acta Radiol*. 1945;26:497–502.
7. Sones FM Jr, Shirey EK. Cine coronary arteriography. *Mod Concepts Cardiovasc Dis*. 1962;31:735–738.
8. Pepine CJ, Allen HD, Bashore TM, et al. ACC/AHA guidelines for cardiac cathetcrization and cardiac catheterization laboratories. *Circulation*. 1991;84:2213–2247.
9. Cameron A, Sheldon WC, Balter S. Cardiac Catheterization Survey. Society for Cardiac Angiography and Interventions Laboratory Performance Standards Committee. *Cathet Cardiovasc Diagn*. 1992;27:267–275.
10. Morris KG. A perspective: designing the all digital cardiac catheterization laboratory. *Am J Card Imaging*. 1988;2:251–258.
11. LeFree MT, Simon SB, Mancini GBJ, Bates ER, Vogel RA. A comparison of 35mm cine-film and digital radiographic image recording: implications for quantitative angiography. *Invest Radiol*. 1988;23:176–183.

12. Reiber HC, Van der Zwet PMJ, von Land CD, et al. Quantitative coronary angiography equipment and technical requirements. In: Reiber JHC, Surruys PW, eds. *Advances in Quantative Coronary Arteriography*. The Netherlands: Kluwer Academic Publishers; 1993:75–111.
13. Simon R. The filmless catheterization laboratory: when will it be a reality? In: Reiber JHC, Surruys PW, eds. *Advances in Quantative Coronary Arteriography*. The Netherlands: Kluwer Academic Publishers; 1993:113–122.
14. Cusma JT, Spero LA, Groshong R, et al. Design and clinical evaluation of a high capacity digital image archival library and high speed network for the replacement of cine-film in the cardiac angiography environment. *SPIE, PACS Design and Evaluation*. 1993;1899:413–422.

Chapter 3

The Hemodynamic Diagnosis of Aortic Stenosis:
New Insights and Issues

Blase A. Carabello, MD

For most patients with aortic stenosis, management and therapy are relatively straightforward because they are based on a well-defined natural history of the disease. This history dictates that asymptomatic patients have nearly normal age-corrected survival and require no specific therapy. However, when symptoms develop, mortality increases precipitously unless aortic valve replacement is performed.[1-3] In most cases, aortic valve replacement greatly improves both survival and quality of life.[4] In fact, aortic stenosis is one of the few cardiac diseases where surgery returns the expected survival rate to that of the general population.[5] Interestingly, improvement in age-corrected survival is most pronounced in patients over the age of 65.[5] Even in patients with advanced ventricular dysfunction, function usually improves dramatically after surgery.[6,7] Thus, in most cases proper management of aortic stenosis includes careful follow-up of the asymptomatic patient followed by prompt aortic valve replacement at the onset of any of the classic aortic stenosis symptoms, ie, angina, syncope, or congestive heart failure.

There are two groups of patients with aortic stenosis, however, for whom the prognosis is not easy to make and for whom management decision making is difficult. These two groups paradoxically are constituted by those patients at the opposite ends of the spectrum of left ventricular performance. Surgical outcome is often poor for those patients who have poor ejection performance and low transvalvular gradient[5]; however, the prognosis is also guarded for those patients with small hyperdynamic ventricles.[8]

From Vetrovec GW, Carabello BA, (eds.) *Invasive Cardiology: Current Diagnostic and Therapeutic Issues.* Armonk, NY: Futura Publishing Company, Inc.: © 1996.

Patients with Low Gradients and Reduced Ejection Fraction

Figure 1 illustrates ejection fraction and transvalvular gradient for 14 patients with severe aortic stenosis and a subnormal ejection fraction who underwent aortic valve replacement.[6] Ten patients had a good clinical outcome with a marked improvement in symptoms. Four patients had a poor outcome and either died or remained severely symptomatic. As can be seen in Figure 1A, there was substantial overlap of ejection fraction in both groups. However, as shown in Figure 1B transvalvular gradient separated the patients into two distinct groups. Those patients with a small gradient had a poor result, while patients with higher gradients had a good result. Figure 2 amplifies the importance of preoperative gradient in predicting outcome for patients with aortic stenosis undergoing aortic valve replacement.[9] This much larger study confirms that the lower the gradient the worse the outcome. These data regarding low gradient and outcome can readily be explained. The function of any muscle is to generate force: force = pressure/area. A low transvalvular gradient almost always coexists with low systolic left ventricular pressure despite the presence of aortic valve obstruction. In turn, this indicates that the weakened left ventricle is incapable of generating the increased left ventricular force needed to overcome the obstruction. Therefore, it is ventricular muscle dysfunction that is in part responsible for the poor outcome in aortic stenosis patients with low transvalvular gradients. A second explanation for the poor outcome in these patients concerns left ventricular afterload. During aortic valve replacement, the surgeon performs acute afterload reduction by increasing the valve orifice area and ablating the transvalvular gradient.[10] This acute reduction in afterload enhances postoperative ventricular performance and is one of the reasons why most patients with severe aortic stenosis and left ventricular dysfunction improve rapidly after surgery. Conversely, if the transvalvular gradient is low, the amount of afterload reduction that the surgeon can effect is limited and therefore improvement is limited.

If the outcome for this group of patients was as clear-cut as is shown in Figure 1, the best strategy would probably be to avoid surgery in patients with low gradients. However as demonstrated in Figure 3, the management decision is not simple to make.[11] Brogan and colleagues reported on 18 patients with a low transvalvular gradient, all of whom were in either New York Heart Association Class III or Class IV and most of whom had severely impaired pre-

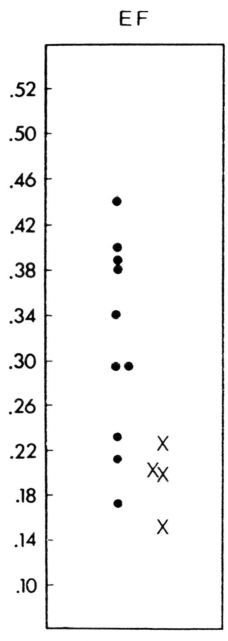

FIGURE 1A. *Ejection fraction (EF) is shown for patients with aortic steno-sis who had a good postoperative outcome (●) and for patients who had a poor postoperative outcome (X). Although ejection fraction is lower in those patients with a poor outcome, there is substantial overlap between the two groups. (Reproduced with permission from Reference 6.)*

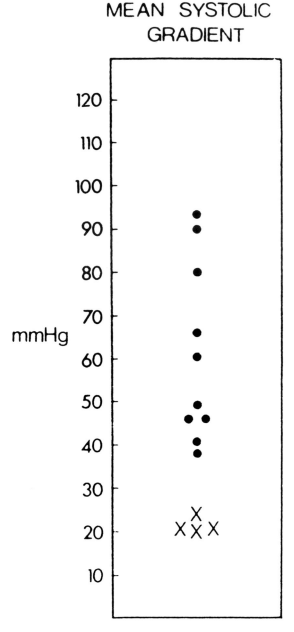

FIGURE 1B. *Mean systolic pressure gradient for the same patients shown in Figure 1A. The patients with a poor outcome had much lower transvalvular gradients that did not overlap with the higher gradients of patients who had a good outcome in this small study. (Reproduced with permission from Reference 6.)*

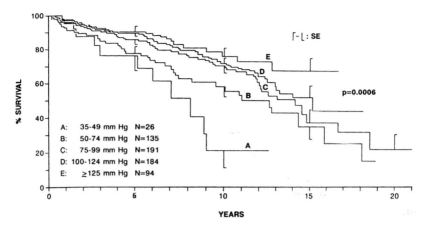

FIGURE 2. *Postoperative survival is shown in relation to preoperative transvalvular gradient. Outcome was best for those patients with a high gradient and worst for those patients with a low gradient. (Reproduced with permission from Reference 9.)*

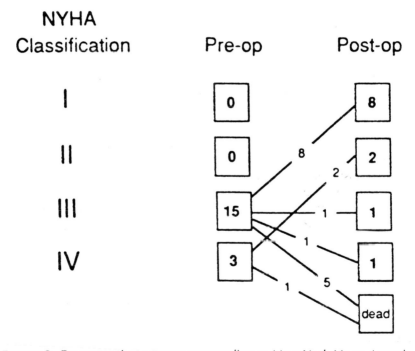

FIGURE 3. *Postoperative outcome according to New York Heart Association (NYHA) classification is demonstrated for patients with aortic stenosis and transvalvular gradients <30 mm Hg. While overall prognosis is poor compared with the known outcome for other patients with aortic stenosis, many patients with a low gradient improved. (Reproduced with permission from Reference 11.)*

operative left ventricular performance. Forty-four percent either died or remained severely symptomatic, confirming the poor prognosis in patients with a low transvalvular gradient. However, 56% improved substantially after valve replacement. Obviously it would be important to know preoperatively which of these patients could be predicted to do well versus which would have a poor outcome. Brogan's study indicates approximately a 50–50 risk of making the management error of either performing surgery that results in a poor outcome versus failing to operate on a group of patients who would greatly benefit from surgery. In that study, however, no specific clinical or hemodynamic factors could discriminate between the two groups. Indeed, currently no such distinguishing marker is available. How then can the clinician manage these patients properly?

Distinguishing Aortic Stenosis from Aortic Pseudostenosis

While there is no simple approach to the management of this group of patients, it seems reasonable to assume that if aortic stenosis is the cause of the patient's left ventricular dysfunction and symptoms, then correction of aortic stenosis might yield improvement. If, however, the patient has left ventricular dysfunction secondary to another cause and incidentally has mild to moderate aortic stenosis, then correction of aortic stenosis will probably not benefit the patient because the aortic stenosis was not the etiology of the patient's symptoms. At first, it would seem easy to make this distinction based on the severity of the aortic valve stenosis itself. If the stenosis were severe, it would be assumed that stenosis was the primary etiology, whereas if the stenosis were mild it would be assumed that the aortic stenosis was a secondary problem. Unfortunately, as demonstrated by data presented in Table 1, this distinction is not easily made.[12] At baseline, this patient's low cardiac output and small transvalvular gradient produced a calculated valve area of 0.6 cm^2. Thus, it appeared that the patient had severe aortic stenosis. However, when cardiac output was increased by 50% with the infusion of nitroprusside, the gradient actually fell and the newly calculated valve area of 1.0 cm^2 suggested that the patient only had mild or moderate aortic stenosis rather than severe aortic stenosis. Furthermore, the hemodynamic improvement with nitroprusside infusion led us to attempt long-term vasodilator therapy, which is usually contraindicated in truly severe aortic stenosis.[13] With long-term vasodilator therapy, the patient im-

TABLE 1

	Baseline	Nitroprusside (0.5 μg/kg per minute)
Cardiac output (L/min)	3.0	4.5
Left ventricular pressure (mm Hg)	130/30	120/20
Aortic pressure (mm Hg)	90/60	90/50
Aortic valve area (cm^2)	0.6	1.0
Valve resistance (dynes sec cm^{-5})	200	160

Reproduced with permission from Reference 12.

proved clinically. Thus, this patient probably had aortic pseudo-stenosis, a situation in which low cardiac output caused the calculated valve area to be small, but in fact severe aortic stenosis did not exist.[14] There is no way to know how this patient would fit into Brogan's series. However, it is likely that this patient would not have improved after surgery because severe aortic stenosis was not the cause of this patient's underlying left ventricular dysfunction.

The Gorlin Formula and Aortic Valve Resistance in Assessing Stenosis Severity

In 1951, Gorlin and Gorlin combined Torricelli's and Bernoulli's principles to derive a formula for calculating the orifice of the stenotic heart valve.[15] The Gorlins' formula was validated for stenotic mitral valves and has become the gold standard for assessing stenosis severity. While the principles supporting the use of this formula are clearly correct, problems exist in using it, especially when calculating aortic valve orifice area. Use of the Gorlin formula to calculate aortic valve area may be complicated because the formula was not validated for this valve, and discharge coefficients for the aortic valve were never developed. Most studies that have examined the relation of transvalvular flow to calculated aortic valve orifice area have found that calculated orifice area is flow-dependent.[16–19] As transvalvular flow increases, the calculated aortic orifice area increases. This is unsettling because it means that valve area may vary by happenstance depending on a given patient's cardiac output on the day of catheterization.

The mechanisms by which calculated orifice area could increase with increased flow are: 1) that the formula itself is flow-dependent, incorrectly indicating that the valve area is getting larger when in fact it is not, or 2) that as cardiac output increases, the aortic valve leaflets are physically forced apart to greater separation, thus creating a true increase in aortic valve area. These issues have recently been partially clarified. At low transvalvular flows (<150 mL/sec), calculated orifice area is flow-dependent. For example, in a patient with a cardiac output of 3 L/min who has a heart rate of 75 and a systolic ejection period of 280 msec, valvular flow is 142 mL/sec and flow dependence of the formula creates a problem in evaluating orifice size.[20] However, at higher flows, the Gorlin formula becomes much less flow dependent.[21] At the University of Chicago, Marcus and colleagues altered cardiac output with a dobutamine infusion in patients with prosthetic valves of known fixed orifice area. At normally high cardiac outputs, calculated orifice area remained remarkably constant throughout a wide range of valve flows. These data suggest that if calculated aortic orifice area increases with increased flow within the normal range of cardiac output, the increased calculated area reflects an actual increase in leaflet separation. Unfortunately, this reassurance about the accuracy of the formula at higher flows is of little help in clinical decision making about the severity of stenosis in the patient with a low cardiac output and low transvalvular gradient where flow dependence of calculated valve area is still a problem. We have advocated two approaches that we believe are helpful in such cases. The first approach is demonstrated in the patient shown in Table 1. If a pharmacologically produced increase in cardiac output causes little change in gradient, a new significantly larger valve area will be calculated, which is usually >0.7 cm², a value often considered the benchmark of critical aortic stenosis. The larger calculated orifice area stems from the Gorlin formula flow dependence at low flows and might also reflect wider leaflet separation of a valve that is in fact only mildly stenotic. Such patients do not have severe aortic stenosis. However, if increased flow produces a substantial increase in gradient (even though valve area increases slightly), the likely diagnosis is true aortic stenosis and the likely outcome is benefit from aortic valve replacement.

An adjunct to the Gorlin formula in assessing stenosis severity in patients with a low transvalvular gradient is the use of valve resistance.[22,23] Valve resistance (R) is the simple quotient of gradient and transvalvular flow. The formula, taking into account conversion of flow in liters per minute to systolic milliliters per second is given below.

$$R = \frac{\text{Heart rate} \times \text{mean gradient} \times \text{systolic ejection period (sec)} \times 1.33}{\text{cardiac output L/min}}$$

There are two potential advantages to using aortic valve resistance to assess stenosis severity. First, the data used are measured directly and do not involve the discharge coefficients of the Gorlin formula, which as noted above were never developed for the aortic valve. Second, in a simplistic sense, aortic valve resistance is the inverse of the Gorlin formula with the square root sign removed. In effect, this gives greater weight to the gradient and less weight to the cardiac output making the formula less flow-dependent. In recent studies[23] (Figure 4), we found that aortic valve resistance could correctly predict that aortic stenosis was mild in patients with low cardiac output when the Gorlin formula indicated that it was severe. However, before aortic valve resistance can be used routinely in making clinical decisions, larger studies must be performed.

In conclusion, patients with a low transvalvular aortic gradient combined with left ventricular dysfunction and low cardiac output are at high risk for aortic valve replacement. However, roughly half of these patients have a good outcome despite the low transvalvular gradient. Currently there is no definite method for separating those low-gradient patients who will do well from those who will not. However, it is probable that some high-risk patients are those who, despite having a valve that is calculated to be severely stenotic, actually only have mild to moderate aortic stenosis, and therefore, are unlikely to benefit from surgery. This group can be

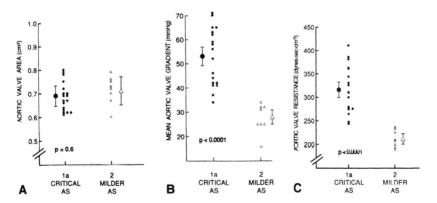

FIGURE 4. Data from patients with truly severe aortic stenosis confirmed at surgery (●) and patients whose valve area initially suggested that they had severe aortic stenosis but who subsequently were found to have mild stenosis (△) are shown. As shown in **Panel A,** calculated valve areas in the two groups were similar. However both mean aortic gradient (**Panel B**) and aortic valve resistance (**Panel C**) were substantially lower in the group with milder aortic stenosis. (Reproduced with permission from Reference 23.)

discerned by the use of maneuvers in the cardiac catheterization laboratory that increase forward output and also by using aortic valve resistance as an adjunct to the Gorlin formula.

Patients With Hyperdynamic Left Ventricles

Concentric left ventricular hypertrophy is viewed as a compensatory mechanism that helps reduce afterload on a given myofibril.[24] Afterload can be quantified as wall stress and is defined by the LaPlace equation,

$$\text{stress} = \frac{\text{pressure} \times \text{radius}}{2 \times \text{thickness}}. \tag{1}$$

In pressure overload, increased pressure in the numerator is offset by concentric hypertrophy that increases wall thickness in the denominator; thus, stress is normalized. If regulation of the amount of compensatory hypertrophy that developed were precise, there would be just enough of an increase in wall thickness to offset the increase in pressure. However, in some patients with aortic stenosis, the change in wall thickness is either too little or too great to normalize stress. If the increase in thickness is too little, wall stress (afterload) increases and ejection fraction becomes depressed.[5,25] Conversely, a group of aortic stenosis patients that has recently attracted attention is a group in which wall thickness is actually greater than it needs to be to normalize stress. Thus, wall stress is subnormal and ejection fraction is supernormal. Originally noted in children with congenital aortic stenosis,[26] this pattern has recently been described in elderly adults with acquired aortic stenosis.[27] As shown in Figure 5, those patients with subnormal stress have high shortening fraction and most of these patients are women.

Aurigemma and colleagues[8] defined this hyperdynamic state as rapid intraventricular acceleration of blood during contraction, producing a scythe-like Doppler flow pattern. Seen postoperatively, this pattern occurred in patients with pronounced hypertrophy and small left ventricular cavities similar to those described by Carroll et al.[26] The group manifesting this pattern had a higher risk of postoperative mortality than did patients without the hyperdynamic findings. As in Carroll's study, most hyperdynamic patients in Aurigemma's study were women. While not all investigators have found increased mortality in patients with hyperdynamic ventricles, at the current time such patients must be viewed as potentially at high risk. The mechanism by which risk is increased is not clear.

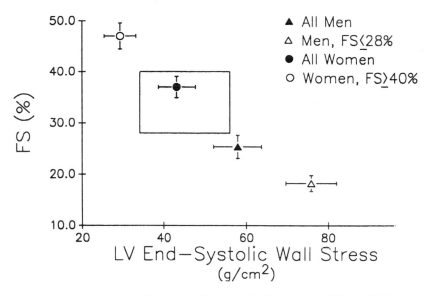

FIGURE 5. *The relation between fractional shortening (FS) and left ventricular (LV) end-systolic wall stress for patients with aortic stenosis is shown. There is an inverse relation with low wall stress allowing high fractional shortening. This pattern predominated in women. (Reproduced with permission from Reference 26.)*

It may be that the thick-walled myocardium is more susceptible to arrhythmias and ischemia. Or it may be that the small stiff chamber offers little preload reserve if decompensation develops postoperatively. Because ejection fraction is close to 100% in these patients, no improvement can be gained by pressor agents or afterload reducing agents that act by enhancing ejection. If ejection cannot be increased (because it is already nearly total) and preload reserve is reduced, there is limited ability for the ventricle to increase its cardiac output when reserve is needed postoperatively.

In summary, patients with aortic stenosis can be followed safely until symptoms develop, at which time prompt surgery affords relief of symptoms and enhances longevity. Even patients with severe left ventricular dysfunction usually benefit from surgery, unless the gradient is <40 mm Hg. In patients with low gradients and low cardiac outputs, maneuvers to increase output may help to discriminate patients who will benefit from surgery from those who will not. Patients with small hyperdynamic ventricles, many of whom are elderly women, may also have increased surgical risk. The best management strategy for minimizing risk in these patients awaits further definition.

References

1. Ross J Jr, Braunwald E: Aortic stenosis. *Circulation*. 1968;38(Suppl V): V61–V67.
2. Kelly TA, Rothbart RM, Cooper CM, et al Comparison of outcome of asymptomatic to symptomatic patients older than 20 years of age with valvular aortic stenosis. *Am J Cardiol*. 1988;61:123–130.
3. Pellikka PA, Nishimura RA, Bailey KR, et al. The natural history of adults with asymptomatic, hemodynamically severe aortic stenosis. *J Am Coll Cardiol*. 1990;15:1012–1017.
4. Schwarz F, Baumann P, Manthey J, et al. The effect of aortic valve replacement on survival. *Circulation*. 1982;66:1105–1110.
5. Lindblom D, Lindblom U, Qvist J, et al. Long-term relative survival rates after heart valve replacement. *J Am Coll Cardiol*. 1990;15:566–573.
6. Carabello BA, Green LH, Grossman W, et al. Hemodynamic determinants of prognosis of aortic valve replacement in critical aortic stenosis and advanced congestive heart failure. *Circulation*. 1980;62:42–48.
7. Smith N, McAnulty JH, Rahimtoola SH: Severe aortic stenosis with impaired left ventricular function and clinical heart failure: results of valve replacement. *Circulation*. 1978;58:255–264.
8. Aurigemma G, Battista S, Orsinelli D, et al. Abnormal left ventricular intracavitary flow acceleration in patients undergoing aortic valve replacement for aortic stenosis. A marker for high postoperative morbidity and mortality. *Circulation*. 1992;86:926–936.
9. Lund O. Preoperative risk evaluation and stratification of long-term survival after valve replacement for aortic stenosis. Reasons for earlier operative intervention. *Circulation*. 1990;82:124–139.
10. St. John Sutton M, Plappert T, Spiegel A, et al. Early post-operative changes in left ventricular chamber size, architecture, and function in aortic stenosis and aortic regurgitation and their relation to intraoperative changes in afterload: a prospective two-dimensional echocardiographic study. *Circulation*. 1987;76:77–89.
11. Brogan WC III, Grayburn PA, Lange RA, et al. Prognosis after valve replacement in patients with severe aortic stenosis and a low transvalvular pressure gradient. *J Am Coll Cardiol*. 1993;21:1657–1660.
12. Carabello BA, Ballard WL, Gazes PC. *Cardiology Pearls*. Sahn SA, Heffner JE, Series eds. Philadelphia: Hanley & Belfus, Inc.; 1994:142.
13. Greenberg BH, Massie BM. Beneficial effects of afterload reduction therapy in patients with congestive heart failure and moderate aortic stenosis. *Circulation*. 1980;61:1212–1216.
14. Carabello BA: Do all patients with aortic stenosis and left ventricular dysfunction benefit from aortic valve replacement? *Cathet Cardiovasc Diagn*. 1989;17:131–132. Editorial.
15. Gorlin R, Gorlin SG: Hydraulic formula for calculation of the area of the stenotic mitral valve, other cardiac valves, and central circulatory shunts. I. *Am Heart J*. 1951;41:1–29.
16. Cannon SR, Richards KL, Crawford M: Hydraulic estimation of stenotic orifice area: a correction of the Gorlin formula. *Circulation*. 1985;71:1170–1178.
17. Bache RJ, Wang Y, Jorgensen CR: Hemodynamic effects of exercise in isolated valvular aortic stenosis. *Circulation*. 1971;44:1003–1013.

18. Wyman RM, Diver DJ, Lorell BH: The effects of increasing inotropy and transvalvular flow on Gorlin formula aortic valve area calculations in aortic stenosis. *Circulation*. 1988;78(suppl II):II-124. Abstract.
19. McCriskin JW, Herman RL, Spaccavento LJ, et al. Isoproterenol infusion increases Gorlin formula aortic valve area in isolated aortic stenosis. *J Am Coll Cardiol*. 1988;11:63A. Abstract.
20. Voelker W, Raczynsky A, Schmitz B, et al. Effect of flow on valve area calculations in mitral stenosis—an in-vitro study in a pulsatile flow model. *Circulation*. 1993;88(suppl I):I-207. Abstract.
21. Marcus R, Bednarz J, Abruzzo J, et al. Mechanism underlying flow-dependency of valve orifice area determined by the Gorlin formula in patients with aortic valve obstruction. *Circulation*. 1993;88(suppl I):I-103. Abstract.
22. Ford LE, Feldman T, Chiu YC, Carroll JD. Hemodynamic resistance as a measure of functional impairment in aortic valvular stenosis. *Circ Res*. 1990;66:1–7.
23. Cannon JD Jr, Zile MR, Crawford FA Jr, et al. Aortic valve resistance as an adjunct to the Gorlin formula in assessing the severity of aortic stenosis in symptomatic patients. *J Am Coll Cardiol*. 1992;20:1517–1523.
24. Grossman W, Jones D, McLaurin LP: Wall stress and patterns of hypertrophy in the human left ventricle. *J Clin Invest*. 1975;56:56–64.
25. Gunther S, Grossman W: Determinants of ventricular function in pressure-overload hypertrophy in man. *Circulation*. 1979;59:679–688.
26. Carroll JD, Carroll EP, Feldman T, et al. Sex-associated differences in left ventricular function in aortic stenosis of the elderly. *Circulation*. 1992;86:1099–1107.
27. Donner R, Carabello BA, Black I, et al. Diminished wall stress in compensated aortic stenosis. *Am J Cardiol*. 1983;51:946–951.

Chapter 4

Invasive and Noninvasive Assessment of Ventricular and Valvular Function

Geoffrey A. Rose, MD and
Arthur E. Weyman, MD

Since the time of Laennec, the practice of cardiology has been repeatedly challenged by the introduction of new tools and methods that enhance the clinician's ability to assess cardiac structure and function. While there are a variety of ways to classify any new technology, one distinction commonly used in assessing applicability is whether the technology is invasive or noninvasive. In general, noninvasive techniques such as echocardiography and magnetic imaging delineate cardiac structure in a manner unparalleled by catheter-based methods. However, these modalities have had an ancillary role in the assessment of functional performance, as compared with invasive methods. This has largely been due to the inability of noninvasive techniques to measure intracardiac pressures directly or to derive indices of cardiac function based on pressure or pressure change. Moreover, because invasive techniques were developed before noninvasive methods reached their current level of sophistication, most established treatment algorithms for cardiac disease involve the use of invasively derived indices of cardiac function. For these reasons, when making critical clinical decisions, clinicians have for the most part used noninvasive methods to determine cardiac anatomy, but have relied on invasive methods to obtain the corresponding hemodynamic data.

Over the past decade, the ability to derive hemodynamic parameters by noninvasive methods has advanced significantly. In many ways these methods have become comparable, if not superior to invasive methods in providing measures of cardiac function.

From Vetrovec GW, Carabello BA, (eds.) *Invasive Cardiology: Current Diagnostic and Therapeutic Issues.* Armonk, NY: Futura Publishing Company, Inc.: © 1996.

In order to determine the appropriate role of these different approaches in clinical decision making, it is first necessary to understand their present capabilities and limitations. Therefore, this chapter focuses on the use of echocardiography and catheter-based methods in deriving indices of ventricular and valvular function as these are the methods most widely used to assess these aspects of cardiac performance.

Indices of Left Ventricular Systolic Function

Ejection Fraction

The assessment of left ventricular systolic function is of cardinal importance, as the prognosis of virtually all forms of cardiac disease has been shown to correlate strongly with the overall contractile performance of the left ventricle. The index most commonly used to quantitate this aspect of ventricular function is the left ventricular ejection fraction (LVEF). This parameter is classified as an *ejection phase index,* of ventricular poerformance in that it relates systolic function to the degree of emptying achieved by ventricular contraction.

Accurate estimation of the LVEF is predicated on the ability to correctly assess left ventricular volume. The shape of the normal left ventricle during diastole resembles that of a prolate ellipsoid, with a major axis extending from base to apex, and two minor axes extending orthogonally from the midpoint of the major axis (Figure 1). When it contracts, LV shape at end systole becomes somewhat more spherical, but the above approximation remains applicable. Left ventricular volume may thus be calculated using volume formulas based on this or other geometric models.

Left ventricular volume was first measured invasively, using left ventricular area and length as assessed by contrast ventriculography. In experiments using ventricular casts of known volume, left ventricular volume obtained by single plane cineangiographic imaging along the major axis correlated well with actual ventricular volume; as might be expected, biplane imaging improved the accuracy of this estimation.[1] However, despite its relative accuracy, it has been observed that contrast ventriculographic determination of LV volume tends to systematically overestimate true LV volume. This is because this technique relies on the projection of the left ventricle, a three-dimensional structure, onto a two-dimensional medium. The resulting silhouette of the left ventricle thus reflects its maximal area and length. Structures within the left ventricular

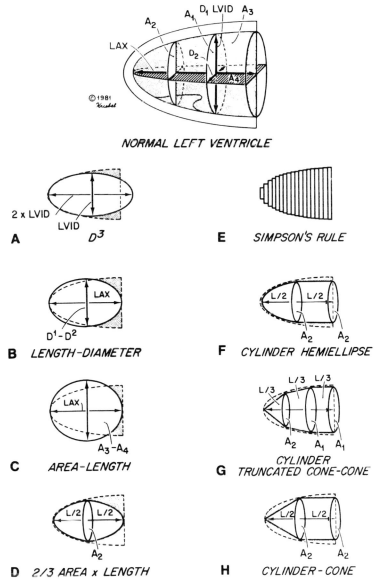

FIGURE 1. *Geometric models of the LV cavity. See text for details. (Reproduced with permission from Reference 4.)*

cavity that reduce its true volume, such as trabeculations and the papillary muscles, are not well visualized, and their effect on LV volume cannot be precisely quantitated. Regression equations have been developed to account for the effect of intracavitary structures on left ventricular volume, and the use of these formulas with ventriculographic data results in a more accurate determination of left ventricular volume.[2]

While area-length methods work well when applied to normal ventricles, such approximations would be expected to be inaccurate as left ventricular shape deviates from that of a prolate ellipsoid, and such distortions in ventricular morphology are commonly encountered in the clinical setting. Aneurysms or regional wall motion abnormalities affecting end-diastolic or end-systolic shape result in left ventricular cavitary volumes that are not easily described by simple models. However, the volume of these complex ventricular shapes can be determined by using Simpson's rule, which relates the total volume of a structure to the sum of individual volume samples (Figure 1). At present, the effort required to perform this type of analysis precludes its routine clinical use.

How does noninvasive assessment of LVEF as determined by echocardiography compare with that of contrast ventriculography? Conceptually, echocardiographic methods might be expected to be more accurate in that the limitations of projection techniques, as described above, are not encountered when viewing the heart in multiple tomographic planes. However, while projection techniques will lead to overestimation of true left ventricular volume, echocardiographic methods tend to underestimate this value.[3] This is because tomographic slices of the left ventricle that are obtained from any location other than from the true apex will represent a foreshortened view of the ventricular cavity. Determining the location of the true left ventricular apex is technically challenging, as there are no fixed external landmarks to guide transducer positioning. Thus, differences exist in the respective manners by which the LV is imaged by echocardiographic and contrast ventriculographic techniques. Each method has inherent limitations in providing accurate measures of true LV volume, and therefore, it is understandable how a discrepancy can occur in the values values obtained by these methods in their measurements of LVEF. When comparing data from these approaches, however, it is important to consider the methods by which these images are then interpreted, as this directly impacts on the accuracy of the individual technique. Implicit in any comparison of echocardiographic and ventriculographic ejection fraction measurements is the use of similar interpretive algorithms. Using biplane Simpson's methods, ejection fraction values by these two methods correlate well, with r values ranging from 0.8 to 0.9.[4] As with ventriculography, numerous simplifications using area-length formulas have been applied to echocardiographic data in order to calculate left ventricular volume, and these methods result in reasonable approximations of left ventricular volume. However, with less data input into left ventricular volume calculations, the accuracy of the results diminishes.

While LVEF is a clinically useful measure, it is nevertheless limited in its ability to characterize left ventricular systolic function because it is strongly influenced by the loading conditions of the heart. The LVEF may vary dramatically solely on the basis of changes in ventricular preload and afterload, without concomitant alteration in the functional properties of individual myocytes. (An example of this phenomenon is the high LVEF often seen in patients with mitral regurgitation, due to the reduction in left ventricular afterload resulting from valvular incompetence.) To better assess the actual contractile properties of the myocardium, other measures of systolic function that are less sensitive to the effects of load have been derived. The basis and use of these indices are discussed below.

Left Ventricular dP/dt

To diminish the effects of the loading conditions of the left ventricle in evaluating systolic performance, investigators have studied the isovolumic period of ventricular systole, as the development of left ventricular pressure during this interval is less influenced by afterload. The peak rate of rise of left ventricular pressure (dP/dt_{max}) has been demonstrated to be a measure of left ventricular function, useful in assessing its contractile function and is classified as an *isovolumic phase index*.[5] To correct for the effects of preload on this parameter, some investigators prefer indexing dP/dt relative to a fixed developed left ventricular pressure, which is the difference between left ventricular cavity pressure and left ventricular end-diastolic pressure.[6] In terms of feasibility, however, these parameters have had limited value. Not only is instrumentation of the left ventricle essential, but also use of micromanometer catheters is required to obtain the high-fidelity pressure signals necessary to derive dP/dt. Moreover, once acquired, dP/dt has been of greater value in monitoring changes in the contractile function of individual patients than in distinguishing differences in systolic performance across groups of patients at large. This is due to the fact that this parameter has not been reliably indexed for variations in myocardial mass. Therefore, assessment of systolic function based on measurements of dP/dt has not had wide clinical applicability.

Noninvasive assessment of dP/dt has recently been described using several different echocardiographic methods, each of which requires assumption of some aspect of intracardiac pressure development. Since the rate of pressure rise during isovolumic contraction is nearly linear, it follows that mean dP/dt over this relatively broad pressure range should correlate with dP/dt_{max}. This concept has been applied to the study of Doppler flow velocities in patients with mitral regurgitation. Because velocity can be related to pressure by the simplified Bernoulli formula ($P = 4V^2$), an approximation of dP/dt_{max} can be determined by measuring the time required for estimated left ventricular pressure to increase by a fixed amount. Typically, these measurement are obtained during the interval that Doppler velocity increases from 1 m/s to 3 m/s (Figure 2, left). Results from this method correlate well with catheter-derived values. However, the absolute value of dP/dt_{max} tends to be underestimated by this technique.[7] Mean dP/dt has also been reported to be reasonably estimated by relating the change in left ventricular pressure (the difference between aortic diastolic pressure and assumed left ventricular end-diastolic pressure) to the isovolumic contraction time, as measured by echo/phonocardiography.[8] Mean dP/dt, as determined by this method, also correlates well with catheterization determined dP/dt_{max}.

In patients with mitral regurgitation, rather than assuming a linear relation between time and the development of left ventricular pressure, the left ventricular left atrial pressure gradient can be continuously assessed by Doppler techniques (Figure 2, right). Assuming that changes in the atrial pressure are insignificant with respect to the changes in the ventricular pressure, all values of left ventricular dP/dt can be thus derived from the continuous wave Doppler profile.[7] Both left ventricular pressure and dP/dt calculated by this method correlate well with those values obtained using micromanometer catheters.

Further clinical experience is needed with echocardiographic assessment of left ventricular dP/dt. The available studies have been performed in small numbers of patients, and the overall LV function to these noninvasive measures of dP/dt remains to be defined. Nevertheless, given the logistical constraints of invasive assessment of dP/dt, these new noninvasive methods hold promise for greater clinical application of this important index of left ventricular systolic function.

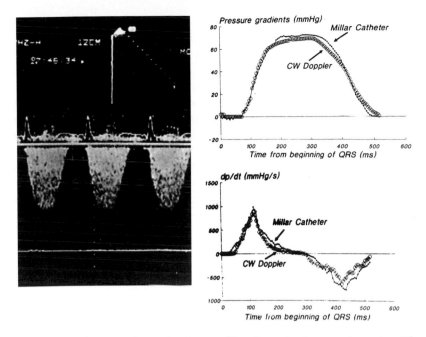

FIGURE 2. *Left: Doppler velocity profile of a mitral regurgitant jet. The peak velocity is >5 m/s. Left ventricular dP/dt can be estimated by dividing the change in pressure as transmitral velocity increases from 1 m/s to 3 m/s by the amount of time over which this pressure develops. Right. Top: Simultaneous high-fidelity and Doppler recording of the left ventriculoatrial pressure gradient. Bottom: Comparison of invasive and Doppler assessment of LV dP/dt. (Reproduced with permission from Reference 13.)*

End-Systolic Pressure/Volume Relation

The pursuit of a measure of left ventricular function uninfluenced by its loading conditions ultimately led to examination of the end-systolic pressure/volume relation, an example of an *end-systolic index* of ventricularperformance. In early observations of isolated muscle preparations, it was noted that the end-systolic length of the muscle strip was almost entirely dependent on the tension at the end of contraction. The initial muscle length, analogous to preload, did not significantly affect this relation.[6] With maintenance of a constant inotropic state, alterations in afterload resulted in a linear relation between end-systolic length and tension. In the intact left ventricle, volume and pressure have been demonstrated to behave in a similar fashion.[9]. Variations in myocardial contractility are reflected by changes in the slope of this end-systolic pressure/volume relation (Figure 3). This parameter has proved useful in hemodynamic studies in characterizing the contractile qualities of the left ventricle. However, its measurement is technically demanding, requiring high-fidelity pressure recording, serial left ventricular volume assessment, and pharmacologic interventions to vary afterload. Nevertheless, this index remains useful when comprehensive evaluation of systolic performance is necessary.

Noninvasive methods have also been used to examine the end-systolic pressure/volume relation. The simplest method has utilized peak systolic pressure by cuff measurement and related this to end-systolic volume, generating a contractility index.[10] This method

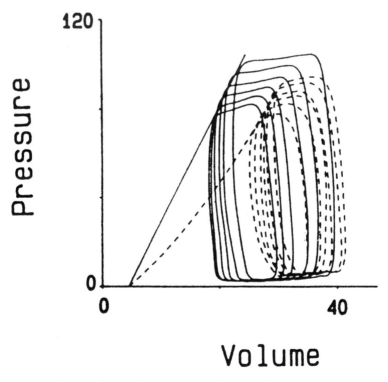

FIGURE 3. *The end-systolic pressure/volume relation. The dashed and solid loops represent pressure/volume loops generated by varying afterload while maintaining a constant inotropic state. Values for end-systolic pressure and volume are linearly related. The steeper slope of the solid line relative to the dashed line reflects greater inotropy. (Reproduced with permission from Reference 9.)*

presumes that peak systolic pressure is equal to the end-systolic pressure, and there is concern as to the applicability of this approximation. More complex methods involve the use of calculating end-systolic wall stress, using a combination of echocardiography, phonocardiography, and calibrated carotid pulse tracings, and relating this to the velocity of fiber shortening.[11] These measures, which reflect force and length, are inversely and linearly related, and their relation is not affected by changes in afterload or preload. However, as with the invasive determination of the end-systolic pressure/volume relation, the technical complexity of this approach has limited its clinical use.

In summary, all of the above indices, provide useful measures of LV systolic performance, but to varying degrees, from an overall sense of global function to a detailed description of its contractile qualities. Whether invasive or noninvasive methods are used to obtain these parameters, detailed quantification of LV function at present requires sophisticated analysis techniques, which limits clinical utility. However, by using insights from the direct measurement of hemodynamic data, the bases for noninvasive assessment of systolic function have been established. Further research is needed to identify noninvasive indices of systolic function that are both easy to apply and insensitive to loading conditions.

Indices of Left Ventricular Diastolic Function

Evaluation of the function of the left ventricle is incomplete without characterization of its diastolic properties. Diastolic function of the left ventricle has long been appreciated to be of importance, but changes in these properties were thought to be adaptive in nature, and thus not subject to acute alteration. It has only been over the past two decades that the complex, interrelated series of events that occur during diastole have been elucidated, and that abrupt changes exclusively in the diastolic function of the left ventricle have been recognized. However, quantifying diastolic function in a simple, reliable fashion remains problematic, whether using either invasive or noninvasive methods. This is due to the fact that available indices reflecting specific diastolic properties of the ventricle are dramatically affected by other diastolic events, and thus cannot be independently interpreted.[12] Despite this limitation, there are several indices commonly used to reflect the diastolic properties of the left ventricle, which are discussed below.

Tau

The isovolumic relaxation constant (T) is perhaps the most commonly used index of the diastolic properties of the left ventricle. After aortic valve closure, the rate of fall in ventricular pressure $(-dP/dt)$ is initially brisk, and the magnitude of $-dP/dt$ is influenced by the peak pressure generated during the previous systolic beat. After reaching peak rate of relaxation early in diastole, the rate of pressure decay during the isovolumic period then becomes exponential in nature, and can be expressed by the formula

$$P(t) = P_o \, e^{-t/T}$$

where P(t) is the pressure at time (t); P_o is the baseline pressure; and T, tau, the time constant of isovolumic relaxation. Tau is typically calculated using data from high-fidelity pressure recordings. Application of the previously described technique of Doppler interrogation of mitral regurgitant velocities has recently been applied to reconstruct the descending portion of the LV pressure curve in attempts to derive tau.[13,14] While correlation has been shown, the absolute value of tau determined by Doppler methods differs significantly from direct hemodynamic measurement. This is likely due to the fact that changes in atrial pressure, which cannot be directly assessed by mitral regurgitant velocities, become important during diastolic events, in contrast to their apparent insignificance during systole. When estimates of left atrial pressure are included in this analysis, Doppler and direct measures of tau correlate more strongly.

Time Course of Left Ventricular Filling

Investigators have examined LV filling as a function of the time course of diastole to further characterize diastolic function. The normal ventricle not only fills most rapidly during early diastole, but can also accommodate further volume after atrial systole. Abnormalities in diastolic function therefore can be detected by alterations in the normal ratio of the early and late contributions to overall LV filling. Whereas invasive techniques have been used to assess the time course of LV filling during diastole, the most experience in applying this principle has been in using Doppler techniques to assess transmitral flow velocities. In the normal heart, the height of the E wave, which corresponds to the rapid ventricular filling phase of diastole, is typically 1.0–1.5 times that of the A wave, which represents atrial contraction (Figure 4). Mild abnormalities

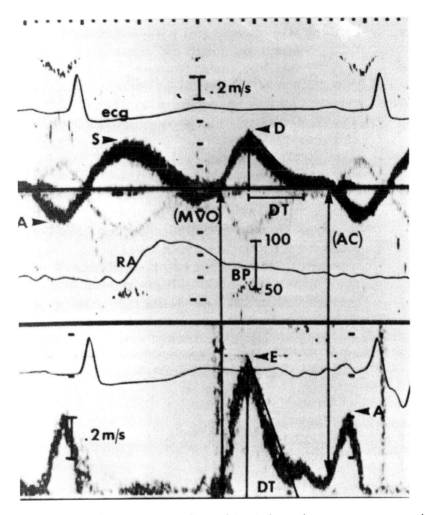

FIGURE 4. *Simultaneous recording of (**top**) the pulmonary venous and (**bottom**) transmitral Doppler velocities. See text for details. (Reproduced with permission from Nishimura RA, Abel MD, Halle LK, et al. Relation of pulmonary vein to mitral flow velocities by transesophageal Doppler echocardiography: effect of different loading conditions. Circulation. 1990;81:1488–1497.)*

in diastolic function become manifest by a reversal of this E/A wave relation. Severe abnormalities are reflected by the development of a tall, accentuated E wave with concomitant blunting of the A wave. However, in progressing from mild to severe diastolic dysfunction, a normal Doppler profile may reappear, as the E wave begins to increase, and A wave decreases. Thus, an isolated measurement of the Doppler mitral inflow profile does not adequately characterize diastolic function. Moreover, not only are these patterns of limited specificity in defining the spectrum of diastolic function, but also these patterns may vary in individual patients as left atrial pressure changes.[15]

Left Atrial Pressure

Left atrial pressure has also been used as an index of overall diastolic function, as impaired diastolic function generally leads to an increase in its magnitude. Left atrial pressure may be estimated invasively by measuring the pulmonary wedge pressure. Echocardiographic methods have centered on combined analysis of pulmonary venous and mitral valve Doppler flow patterns.[16] In general, as left atrial pressure increases, the systolic fraction of pulmonary venous profile diminishes, and the height of the E wave on the mitral inflow profile increases (Figure 4). In addition, the duration of the A wave on the pulmonary venous profile increases relative to its duration on the mitral profile. While these patterns appear to reflect increased left atrial pressure, there is at this time little experience with their clinical utility and correlation with invasive measures of pulmonary wedge pressure.

In summary, noninvasive indices of diastolic function have not yet achieved the same level of accuracy or usefulness as their systolic counterparts. Further investigation is needed to establish methods capable of better assessing this important aspect of LV performance.

Valvular Function

It is in the assessment of valvular heart disease that noninvasive techniques have made their greatest clinical impact. The structural and hemodynamic information provided noninvasively by echocardiography renders it the method of choice for serially quantifying the significance of valvular pathology. That stated, invasive methods are also depended on to assess valvular function, often to confirm the findings of noninvasive studies before definitive treatment is undertaken. At times, discrepancies arise between these two approaches in their quantitative measures of valvular function, and this occasionally leads to confusion as to the importance of the particular valvular abnormality. Understanding the reasons for these differences first requires reviewing the fundamental principles from which these methods have been derived.

Valvular Stenosis

When a valve becomes stenotic, its cross-sectional area decreases, and normal patterns of transvalvular flow are affected. In order for the magnitude of flow to remain constant, the velocity of flow must accelerate as it passes through the narrowed orifice. For total energy to remain constant, this increase in the kinetic energy of the flow stream must result in a decrease in the intraluminal pressure. After passing through the orifice, the flow stream continues to converge. Its point of maximal convergence, and thus the point at which velocity is highest and the magnitude of pressure loss is greatest, is known as the vena contracta. The location of the vena contracta distal to the valve orifice is influenced by the orifice diameter (Figure 5). Beyond the vena contracta, the flow stream diverges, and thus decelerates, which leads to recovery of the initial pressure loss. However in most circumstances, as the flow stream diverges, turbulence develops, dissipating energy and limiting the amount of pressure ultimately recovered.

Given these principles, how accurate are invasive and nonin-

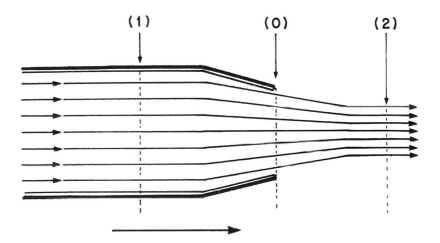

FIGURE 5. *Flow through a stenotic orifice. Flow velocity increases from point (1) to the stenotic orifice (0). Beyond the stenosis, the flow stream continues to converge, resulting in maximal flow velocity at point (2), the vena contracta. See text for details. (Reproduced with permission from Reference 4.)*

vasive methods in providing a quantitative measure of valvular stenosis? Catheter-based methods would be predicted to underestimate the peak transvalvular gradient because these methods typically record pressure beyond the vena contracta. The greater the amount of pressure recovery beyond the vena contracta, the more catheter-based methods will underestimate the peak transvalvular gradient. However, the true hemodynamic burden of a stenosis tends to be more related to the net downstream loss of pressure than to the maximal gradient present in a discrete zone beyond the stenotic orifice. Thus, the true peak transvalvular gradient, which is routinely measured by echocardiographic methods, may not be representative of the hemodynamic importance of a stenosis if significant pressure recovery occurs beyond the stenosis. It is therefore not surprising that catheter and echocardiographic measurements of the transvalvular gradient often differ in their absolute value. However, this difference is typically not clinically important, due to the small recovery of pressure that occurs beyond stenotic valves (Figure 6). The correlation between catheter-based and echocardiographic measurements of peak and mean transvalvular gradients has been excellent.[17]

To calculate valve area, invasive and noninvasive methods rely on the principle of continuity of flow, which states that flow proximal and distal to an orifice must remain constant. Total flow across the orifice can be estimated by the product of orifice cross-sectional area and the velocity of flow. Because flow velocity is proportional to the square root of the pressure gradient, pressure/flow relations may also be used to calculate valve area. However, it should be noted that use of this principle will result in calculation of the effective valve orifice at the vena contracta, rather than the true anatomic orifice. This is due to the further increase in flow velocity, and thus the pressure gradient, which occurs beyond the stenotic orifice.

If based on the same principle, why do invasive and noninvasive methods often differ in their quantitative assessment of valve area? Catheter-based methods use the Gorlin equation to calculate valve area: $A = F/(k\ \Delta p^{1/2})$, where A represents valve area; F represents the transvalvular flow; k represents a derived constant; and Δp represents the mean transvalvular pressure gradient. The constant in the equation was derived so that the formula would generate a value representing the anatomic valvular area, rather than the effective valve area. This is important to recognize because differences in valvular morphology may lead to different effective areas, despite similar anatomic areas. Another aspect of the Gorlin equation that must be recognized is its critical dependence on total transvalvular flow, which may lead to inaccuracy at very high or

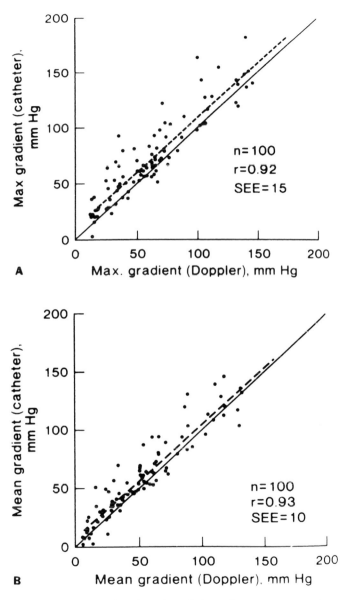

FIGURE 6. *Comparison of catheter and Doppler assessment of the peak transvalvular gradient in patients with aortic stenosis. (Reproduced with permission from Reference 17.)*

very low flow rates. In addition, reliably estimating the total trans-valvular flow is difficult in patients with regurgitant valvular lesions.

Rather than using the pressure gradient and total flow, echocardiographic methods instead calculate the minimal cross-sectional area produced by the stenosis by relating cross-sectional area and flow velocity proximal to the stenotic orifice to the peak velocity recorded distal to the orifice. Using this method, absolute flow does not need to be measured, so valvular regurgitation does not limit use of this technique. Because peak velocities are used, the effective valve area, rather than the anatomic area is calculated by these methods.

Thus, it is evident why catheterization and echocardiographic data may provide different measures of the same degree of valvular stenosis. However, clinical experience has demonstrated that while absolute numbers may vary, in most instances both methods yield information on which clinical decisions can be confidently made.

Valvular Regurgitation

In contrast to valvular stenosis, the current angiographic and echocardiographic methods used in clinical practice provide only qualitative, or at best semiquantitative, measures of the degree of regurgitation. Such measures are helpful at the extreme ends of the spectrum of valvular regurgitation, but they are of little use in patients with moderate forms of disease. Angiographic and echocardiographic techniques do exist to assess either the actual volume of regurgitation or the regurgitant fraction. However, these methods have the same fundamental limitations (described previously) that are encountered when estimating volume using geometric models.

The development of color Doppler has led to renewed efforts to identify echocardiographic methods to quantify valvular regurgitation.[18] With this technique, regurgitant flow produces a jet of color in the recipient chamber. Initial attempts centered on examining the geometric aspects of these jets, hypothesizing that the area or length of the jet might accurately reflect the amount of regurgitant flow. However, subsequent studies have demonstrated that these properties of color jets are also greatly influenced by hemodynamic and instrument factors. Thus, while these simple color jet parameters provide further qualitative information, they do not accurately predict the volume of regurgitation. More recent attempts have focused on using the color Doppler signal either to gauge the momentum of the regurgitant jet or to derive isovolumic surfaces from which regurgitant volume can be calculated (Figure 7). It is hoped

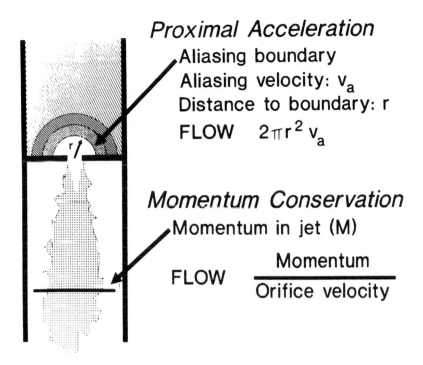

Proximal Acceleration
Aliasing boundary
Aliasing velocity: v_a
Distance to boundary: r
FLOW $2\pi r^2 v_a$

Momentum Conservation
Momentum in jet (M)

$$FLOW \quad \frac{Momentum}{Orifice\ velocity}$$

FIGURE 7. *Bases for color Doppler techniques in assessing transvalvular regurgitant flow. (Reproduced with permission from Reference 4.)*

that these newer techniques will ultimately yield indices to better assess patients with valvular regurgitation, but at present these methods are still being developed.

Conclusions

While noninvasive modalities have been relied on for some time to provide detailed and accurate information of cardiac structure, these methods are increasingly used to quantitate cardiac function, which has previously been the province of invasive methods. The broadest clinical clinical experience has been with the use of echocardiographic methods, but other noninvasive modalities such as radionuclide and magnetic cardiac imaging are also being applied to obtain this type of information. Which approach is preferable when such information is needed? Invasive methods are relatively safe, but are not well suited for screening purposes or for the serial assessment of functional performance. Conversely, obtaining precise hemodynamic data noninvasively requires greater technical skill and the use of analysis techniques more sophisticated than those routinely used in the clinical setting. Thus, rather than considering one approach as ideal, at the present time invasive and noninvasive methods should be viewed as complementary approaches in assessing ventricular and valvular function, each with certain benefits and limitations. However, the increasing ability to obtain detailed hemodynamic information noninvasively represents a significant advance in the clinical care of patients with cardiac disease, and furthering such capabilities should remain an important goal.

References

1. Wynne J, Green LH, Mann T, et al. Estimation of left ventricular volumes in man from biplane cineangiograms filmed in oblique projections. *Am J Cardiol.* 1978;41:726–732.
2. Fifer MA, Grossman W. Measurement of ventricular volumes, ejection fraction, mass, and wall stress, In: Grossman W, Baim DS, eds. *Cardiac Catheterization, Angiography, and Intervention.* Fourth edition. Philadelphia: Lea and Febiger; 1991;300–318.
3. Barrett MJ, Jacobs L, Gomberg J, et al. Simultaneous contrast imaging of the left ventricle by two-dimensional echocardiography and standard ventriculography. *Clin Cardiol.* 1982;5:208–213.
4. Weyman AE. *Principles and Practice of Echocardiography.* Second edition. Philadelphia: Lea and Febiger; 1994:124–142.
5. Mason DT. Usefulness and limitations of the rate of rise of intraventricular pressure (dP/dt) in the evaluation of myocardial contractility in man. *Am J Cardiol.* 1969;23:516–527.
6. Fifer MA, Braunwald E. End-systolic pressure-volume and stress-length relations in the assessment of ventricular function in man. *Adv Cardiol.* 1985;32:36–55.
7. Chen C, Rodriquez L, Guerrero JL, et al. Noninvasive estimation of the instantaneous first derivative of left ventricular pressure using continuous-wave Doppler echocardiography. *Circulation.* 1991;83:2101–2110.
8. Rhodes J, Udelson JE, Marx GR, et al. A new non-invasive method for the estimation of peak dP/dt. *Circulation.* 1993;88:2693–2699.
9. Kass D, Maughan WL. From 'Emax' to pressure-volume relations: a broader view. *Circulation.* 1988;77:1203–1212.
10. Osbakken M, Bove AA, Spann JF. Left ventricular function in chronic aortic regurgitation with reference to end-systolic pressure, volume and stress relations. *Am J Cardiol.* 1981;47:193–198.
11. Colan SD, Borow KM, Neumann A. Left ventricular end-systolic wall stress-velocity of fiber shortening relation: a load-independent index of myocardial contractility. *J Am Coll Cardiol.* 1984;4:715–724.
12. Little WC, Downes TR. Clinical evaluation of left ventricular diastolic performance. *Prog Cardiovasc Dis.* 1990;32:273–290.
13. Chen C, Rodriguez L, Levine RA, et al. Noninvasive measurement of the time constant of left ventricular relaxation using the continuous-

wave Doppler velocity profile of mitral regurgitation. *Circulation*. 1992; 86:272–278.

14. Nishimura RA, Schwartz RS, Tajik AJ, et al. Noninvasive measurement of rate of left ventricular relaxation by Doppler echocardiography: validation with simultaneous cardiac catheterization. *Circulation*. 1993; 88:146–155.

15. Choong CY, Herrman HC, Weyman AE, et al. Preload dependence of Doppler-derived indexes of left ventricular diastolic function in humans. *J Am Coll Cardiol*. 1987;10:800–808.

16. Kuecherer HF, Muhiudeen IA, Kusumoto FM, et al. Estimation of mean left atrial pressure from transesophageal pulsed Doppler echocardiography of pulmonary venous flow. *Circulation*. 1990;82: 1127–1139.

17. Currie PJ, Seward JB, Reeder GS, et al. Continuous-wave Doppler echocardiographic assessment of severity of calcific aortic stenosis: a simultaneous Doppler-catheter correlative study in 100 adult patients. *Circulation*. 1985;71:1162–1169.

18. Cape EG, Skoufis EG, Weyman AE, et al. A new method for noninvasive quantification of valvular regurgitation based on conservation of momentum: in vitro validation. *Circulation*. 1989;79:1343–1353.

Chapter 5

Difficult Hemodynamic Interpretations

Morton J. Kern, MD

To some, the use of hemodynamics in the cardiac catheterization laboratory is considered an antiquated technique. This opinion has become more prevalent as precision diagnostic abilities of noninvasive modalities, such as echocardiography and myocardial perfusion imaging have been introduced. However, the indications for hemodynamic measurements within the cardiac catheterization laboratory remain important and undiminished by the variations in the quality of noninvasive studies performed in the assorted community and university laboratories relative to those results reported within sophisticated academic institutions. The continued use of high-quality hemodynamic data within the cardiac catheterization laboratory is intended to confirm diagnostic impressions, identify new cardiac lesions, and support the use of new interventions. Hemodynamic assessment remains critical to the further understanding of cardiovascular pathophysiology. In the discussion of difficult hemodynamic data, the indications, techniques, and problems discussed are not new, but certainly worth reexaming for clinical practitioners with the emphasis on angiographic and noninvasive rather than physiologic data for decision making.

Indications for Hemodynamic Assessment within the Cardiac Catheterization Laboratory

Table 1 lists the five predominant indications for hemodynamic data collection in the cardiac catheterization laboratory. The

From Vetrovec GW, Carabello BA, (eds.) *Invasive Cardiology: Current Diagnostic and Therapeutic Issues.* Armonk, NY: Futura Publishing Company, Inc.: © 1996.

TABLE 1

Indications for Hemodynamic Assessment in the
Cardiac Catheterization Laboratory

---

1. Dyspnea of uncertain etiology
2. Confirm echocardiographic and other noninvasive evaluation
3. Confirm new clinical findings
4. Routine for teaching center
5. Special studies and research

---

use of routine right heart catheterization as part of every coronary angiographic procedure should be questioned as limited new information is rarely obtained at considerable, and perhaps unnecessary, expense. The indications for right heart catheterization are those that include assessment of valvular heart disease, pulmonary hypertension, and dyspnea of unknown etiology. The routine use of pulmonary capillary wedge pressure in patients with extensive coronary artery disease often can be equally addressed by examination of left ventricular end-diastolic pressure at the beginning and end of a procedure. Should an unstable clinical condition arise, a right heart catheterization can be performed at any time during the evaluation of the coronary angiograms.

Echocardiographic findings often conflict with physical and diagnostic impressions. At times, the presence of systolic high velocities across the aortic valve may be due to either valvular or subvalvular obstruction. The differentiation may require cardiac catheterization to rectify the diagnosis prior to aortic valve replacement. In addition, high-velocity data of severe mitral regurgitation has been mistaken for that of aortic stenosis under certain circumstances when the echocardiographic window has been inappropriately identified. This condition is also easily confirmed within the hemodynamic assessment during coronary angiography prior to aortic valve replacement. In those patients with aortic stenosis in whom the diagnosis is unequivocal, the use of a transvalvular gradient may be superfluous. However, often patients with aortic stenosis have moderate or small transvalvular gradients and, thus, a confirmational hemodynamic study at the time of coronary angiography prior to valve replacement is helpful at little additional time or risk.

Difficult hemodynamic conditions within the catheterization laboratory are often clarified by the application of special techniques. Table 2 lists those special techniques used in hemodynamic assessment for complex cardiovascular conditions.

TABLE 2

Special Techniques for Hemodynamic Data Collection

1. Transseptal catheterization
2. High-fidelity pressure measurement
3. Double lumen catheter systems
4. Sheath and catheter combinations
5. Multiple vessel access
6. Direct left ventricular puncture
7. Pericardial pressure assessment
8. Coronary flow/pressure gradient measurements

The special techniques in the cardiac catheterization laboratory require familiarity with the equipment, methodologic measurements for satisfactory pressure fidelity, and application of the techniques for the appropriate indications. Although transseptal catheterization is no longer in widespread use, its application for mitral valvuloplasty will soon demand its reintroduction into the routine practice. High-fidelity micromanometer-tipped catheters are not routine for clinical practice. However, the most precise and unquestioned pressure gradient measurements of valvular heart disease can be obtained with these catheters. A double transducer high-fidelity aortic-left ventricular pressure sensor catheter eliminates any of the technical questions and disparities identified when using the more readily obtained peripheral (sheath) and central arterial pressure measurements. To date, there are no satisfactory double lumen catheter systems to assess aortic valve disease. A major limitation of the double lumen catheter is a fixed distance between pressure lumens, which may obfuscate rather than clarify the pressure gradient measured across an aortic valve. Although the most widely used hemodynamic pressure measuring system for simultaneous pressure data include those of peripheral sheaths and central catheters, this methodology has recently come under reevaluation. It is suggested that for the most precise transvalvular pressure measurements, aortic pressure at the valve and in the left ventricle be used.

The most recent addition to hemodynamic assessments within the cardiac catheterization laboratory is that of direct translesional coronary artery pressure and flow velocity measurements. These findings have a direct bearing on the selection of patients for coronary interventions. This methodology will be discussed.

The most common problems seen for hemodynamic assessment include those listed in Table 3. The use of high-quality and re-

TABLE 3

Common Difficult Hemodynamic Problems within the Cardiac Catheterization Laboratory

1. Left ventricular relaxation abnormality
2. Mitral gradients
3. Aortic stenosis
4. Constrictive physiology
5. Hypotension of unknown etiology
6. Assessment of 'V' waves
7. Assessment of prosthetic valves
8. Postoperative failure

liable hemodynamic data within the cardiac catheterization laboratory will ameliorate some of the questions surrounding the clinical significance of these common problems. The use of high-fidelity pressure catheters to address whether true left ventricular relaxation abnormality is present has been advocated. Precise mitral gradients may require transseptal technique. Aortic stenosis with low transvalvular gradients and low cardiac output represents a continuing clinical dilemma for which high-quality hemodynamics, as well as precision in cardiac output assessment and valvular resistance are required. Constrictive physiology must be differentiated from that of restrictive myopathy and early pretamponade physiology identified echocardiographically represents a source of confusion for both the experienced and novice hemodynamisist. Hypotension of unknown etiology may be due to many of the above noted pathologic conditions, in addition to occult pericardial effusion, hypovolemia, or a variety of other clinical syndromes in which hemodynamic data can clarify the volume status, as well as valvular function involved in difficult and critical situations. Similarly, the assessment of right or left atrial V waves depends on our understanding of the pressure-volume relation within the chamber of interest. The concepts are important to the assessment of prosthetic valves, as well as postoperative heart failure requiring complete left- and right-sided hemodynamic assessment. The evaluation of pericardial constriction or localized tamponade to the hypotensive postoperative patient is of particular importance for the therapeutic approaches available.

The following case examples are presented as illustrations difficult hemodynamic problems. A more detailed discussion of difficult hemodynamic problems is available elsewhere.[1–3]

Case 1. Constrictive Physiology With Echocardiographic Signs of Tamponade in a Patient with Hypertension

A 53-year-old white female underwent orthotopic cardiac transplantation for dilated cardiomyopathy.[4] Postoperatively, she received cyclosporine, azathioprine, and a tapering dose of steroids. The initial postoperative right atrial pressure was elevated to 19 mm Hg on day 2 and decreased to 10 mm Hg over the next four days. Endomyocardial biopsy on day 4 showed no evidence of rejection. A moderate pericardial effusion was noted without echocardiographic evidence of hemodynamic compromise. Over the next week, physical examination showed increasing jugular venous distension, hepatomegaly, and increasing abdominal girth. Lung fields remained clear. A repeat echocardiogram showed right ventricular enlargement, normal systolic left ventricular function, and larger anterior and posterior pericardial effusions without echocardiographic signs of tamponade. On postoperative day 17, the patient became hypotensive with a systolic blood pressure of 85 mm Hg and a new pulsus paradoxus. Hemodynamic data demonstrated equalization of left and right ventricular end-diastolic pressures with a prominent "dip-and-plateau" configuration to the right ventricular tracing suggestive of constrictive/restrictive physiology (Figures 1 through 3). Pericardiocentesis was then performed. Surprisingly, intrapericardial pressure was elevated to only 10 mm Hg. After removal of 250 mL of serosanguinous pericardial fluid, the pericardial pressure fell to 0 mm Hg (Figure 4) with no change in

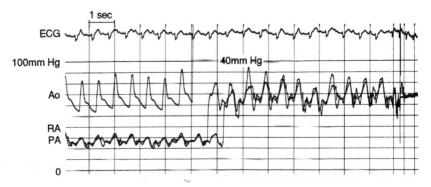

Figure 1. *Aortic (Ao), right atrial (RA), and pulmonary artery (PA) pressures (0–100 mm Hg and 0–40 mm scales). Note pulsus paradoxus of aortic pressure.*

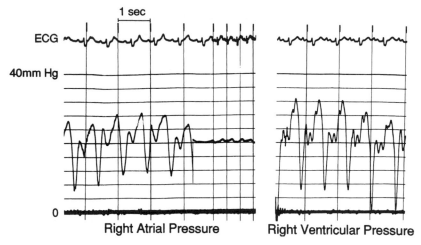

FIGURE 2. *Right atrial and right ventricular pressure waves (40 mm Hg full scale) showing exaggerated Y descents, "M" configuration, and early "dip-and-plateau" on right ventricular tracing. ECG: electrocardiogram. (Reproduced with permission from Reference 4.)*

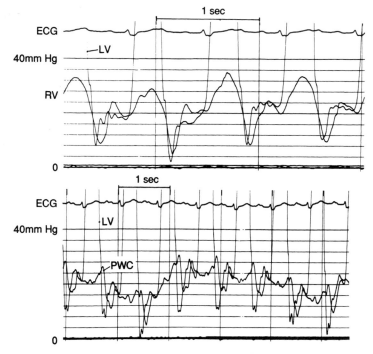

FIGURE 3. ***Top panel:*** *Left (LV) and right ventricular (RV) pressure waves (40 mm Hg full scale).* ***Bottom panel:*** *LV and pulmonary capillary wedge (PCW) pressure waves demonstrating diastolic equalization. (Reproduced with permission from Reference 4.)*

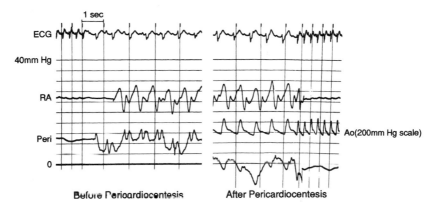

FIGURE 4. *Right atrial (RA) and intrapericardial (Peri) pressure before (**left panel**) and after (**right panel**) pericardiocentesis. Note absence of change in RA waveform and low atrial pressure after pericardial fluid was removed. (Reproduced with permission from Reference 4.)*

right atrial or arterial blood pressure, cardiac output, or other hemodynamic parameters. Endomyocardial biopsy was also performed and confirmed moderately severe transplant rejection. With a vigorous course of antirejection therapy including antilymphocyte globulin, the patient was discharged on day 43 after resolution of her rejection episode. Outpatient right heart catheterization 2 months later showed mild persistent elevation of right heart pressures without diastolic equalization.

The hemodynamic data was consistent with constrictive/restrictive physiology in association with a pericardial effusion and hypotension after orthotopic cardiac transplantation.

Was pericardiocentesis necessary? Although the pericardiocentesis did not alter the hemodynamic findings, the confirmation of another etiology of hypotension could now be established and treated. With treatment of rejection, the hemodynamics reverted to normal. Constrictive physiology, thus, represented an early and reversible manifestation of acute allograft rejection. While restrictive physiology has been reported both early and late after cardiac transplantation, the onset of classical restrictive physiology has not been previously described as predicting allograft rejection.

Case 2. Arterial Pressure Generation Without Electrocardiographic QRS Complexes

A 37-year-old male had surgery for longstanding refractory Class IV congestive heart failure due to idiopathic cardiomyopathy.[5] The surgical treatment for refractory idiopathic congestive heart failure was successful. The arterial pressure and electrocardiogram are shown in Figure 5 and demonstrate a highly irregular arterial pulse pattern with a more regular electrocardiogram. Explain the systolic arterial pressure wave in the absence of apparent high-grade atrial or ventricular ectopy.

This puzzling tracing represents an unusual example of pressure generation occurring from two ventricles in a patient after heterotopic heart transplant (Figure 6). Although 95% of all heart transplantations performed in 1993 have been orthotopic replacements, heterotopic heart transplantation is indicated in patients with pulmonary hypertension who need left ventricular assistance. Orthotopic replacement of a "new" donor heart, unaccustomed to high pulmonary artery pressures would result in severe, potentially fatal

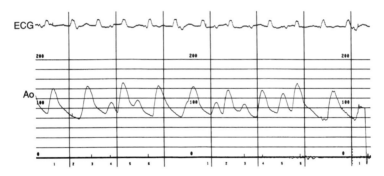

FIGURE 5. *Aortic (Ao) pressure with electrocardiography. Why is pressure generated without corresponding QRS complexes? (Reproduced with permission from Reference 5.)*

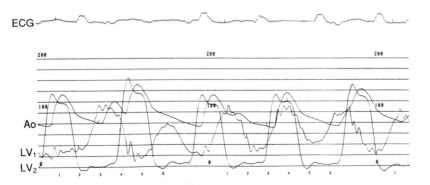

FIGURE 6. *Simultaneous aortic (Ao) and left ventricular (LV$_1$, LV$_2$) pressures (200 mm Hg scale). LV$_1$: native left ventricle; LV$_2$: donor left ventricle. (Reproduced with permission from Reference 5.)*

right ventricular failure after transplantation. The vascular communications of heterotopic transplantation used in this patient were as follows: the aorta of the accessory (donor) heart is attached end-to-side directly to the aorta of the recipient heart and the donor pulmonary artery by graft to the native pulmonary artery. A communication between both left atria is created (large "atrial" septal defect) to allow filling of the donor left ventricle. The donor right ventricle is filled by right atrial flow from the recipient heart. Because the function of the native left ventricle is generally very poor and, at times, insufficient to influence systemic pressure, the arterial pulse depends principally on the Frank-Starling mechanism of filling of the donor heart. However, the electrocardiographic complex that is most prominent may be that of the recipient heart, often accounting for the disparity between electrocardiographic rhythm and pressure waves.

Hemodynamically, the donor heart acts as a built-in left ventricular assist device and maintains the systemic circulation. The customary hemodynamic pressure waveforms may be significantly affected by the dysrhythmic activity of the recipient heart, occasionally requiring high doses of antiarrhythmic agents. Abnormal hemodynamic patterns of donor left ventricular pressure may indicate early transplant rejection. Failing function of the heterotopic transplant often appears as a significant decline in the magnitude of systemic pressure and a slowed and diminished pattern of the peripheral pressure wave. The ratio of the arterial pulse of each of the two contracting ventricles is thought to be an indicator of impending cardiac rejection.

Acting as a pressure "assist" pump, the donor heart influences the systemic pressure in two ways: 1) copulsation: contracting in time with the recipient heart, or 2) counterpulsation: contracting during the recipient heart's diastole. These coincident or counterpoint beats are evidenced by the changing waveform of aortic pressure. The timing of the two left ventricular pressures and influence on aortic pressure can be seen in Figure 6. The subtle small waves in the electrocardiogram mistakenly appearing as P waves are the electrocardiographic complexes of the donor heart with the largest complexes being the recipient heart. This rhythm is more complicated because a ventricular premature contraction in the donor heart may not be detected electrocardiographically and further confuse the pressure wave interpretation. However, in patients with reduced native left ventricular function, left ventricular pressure may be insufficient to exceed systemic pressure, thus, the magnitude of arterial pressure is dependent on donor heart R-R interval and Frank-Starling filling-force relation.

The effect of donor heart copulsation on coronary blood flow can be seen in Figure 7. The left anterior descending coronary artery

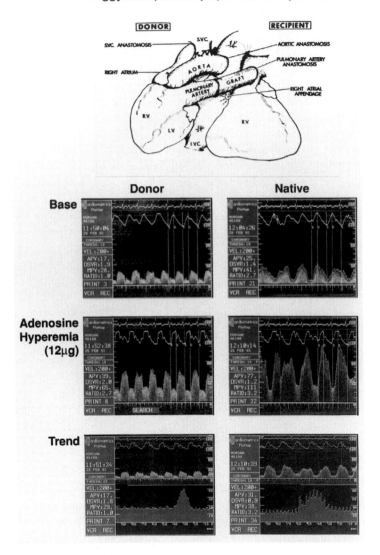

FIGURE 7. *Top: Graphic representation of heterotopic heart transplant surgical anastomoses. SVC: superior vena cava; IVC: inferior vena cava; RV: right ventricle; LV: left ventricle.* **Bottom:** *Coronary flow velocity in each of the left anterior descending coronary arteries is displayed in a spectral format (0–200 cm/sec velocity scale). Electrocardiogram and aortic pressure are displayed at top of each tracing. APV: average peak velocity. Trend shows 90-second continuous APV during hyperemia with adenosine.*

blood flow velocity in each heart was measured at the time of diagnostic angiography with a 0.018-inch Doppler-tipped flow velocity guidewire (FloWire™, Cardiometrics, Inc., Mountain View, CA). The normal phasic coronary flow pattern is shown in the donor heart. The coronary flow pattern is disrupted and intermittently augmented in the recipient heart when donor systole corresponds to recipient heart diastole. This copulsation augments diastolic pressure and flow in the recipient heart much like the effects of intra-aortic balloon pumping on coronary flow in normal arterics.[6]

Case 3. Translesional Coronary Hemodynamics: Decision Making Based on Pressure and Flow in Coronary Arteries

A 43-year-old male who had chest pain syndrome and an abnormal stress test with reversible scintigraphic perfusion defects in the anterior and anteroapical regions was scheduled for angioplasty.[7] Coronary arteriography in the left anterior oblique projection revealed a 58% diameter stenosis (82% area stenosis) of the left anterior descending (Figure 8). Flow velocity and translesional pressure gradients were obtained using a 2.2F fluid-filled tracking catheter and a 0.018-inch Doppler-tipped angioplasty guide wire as previously described (Figure 9).[8] Proximal mean flow velocity was approximately 30 cm/sec, distal velocity was 25 cm/sec with a proximal to distal velocity ratio of 1.2 (Figure 10A). The translesional pressure gradient was approximately 20 mm Hg. Distal coronary flow velocity after 18 µg of intracoronary adenosine increased to 2.9 × basal flow with distal mean velocity reaching 87 cm/sec. Of note, during hyperemia the resting gradient increased to approximately 46 mm Hg (Figure 10A, bottom right). Although flow velocity was normal, the resting translesional gradient was marginal. Coronary angioplasty was successfully performed (Figure 8, bottom). The residual stenosis was 33% diameter (55% area stenosis) by quantitative angiography, a satisfactory angiographic result. Distal flow velocity after the angioplasty was recorded at 5 and 15 minutes after the procedure to assess immediate physiologic results as well as alterations in coronary vasodilatory reserve after a successful dilation (Figure 10B). Five minutes after angioplasty, distal basal mean velocity was 27 cm/sec, unchanged from before the procedure. Distal hyperemia at 5 minutes was 53 cm/sec for a coronary vasodilatory reserve of 2.1. After 15 minutes, baseline flow velocity had fallen slightly to a mean value of 18 cm/sec and hyperemia remained unchanged at 52 cm/sec for a coronary re-

43 yr old Male, LAD, Pre PTCA

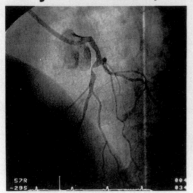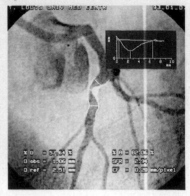

43 yr old Male, LAD, Post PTCA

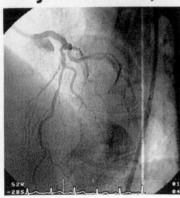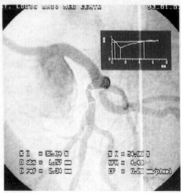

FIGURE 8. *Angiographic frames of a left anterior descending lesion (58% diameter narrowed) with an abnormal stress test. Before (**top**) and after (**bottom**) angioplasty. (Reproduced with permission from Reference 7.)*

serve value of 2.7, nearly identical to that observed before angioplasty. The pressure gradient after the procedure was 5 mm Hg with maximal hyperemic flow velocity increasing the gradient to 25 mm Hg. Basal and hyperemic flow were unchanged by this angiographically successful procedure. The thallium scan, however, remained abnormal. Clinically, the patient has done well.

The translesional coronary hemodynamic data highlight the clinically important questions of which of the major physiologic indicators should be accepted in determining the need for angioplasty and the success after a mechanical intervention. The thallium scan

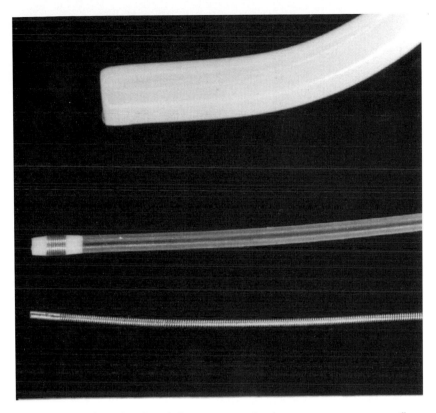

FIGURE 9. *Catheterization laboratory methods to assess coronary flow.* ***Top:*** *8F angiographic (Doppler) catheter.* ***Middle:*** *2.7F pressure gradient catheter (Target Therapeutics, Fremont, CA).* ***Bottom:*** *Doppler FloWireTM 0.014-inch diameter (Cardiometrics, Inc., Mountain View, CA). (Reproduced with permission from Reference 7.)*

remained positive after the angioplasty, despite the fact that the gradient was relieved. Normal distal flow before angioplasty was unchanged after angioplasty. The marginal pressure gradient of 20 mm Hg was reduced to 5 mm Hg without any alteration in distal flow. Without improvement in distal flow or distal hyperemia, it is difficult to say that reduction of the translesional gradient was significant. Likewise, a hyperemic gradient of 45 mm Hg in view of a distal flow velocity that can increase 3 times basal values also likely had little physiologic significance in this particular patient. Studies assessing improvement in the translesional pressure-velocity relation (Figure 11) are underway to improve our understanding of lesion significance leading to more refined appropriate selection of patients for coronary intervention. Since augmentation of distal

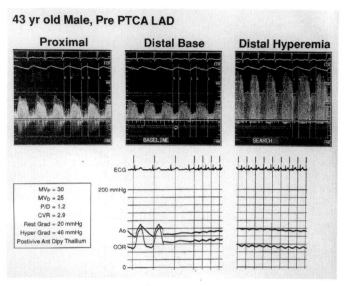

FIGURE 10A. *Translesional flow velocity and pressure gradient before angioplasty. Proximal and distal flow are nearly equivalent with proximal/distal ratio 1.2. Distal hyperemia is 2.9 × basal flow. The mean resting gradient of 20 mm Hg increases to 46 mm Hg during hyperemia. (Reproduced with permission from Reference 7.)*

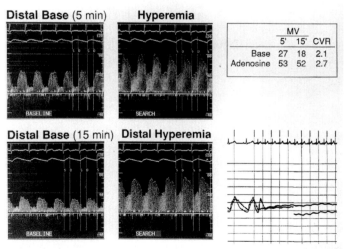

FIGURE 10B. *After angioplasty, distal flow is similar both at rest and during hyperemia. The resting gradient of 2 mm Hg increases to 20 mm Hg with 2.7 × basal flow increase. The thallium scan remained positive. Did angioplasty improve blood flow? See text. (Reproduced with permission from Reference 7.)*

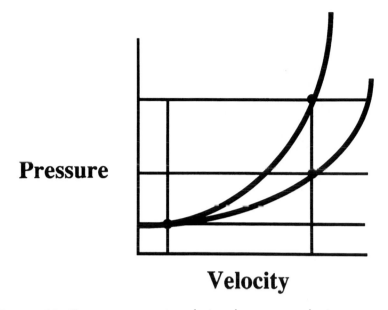

Pressure

Velocity

FIGURE 11. *Coronary artery translesional pressure-velocity curves. Two lesions can have the same resting pressure, but different flow velocity responses. Which would benefit by intervention?*

flow is the objective of anti-ischemic interventions, this parameter may be the most significant indicator of lesion significance.

Summary

Hemodynamic data remain integral components of cardiac catheterization. Hemodynamic data can validate clinical findings, but may confuse the issue if imprecisely examined or collected. Translesional coronary hemodynamics may provide more objective data to make decisions regarding future coronary interventions.

Acknowledgment

The author wishes to thank the J.G. Mudd Cardiac Catheterization Laboratory Team, and Donna Sander for manuscript preparation.

References

1. Grossman W (ed). *Cardiac Catheterization and Angiography.* 3rd Edition. Philadelphia: Lea & Febiger; 1986.
2. Pepine CJ, Hill JA, Lambert CR (eds). *Diagnostic and Therapeutic Cardiac Catheterization.* Baltimore: Williams & Wilkins; 1989.

3. Kern MJ (ed). *Hemodynamic Rounds: Interpretation of Cardiac Pathophysiology from Pressure Waveform Analysis.* New York: Wiley-Liss; 1992:1–218.
4. Seacord LM, Miller LW, Pennington DG, McBride LR, Kern MJ. Reversal of constrictive/restrictive physiology with treatment of allograft rejection. *Am Heart J.* 1990;120:455–459.
5. Kern MJ, Deligonul U, Miller L. Interpretation of cardiac pathophysiology from pressure waveform analysis: extra hearts, Part I. *Cathet Cardiovasc Diagn.* 1991;22:197–204.
6. Kern MJ, Aguirre F, Bach R, Donohue T, Segal J. Augmentation of coronary blood flow by intra-aortic balloon pumping in patients after coronary angioplasty. *Circulation.* 1993;87:500–511.
7. Kern MJ, Flynn MS, Caracciolo EA, Bach RG, Donohue TJ, Aguirre FV. Use of translesiona coronary flow after velocity for interventional decisions in a patient with multiple intermediately severe coronary stenoses. *Cathet Cardiovasc Diagn.* 1993;29:148–153
8. Donohue TJ, Kern MJ, Aguirre FV, et al. Assessing the hemodynamic significance of coronary artery stenoses: analysis of translesional pressure-flow velocity relations in patients. *J Am Coll Cardiol.* 1993;22: 449–458.

Chapter 6

Can Coronary Angiography Define the Extent and Morphology of Coronary Disease and Predict the Site of a Subsequent Myocardial Infarction?

William C. Little, MD,
Robert J. Applegate, MD, and
Gregory Braden, MD

Coronary angiography plays a pivotal role in the evaluation and management of patients with ischemic heart disease. It is used to define the presence, extent, and severity of coronary artery disease, and to guide mechanical therapy (percutaneous transluminal coronary angioplasty [PTCA] and coronary artery bypass graft [CABG]). The interpretation of the coronary angiogram has focused on the presence of "significant" stenoses of more than 50% to 70% diameter narrowing. These stenoses limit coronary flow, may produce ischemia, and can be targeted for "revascularization."

In spite of the well-recognized role of the coronary angiogram in management of patients with coronary artery disease, there is a growing body of data indicating that coronary angiography: 1) cannot predict the site of subsequent intracoronary thrombosis development producing unstable angina or myocardial infarction (MI); 2) is insensitive in determining the extent of coronary atherosclerosis; and 3) is not able to evaluate coronary artery morphology accurately.[1] Furthermore, minor angiographically insignificant changes in luminal diameter have prognostic importance.[2] These recent observations merit close consideration because they have important implications for the understanding of the pathophysiol-

From Vetrovec GW, Carabello BA, (eds.) *Invasive Cardiology: Current Diagnostic and Therapeutic Issues.* Armonk, NY: Futura Publishing Company, Inc.: © 1996.

ogy of coronary artery disease and the clinical management of patients with this disease.

Coronary Angiography: Limitations in Detection of Atherosclerosis

Coronary angiography provides information concerning the presence and severity of obstructive coronary disease by imaging a shadow of the arterial lumen. Most frequently, coronary artery disease is apparent angiographically as focal areas of luminal narrowing. Thus, based on clinical interpretation of angiograms, coronary artery disease is perceived to be a focal process. However, pathologic examination and studies using intraoperative or intravascular ultrasound indicate that coronary artery disease is diffuse rather than focal.[3-8] Early in the atherosclerotic process, the coronary lumen appears to be preserved by a compensatory dilation of the external arterial diameter as the arterial wall thickens.[8-11] Thus, there is usually a substantial amount of atherosclerosis in the coronary artery wall before there is any significant narrowing of the lumen. This suggests that the presence of even a single stenosis on coronary angiography may be a marker of diffuse atherosclerotic involvement of the coronary arteries. Consistent with this concept, recent studies demonstrate abnormal endothelial function, indicative of atherosclerotic involvement, in angiographically normal coronary artery segments in patients with stenoses in another coronary artery,[12] and these sites have been found by intracoronary ultrasound imaging to generally contain angiographically unapparent atherosclerosis.[13] Additionally, intravascular ultrasound has also been shown to demonstrate significant atherosclerosis in patients whose coronary angiograms are normal or contain only minimal luminal narrowing.[14] Thus, by detecting reductions in luminal diameter, coronary arteriography severely underestimates the overall extent of coronary atherosclerosis.

Coronary Angiography Before Myocardial Infarction

Myocardial infarction is usually caused by the sudden, thrombotic occlusion of a coronary artery at the site of a fissured atherosclerotic plaque.[15-17] Pathologic studies indicate that the underlying atherosclerotic plaque typically reduces the luminal cross-sectional area by 80% to 90%.[18,19] Furthermore, the presence of a high-grade stenosis (>80% or 90% angiographic diameter narrowing) is an angiographic risk factor for subsequent occlusion of a coronary artery.[20,21] Thus, stenotic sites identified by coronary angiograms are assumed to be at risk for thrombotic occlusion, while coronary arteries that do not contain obstructive stenoses (<50%) are considered to be nearly free of the risk of occlusion.[21]

In a review of 313 patients who had undergone two coronary angiograms, Moise et al[20] found 116 newly occluded coronary vessels at the time of the second angiogram. The presence of a high-grade (>80%) coronary stenosis, the extent of coronary disease, smoking, and male gender were the factors most predictive of the development of a new coronary artery occlusion. Coronary artery segments that contained a stenosis were more likely to subsequently occlude than were segments free of stenotic lesions. Similarly, Ellis et al[21] found that the more severe the stenosis in the left anterior descending coronary artery, the higher the risk for anterior MI. However, nonstenotic coronary artery segments are not risk-free, and segments without high-grade stenoses are much more numerous than critically narrowed segments. Thus, the majority (72%) of the coronary occlusions in Moise's study occurred in segments that were previously free of high-grade stenoses. Furthermore, the number of coronary artery segments with any abnormality (wall irregularities or stenoses) independent of the severity or numbers of severe stenoses, was the strongest predictor of future coronary events in these patients.[22]

We analyzed 58 patients who had undergone coronary angiography before and after suffering an MI.[23-25] The second coronary angiogram was used to define the location of the new total or subtotal coronary occlusion producing the MI, and was compared with the prior angiogram to assess its predictive value (Figure 1). The severity of stenosis was assessed using a computerized quantitative coronary angiographic system. On the initial angiogram, taken before MI, the location of the most severe angiographic stenosis did not accurately predict the site of the subsequent MI. In only 38% of patients was the most severe angiographic stenosis found to be responsible for the subsequent MI. Furthermore, in 35 (60%) of our patients, the most severe luminal diameter stenosis existing in the infarct-related artery prior to the MI was <50%. Similar results were obtained when the analysis was limited to the 25 patients who had experienced MI within 1 year after the initial angiogram. Thus, an angiographically severe coronary artery stenosis was infrequently present in the infarct-related artery on the initial angiogram, while the other arteries that did contain high-grade stenoses often remained patent.

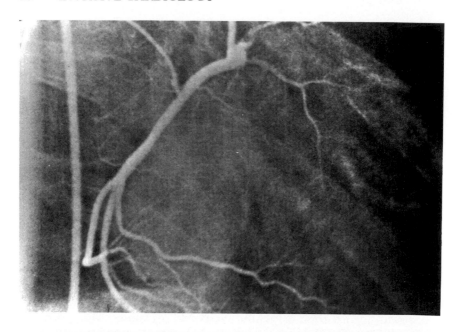

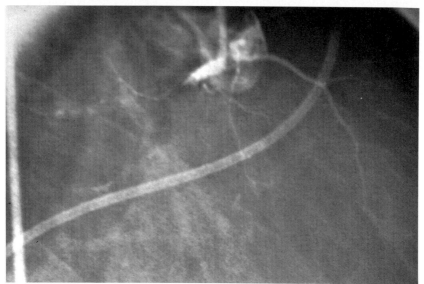

FIGURE 1. **Top.** *Right coronary angiogram taken within 1 year of the development of acute myocardial infarction, demonstrating no stenotic areas in the right coronary artery.* **Bottom.** *Coronary angiogram taken soon after onset of acute inferior myocardial infarction, demonstrating total obstruction of the proximal right coronary artery. (Reproduced with permission from Reference 24.)*

These findings have been confirmed by other studies. Ambrose et al[26] performed a similar analysis of 23 patients who had undergone serial coronary angiograms before and after suffering MI, with nearly identical results. Only 22% of the infarct-related arteries contained a >75% diameter stenosis before MI. Similarly, Hacket et al[27] and Giroud et al[28] found that in the overwhelming majority of patients with MI, the infarct artery contained <50% stenosis in an angiogram obtained prior to the MI, and that the most severely stenosed artery was the site of the subsequent occlusion in only one third of patients. A prospective, serial angiographic study by Webster et al[29] at the Mayo Clinic also found that the majority of MIs occurred due to occlusion of arteries that previously contained <50% stenosis. These studies indicate that MI often arises from vessels that did not contain angiographically apparent stenoses, and that coronary angiography cannot adequately predict the site of a subsequent occlusion that will produce an MI.

Patients who were treated with CABG or PTCA were not included in the serial angiographic studies of MI. Accordingly, we have also evaluated patients who suffered an MI at least 1 month after successful CABG or PTCA.[30,31] Coronary angiography performed within 2 weeks of the MI was used to define the infarct-related artery. The angiogram obtained before CABG or at the time of PTCA was used to assess the preexisting coronary disease. One third of the MIs occurring after successful CABG were found to be caused by an occlusion of an artery that had not been bypassed. This artery had not received a bypass graft because in all patients except one, it did not obtain an obstructive (>50% diameter narrowing) stenosis. Similarly, 57% of MIs after successful PTCA were due to an occlusion of an artery that had not received PTCA because it did not contain an obstructive stenosis.[31]

In addition to the serial angiographic data, several lines of evidence indicate that MI can occur in the absence of severe atherosclerotic obstruction of the coronary lumen. First, in many patients, MI (or sudden death) is the initial manifestation of coronary artery disease.[32,33] The absence of exertional angina in these patients prior to the catastrophic event suggests that functionally obstructive atherosclerotic lesions may not have been present prior to the development of catastrophic coronary thrombosis.

Second, serial angiographic observations in patients with unstable angina indicate that a thrombus overlying an atheroma abruptly increases the severity of coronary artery obstruction without totally obstructing the artery.[34-36] In agreement with the results of serial angiographic studies of patients with MI, the artery responsible for unstable ischemic syndromes frequently does not contain a high-grade stenosis prior to the onset of symptoms.[37,38]

Third, the use of thrombolytic agents has also provided evidence that the atheroma inciting MI may not always be stenotic prior to formation of the thrombus. After coronary flow is restored by thrombolytic therapy in patients with MI, only minor, nonstenotic lesions (<50% diameter narrowing) are present in some patients.[27,39–41] Frequently, however, there is a high-grade residual stenosis present after thrombolysis. This may represent a preexisting severe stenosis at the site of coronary occlusion or a combination of residual thrombi overlying the atheroma, making the lesion appear much more severe than it was immediately prior to the infarct. The study of Brown et al[42] suggests the latter is a common occurrence. These investigators used angiographic magnification and computerized measurements to separate the coronary atheroma from the overlying thrombus in 32 patients who had received intracoronary streptokinase. The underlying atherosclerotic lesion produced on average only a 56% diameter stenosis. Similar results using quantitative angiography after thrombolytic therapy have been reported by Serruys et al[39,40] and Hacket et al[27,41] Thus, studies performed after thrombolytic therapy for myocardial infarction provide evidence that the culprit stenosis was not severe.

Finally, analysis of the TAMI data by Ellis et al[43] is also consistent with the hypothesis that a severe stenosis is not necessary for thrombus formation. They evaluated the ability of coronary angiography performed soon after successful thrombolytic therapy to predict subsequent episodes of ischemia. No angiographic variable predicted recurrent ischemia. Such ischemic episodes, which usually result from rethrombosis, occurred with nearly equal frequency in patients with mild and severe residual stenoses after thrombolytic therapy.

Angiographic Morphology

It has been suggested that the morphology of a stenosis can be used to predict the site of future coronary occlusions. At the time of onset of MI or unstable angina, the endothelium of the plaque underlying the coronary thrombosis is disrupted, exposing the thrombogenic components of the plaque to the blood stream. This fissured plaque with overlying thrombus may be angiographically apparent as a convex, intraluminal obstruction with convex edges, irregularities, and/or intraluminal defects.[37,44] The culprit lesions frequently exhibit these angiographic characteristics after the development of MI or unstable angina.[44,45] It is possible that stenoses with these characteristics in patients without MI or angina may have a higher risk of subsequent occlusion. However, we recently found that on angiograms performed prior to MI, the culprit plaque does not usually appear complex in the majority of patients.[46] In addition, the angiographic morphology of the culprit lesion after thrombolytic therapy does not predict subsequent reocclusion.[47] Prior to MI, the future infarct site may have only minor wall irregularities or a scalloped area.[46] Similarly, analysis of patients in the CASS study with left anterior descending lesions suggested that lesion roughness was a predictor of subsequent occlusion.[47] These data indicate that complex angiographic morphology may be present in unstable coronary syndrome after a plaque has been disrupted and triggered thrombus formation. However, this complex angiographic morphology need not be present prior to the event.

Two new techniques, intracoronary angioscopy and intracoronary ultrasound, allow evaluation of coronary morphology in vivo that can be compared with coronary angiography.[48] Angioscopy usually identifies ruptured plaques with overlying thrombosis in patients with unstable angina.[49] The complex morphology of these culprit lesions is not always apparent on the coronary angiogram. After balloon angioplasty, angioscopy visualizes small tears and disruption of the arterial endothelium.[50] These same areas may appear smooth on the coronary angiogram. Thus, angioscopy demonstrates limitations of coronary angiography in defining endothelial morphology of coronary artery lesions. Intracoronary ultrasound provides a cross-sectional image of the vessel wall.[51,52] Intracoronary ultrasound is more sensitive in detecting coronary calcification than coronary angiography.[53] Furthermore, coronary angiography is a poor predictor of lesion eccentricity based on determination of arterial wall thickness defined with ultrasound.[51]

Comparison With Autopsy and Natural History Studies

We have reviewed evidence suggesting that coronary angiography is insensitive in the early detection and quantitation of the extent of coronary atherosclerotic disease and that an angiographically apparent stenosis is not a prerequisite to the development of thrombus formation and MI. How can these ideas be reconciled with: 1) the autopsy data that indicate that occlusive coronary artery thrombi frequently develop at the site of severe (80% to 90%) stenoses[54]; and 2) studies demonstrating that the prognosis of patients with stable angina is related to the number of angiographically stenosed coronary arteries.[55]

First, in pathologic studies, an area stenosis rather than a diameter stenosis is determined. Because a cross-sectional area is proportioned to the square of the diameter, a 90% area stenosis is equivalent to a 68% diameter stenosis (Figure 2). The pathologist uses the entire area within the internal elastic lamina as the denominator. Angiographers use an angiographically normal adjacent segment as the reference. However, this angiographically normal segment generally has atherosclerosis within the vessel wall[56]and thus may be substantially more narrow than the internal elastic lamina. Because of these considerations, the culprit lesion in MI, quantitated as a 90% reduction in cross-sectional area in a pathologic study, may have been apparent only as a 40% or smaller diameter stenosis on an angiogram (Figure 2). Therefore, the observation that MI can occur in the absence of an angiographically

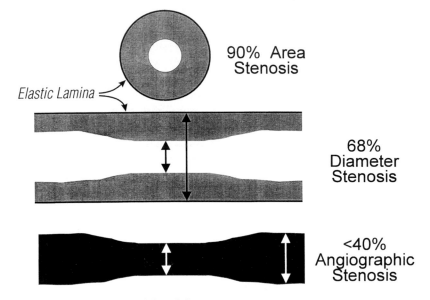

FIGURE 2. *Illustration of the difference in the severity of stenosis quantitated as a percent area stenosis in pathologic studies and percent diameter stenosis determined angiographically. A 90% reduction in luminal cross-sectional area is equivalent to only a 68% reduction in diameter. In pathologic studies, the normal reference cross-sectional areas are defined by the internal elastic lamina. This landmark is not visible angiographically. Thus, the reference diameter is measured from an adjacent normal segment. Since coronary angiography underestimates the extent of coronary atherosclerosis, this normal segment may, in fact, be narrowed. Thus, a 90% area stenosis in an autopsy study may have produced a 40% or less diameter stenosis angiographically.*

apparent stenosis, and the autopsy data suggesting severely athero-sclerotic vessels are not in conflict. Moreover, because of the limi-tations of coronary angiography in detecting the extent of atherosclerosis, the occlusion of an area of angiographically in-significant narrowing is actually thrombosis at a site of advanced atherosclerosis, albeit without narrowing of the lumen.

The prognosis of patients with stable angina is related to the number of stenosed coronary arteries and the left ventricular ejec-tion fraction.[55] However, patients with irregularities of the coro-nary artery walls, but without any angiographically significant stenosis (<50% diameter narrowing), have a substantially lower survival rate than patients with completely normal coronary arter-ies.[55] The impaired survival of patients with insignificant coronary artery disease is most likely due to the development of thrombotic coronary artery occlusion. Because patients with "insignificant" coronary artery disease usually have normal left ventricular ejec-tion fractions, their survival should be compared with that of pa-tients with "severe" coronary artery disease with similar left ventricular function.[57] Interestingly, the survival curve of patients from the CASS registry with nonstenotic coronary artery disease is superimposable with the survival curve of patients with severe coronary artery disease with >70% diameter stenoses of all three arteries (ie, three-vessel disease) and normal left ventricular func-tion who were randomized to initial medical therapy in the CASS trial (Figure 3).[57-59] This observation suggests that the presence of atherosclerosis in the coronary arterial wall, whether or not it sig-nificantly narrows the lumen, places a patient at increased risk for MI or death.

Prognostic Importance of Small Changes in Luminal Diameter

Although stenosis severity and morphology per se do not ap-pear sensitive in predicting the site of future coronary occlusions, recent data indicate that small changes in coronary luminal diam-eter, which would not be considered clinically significant, are asso-ciated with a significant increase in cardiac events. As part of a clinical trial of nicardipine, Waters et al[60] performed coronary an-giograms 2 years apart in 335 patients. The patients were then prospectively followed for a mean of 44 ± 10 months after the sec-ond arteriogram.[61] Progression of coronary artery disease was de-fined as a >15% increase in stenosis severity at one or more sites. Much of the progression seen was relatively minor and previously

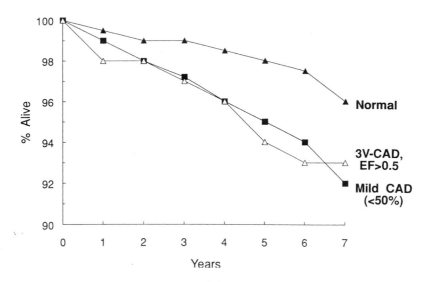

FIGURE 3. *Diagram comparison of the survival of patients with normal coronary arteries (normal) and patients with mild coronary artery disease without any stenotic lesions (>50%) stenosis) from the CASS Registry,58 and the survival of patients with severe three vessel coronary artery disease and normal left ventricular ejection fractions (3V-CAD, EF>0.5).55 Note that the survival rate of patients with mild, angiographically insignificant coronary artery disease is superimposable on the survival rate of patients with severe three-vessel coronary artery disease. (Modified with permission from Reference 1.)*

would not have been considered clinically important. However, patients with progression were 7.3 times more likely to have cardiac death and 2.3 times as likely to have death or infarction during the subsequent follow-up. Although half of these patients, had been randomized to receive nicardipine during the 2 years between angiograms, it had no effect on progression or regression of established coronary atherosclerosis. Similar findings have also been recently reported from the placebo group of the Program on the Surgical Control of Hyperlipidemias (POSCH) Group.[62] In follow-up of the patients in this study, changes from a baseline angiogram, to 1 performed 3 years later, were strongly and significantly associated with subsequent overall and atherosclerotic coronary heart disease mortality. Thus, these prospective studies of the natural history of coronary artery disease, demonstrate that even minor progression of angiographic luminal narrowing is a strong predictor of future cardiac events.

In addition to these clinical observations, there are theoretical reasons to support the concept that small changes in coronary artery lumen diameter, such as observed in these serial angiographic trials, may be associated with a substantial alteration in plaque stress. Loree et al [63] and Richardson et al[64] evaluated the stresses in atherosclerotic vessels. They found that small changes in thickness of the fibrous cap have a much stronger effect on its circumferential stress than does the caliber of the coronary lumen. The highest levels of stress occurred in thin caps at the site of only minimal stenosis. These data provide a mechanistic explanation why plaque rupture and coronary occlusion may occur in areas that do not contain an angiographically apparent stenosis. Therefore, it is plausible that small changes in the coronary artery diameter may reflect the activity of the underlying atherosclerotic process; areas of progression may identify sites prone to sudden catastrophic changes in lumen patency.

Clinical Implications

Based on the data reviewed in this chapter, we have proposed[24] that atherosclerotic coronary artery lesions can have two important characteristics. They may be obstructive and/or have thrombogenic potential (Figure 4). Obstructive plaques cause luminal encroachment and are recognizable on coronary angiograms. By limiting coronary flow, they may produce exertional angina. Thrombogenic plaques are vulnerable to fissuring if exposed to an appropriate triggering stimuli and result in thrombosis formation. Nonobstructive plaques containing eccentric pools of lipid with a thin cap may be most prone to fissuring.[63,64] If a plaque expresses its thrombogenic potential, it may cause an MI if the resulting thrombus occludes the artery, or may produce unstable angina if the thrombus is not totally obstructive. Thrombus formation may also produce sudden death. Plaques with thrombogenic potential do not need to be obstructive and thus may not be recognized on a coronary angiogram.

An angiographically obstructive stenosis indicates the presence of coronary atherosclerosis and the potential for development of MI, but the coronary stenosis does not necessarily indicate the location at which the thrombotic occlusion will occur.[23,24] The presence of high-grade stenosis is a marker for advanced atherosclerotic coronary artery disease. It is important to recognize that localized areas of angiographic stenosis underestimate the extent of atherosclerotic involvement of the coronary arteries. In the patients whose

CORONARY ARTERY LESIONS

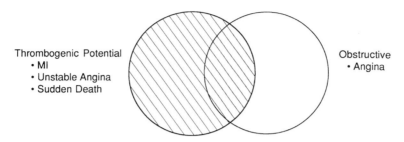

Thrombogenic Potential
• MI
• Unstable Angina
• Sudden Death

Obstructive
• Angina

FIGURE 4. *Diagram illustrating clinically important characteristics of coronary atherosclerotic lesions. The plaque can be obstructive and/or have thrombogenic potential. Obstructive plaques produce angina. If a plaque expresses its thrombogenic potential, it may cause myocardial infarction (MI), unstable angina, or death. Not all plaques with thrombogenic potential are obstructive, and not all obstructive plaques are vulnerable to becoming thrombogenic. (Modified with permission from Reference 24.)*

angiogram demonstrates only nonobstructive atherosclerosis, the possibility of the future occurrence of MI cannot be ruled out, since potentially thrombogenic plaques need not be obstructive.

CABG and PTCA are appropriately directed only at the angiographically significant (ie, stenotic or flow limiting) lesions. Since it is difficult to predict the site of the subsequent occlusion from a coronary angiogram, these interventions may not be effective in preventing subsequent MI. This does not indicate that coronary arteries that do not have obstructive lesions should be dilated.[65] Instead, effective therapy to prevent MI may need to be directed at the entire coronary tree, and not just at obstructive lesions. Although mechanical treatment of high-grade coronary stenoses relieves angina and improves exercise tolerance, slowing or reversing the progression of atherosclerosis in the walls of the coronary arteries may be a more powerful intervention to prevent the catastrophic complications of coronary artery disease (unstable angina, MI, and death).

Conclusion

Coronary atherosclerosis is a disease of the arterial wall. The initial response to thickening of the wall with atherosclerosis is a compensatory enlargement of the artery, that preserves the lumen[9] while potential thrombogenic plaques are developing in the wall of the artery. Thus, imaging the lumen with coronary angiography is an inaccurate means of quantitating the severity and extent of coronary disease and its morphology, and, thus provides inadequate information to predict the site of subsequent occlusion that will produce myocardial infarction.

Acknowledgments

We appreciate Judy Fleurant's excellent secretarial assistance in preparation of this manuscript.

References

1. Little WC, Downes TR, Applegate RJ. The underlying coronary lesion in myocardial infarction: implications for coronary angiography. *Clin Cardiol.* 1991;14:868–874.
2. Applegate RJ, Herrington DM, Little WC. Coronary angiography: more than meets the eye. *Circulation.* 1993;87:1399–1401.
3. Roberts WC, Jones AA. Quantitation of coronary arterial narrowing at necropsy in sudden coronary death: analysis of 31 patients and comparison with 25 control subjects. *Am J Cardiol.* 1979;44:39–45.
4. Roberts WC, Jones AA. Quantification of coronary arterial narrowing at necropsy in acute myocardial infarction: analysis and comparison of findings in 27 patients and 22 control subjects. *Circulation.* 1980;61:786–790.
5. Waller BF. The eccentric coronary atherosclerotic plaque: morphologic observations and clinical relevance. *Clin Cardiol.* 1989;12:14–20.
6. Vlodaver Z, Frech R, Van Tassel RA, Edwards JE. Correlation of the antemortem coronary arteriogram and the postmortem specimen. *Circulation.* 1973;47:162–169.
7. Downes TR, Braden GA, Herrington DM, Applegate RJ, Kutcher MA, Little WC. Mechanism of PTCA dilatation in coronary vessels: intravascular ultrasound assessment. *J Am Coll Cardiol.* 1991;17:126A. Abstract.
8. Dietz WA, Tobis JM, Isner JM. Failure of angiography to accurately depict the extent of coronary artery narrowing in three fatal cases of percutaneous transluminal coronary angioplasty. *J Am Coll Cardiol.* 1992;19:1261–1270.
9. Glagov S, Weisenberg E, Zarins CK, Stankunavicius R, Kolettis GJ. Compensatory enlargement of human atherosclerotic coronary arteries. *N Engl J Med.* 1987;316:1137l–11375.
10. Stiel GM, Ludmill LSG, Schofer J, Donath K, Mathey DG. Impact of compensatory enlargement of atherosclerotic coronary arteries on angiographic assessment of coronary artery disease. *Circulation.* 1989;80:1603–1609.
11. McPherson DD, Sirna SJ, Hiratzka LF, et al. Coronary arterial remodeling studied by high-frequency epicardial echocardiography: an early

compensatory mechanism in patients with obstructive coronary atherosclerosis. *J Am Coll Cardiol.* 1991;17:79–86.

12. Ludmer PL, Selwyn AP, Shook TL, et al. Paradoxical vasoconstriction induced by acetylcholine in atherosclerotic coronary arteries. *N Engl J Med.* 1986;315:1046–1051.

13. Yamagishi M, Miyatake M, Tamai J, Nakatani S, Koyama J, Nissen SE. Intravascular ultrasound detection of atherosclerosis at the site of focal vasospasm in angiographically normal or minimally narrowed coronary segments. *J Am Coll Cardiol.* 1994;23(2):352–357.

14. Porter TR, Sears T, Feng X, Michels A, Welsh D, Shumer S. Intravascular ultrasound study of angiographically mildly diseased coronary arteries. *J Am Coll Cardiol.* 1993;22:1858–1865.

15. Constantinidines P. Plaque hemorrhages, their genesis, and their role in supra-plaque thrombosis and atherogenesis. In: Glagov S, Newman WP, Schaeffer SA, eds. *Pathobiology of the Human Atherosclerotic Plaque.* New York: Springer-Verlag; 1989:393–411.

16. DeWood A, Spores J, Notske R, et al. Prevalence of total coronary occlusion during the early hours of transmural myocardial infarction. *N Engl J Med.* 1980;303:897–902.

17. Gorlin R, Fuster V, Ambrose JA. Anatomic physiologic links between acute coronary syndromes. *Circulation.* 1986;74:6–9.

18. Davies MJ. Successful and unsuccessful coronary thrombolysis. *Br Heart J.* 1989;61:381–384.

19. Falk E. Plaque rupture with severe pre-existing stenosis precipitating coronary thrombosis. *Br Heart J.* 1983;50:127–134.

20. Moise A, Lesperance J, Therous P, Tayemans Y, Goulet C, Bourassa MG. Clinical and angiographic predictors of new total coronary occlusion in coronary artery disease: analysis of 313 nonoperated patients. *Am J Cardiol.* 1984;54:1176–1181.

21. Ellis S, Alderman E, Cain K, et al. Prediction of risk of anterior myocardial infarction by lesion severity and measurement method of stenoses in the left anterior descending coronary distribution: a CASS Registry Study. *J Am Coll Cardiol.* 1988;11:908–916.

22. Moise A, Clement B, Saltiel J. Clinical and angiographic correlates and prognostic significance of the coronary extent score. *Am J Cardiol.* 1988;61:1255–1259.

23. Little WC, Constantinescu M, Applegate RJ, et al. Can coronary angiography predict the site of a subsequent myocardial infarction in patients with mild to moderate coronary artery disease? *Circulation.* 1988;78:1157–1166.

24. Little WC. Angiographic assessment of the culprit coronary artery lesion before acute myocardial infarction. *Am J Cardiol.* 1990;66:44G–47G.

25. Little WC, Workman R, Burrows M, et al. Coronary anatomy preceding non-Q wave myocardial infarction. *J Am Coll Cardiol.* 1989;13:6A. Abstract.

26. Ambrose JA, Tannenbaum MA, Alexopoulos D, et al. Angiographic progression of coronary artery disease and the development of myocardial infarction. *J Am Coll Cardiol.* 1988;12:56–62.

27. Hacket D, Verwilghen J, Davies G, Maseri A. Coronary stenoses before and after acute myocardial infarction. *Am J Cardiol.* 1989;63:1517–1518.

28. Giroud D, Li JM, Urban P, Meier B, Rutishauser W. Relation of the site

of acute myocardial infarction to the most severe coronary arterial stenosis at prior angiography. *Am J Cardiol.* 1992;69:729–732.

29. Webster M, Chesebro JH, Smith HC, et al. Myocardial infarction and coronary artery occlusion: a prospective 5-year angiographic study. *J Am Coll Cardiol.* 1990;15:218A. Abstract.

30. Little WC, Gwinn NS, Burrows MT, Kutcher MA, Kahl FR, Applegate RJ. Cause of acute myocardial infarction late after successful coronary artery bypass grafting. *Am J Cardiol.* 1990;65:808–810.

31. Kerensky RA, Kutcher MA, Mumma M, Applegate R, Little WC. Myocardial infarction late after successful PTCA: progression of disease versus reoccurrence. *J Am Coll Cardiol.* 1991;17:304A. Abstract.

32. Alonzo AA, Simon AB, Feinleib M. Prodromata of myocardial infarction and sudden death. *Circulation.* 1975;52:1056–1062.

33. Turner SA, Rufty AJ, Hackshaw BT, Applegate R, Little WC. Myocardial infarction as the presenting manifestation of coronary artery disease. *Clin Res.* 1989;37:303A. Abstract.

34. Ambrose JA, Winters SL, Arora RR, et al. Coronary angiographic morphology in myocardial infarction: a link between the pathogenesis of unstable angina and myocardial infarction. *J Am Coll Cardiol.* 1985;6:1233–1238.

35. Wilson RF, Holida MD, White CW. Quantitative angiographic morphology of coronary stenoses leading to myocardial infarction or unstable angina. *Circulation.* 1986;73:286–293.

36. Sherman CT, Litvack F, Grundfest W, et al. Coronary angioscopy in patients with unstable angina pectoris. *N Engl J Med.* 1986;315:913–919.

37. Ambrose JA, Winters SL, Arora RR, et al. Angiographic evolution of coronary artery morphology in unstable angina. *J Am Coll Cardiol.* 1986;7:474–478.

38. Moise A, Theroux P, Taycmans Y, et al. Unstable angina and progression of coronary atherosclerosis. *N Engl J Med.* 1983;309:685–690.

39. Serruys PW, Wijns W, Van Den Brand M, et al. Is transluminal coronary angioplasty mandatory after successful thrombolysis?. *Br Heart J.* 1983;50:257–265.

40. Serruys PW, Arnold AER, Brower RW, et al. Effect of continued rt-PA administration on the residual stenosis after initially successful recanalization in acute myocardial infarction: a quantitative coronary angiography study of a randomized trial. *Eur Heart J.* 1987;8:1172–1181.

41. Hacket D, Davies G, Maseri A. Pre-existing coronary stenoses in patients with first myocardial infarction are not necessarily severe. *Eur Heart J.* 1988;9:1317–1323.

42. Brown BG, Gallery CA, Badger RS, et al. Incomplete lysis of thrombus in the moderate underlying atherosclerotic lesion during intracoronary infusion of streptokinase for acute myocardial infarction: quantitative angiographic observations. *Circulation.* 1986;73:653–661.

43. Ellis SG, Topol EJ, George BS, et al. Recurrent ischemia without warning. Analysis of risk factors for in-hospital ischemic events following successful thrombolysis with intravenous issue plasminogen activator. *Circulation.* 1989;80:1159–1165.

44. Nakagawa S, Hanada Y, Koiwaya Y, Tanaka K. Angiographic features in the infarct-related artery after intracoronary urokinase followed by prolonged anticoagulation. *Circulation.* 1988;88:1335–1344.

108   *INVASIVE CARDIOLOGY*

45. Ambrose JA. Coronary arteriographic analysis and angiographic morphology. *J Am Coll Cardiol.* 1989;13:1492.
46. Nierste D, Little WC. Morphology of the culprit coronary artery lesion preceding myocardial infarction. *Circulation.* 1989;80:II-349. Abstract.
47. Ellis S, Alderman EL, Cain K, Wright A, Bourassa M, Fisher L. Morphology of left anterior descending coronary territory lesions as a predictor of anterior myocardial infarction: a CASS registry study. *J Am Coll Cardiol.* 1989;13:1481–1491.
48. Siegel RJ, Mehrdad A, Fishbein MD, et al. Histopathologic validation of angioscopy and intravascular ultrasound. *Circulation.* 1991;84:109–117.
49. Sherman CT, Litvack F, Grundfest WS, et al. Demonstration of thrombus and complex atheroma by in-vivo angioscopy in patients with unstable angina pectoris. *N Engl J Med.* 1986;315:913–919.
50. Ichido Y, Hasegawa K, Kawamura J, Shibaya I. Angioscopic observation of the coronary luminal changes induced by percutaneous transluminal coronary angioplasty. *Am Heart J.* 1989;117:769–776.
51. Braden GA, Herrington DM, Kerensky RA, Kutcher MA, Little WC. Angiography poorly predicts actual lesion eccentricity in severe coronary stenoses: confirmation by intracoronary ultrasound imaging. *J Am Coll Cardiol.* 1994;23(1):40–48.
52. Hodgson JM, Reddy KG, Suneja R, Nair R, Lesnefsky EJ, Sheehan HM. Intracoronary ultrasound imaging: correlation of plaque morphology with angiography, clinical syndrome and procedural results in patients undergoing coronary angioplasty. *J Am Coll Cardiol.* 1993;21:35–44.
53. Honye J, Mahon DJ, Jain A, et al. Morphological effects of coronary balloon angioplasty in vivo assessed by intravascular ultrasound imaging. *Circulation.* 1992;85:1012–1025.
54. Qiao JH, Fishbein MC. The severity of coronary atherosclerosis at sites of plaque rupture with occlusive thrombosis. *J Am Coll Cardiol.* 1991;17:1138–1142.
55. Mock MB, Ringqvist I, Fisher LD, et al. Survival of medically treated patients in the coronary artery surgery study (CASS) registry. *Circulation.* 1982;66:562.
56. Braden GA, Downes TR. Intravascular ultrasound detection of coronary artery "disease" rather than "lumens". *Clin Res.* 1990;38:963. Abstract.
57. Alderman EL, Bourassa MG, Cohen LS, et al. Ten-year follow-up of survival and myocardial infarction in the randomized coronary artery surgery study. *Circulation.* 1990;82:1629–1646.
58. Kemp HG, Kronmal RA, Vlietstra RE, Frye RI, and participants in the Coronary Artery Surgery Study. Seven year survival of patients with normal or near normal coronary arteriograms: a CASS registry study.. *J Am Coll Cardiol.* 1986;7:479–483.
59. Epstein SE, Quyyumi AA, Bonow RO. Sudden cardiac death without warning. *N Engl J Med.* 1989;321:320–324.
60. Waters D, Lesperance J, Francetich M, et al. A controlled clinical trial to assess the effect of a calcium channel bocker on the progression of coronary atherosclerosis. *Circulation.* 1990;82:1940–1953.
61. Waters D, Craven TE, Lesperance J. Prognostic significance of progression of coronary atherosclerosis. *Circulation.* 1993;87:1067–1075.
62. Buchwald H, Matts JP, Fitch LL, et al. Changes in sequential coronary

anteriograms and subsequent coronary events. *JAMA*. 1992;268:1429–
1433.

63. Loree HM, Kamm RD, Stringfellow RG, Lee RT. Effects of fibrous cap
thickness on peak circumferential stress in model atherosclerotic vessels. *Circ Res*. 1992;71:850–858.

64. Richardson PD, Davies MJ, Born GVR. Influence of plaque configuration and stress distribution on fissuring of coronary atherosclerotic
plaques. *Lancet*. 1989;2:941–944.

65. Ischinger T, Gruentzig AR, Hollman J, et al. Should coronary arteries
with <60% diameter stenosis be treated by angioplasty?. *Circulation*.
1983;68:148–154.

Chapter 7

Coronary Angioscopy:
Assessment of Lesion Morphology

Christopher J. White, MD and
Stephen R. Ramee, MD

Angiographic atherosclerotic coronary lesion morphology is an important determinant of a successful coronary angioplasty (PTCA).[1-5] However, a major limitation of these studies is the documented insensitivity of angiography for detecting subtle changes in coronary artery surface morphology, such as plaque fractures, dissections, intracoronary thrombi, and the assessment of residual stenosis after angioplasty.[6-8]

Rapid advancements in angioplasty catheter design have led to the development of many new technologies for therapeutic and diagnostic applications. One of these new devices is the angioscope.[9-11] The angioscope is a percutaneous catheter-based system designed to allow direct visual inspection of the endoluminal surface of the coronary arteries. The promise of the angioscope is that direct visual examination of the surface morphology of a diseased coronary artery will provide more specific, more sensitive, and more accurate information than angiography for identifying details of atherosclerotic plaque morphology.

Angioscope Equipment and Procedure

The imaging system is made up of components including illumination fibers, imaging fibers, a video camera and monitor, and a videotape recorder. The angioscope (Imagecath™, Baxter Edwards, Irvine, CA) contains 3000 image fibers and is designed as a rapid exchange catheter using a 0.014-inch angioplasty guide wire. The angioscope measures 4.5F in diameter and has a lumen for in-

From Vetrovec GW, Carabello BA, (eds.) *Invasive Cardiology: Current Diagnostic and Therapeutic Issues.* Armonk, NY: Futura Publishing Company, Inc.: © 1996.

flating and deflating the occlusion balloon at its distal tip. The occlusion balloon is very compliant and achieves a variable final diameter up to a maximum diameter of 5.0 mm. An optically clear flush solution is infused through the angioscope's distal lumen to clear the field of view during inflation of the occlusion balloon. The image bundle may be advanced or withdrawn independently of the outer catheter a distance of approximately 5 cm, allowing examination of a large segment of the artery or lesion of interest.

An 8F conventional angioplasty guiding catheter is placed in the coronary ostium of interest, and 10,000 units of heparin are administered. A 0.014-inch angioplasty guide wire is advanced across the target lesion and into the distal segment of the vessel. The angioscope has three umbilical connections for the light source, the video camera, and the flush lumen, which are connected when the scope is outside of the body. The scope is "white balanced", focused, and flushed before introduction into the guiding catheter.

The angioscope is then advanced over the guide wire and positioned proximal to the region to be examined. Optically clear flush solution (warmed Ringer's lactate) is infused through the distal lumen of the scope with a power injector at a rate 0.5–1.0 cc per second. The occlusion balloon is hand-inflated with a 1-cc syringe filled with a 50:50 mixture of saline and radiographic contrast. Special care is taken not to overinflate the balloon, which may damage the vessel. The imaging bundle is then advanced over the guide wire to view the intraluminal surface of the vessel. Each imaging sequence lasts approximately 30 to 45 seconds after which the occlusion balloon is deflated, and antegrade blood flow restored. These steps can be repeated several times until the region of interest has been adequately investigated.

Saphenous Vein Bypass Grafts

The angiographic appearance of "friable" or loosely adherent plaque lining saphenous vein coronary bypass grafts has been suggested by some investigators to be a relative contraindication to balloon angioplasty due to the increased risk of distal embolization of atherosclerotic material.[12] Histological studies of saphenous vein bypass graft stenoses demonstrate the progression from fibrointimal proliferation in early graft lesions (<1 year old) to the development of typical atherosclerotic plaque in grafts ≥3 years old.[13,14] These plaques differ very little in their composition from native coronary artery atherosclerotic lesions except that the plaques may be larger in ectatic saphenous vein grafts and because of their bulk may be more likely to cause clinically significant embolization during angioplasty. It has been reported that angioplasty of saphenous vein bypass grafts >3 years old have been associated with increased risk of distal embolization.[15] However, other investigators have not confirmed the increased association of angioplasty complications with any specific angiographic lesion morphology in bypass grafts or that older vein grafts are associated with an increased risk of procedural complications.[16–18]

We compared angiographic and angioscopic lesion morphology in 21 saphenous vein bypass grafts.[9] All but one of the patients had unstable angina. The mean age of the saphenous vein coronary bypass grafts was 10.1 ± 2.4 years (range 5 to 15 years). Restenosis, at a prior angioplasty site, was present in seven patients.

Intravascular thrombi were detected by angioscopy in 71% (15/21) grafts while only 19% (4) had thrombi detected by angiography ($P<0.001$). We found no difference in the angioscopic incidence of intracoronary thrombi in restenosis graft lesions 71% (5/7) compared with the de novo graft lesions 71% (10/14). We also found no correlation between the age of a bypass graft and the presence of angioscopic thrombus.

Intimal dissection was seen in 66% (14) of grafts by angioscopy versus only 9.5% (2) grafts by angiography ($P<0.01$). None of the patients had angiographic evidence of dissection prior to PTCA, whereas seven patients had intimal tears seen with angioscopy before angioplasty. After PTCA there were 2 (9.5%) angiographic dissections versus 11 (52.3%) that were seen with the angioscope. The identification of angioscopic dissection did not correlate with the age of the bypass graft.

Graft friability was detected before PTCA by angioscopy in 11 (52.3%) versus only 4 (19%) grafts by angiography ($P<0.05$). Interestingly, graft age did not correlate with the presence of friable plaque. Angioscopy confirmed the presence of friable plaque in 3 of the 4 grafts identified by angiography as having friable plaque. The vein graft incorrectly identified as friable by angiography had a lesion with a white fibrotic-appearing nonshaggy intimal lining identified by angioscopy.

Our data demonstrate the superior ability of angioscopy to detect features of lesion morphology that are frequently not seen by angiography in saphenous vein coronary bypass grafts. This uncertainty regarding the risk of embolization and the uncertain ability of angiography to identify a high-risk subgroup for complications of angioplasty may be related to the insensitivity of angiography for detecting friable lesions as we have shown. None of our patients experienced embolization associated with angioplasty of these older vein grafts including the 11 patients with friability of the luminal surface as identified by angioscopy.

Angioscopic identification of friable plaque does not preclude an uncomplicated angioplasty procedure. In these older grafts there is no correlation between their absolute age and the presence of friable or loosely adherent plaque. Whether the angioscopic appearance of plaque can predict in which grafts atheroembolism is more likely to occur will require the study of a larger patient population.

Abrupt Vessel Closure After PTCA

Abrupt vessel closure is the major cause of in-hospital morbidity and mortality associated with percutaneous angioplasty.[1-5] Prompt restoration of blood flow is essential to avoid irreversible myocardial damage. Therapeutic options for reopening abruptly occluded vessels include the administration of intracoronary nitroglycerin, repeat (long duration) balloon dilation, intracoronary thrombolysis, directional atherectomy, stent placement, and emergency coronary bypass surgery. Currently, the treatment of abrupt occlusion is guided by the angiographic appearance of the lesion. Given the documented insensitivity of angiography for detecting specific lesion morphologies (thrombi vs. dissection), the clinician is at a disadvantage when attempting to apply lesion specific therapy.

The restoration of patency after abrupt closure might be improved if specific information regarding the cause of the occlusion were known to the operator. For example, thrombolytic therapy would be expected to be much more effective in recanalizing a thrombosed vessel, but would be ineffective in reestablishing patency in a vessel occluded with tissue fragments or by dissection.

We performed percutaneous coronary angioscopy in 10 patients with abrupt closure of a dilated vessel. Intravascular thrombi were present at the lesion site in 9 (90%) of 10 patients and directly responsible for the occlusion in 2 patients (20%). Fragmented plaque and tissue flaps secondary to dissection of the artery wall were present in all 10 patients and were responsible for occlusing the vascular lumen in 8 patients (80%).

The endovascular morphology we observed in these patients clearly demonstrated the primary cause of the vascular obstruction. It is interesting to note that although the majority of the patients had unstable angina, a condition that has been associated with a high incidence of intracoronary thrombi,[19,20] the majority of occlusions after PTCA were due to dissection and obstructive tissue flaps, and not due to vessel thrombosis.

We were able to determine a "primary cause" of the abrupt occlusion with the angioscope when both thrombi and dissections were present. Angioscopic information was used in these patients to select specific treatment modalities directed at the underlying cause of the failed angioplasty attempt, ie, thrombolytic therapy for thrombus and repeat balloon dilation, directional atherectomy, or stent placement for occlusive dissections (tissue flaps).

We believe that specific information regarding the causes of the occlusion will allow the physician to select the most appropriate treatment strategy. If this knowledge can be gained rapidly and safely by angioscopy, it should expedite the reestablishment of coronary flow and avoid inappropriate (thrombolysis for tissue obstruction) or unattractive (stents in thrombus-filled arteries) therapeutic choices.

Risk Stratification for Coronary Angioplasty

There are conflicting reports regarding the significance of intracoronary thrombus as a harbinger of potential complications associated with coronary angioplasty.[1-5] The presence of intracoronary thrombus may serve as a nidus for further thrombus formation, predisposing a traumatized endovascular surface to thrombotic occlusion. The inability of angiography to convincingly demonstrate a relation between intracoronary thrombi and angioplasty complications may be related to angiography's documented insensitivity for coronary thrombus.[21]

We have performed angioscopy in 122 patients before and/or after coronary angioplasty. Angioscopy was better able to detect intracoronary thrombus than angiography was detecting coronary thrombi in 61% (74/122) of vessels by angioscopy versus 20% (24/122) of patients by angiography ($P<0.001$) (Figure 1). Angioscopic thrombus was visualized in 74% (70/95) of the unstable angina patients compared with 15% (4/27) of the stable angina patients ($P<0.001$). In the 24 vessels with angiographic evidence of thrombus, angioscopy confirmed the presence of thrombus in 20 (83%). The sensitivity of angiography for detecting intracoronary thrombi was 27% and the specificity was 92% when compared with angioscopy.

In-hospital complications (death, myocardial infarction, recurrent ischemia, or emergency coronary bypass surgery) occurred in 32.4% (24/74) of patients with angioscopic thrombus as opposed to

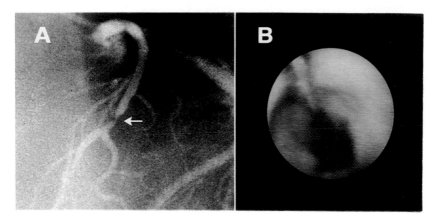

FIGURE 1. A: *Angiography of a left anterior descending coronary artery stenosis in a patient with unstable angina. There is no evidence of intra-coronary thrombus.* **B,** *Angioscopy of the lesion before PTCA. The guide wire is visible at 11 o'clock. A red thrombus is visible at the lesion site, easily seen against the background of yellow plaque.*

10.4% (5/48) of those without thrombus (P=0.01). The relative risk, or odds ratio, of a complication occurring when angioscopic thrombus was present was 3.11, (95% CI 1.28–7.60, P=0.01) versus 0.85 (95% CI 0.36–2.00, P=0.91) when angiographic thrombus was detected. Multivariate analysis of clinical (age, sex, unstable/stable angina), angiographic (AHA/ACC lesion type, minimal lumen diameter before or after PTCA, and thrombus) and angioscopic thrombus demonstrated that only angioscopic thrombus was significantly related to any in-hospital complication.

The specificity of angiography for detecting intracoronary thrombi is also weakened when one realizes that not all angiographic filling defects are thrombi. By depicting both color and texture, angioscopy can readily distinguish white or yellow plaque fragments protruding into the vessel lumen from red thrombus. However, one limitation of angioscopy is the difficulty in differentiating "white" thrombus from white tissue elements that may be present in the vessel lumen. The angioscopic distinguishing feature of these white intraluminal masses is their shape and texture. Tissue fragments or dissection flaps usually demonstrate sharp, angular margins analogous to tattered white bedsheets on a clothesline blowing in the wind, whereas white thrombi (platelet aggregates and fibrin strands) are globular masses with fuzzy, indistinct borders.

Patients who had unstable angina had a significantly increased incidence of intracoronary thrombi compared with stable angina patients, which is in agreement with prior angioscopic studies.[9,21] Intracoronary thrombus was also more commonly associated with the more complex AHA/ACC type B and C lesions compared with the less complex type A lesions.[22] Univariate analysis of these angiographic lesion morphologies did not demonstrate a significant association with in-hospital complications of angioplasty.

Prior studies have demonstrated an increased incidence of angioplasty complications associated with unstable angina and complex coronary lesion morphology.[23] Some studies have demonstrated an association of angiographic intracoronary thrombi with angioplasty complications[4,5] while others have not.[1]

Thrombi detected by angioscopy, but too small to be identified by angiography, appear to have clinical significance and be related to adverse outcomes after angioplasty. Multivariate analysis demonstrated that when compared with clinical variables (age, sex, unstable angina, and stable angina) or angiographic morphology (angiographic thrombus or lesion complexity), angioscopic intracoronary thrombus was most strongly associated with in-hospital adverse events after PTCA.

Conclusion

Our experience suggests that angioscopic lesion morphology may have definite clinical utility in guiding interventional therapy in selected patients. The angioscope may prove useful in identifying vein grafts with friable plaque likely to embolize with intervention, to select a treatment strategy for an abruptly occluded artery after angioplasty, or to visualize and identify an angiographic filling defect to determine if it is thrombus or a tissue flap protruding into the lumen (Figure 2).

The greatest potential clinical impact for angioscopy will be the ability of angioscopy to stratify patients at high risk for having a complication after coronary angioplasty. Although the risk of complications appears to be strongly related to the presence of intracoronary thrombus, we have yet to demonstrate a cause-and-effect relation between the intracoronary thrombi visualized by angioscopy and the occurrence of an angioplasty complication. Thrombus may occur in association with lesions more likely to fail angioplasty rather than directly contributing to the failure. Alternatively, a small amount of red thrombus may serve as a nidus for subsequent growth of a thrombus directly contributing to vessel closure or recurrent ischemia. To determine the answer to this

question, a trial demonstrating that patients receiving angioscopically directed therapy have better outcomes than a comparable
group of patients undergoing angioplasty guided by angiography
alone is needed.

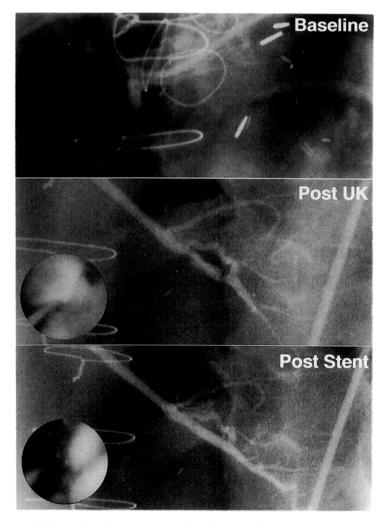

FIGURE 2. Top: *Baseline angiography of an occluded saphenous vein bypass graft to a right coronary artery.* **Middle:** *Angiography of the distal
anastomosis of the recanalized graft after a urokinase infusion. Note the
filling defect, which suggested the possibility or residual thrombus. Angioscopy of the distal anastomosis is shown in the insert and shows that
the angiographic filling defect is due to plaque, not thrombus.* **Bottom:**
*Angiography after placement of the stent. The insert shows the angio-
scopic appearance of the lumen following stent placement.*

References

1. de Feyter PJ, van den Brand M, Jaarman G, et al. Acute coronary occlusion during and after percutaneous transluminal coronary angioplasty. Frequency, prediction, clinical course, management, and follow-up. *Circulation.* 1991;83:927–936.927–936.
2. Ellis SG, Roubin GS, King SB III, et al. Angiographic and clinical predictors of acute closure after native vessel coronary angioplasty. *Circulation.* 1988;77:372–379.
3. Detre KM, Holmes DR Jr, Holubkov R, et al. Incidence and consequences of periprocedural occlusion. The 1985–1986 National Heart Lung and Blood Institute Percutaneous Transluminal Coronary Angioplasty Registry. *Circulation.* 1990;82:739–750.
4. Sugrue DD, Holmes DR Jr, Smith HC, et al. Coronary artery thrombus as a risk factor for acute vessel occlusion during percutaneous transluminal coronary angioplasty: improving results. *Br Heart J.* 1986;56:62–66.
5. Mabin TA, Homes DR, Smith HC, et al. Intracoronary thrombus: role in coronary occlusion complicating percutaneous transluminal coronary angioplasty. *J Am Coll Cardiol.* 1985;5:198–202.
6. Katritsis D, Webb-Peploe M. Limitations of coronary angiography: an underestimated problem? *Clin Cardiol.* 1991;14:20–24.
7. Block PC, Myler RK, Stertzer S, et al. Morphology after transluminal angioplasty in human beings. *N Engl J Med.* 1981;305:382–385.
8. Duber C, Jungbluth A, Rumpelt HJ, et al. Morphology of the coronary arteries after combined thrombolysis and percutaneous transluminal coronary angioplasty for acute myocardial infarction. *Am J Cardiol.* 1986;58:698–703.
9. Ramee SR, White CJ, Collins TJ, et al. Percutaneous angioscopy during coronary angioplasty using a steerable microangioscope. *J Am Coll Cardiol.* 1991;17:100–105.
10. White CJ, Ramee SR, Collins TJ, et al. Percutaneous angioscopy of saphenous vein coronary bypass grafts. *J Am Coll Cardiol.* 1993;21:1181–1185.
11. White CJ, Ramee SR, Collins TJ, et al. Percutaneous coronary angioscopy: applications in interventional cardiology. *J Intervtional Cardiol.* 1993;6:61–67.
12. Cote G, Myler RK, Stertzer SH, et al. Percutaneous transluminal angioplasty of stenotic coronary artery bypass grafts: 5 years experience. *J Am Coll Cardiol.* 1987;9:8–17.
13. Saber RS, Edwards WD, Holmes DR, et al. Balloon angioplasty of aortocoronary saphenous vein bypass grafts: a histopathologic study of six grafts from five patients, with emphasis on restenosis and embolic complications. *J Am Coll Cardiol.* 1988;12:1501–1509.
14. Waller BF, Rothbaum DA, Gorfinkel JH, et al. Morphologic observations after percutaneous transluminal baloon angioplasty of early and late aortocoronary saphenous vein bypass grafts. *J Am Coll Cardiol.* 1984;4:784–792.
15. Platko WP, Hollman J, Whitlow PL, et al. Percutaneous transluminal angioplasty of saphenous vein graft stenosis: long-term follow-up. *J Am Coll Cardiol.* 1989;14:1645–1650.
16. Dorros G, Lewin RF, Mathiak LM, et al. Percutaneous transluminal coronary angioplasty in patients with two or more previous coronary artery bypass grafting operations. *Am J Cardiol.* 1988;61:1243–1247.

17. Marquis JF, Schwartz L, Brown R, et al. Percutaneous transluminal angioplasty of coronary saphenous vein bypass grafts. *Can J Surg.* 1985;28:335–337.
18. Jost S, Gulba D, Daniel WG, et al. Percutaneous transluminal angioplasty of aortocoronary venous bypass grafts and effect of the caliber of the grafted coronary artery on graft stenosis. *Am J Cardiol.* 1991;68:27–30.
19. Breshnahan DR, Davis JL, Holmes DR, et al. Angiographic occurance and clinical correlates of intraluminal coronary artery thrombus: role of unstable angina. *J Am Coll Cardiol.* 1985;6:285–289.
20. Ambrose JA, Hjemdahl-Monsen CE, Borrico S, et al. Angiographic demonstration of a common link between unstable angina pectoris and non-Q wave myocardial infarction. *Am J Cardiol.* 1988;61:244–247.
21. Sherman CT, Litvack F, Grundfest W, et al. Coronary angioscopy in patients with unstable angina pectoris. *N Engl J Med.* 1986;315:913–919.
22. Ellis SG, Vandormael MG, Cowley MJ, et al. Coronary morphologic and clinical determinants of procedural outcome with angioplasty for multivessel coronary disease: implications for patient selection. *Circulation.* 1990;82:1193–1202.
23. de Feyter PJ, Suryapranata H, Serruys PW, et al. Coronary angioplasty for unstable angina: immediate and late results in 200 consecutive patients with identification of risk factors for unfavorable early and late outcome. *J Am Coll Cardiol.* 1988;12:324–333.

Chapter 8

Newer Approaches to the Noninvasive Diagnosis of Coronary Artery Disease

Mark A. Lawson, MD and Gerald M. Pohost, MD

Introduction

Clinicians are faced with two questions when evaluating a patient with chest pain syndrome: does the patient have coronary artery disease (CAD), and if so, how accurately can the severity and extent of disease be determined without coronary angiography? Patients with CAD are at risk for a broad spectrum of future events, such as myocardial infarction or sudden death. The ultimate goal of noninvasive diagnosis of CAD should be to identify the high-risk patient in whom revascularization would be beneficial. Accordingly, risk stratification depends on a quantitative determination of left ventricular (LV) function and on the amount of ischemic myocardium likely to be affected by the next occlusive event. This chapter provides selected information regarding conventional and newer approaches to noninvasive diagnosis of CAD. For further information on any procedure, the reader is referred to a number of relevant references listed in the bibliography.

Cardiovascular Response to Exercise and Pharmacologic Intervention

Noninvasive approaches to the diagnosis of CAD disease rely on the distribution of a tracer or on the pathophysiologic function

From Vetrovec GW, Carabello BA, (eds.) *Invasive Cardiology: Current Diagnostic and Therapeutic Issues.* Armonk, NY: Futura Publishing Company, Inc.: © 1996.

of ischemic myocardium. Myocardium supplied by an obstructed vessel may have normal perfusion and function under resting conditions. Therefore, stenotic lesions are identified, usually after some cardiovascular provocation, either by exercise or pharmacologic manipulation.

Exercise Intervention

Dynamic changes experienced during exercise include elevations in heart rate, blood pressure, and cardiac output, all of which affect myocardial oxygen consumption. In addition, coronary blood flow increases due to an elevation in myocardial oxygen consumption. A mismatch in supply and demand occurs when the increase in myocardial metabolic requirements during exercise exceed the ability of the vasculature to supply adequate oxygen and substrate. Myocardial ischemia results in diastolic and systolic LV dysfunction, ischemic electrocardiographic (ECG) changes, and ultimately angina pectoris. Upright treadmill exercise testing is most commonly used to induce stress.

Pharmacologic Intervention

Many patients are unable to exercise because of arthritis, claudication, paralysis, or other medical problems. As a substitute for exercise, pharmacologic agents can be used either to increase myocardial work (eg, dobutamine or isoproterenol) or to increase myocardial blood flow (eg, dipyridamole or adenosine). Dobutamine is a positive inotropic agent with both α- and β-adrenergic receptor stimulation. When infused, dobutamine produces a marked increase in contractility, a modest increase in heart rate, and consequently a significant increase in myocardial oxygen consumption. Dipyridamole is a coronary vasodilator that acts either to inhibit adenosine uptake and/or to stimulate the adenosine receptor located on the coronary endothelium. Adenosine also has been used for this purpose. Both of these vasodilators may cause a mild increase in myocardial oxygen demand because of a mild increase in heart rate and a decrease in blood pressure. In the normal vasculature, dipyridamole will cause up to a fivefold increase myocardial blood flow, whereas diseased vasculature will rise to a lesser extent or even decrease. Occasionally, the resulting maldistribution in flow may cause a "steal" phenomenon leading to ischemia. Agents used in perfusion imaging distribute throughout the myocardium in proportion to blood flow delivery.

Approaches for Detecting Coronary Artery Disease

Exercise Treadmill Testing

Exercise treadmill testing probably remains the most widely used noninvasive diagnostic test for CAD. A patient with CAD often cannot produce sufficient coronary blood flow to maintain the metabolic demand of the myocardium during exercise, and as a consequence, the myocardium becomes ischemic. The most widely used noninvasive test for detecting CAD is the graded treadmill exercise test. Exercise begins at a low workload with progressive increments in workload while ECG and blood pressure are monitored. Patients exercise to their maximal exercise capacity. A recovery period follows exercise until the patients' ECG and blood pressure return to the preexercise conditions. This approach is advantageous to the physician not only as a test for exercise-induced ischemia, but also as an estimate of cardiac reserve. Interpretation of the results of this test includes clinical observations (eg, angina, dyspnea), blood pressure responses (rise or fall), and ECG evaluation (ST segment changes or arrhythmia). Angina pectoris induced by exercise is highly predictive of CAD. Clinical signs of inadequate cardiac output include a drop in skin temperature, peripheral cyanosis, lightheadedness, and vertigo. Development of a ventricular gallop during postexercise auscultation usually results from LV dysfunction. The patient should be examined for transient mitral regurgitation due to ischemic papillary dysfunction. The systolic blood pressure should increase at least 10 mm Hg with each progressive stage of the standard Bruce protocol. A hypotensive or blunted blood pressure response, when associated with CAD, is generally a poor prognostic sign. Heart rate increases during exercise. The common use of beta-blockers has complicated the interpretation of heart rate response during exercise. The product of peak heart rate and systolic blood pressure, the so-called pulse-pressure product, estimates myocardial oxygen demand, which parallels coronary blood flow. The literature on ECG interpretation during exercise is voluminous; however, most would agree that the probability of CAD is related to the extent of ST segment depression. Thus, patients with >1 mm of horizontal or downsloping ST segment depression (usually measured at 80 msec after the J-point) are thought to have a positive ischemic ECG response. ST segment depression that persists for at least 1 minute into the recovery phase is even more indicative of ischemia. The specificity and sensitivity of exercise-induced ST segment depression using the ECG criteria described above is 84% and 66%, respectively.[1]

Radionuclide Studies

Nuclear cardiology techniques use radionuclide tracers to assess either myocardial perfusion, ventricular function, or myocardial viability.

Myocardial Perfusion Imaging

There are several approaches for myocardial perfusion imaging with radionuclides. They can be divided between single-photon methods and positron emission tomographic methods. For single-photon methods, there are three main tracers for myocardial perfusion imaging: [201]Tl, ^{99m}Tc–sestamibi, and ^{99m}Tc-teboroxime.

Thallium-201

Thallium-201 is the single-photon radionuclide with which there is the most experience and the best understanding; it also continues to be the most widely used. [201]Tl has a half-life of approximately 73 hours and a photo peak in the range of 70–80 keV. As the Tl[+] ion, thallium behaves as a potassium analog and is actively transported across cell membranes by the Na^+–K^+ adenosine triphosphatase (ATPase) pump. Only viable myocardial tissue can extract [201]Tl. The distribution of ^{201}Tl depends on myocardial blood flow. Because it is extracted by myocardial cells with high efficiency, it is an ideal agent for studying perfusion patterns during exercise and with coronary vasodilators such as dipyridamole and adenosine. [201]Tl is administered at peak exercise or during the peak vasodilatory effect of dipyridamole or adenosine. Peak myocardial activity distal to a physiologically significant coronary stenosis is delayed relative to the normally perfused tissue. Thus, defects are observed in the territories supplied by such stenotic vessels or in nonviable territories, such as acutely infarcted myocardium or myocardial scar. Of all the perfusion agents, thallium is unique in that it demonstrates the phenomenon of redistribution. Redistribution involves the observation of a defect on initial images resulting from reduced perfusion during stress, with dipyridamole or adenosine, or even at rest. If the defect is related to hypoperfused yet viable myocardium, it will "fill-in" because of the continued bathing of the tissue in blood containing thallium, albeit at relatively low levels. Over time, the activity of normal and hypoperfused myocardium approaches one another. ^{201}Tl can improve the accuracy of the exercise treadmill test for diagnosing CAD. The sensitivity and specificity of the exercise technique is approximately 83% and 88%, respectively. These are similar for the dipyridamole and adenosine-thallium approaches.

Increased lung uptake of ^{201}Tl during exercise presumably reflects ischemia-induced LV dysfunction. Stress-induced increases in pulmonary capillary wedge pressure and decreases in cardiac output correlate with increased ^{201}Tl lung uptake. However, patients with chronic obstructive pulmonary disease may also demonstrate increased ^{201}Tl lung activity, and it should be present both on the stress and delayed scans.[2-4]

Newer Thallium Approaches

When a stress perfusion defect demonstrates redistribution, it can be said to be viable with a high degree of confidence. Conversely, if the defect persists over a 3–4 hour interval, it may either be nonviable or viable with an inadequate time provided for redistribution. Imaging at a substantially later time (eg, 24 hours) evaluates ischemic but viable myocardium in what appears to be an irreversible fixed abnormality on the 4-hour delayed images. The redistribution of thallium depends not only on the severity of the perfusion abnormality but also on subsequent thallium blood levels. A "reinjection" method has been recently reported where a second dose of thallium (usually 1 mCi) is given after the delayed (4-hour) images to augment the thallium blood levels. Reinjection images are obtained 15 minutes later. If the early persistent defect fills in after either of these approaches, viability has been documented. Approximately one half of irreversible defects observed on 4-hour delayed images may have further uptake of ^{201}Tl with reinjection. When the reinjection method is used, the study can be completed in 1 day.[5]

^{99m}Tc–sestamibi (MIBI)

Agents labeled with ^{99m}Tc take advantage of ^{99m}Tc single-photon peak of 140 keV (ideal for the Anger camera) and relatively short half-life, permitting higher doses to be administered. These characteristics provide images with higher resolution. MIBI belongs to a chemical family called isonitriles, which have varying abilities to enter and remain within the myocardial cell. MIBI passively diffuses into the myocardial cell where it is sequestered within mitochondria due to a large negative transmembrane potential. Similar to thallium, the distribution of MIBI correlates well with regional myocardial blood flow. However, in contrast to thallium, it exhibits minimal redistribution and may not be as useful for evaluating viability. Because MIBI localizes to splanchnic visceral tissue adjacent to the heart, optimal image acquisition is delayed after administration once the splanchnic visceral activity has substantially diminished. Nevertheless, a two-injection protocol can be used with MIBI to obtain data largely similar to that of thallium. For example, a 1-day rest-stress study can be completed with 10 mCi of MIBI administered while the patient is in the resting state, and 20–25 mCi in the exercise state. The sensitivity and specificity of MIBI to detect CAD is 94% and 77%, respectively.[3,6]

Newer Approaches using MIBI

A combination of thallium and MIBI is ideal for radionuclide myocardial perfusion imaging with a complete study being completed within 2 hours. Initially, the patient receives thallium in the resting state and images are taken. Then, the patient exercises, is injected with MIBI, and images are again taken. The exercise (MIBI) and rest (thallium) images are compared to determine the fate of exercise-induced defects. If an exercise MIBI defect is not present on the resting thallium study, the defect represents a zone of ischemia in viable myocardium. This so-called "hybrid" technique optimally uses both radiotracers in a convenient, efficient, and practical manner with an overall sensitivity of >90% and specificity of 75%.[7]

^{99m}Tc–Teboroxime

^{99m}Tc-teboroxime is not widely used at present because of its very short biological half-life (6 minutes). Another limitation of this tracer is slow hepato-biliary clearance that interferes with evaluation of the inferior myocardial wall. Optimal imaging with this agent is accomplished using a multiple-head camera so that sufficient counts can be obtained prior to decay. Administration of teboroxime in concert with a short-lived pharmacologic coronary vasodilator such as adenosine will allow a complete perfusion study (both rest and stress) to be completed within 1 hour. With appropriate instrumentation, teboroxime may gain further popularity.[3,6]

Positron Emission Tomography Perfusion Agents

While positron emission tomography (PET) is not widely available at present, its theoretical advantages have made enthusiasts of many investigators. There are two agents used in myocardial perfusion imaging with PET: rubidium-82 (^{82}Rb) and ^{13}NH$_3$. Rubidium-82 is a generator-produced radionuclide with a very short half-life of 75 seconds. The agent is injected with a bolus of saline, which removes the appropriate amount of rubidium from the generator and then infuses it into the patient. Since the half-life is short, numerous injections that can reflect responses in perfusion to a number of interventions are possible. The other positron agent, ^{13}NH$_3$, requires a cyclotron to produce the ^{13}N. The physical half-life of the ^{13}N is 10 minutes. Due to the short half-life of this agent, multiple injections can be made over a short duration. Both of these agents can be used with the two-injection approach, one at rest and one following the administration of dipyridamole or adenosine. The disadvantage of PET imaging is its cost. The camera, cyclotron, and particularly the operations of these require substantial space and technical expertise. In consideration of health care reform issues, it appears most likely that the single-photon methods will prevail.[3]

Ventricular Function

^{99m}Tc-pertechnetate binds to red blood cells in the presence of stannous pyrophosphate. Thus, ^{99m}Tc remains in the blood pool, and because the heart is the largest blood pool within the chest, the chambers can be imaged with a scintillation camera. The cardiac cycle is divided into 28–30 segments from which static images are sequentially obtained and reviewed in a cinegraphic mode (radionuclide cineangiography [RNA]). The left ventricular ejection fraction (LVEF) is calculated from the difference in end-systolic and end-diastolic counts, and regional wall motion abnormalities can be detected by asymmetric contraction of the chamber silhouette. If regional wall motion abnormalities are present on a resting RNA study, CAD is suspected. Exercise can be combined with serial RNA measurements. The most widely performed exercise test is semisupine bicycle exercise (with progressing exercise similar to treadmill testing) with RNA obtained at the end of each stage. Worsening of segmental wall motion from ischemic myocardium suggests CAD with an overall sensitivity of 86% to 90% and specificity of 79% to 84%. An abnormal fall or blunting of LVEF is sensitive, but not specific to CAD. This exercise technique is limited to one view, and thus, all myocardial regions cannot be evaluated.[3,8]

Newer Radionuclide Approaches to Determine LV function

The addition of LV function to myocardial perfusion imaging can increase the sensitivity to detect CAD without losing specificity. MIBI can be used to assess LV function by first-pass and gated techniques. The first-pass technique requires the use of a high count rate camera mounted at the front of the exercise treadmill. At peak exercise, the patient is injected with a bolus of MIBI, and images are recorded during the first pass of the MIBI through the central circulation and the left ventricle. Perfusion imaging then is initiated at the usual time for MIBI. From these data, an LVEF can readily be determined and is an important variable for predicting survival. In a second technique, SPECT images may be gated to the cardiac cycle with the appropriate software. Reconstructed tomographic slices are viewed as a continuous loop of contraction and relaxation. The myocardium will thicken and appear brighter during systole in normal myocardium. This approach provides information on perfusion at the time of peak exercise when the MIBI is administered and on regional wall motion at the time of imaging. Perfusion defects that demonstrate normal wall motion represent ischemic yet viable myocardium. These approaches provide an assessment of regional and global LV function as well as myocardial perfusion.[3]

Myocardial Viability

Newer techniques to assess viability with thallium (late redistribution and second injection) and potentially MIBI have been described. While not a new method, a PET approach for evaluating myocardial viability should be noted. The approach involves the use of myocardial perfusion imaging with $^{13}NH_3$ or ^{82}Rb coupled with imaging of glycolysis with ^{18}F-fluorodeoxyglucose (FDG). Uptake of FDG in perfusion defect zones implies viability, while lack of FDG uptake implies nonviablity. This PET technique has become the gold standard for evaluating viability although the thallium reinjection approach closely corresponds to the PET approach.

Echocardiography

As with radionuclide perfusion imaging, dynamic and pharmacologic stress have been used in conjunction with echocardiography to assess wall motion. Echocardiographic evaluation is obtained in the parasternal long axis, parasternal short axis, and apical two- and four-chamber views. The images at rest are compared with those at peak stress. With the aid of a computer, rest and stress images can be digitized and viewed next to each other in a continuous loop display. Development of new segmental wall motion abnormalities or worsening of resting abnormalities suggest obstructive CAD.

Exercise Echocardiography

Exercise echocardiography is performed on either a treadmill or a bicycle. With treadmill echocardiography, the patient exercises maximally, and immediately after exercise, the patient is placed in the left lateral decubitus position and an echocardiogram is obtained. However, stress-induced wall motion abnormalities can quickly return to normal before all four echocardiographic views can be completed. Bicycle echocardiography overcomes this limitation by acquiring the echocardiogram *during* exercise; however, motion and respiratory artifacts may affect image quality.[9]

Pharmacologic Stress Echocardiography

Dobutamine stress echocardiography has been used as an alternative to exercise. Dobutamine is infused intravenously beginning at 5 µg/kg per minute and is increased every 3–5 minutes by 10 µg/kg per minute to a total dose of 40–50 µg/kg per minute to maximize cardiac work. If the heart rate does not reach 85% of the maximum predicted heart rate, 0.5–1.0 mg of atropine may be given during the last stage. Left ventricular regional wall motion progressively increases with increasing doses of dobutamine in the absence of CAD. An abnormal response is manifested by a reduction in wall thickening or motion at any stage of the dobutamine infusion compared with the previous stage. Dipyridamole given intravenously at 0.56 mg/kg and at higher doses of up to 0.84 mg/kg has been used with echocardiography to induce ischemia. However, coronary flow reduction sufficient to induce a wall motion abnormality usually requires the higher doses, which are not well tolerated by patients. Likewise, high-dose adenosine is poorly tolerated by patients. Accordingly, dobutamine is the only pharmacologic agent that can be recommended. Table 1 lists the sensitivity and specificities of these stress echocardiographic methods.[9–12]

TABLE 1

Comparison of Exercise and Nonexercise Stress Echocardiography[9–12]

Type of Stress	Sensitivity (%)	Specificity (%)
Dobutamine	76–89	83–89
Dipyridamole	56–60	67–96
Adenosine	40	93
Exercise	86–97	64–88

Newer Echocardiographic Approaches

While the above mentioned approaches use transthoracic echocardiography, these approaches can be used in conjunction with transesophageal echocardiography. Transesophageal echocardiography is the preferred method for patients with poor acoustic windows. Dipyridamole, dobutamine, and adenosine infusions as well as transesophageal pacing have been studied with transesophageal echocardiography. New wall motion abnormalities that develop are easily visualized by transesophageal echocardiography independent of body habitus. Transesophageal echocardiography is unique in its ability to evaluate coronary blood flow velocity with Doppler, and investigations continue in characterizing coronary flow reserve before and after pharmacologic intervention.[13,14]

Ultrafast Computed Tomography

Ultrafast computed tomography can be used to assess regional myocardial perfusion. Radiopaque contrast medium is injected as a bolus and tracked through the heart chambers and the myocardium. Regional and global ventricular function can be measured after injecting a bolus of contrast medium at rest or during stress. In addition, CAD can be diagnosed by the detection of calcification within the coronary artery; however, the severity cannot be quantified. Although the presence of calcification has a sensitivity of 100%, the specificity ranges between 60% and 90%. While ultrafast computed tomography systems are technically advanced, they are expensive, not widely available, and require potentially harmful iodinated contrast media.[15–17]

Magnetic Resonance Imaging

Magnetic resonance imaging (MRI) provides excellent spatial resolution and is well suited for the detection of CAD. There are several MRI techniques that may be useful in diagnosing CAD: dobutamine stress MRI, magnetic resonance perfusion imaging, ^{31}P magnetic resonance spectroscopy with exercise, and magnetic resonance coronary angiography. Left ventricular function is easily obtained from cine-MRI methods. Magnetic resonance systems are widely available and can be used to obtain cardiac imaging studies with appropriate software. This technique is contraindicated in patients with implanted metallic matter such as pacemakers and cerebral aneurysm clips.

Wall Motion Assessment by Dobutamine Stress MRI

In a manner similar to dobutamine stress echocardiography, ischemic wall motion changes can be detected by cine-MRI. The sensitivity of this approach to detect multivessel disease has been reported at 100%, and at 88% for single vessel disease. There is excellent matching of the site and extent of perfusion defects when compared with ^{201}Tl imaging with 90% to 95% agreement. The relatively long time required to obtain images is the current disadvantage to this technique. However, as faster MRI methods become available, this disadvantage will disappear. For example, new ultrafast methods, known as echo planar methods, can acquire an image in 40 msec.[18,19]

Myocardial Perfusion Imaging by MRI

Changes in myocardial blood flow are generally not visualized by MRI without the use of paramagnetic contrast agents (eg, gadolinium-based agents). Signal intensity increases in myocardium that is perfused by a paramagnetic contrast agent. Contrast-enhanced MRI uses a first-pass technique during which a bolus of contrast is injected intravenously, and serial magnetic resonance images obtained track the bolus through the cardiac chambers, and finally into the myocardium. Inhomogeneities in myocardial perfusion are accentuated after an infusion of dipyridamole, and the distribution of contrast is proportional to myocardial blood flow. Myocardial territories supplied by a stenotic coronary artery will show a lower peak signal intensity as well as a delay in the appearance of contrast. To date, only a few studies with small numbers of patients have investigated contrast-enhanced MRI for the detection of CAD. The current techniques are only capable of acquiring a single tomographic plane through the ventricle. Newer, high-speed acquisition methods should allow multislice imaging.[20,21]

Myocardial Perfusion Imaging by MRI without Contrast

Magnetic resonance imaging that does not require the use of magnetic resonance contrast agents and nor relies on indirect indications (eg, regional wall motion abnormality) of ischemic myocardium are currently under investigation. These methods include imaging the paramagnetic deoxyhemaglobin generated during myocardial ischemia or using a technique called magnetization transfer.

Magnetic Resonance Spectroscopy

During myocardial ischemia, there is a change in high-energy phosphate metabolism with a decrease in phosphocreatine and the phosphocreatine:adenosine triphosphate ratio. Quantification of high-energy phosphates is possible with ^{31}P magnetic resonance spectroscopy. Using isometric hand-grip exercise, a transient imbalance in phosphate metabolism can be detected in ischemic myocardium. A limitation of this approach is the length of time necessary to complete a metabolic study.[22]

Magnetic Resonance Coronary Angiography

One of the most intriguing possibilities of MRI for detecting CAD is magnetic resonance coronary angiography. This approach will be helpful for screening proximal or mid-vessel CAD in patients who might otherwise be referred for conventional x-ray coronary angiography (eg, those patients with atypical chest pain or asymptomatic individuals with multiple risk factors). The coronary arteries can be imaged either in-plane or viewed after computer-assisted three-dimensional reconstruction of multiple overlapping transverse planes. Magnetic resonance coronary angiography currently is limited by artifacts and misalignment resulting from cardiac and respiratory motion, and by the presence of epicardial fat that decreases artery contrast. The degree of coronary stenosis may be exaggerated due to signal loss from turbulence or sluggish flow. This approach requires further development and will improve over time.[23]

Proper Selection of Diagnostic Test

Many modalities are available to help diagnose CAD and risk stratify those patients with disease. Table 2 summarizes the relative utility of each of the conventional and newer approaches in evaluating myocardium at risk and LV function. Additional considerations must be weighed before deciding which test would be most appropriate. These include: 1) limitation of each study; 2) the question to be answered in a particular patient; 3) additional information that may be obtained from a particular study; 4) cost and incremental information per dollar spent; 5) availability of equipment; 6) expertise of the laboratory and interpreting physicians; 7) patient preference; 8) sensitivity, specificity, predictive value, and accuracy of each modality; 9) patient's age; and 10) other comorbid conditions (eg, obstructive lung disease, arthritis, etc.). Some advantages and disadvantages of the most commonly studied approaches are summarized in Table 3. In this new age of health care reform and managed care, increasing attention will be placed on cost effectiveness.

TABLE 2

Comparison of Noninvasive Approaches

Approach	Myocardium at Risk	LV Function
Exercise ECG	+/−	+/−
^{201}Tl/^{99m}Tc Exercise	++	+/−
^{201}Tl/^{99m}Tc Dipyridamole	+++	−
Exercise RVG	+	|||
Dobutamine ECHO	+	+++
Dobutamine Ultrafast CT	|+	++
Dobutamine MRI	++	+++
Perfusion MRI	+++	−*

*Can be combined with LV functional study.

TABLE 3

Comparison of the Advantages and Disadvantages Approaches

Approach	Advantages	Disadvantages
Exercise ECG	Measures cardiac reserve Readily available	Requires adequate exercise
^{201}Tl or ^{99m}Tc Exercise	Measures cardiac reserve Test for viability Improved sensitivity/ specificity	Hours to complete Minute radiation exposure
^{201}Tl or ^{99m}Tc Dipyridamole	Used in patients who cannot exercise Fewer false positive with LBBB Test for viability	Minor side effects Hours to complete Minute radiation exposure
Dobutamine ECHO	Complete within 1/2 hour "Physiologic" stress Used in patients who cannot exercise Inherent exam of LV size, function, and valves Readily available	Minor side effects Hyperdynamic motion impairs interpretation Limited by "acoustic window"
Ultrafast CT	High-speed acquisition High resolution Detects calcium in coronary arteries Inherent exam of LV size, function	Radiation exposure Use of iodinated contrast Not widely available
Dobutamine MRI	High resolution "Physiologic" stress Inherent exam of LV size, function, and valves Used in patients who cannot exercise	Requires prolonged infusion to complete scan
Perfusion MRI	High resolution Inherent exam of LV size, function, and valves Used in patients who cannot exercise	Minor side effects Requires continued development
MR coronary angiography	High resolution Inherent exam of LV size, function, and valves	Requires continued development

References

1. Fletcher GF, Froelicher VF, Hartley LH, et al. Exercise standards: a statement for health professionals from the American Heart Association. *Circulation.* 1990;82:2286–2322.
2. Maddahi J, Rodrigues E, Berman JS. Assessment of myocardial perfusion imaging by single-photon agents. In: Pohost GM, O'Rourke RA, eds. *Principles and Practice of Cardiovascular Imaging.* Boston, MA: Little Brown; 1991:202–204.
3. Johnson LL, Pohost GM. Nuclear cardiology. In: Schlant RC, Alexander RC, eds. *Hurst's: The Heart.* New York: McGraw-Hill; 1993:2339–2360.
4. Gould KL. Noninvasive assessment of coronary stenosis by myocardial perfusion imaging during pharmacologic coronary vasodilation. *Am J Cardiol.* 1978;41:267–278.
5. Dilsizian V, Rocco TP, Nanette MT, et al. Enhanced detection of ischemic but viable myocardium by the reinjection of thallium after stress-redistribution imaging. *N Engl J Med.* 1990;323:141–146.
6. Berman DS, Kiat H, Maddahi J. The new [99mTc] myocardial perfusion imaging agents: [99mTc]–sestambil and [99mTc]-teboroxime. *Circulation.* 1991;84(suppl I):I-7-I-21.
7. Berman DS, Kiat H, Friedman JD, et al. Separate acquisition rest thallium-201/stress technetium-99m sestamibi dual-isotope myocardial perfusion single-photon emission computed tomography: a clinical validation study. *J Am Coll Cardiol.* 1993;22:1455–1464.
8. Gibbons RJ, Fyke FE III, Clements IP, et al. Noninvasive identification of severe coronary artery disease using exercise radionuclide angiography. *J Am Coll Cardiol.* 1988;11:28–34.
9. Presti CF, Armstrong WF, Feigenbaum H. Comparison of echocardiography at peak exercise and after bicycle exercise in evaluation of patients with known or suspected coronary artery disease. *J Am Soc Echocardiogr.* 1988;1:119–126.
10. Sawada SG, Segar DS, Ryan T, et al. Echocardiographic detection of coronary artery disease during dobutamine infusion. *Circulation.* 1991;83:1605–1614.
11. Martin TW, Seaworth JF, Johns JP, et al. Comparison of adenosine, dipyridamole, and dobutamine stress echocardiography. *Ann Intern Med.* 1992;116:190–196.
12. Previtali M, Lanzarini L, Fetiveau R, et al. Comparison of dobutamine stress echocardiography, dipyridamole stress echocardiography, and exercise stress testing for diagnosis of coronary artery disease. *Am J Cardiol.* 1993;72:865–870.
13. Flachskampf FA, Hoffman R, Hanrath P. Transesophageal stress echocardiography. *Coronary Artery Dis.* 1992;3:364–368.
14. Hutchison SJ, Shen A, Soldo S, et al. Transesophageal monitoring during "regular" and "high" dose dipyridamole stress testing: comparative value of coronary flow reserve versus other parameters. *Circulation* 1993;88:I-67.
15. Chomka EV, Wolfkiel CJ, Claudio J, et al. Combined perfusion and functional imaging of the left ventricle in patients with recent myocardial infarction by ultrafast computed tomography. *J Am Coll Cardiol.* 1987;9:151A.

16. Rumberger JA, Feiring AJ, Lipton MJ, et al. Use of ultrafast computed tomography to quantitate regional myocardial perfusion. *J Am Coll Cardiol.* 1987;9:59–69.
17. Tannenbaum SR, Kondos GT, Veselick KE, et al. Detection of calcific deposits in coronary arteries by ultrafast computed tomography and correlation with angiography. *Am J Cardiol.* 1989;63:870–871.
18. Pennell DJ, Underwood R, Manzara CC, et al. Magnetic resonance imaging during dobutamine stress in coronary artery disease. *Am J Cardiol.* 1992;70:34–40.
19. van Rugge FP, van der Wall EE, de Roos A, et al. Dobutamine stress magnetic resonance imaging for detection of coronary artery disease. *J Am Coll Cardiol.* 1993;22:431–439.
20. Manning WJ, Atkinson DJ, Grossman W, et al. First pass nuclear magnetic resonance imaging studies using gadolinium-DTPA in patients with coronary artery disease. *J Am Coll Cardiol.* 1991;18:959–965.
21. Schaefer S, van Tyen R, Saloner D. Evaluation of myocardial perfusion abnormalities with gadolinium-enhanced snapshot MR imaging in humans. *Radiology.* 1992;185:795–801.
22. Weiss RG, Bottomley PA, Hardy CJ, et al. Regional myocardial metabolism of high-energy phosphates during isometric exercise in patients with coronary artery disease. *N Engl J Med.* 1990;323:1593–1600.
23. Manning WJ, Li W, Edelman RR. A preliminary report comparing magnetic resonance coronary angiography with conventional angiography. *N Engl J Med.* 1993;328:828–832.

Chapter 9

Perspectives on Percutaneous Transluminal Coronary Angioplasty:
Limitations and Comparison with Surgery

Spencer B. King III, MD

Coronary angioplasty, which was developed by Gruentzig and first used in patients in 1977, has taken its place as a major therapeutic intervention for coronary artery disease in the 1990s.[1] By 1986, 133,000 procedures had been performed[2] and by 1993 it was estimated that over 350,000 procedures had been performed. In addition to the original application in single vessel disease, angioplasty is now used in patients with multivessel disease, multiple lesions in the same vessel, chronic total occlusions, vein graft and internal mammary artery graft stenoses, and in total thrombotic occlusions accompanying acute myocardial infarction. Despite the increased use of angioplasty, significant limitations exist that have led to the development of many new devices, some of which have been tested against balloon angioplasty. Restenosis continues to be the principal obstacle to the application of interventional cardiology techniques. Results of the first trials to compare angioplasty with bypass surgery are now becoming available. In this chapter, we examine the results with angioplasty, the efforts to control restenosis, the comparisons with bypass surgery, and the current guidelines for the use of angioplasty.

Status of Balloon Angioplasty

The original series of cases treated by Gruentzig from 1977 to 1980 constitutes the longest follow-up. Even though the equipment

From Vetrovec GW, Carabello BA, (eds.) *Invasive Cardiology: Current Diagnostic and Therapeutic Issues.* Armonk, NY: Futura Publishing Company, Inc.: © 1996.

available at that time allowed success in only 133 of the 169 patients treated, the course of those patients provides insight into the long-term outcome of patients undergoing successful angioplasty with relatively ideal lesions and clinical settings for the technique. The follow-up, which is now complete at 10 years,[3] showed that patients who had involvement of only one artery had a 95% survival, whereas a smaller group of patients with multivessel disease had an 81% 10-year survival. Bypass surgery was subsequently performed in 23 of these 133 patients. Another series from Emory University Hospital has also been followed for 10 years.[4] Four hundred and twenty-seven patients treated in 1981 had predominantly single vessel disease. Ten-year survival was 91%, additional angioplasty was required in 30%, and bypass surgery in 23%. Freedom from death, myocardial infarction, or bypass surgery occurred in 55% of the 427 patients. In the mid-1980s, multivessel disease was approached more often. Reports from Vetrovec's group[5] and from Hartzler's group showed good initial results with angioplasty in multivessel disease, however, long-term survival has not been as good.

Results of the NHLBI Registries

The need for surveillance of angioplasty results was recognized from the beginning, and therefore, the NHLBI established a registry of 16 centers that entered all angioplasty patients treated during the period 1979–1981. One thousand three hundred and forty-five patients were treated in that registry and if a strict definition of success is applied (ie, ≥20% reduction in stenosis and <50% residual stenosis), one finds that only 58% of the patients had at least one lesion successfully opened. These same centers reconstituted the NHLBI registry in 1985 and 1986 entering 2,136 patients. Using the same definition, the success rate increased to 87%. The short-term outcome of the registry patients also changed significantly. Although mortality was approximately 1% in both registries and nonfatal infarction approximately 5%, the use of bypass surgery during the initial hospitalization, which had been high in the initial registry (25%), dropped to 6% in the 1985–1986 registry. Because the baseline characteristics of the patients were quite different between the two registries, a raw comparison of the long-term outcome is not possible. However, for the initial registry patients who had predominantly single vessel disease and were an average of 53 years of age, there was a 5-year survival rate of 93.6%. The second registry group, treated in 1985–1986 who were an average of 58 years of age and half of whom had multivessel disease, had a 5-year survival of 90.2%. Those 1985–1986 registry patients with single vessel disease had a 93% survival versus 87% for those with multivessel disease.

The continued development of more sophisticated angioplasty equipment and the increasing experience of operators have led to an expansion of the use of angioplasty to more complex patient groups and to continuing changes in short-term outcomes. At Emory University Hospital, the current success rate (using the definition given earlier) is 96% with the use of in-hospital bypass surgery dropping below 2%. In our experience, mortality continues to be greater in multivessel disease patients (0.8%) than for those patients with single vessel disease (0.2%).

Complications of Angioplasty

The primary complications of angioplasty are the inability to open the lesion due to the severity of the stenosis, the hardness of the lesion, the length of the lesion, the tortuosity of the vessels or other technical considerations, or the abrupt closure of the vessel after the angioplasty procedure. Factors that predict acute closure are listed in Table 1. Should acute closure occur, there are certain features that put the patient at greater risk for fatal outcome (Table 2).

TABLE 1

Factors Predictive of Abrupt Vessel Closure

Preprocedure
    Clinical factors
        Female gender
        Unstable angina
        Insulin-dependent diabetes mellitus
        Inadequate antiplatelet therapy
    Angiographic factors
        Intracoronary thrombus
        >90% stenosis
        Stenosis length two or more luminal diameters
        Stenosis at branch point
        Stenosis on bend ($\geq 45°$)
        Right coronary artery stenosis

Postprocedure
    Intimal dissection >10 mm
    Residual stenosis >50%
    Transient in-lab closure
    Residual transstenotic gradient ≥ 20 mm Hg

TABLE 2

Factors Associated with Increased Mortality for Angioplasty

Clinical Factors
Female gender
Age >65 years
Unstable angina
Congestive heart failure
Chronic renal failure

Angiographic Factors
Left main coronary disease
Three-vessel disease
Left ventricular ejection fraction <0.30
Risk index
Myocardial jeopardy score
Proximal right coronary stenosis
Collaterals originate from dilated vessel

Restenosis

The major limitation of angioplasty continues to be restenosis after the procedure. The mechanism of restenosis is complex and involves mechanical recoil at the time of the procedure, varying degrees of thrombosis, smooth muscle cell proliferation, migration and extracellular matrix formation, and perhaps chronic vascular retraction in the late follow-up period. A number of clinical variables have been correlated with restenosis including: male gender, diabetes, elevated blood insulin levels, renal failure, and unstable angina. Angiographic correlates of restenosis are: lesion severity, proximal left anterior descending coronary (LAD) artery location, chronic total occlusions, vessel origin lesions, branch point stenoses, long lesions, thrombotic lesions, and the body of vein grafts. Restenosis continues to occur in 30% to 50% of patients,[7] however, 15% to 30% of patients with angiographic restenosis will remain asymptomatic. In a study from Emory University Hospital of 3,363 patients undergoing repeat angiography,[8] those with restenosis were found to have a low incidence of myocardial infarction. Most presented with symptoms quite similar to their original presentation, and therefore, the consequences of developing restenosis remain relatively benign. When repeat angioplasty was performed, it was successful in 96% with low complication rates: Q wave infarction <2%; mortality <0.3%; and bypass surgery <2.5%.

Attempts to control restenosis have focused on pharmacologic therapies and new devices.

Pharmacologic Approaches

Many clinical trials have been conducted on antiplatelet drugs, antithrombotic drugs, anti-inflammatory and antiproliferative drugs, and lipid lowering agents. None of these have shown a convincing positive result. The Lovastatin restenosis trial[9] recently demonstrated a dramatic lowering of the low-density lipoprotein cholesterol from 125 to 75 in the treatment group, yet there was no effect on the restenosis rate. Angiopeptin, a somatostatin analog, showed encouraging results in a Scandinavian pilot study, but larger studies have not yet confirmed those results. Future efforts at controlling restenosis will focus on achieving high tissue concentration through local delivery systems. Local endovascular therapy ranging from antiplatelet agents to antithrombotic agents and antineoplastic agents will be tried. Transfer of genetic signals including antisense oligonucleitides can be targeted to growth factors or to various mediators of cell growth. Genetic transfer to achieve stimulation of nitric oxide synthetase, tissue plasminogen activator, tumor suppressing factors, and others will likely be developed.

New Devices

The mechanism of angioplasty, which disrupts plaque, creates an irregular surface that may be a significant factor in the restenosis process.[10] New devices that open the artery by different mechanisms might achieve a vascular geometry that would be more compatible to long-term patency. Several new devices have been evaluated for their effect on the restenosis process. Among the mechanisms by which new devices might influence restenosis are: 1) opening the artery without creating stretch injury; 2) achieving a smoother internal surface; 3) creating a larger posttreatment lumen.[11] Creating the larger lumen appears to be the most likely method by which improvement in restenosis can be achieved because no device appears to interfere with the new cell growth. Bigger lumens can be achieved using stents and atherectomy devices. The larger lumen achieved with directional atherectomy has not reduced the restenosis rate in two major trials (CAVEAT and C-CAT),[12,13] and more recently trials of intracoronary stents in the United States (STRESS trial)[14] and in Europe (Benestent trial)[15] have created the largest lumens, and therefore, have the greatest potential to reduce restenosis. Different problems are inherent in each of these new interventional devices and will be discussed in other chapters.

Comparison of Angioplasty with Other Therapies

Comparison of angioplasty with medical therapy has been done in only one randomized trial. The Angioplasty Compared to Medicine (ACME) trial[16] examined patients with predominantly single vessel disease, who could be treated medically or with angioplasty. The investigators concluded that angioplasty was not different from medical therapy in terms of survival at 6 months; however, there was an improvement in angina and exercise performance with angioplasty. Of the angioplasty patients, 25% required additional procedures, primarily angioplasty. In this trial, percutaneous transluminal coronary angioplasty (PTCA) was a more costly strategy than medical therapy.

Trials comparing angioplasty with bypass surgery have just begun to be released. These include the EAST (Emory Angioplasty vs. Surgery trial),[17] RITA (The Randomized Intervention Treatment of Angina Trial),[18] CABRI (Coronary Angioplasty vs. Bypass Revascularization Investigation),[19] GABI (German Angioplasty Bypass Investigation),[20], and BARI (Bypass Angioplasty Revascularization Investigation).[21]

The first trial to be completed is the EAST trial. This single center investigation, sponsored by the NHLBI and carried out at Emory University, enrolled 392 patients with multivessel disease and no prior procedures. The primary end point is a composite of death from any cause, new Q wave infarction, or a large ischemic defect detected by thallium scanning at 3-year follow-up. Other end points included success of revascularization demonstrated angiographically and by thallium scanning, the need for future revascularization procedures, quality of life, and economic impact. Patients were enrolled between 1987 and 1990 and the 3-year follow-up was completed in April, 1993. The patients averaged 63 years of age and 40% had triple vessel disease, while the other 60% had double vessel disease. Overall survival at 3 years was 93.4% with no difference between the treatment arms. The primary composite end point was not different at 3 years. The angioplasty patients, however, required many more repeat procedures, with 22% requiring bypass surgery and 40% requiring angioplasty by the

3-year follow-up. Overall, slightly more than half of the angioplasty group required an additional procedure.

The RITA trial randomized approximately 1,000 patients from 16 medical centers in the United Kingdom. The primary end point is freedom from death or nonfatal infarction at 5 years. This trial is structured so that to be eligible, patients must have all lesions suitable for both angioplasty and bypass surgery. For that reason approximately half of the patients in the RITA trial had single vessel disease. The 2.5-year follow-up shows no difference in the primary end point of death or nonfatal infarction between the groups. The number of repeat procedures was significantly greater in the PTCA group, with relief of angina favoring the surgery group.

The CABRI study is a European multicenter trial of approximately 1,000 patients from institutions throughout Europe. End points include death, myocardial infarction, repeat revascularization, angina, quality of life, and exercise performance. A 1-year interim report showed 2.1% mortality in the coronary artery bypass graft (CABG) group and 3.9% in the PTCA group. This difference was not significant. Freedom from death, myocardial infarction or coronary bypass surgery at one year was 92% in the CABG group and 78% in the PTCA group. Repeat bypass surgery was required in 20% at 1 year. Approximately 40% of the patients had triple vessel disease.

The GABI trial is a multicenter randomized trial in Germany. One hundred and fifty-nine patients were randomized, approximately 20% of whom had triple vessel disease. Hospital and 1-year mortality was not different between the groups, however, repeat interventions were required in >40% of the angioplasty group and was rare in the surgery group. Of the angioplasty group, 21% required bypass surgery by 1 year.

BARI is the second study funded by the NHLBI. This is a large multicenter study of over 1,800 patients randomized from 16 centers. The primary end point is all-cause mortality at 5 years. Baseline characteristics of the BARI patients are similar to those in the EAST trial. Results from the BARI trial will become available in late 1995.

Primary Angioplasty for Acute Myocardial Infarction

Thrombolytic therapy in the setting of acute myocardial infarction is now an established technique. Balloon angioplasty opens coronary arteries quickly and can restore a nutrient flow in more than 90% of acute myocardial infarction patients. Whether angioplasty would be superior to medical therapy was recently investigated in the PAMI (Primary Angioplasty for Myocardial Infarction) trial.[22] This trial showed that angioplasty could be performed safely and showed that the combined occurrence of death and nonfatal infarction was reduced in the patients treated with angioplasty compared with those treated with thrombolytic therapy. Those patients treated with angioplasty also had a shorter hospital stay. It is important to note that the differences shown in this trial were due to differences in certain high-risk subgroups. Patients who benefited most were those with anterior myocardial infarction and those over 65 years of age. It should be emphasized that this study was conducted in centers with angioplasty expertise that were equipped for immediate 24-hour response to acute infarct patients.

Guidelines for Performing Angioplasty

The American Heart Association and the American College of Cardiology Task Force on New Technology Assessment have published an updated version of the guidelines for indications for PTCA.[23] Prior to selecting angioplasty as a therapy, several criteria should be met. Will angioplasty have a reasonable chance of addressing the problem at hand if successful? Is the chance of angioplasty success with the available devices and experience high? What is the risk of acute closure of the artery or arteries treated? What are the risks of serious complications including death or myocardial infarction should the vessel close? What is the chance for long-term success with the procedure or with additional procedures? Finally, what results would be expected from alternative therapies such as bypass surgery or medical therapy?

The indications are divided for single vessel disease and multivessel disease and are further divided according to whether the patient is asymptomatic, mildly symptomatic, or significantly symptomatic. Guidelines are also given for patients in the setting of acute myocardial infarction. Angioplasty indications are divided into three classes: class I is those conditions for which it is generally agreed that coronary angioplasty is justified. A class I indication does not mean that angioplasty is the only acceptable therapy; class II is those conditions for which there is a divergence of opinion regarding the justification for coronary angioplasty in terms of value and appropriateness; class III is those conditions for which there is general agreement that angioplasty is ordinarily not indicated.

The indications listed for symptomatic patients include those who have lesions that are amenable to angioplasty and in addition have ischemia on therapy, angina unresponsive to therapy, or are intolerant of therapy side effects and who have a high to moderate chance of angioplasty success with a low to moderate risk of mortality or morbidity. Asymptomatic patients or those with mild symptoms should show more severe ischemia on laboratory testing or have been resuscitated from cardiac arrest or be in need for high risk noncardiac surgery. The likelihood of successful angioplasty should be high with a low risk of mortality and morbidity.

For acute myocardial infarction, angioplasty is recommended in patients with infarction and a pain duration <6 hours, or those with persisting or recurrent pain within 12 hours of the infarction or cardiogenic shock, or continued ischemia after thrombolysis. Angioplasty after the acute phase of myocardial infarction can be recommended for recurrent pain, recurrent ischemia on laboratory testing, or refractory ventricular tachycardia, or for severe lesions in arteries serving viable myocardium. However, as shown in the TIMI II study, elective angioplasty immediately after thrombolysis is currently not recommended because of adverse results of this strategy.

These guidelines reemphasized the need for a surgical program within the institution where angioplasty is performed. This recommendation was made in recognition of the important role of backup surgery when angioplasty fails or complications occur and so that onsite consultation can be obtained for high-risk cases. Surgery within the institution is also important in that it provides an opportunity for patients to access the full range of revascularization procedures.

Summary

Although new devices are increasingly used to perform angioplasty, balloon technology remains the predominant method used in interventional cardiology. Many of the lesions addressed with balloon techniques are not suitable for other new devices and in general the new devices have not shown superior long-term results. It is hoped that this will not always be the case and that improvements in technology will result in improved long-term outcomes. In the meantime, balloon angioplasty remains a viable tool, especially when applied in patients with discrete lesions in accessible portions of the coronary tree and patients with significant symptoms or objective signs of ischemia.

The choice between angioplasty and surgery cannot be simplified into a choice between single and multivessel disease. As the randomized trials will probably demonstrate, patients with the most diffuse forms of multivessel disease will likely continue to be best served by surgical therapy, whereas many patients with lesions treatable by interventional cardiology techniques in multiple sites can be effectively managed with that approach. The marked superiority of surgery in terms of repeat procedures is being well documented. Surgery will probably also result in improved degree of revascularization and therefore, long-term results of the randomized trials are crucial to judge whether late events will be driven by this less complete revascularization in the angioplasty group or late graft closure in the surgery group.

It has become clear that angioplasty and surgery are complementary techniques and it is hoped as further knowledge is gained that the optimum selection of each procedure can be made for those patients in need of these procedures.

References

1. Gruentzig AR, Senning A, Siegenthaler WE. Nonoperative dilation of coronary artery stenosis: percutaneous transluminal coronary angioplasty. *N Engl J Med.* 1979;301:61–68.
2. National Center for Health Statistics: 1986 Summary: *National Hospital Discharge Survey.* Hyattsville, MD: National Center for Health Statistics, 1987: DHHS Publication No. (PHS) 87–1250, Public Health Service (advance data from vital and health statistics: no. 145).
3. King SB, Schlumpf M. Ten year completed follow-up after percutaneous transluminal coronary angioplasty: the early Zurich experience. *J Am Coll Cardiol.* 1993;22:353–360.
4. Talley JD, Hurst JW, King SB, et al. Clinical outcome 5 years after attempted percutaneous transluminal coronary angioplasty in 427 patients. *Circulation.* 1988;77:820–829.
5. Cowley MJ, Vetrovec GW, DiSciasio G, et al. Coronary angioplasty of multiple vessels: short term outcome and long-term results. *Circulation.* 1985;72:1314–1320.
6. O'Keefe JH Jr, Rutherford BD, McConahay DR, et al. Multivessel coronary angioplasty from 1980–1989: procedural results and long-term outcome. *J Am Coll Cardiol.* 1990;16:1079–1102.
7. Serruys PW, Luijten HE, Beatt KJ, et al. Incidence of restenosis after successful coronary angioplasty: a time-related phenomenon. A quantitative angiographic study in 342 consecutive patients at 1, 2, 3, and 4 months. *Circulation.* 1988;77:361–371.
8. Weintraub WS, Ghazzal ZM, Douglas JS Jr, et al. Initial management and long-term clinical outcome of restenosis after initially successful percutaneous transluminal coronary angioplasty. *Am J Cardiol.* 1992;70:47–55.
9. Lovastatin restenosis trial study group. Lovastatin restenosis trial: final results. *Circulation.* 1993;88:I-506. Abstract.

10. Liu MW, Roubin GS, King SB III. Restenosis after coronary angioplasty. Potential biologic determinants and role of intimal hyperplasia. *Circulation.* 1989;79:1374–1387.
11. King SB III. Role of new technology in balloon angioplasty. *Circulation.* 1991;84:2574–2579.
12. Topol EJ, Leya F, Pinkerton CA, et al. A comparison of directional atherectomy with balloon angioplasty in patients with coronary artery disease. *N Engl J Med.* 1993;329:221–227.
13. Adelman AG, Cohen EA, Kimball BP, et al. A comparison of directional atherectomy with balloon angioplasty for lesions of the left anterior descending coronary artery. *N Engl J Med.*1993;329:228–233.
14. Schatz RA, Baim DS, Leon NB, et al. Clinical experience with the Palmaz-Schatz coronary stent. Initial results of a multi-center study. *Circulation.* 1991;83:148–161.
15. Serruys PW, DeJaegere PP, Kiemeneij F, et al. Clinical events and angiographic results of the first 120 patients randomized in the Benestent study. *Circulation.* 1992;86:373. Abstract.
16. Parisi AF, Folland ED, Hatigan PA. Comparison of angioplasty with medical therapy in the treatment of single vessel coronary artery disease. *N Engl J Med.* 1992;326:10–16.
17. King SB III, Lembo NJ, Hall EC, and the EAST investigators. The Emory angioplasty vs. surgery trial (EAST): analysis of baseline patient characteristics. *Circulation.* 1992;82(Suppl I):I-508. Abstract.
18. RITA trial participants. Coronary angioplasty vs. coronary artery bypass surgery: the randomized intervention trial of angina (RITA). *Lancet.* 1993;341:573–580.
19. Lembo NJ, King SB III. Randomized trials of percutaneous transluminal coronary angioplasty, coronary artery bypass grafting surgery, or medical therapy in patients with coronary artery disease. *Coronary Artery Dis.* 1990;1:449–454.
20. Hamm CW, Reimers J, Rupprecht H, et al. Angioplasty vs bypass surgery in patients with multivessel disease: Re-interventions and complications during 6 months follow up. *J Am Coll Cardiol.* 1993; 21:72A. Abstract.
21. Frye R. Protocol for the bypass angioplasty revascularization investigation. *Circulation.* 1991;84(suppl V):V1-V27.
22. Grines CL, Browne KF, Marco J, et al. A comparison of immediate angioplasty with thrombolytic therapy for acute myocardial infarction. *N Engl J Med.* 1993;328:673–679.
23. Ryan TJ, Bauman WB, Kennedy WJ, et al. Guidelines for percutaneous transluminal coronary angioplasty. A report of the American Heart Association/American College of Cardiology Task Force on Assessment of Diagnostic and Therapeutic Cardiovascular Procedures (Committee on Percutaneous Transluminal Coronary Angioplasty). *Circulation.* 1993;88:2987–3007.

Chapter 10

Lesion Morphology and Acute Outcome After Excimer Laser Angioplasty:
A Prospective Evaluation

David R. Holmes, Jr, MD,
Lloyd W. Klein, MD, and Frank Litvack, MD,
for the Excimer Laser Coronary Angioplasty
Registry Investigators*

The relation between lesion morphology and the acute outcome of conventional percutaneous transluminal coronary angioplasty (PTCA) remains a controversial issue that has been the subject of several clinical studies.[1-5] A coding system advanced by a combined ACC/AHA Task Force in 1988 grouped various morphologic characteristics into A, B, and C categories in order to objectively quantitate the risks and expected outcome of PTCA. The original criteria have been shown to be generally predictive, but also to have certain flaws in estimating relative risk in the rather broad, moderate risk (B) category. A modification of these criteria, proposed by Ellis and colleagues,[3] addressed these problems and is now commonly accepted as the standard morphologic classification with reasonable predictive power for PTCA outcome.

However, the relation between lesion morphology and outcome with the newer percutaneous revascularization devices such as excimer laser coronary angioplasty (ELCA) has not been established.[6,7] Because these technologies were developed, at least in part to circumvent the problems posed by balloon dilatation of complex stenoses, this is an important issue.

*A list of the participating centers is found at the end of this chapter.

From Vetrovec GW, Carabello BA, (eds.) *Invasive Cardiology: Current Diagnostic and Therapeutic Issues.* Armonk, NY: Futura Publishing Company, Inc.: © 1996.

In this chapter, a prospective multicenter experience is presented that evaluates whether or not the AHA/ACC criteria proposed for predicting outcome after balloon dilatation retains its predictive capabilities with ELCA. Lesion morphology was prospectively characterized at 36 centers, and the short-term outcome analyzed with respect to specific morphologic descriptors and the ACC/AHA classification.

Materials and Methods

Laser System

The laser system used for this registry has been previously described.[8-11] It is a 308-nm xenon chloride pulsed excimer laser that is magnetically switched with a pulse duration of ≥200 nsec (Advanced Interventional Systems, Irvine, Ca). The system operates with a laser output of ≥200 mJ per pulse at 20–30 Hz, using catheter distal tip energies of 35–60 mJ/mm². During this registry study, over-the-wire multifiber catheters were used with diameters of 1.3, 1.6, 2.0, and 2.2 mm. The original catheters used 200 μm fibers while the more recent experience used 50 μm fibers. Both were included in this analysis. The data from the recently introduced directional excimer laser coronary angioplasty (DELCA) catheter were not used for this study.[12]

Study Patients

All studies were carried out using an investigational protocol that had received institutional review board approval at each center. Patient selection criteria included symptomatic or exercise-induced myocardial ischemia in the setting of coronary arterial stenoses that could be accessed by the guide wire and laser catheter.

All patients at each of the 36 investigative centers who underwent laser therapy from May 3, 1989 to June 30, 1993 were included in this study. For each patient, the clinical and anatomical data and procedural details were collected and collated into the central ELCA registry. This study compared the relation between lesion classification and outcome of laser angioplasty.

Angiographic Assessment

Orthogonal views of the coronary arterial stenoses were obtained at baseline, after laser angioplasty, and after adjunctive dilatation when required. An attempt was made to use identical projections at the time of each angiogram. Dimensions of the target vessel and stenosis were usually made with electronic or manual calibers at each center. There was, however, no central angiographic laboratory.

The stenoses were assessed prospectively prior to the procedure for length, lesion angulation, bifurcation lesion, lesion calcification, eccentricity, the presence of a chronic total occlusion, ostial location, friable graft lesion, irregular stenosis contour, thrombus present, or tortuous vessel contour. The modified ACC/AHA classification of Ellis et al[3] was used (Table 1).

TABLE 1

Characteristics of Type A, B, and C Lesions Influencing Successful Percutaneous Transluminal Coronary Angioplasty

Type A Lesions (high success, >85%; low risk)

Discrete (<10 mm length)	Little or no calcification
Concentric	Less than totally occlusive
Readily accessible	Not ostial in location
Nonangulated segment (<45°)	No major branch involvement
Smooth contour	Absence of thrombus

Type B Lesions (moderate success, 60–85%; moderate risk)*

Tubular (10–20 mm long)	Moderate to heavy calcification
Eccentric	Total occlusions <3 months old
Moderate tortuosity of proximal segment	Ostial location
Moderate angulated segment (>45° but <90°)	Bifurcation lesions requiring double guide wires
Irregular contour	Some thrombus present
B1 lesions—one characteristic	
B2 lesions—one characteristic	

Type C Lesions (low success, <60%; high risk)

Diffuse (>20 mm length)	Total occlusion >3 months old
Excessive tortuosity of proximal segment	Inability to protect major side branches
Extremely angulated segments (>90°)	Degenerated vein grafts with friable lesions

*Although the risk of abrupt vessel closure is moderate, in certain instances the likelihood of a major complication may be low, such as in dilation of total occlusions <3 months old or when abundant collateral channels supply the distal vessel.

Definitions

A short-term laser success was defined as a ≥20% reduction in the stenosis luminal diameter or a minimal luminal diameter of >0.8 mm with a 1.3-mm catheter, >1 mm with a 1.6-mm catheter, or >1.5 mm with a 2.0-mm catheter. A procedural success was defined as a diameter stenosis <50% at the end of the procedure irrespective of whether PTCA was used with no in-hospital death, need for coronary bypass graft surgery (CABG), Q wave myocardial infarction, or need for a repeat catheterization-based procedure. Acute or threatened closure was defined as TIMI 0 or 1 when associated with pain or electrocardiographic changes consistent with myocardial ischemia. For chronic total occlusions, passage of the guide wire through the occlusion was required before the patient could be enrolled in the laser protocol.

Although follow-up angiography was strongly recommended, it was not mandatory; therefore, follow-up angiographic data is incomplete and is not reported.

Procedural Details

Details of the laser angioplasty procedure have been previously described. Selection of the specific catheter size was not mandated, but was based on consideration of the size of the target vessel and lesion to be treated. Typically, a 1.3-mm catheter was used in a vessel of at least 2.0 mm in diameter. After this catheter became widely available, it was often used as the primary catheter and then followed with adjunctive dilatation. Prior to wide availability of this catheter, 1.6-mm catheters were used and usually required a vessel of ≥2.3 mm, while a 2.0-mm catheter was used in vessels of at least 3.0 mm in diameter. After the stenosis or occlusion was crossed, the catheter was advanced up to 5 mm proximal to the lesion and lasing was initiated. Typically, during lasing, the catheter was advanced at approximately 1 mm/s. After assessment of the results of the initial pass, operators could perform adjunctive dilatation or sequentially increase the laser catheter size.

Medications included aspirin, usually administered 24 hours prior to and continued after the procedure, nitrates, and calcium channel blockers. Heparin was given as a bolus of 10,000–15,000 units during the procedure.

Statistical Analysis

Continuous variables were expressed as mean ± standard deviation (SD). Dichotomous variables were expressed as frequencies.

Differences between groups were assessed with unpaired Student's *t* test for continuous variables and Pearson's γ^2 analysis for dichotomous variables. *P* values <0.05 were considered statistically significant.

Results

Two thousand five hundred and nine lesions were treated in 2,183 patients. One thousand five hundred forty-three patients were male (Table 2). The majority were severely symptomatic; 72% were Canadian Cardiovascular Society III or IV. Of these patients, 34% had undergone prior CABG, 40% had been previously treated with PTCA, and 10% had undergone prior ELCA.

The left anterior descending artery was the most commonly treated vessel (862 lesions, 34%) followed by the right coronary artery (832 lesions, 33%), the circumflex (375 lesions, 15%), and saphenous vein bypass grafts (331 lesions, 13%). In addition, 108 patients (4%) underwent ELCA of the left main coronary artery. The mean energy density used for the entire group was 53 ± 8 mJ/mm² and ranged from 13 to 95 mJ/mm².

The modified ACC/AHA lesion classification is shown in Figure 1. As documented, only 6% were type A lesions. B2 and C lesions were most commonly treated in 46% and 33%, respectively. The specific frequency of adverse lesion characteristics is shown in Table 3. Lesion eccentricity, lesion irregularity, calcification, vessel tortuosity and lesion length >20 mm were the most common lesion characteristics treated with 1,365, 947, 921, 614, and 557 lesions, respectively.

TABLE 2

Patient Demographics (*n* = 2,183)

Mean age (yrs)	63 ± 11
Male gender (%)	71
CCVS (%)	
0–2	28
3–4	72
Ejection fraction	52 ± 14
Prior treatment (%)	
CABG	34
PTCA	40
ELCA	10

CCVS, Canadian Cardiovascular Society class; CABG, coronary artery bypass graft surgery; PTCA, percutaneous transluminal coronary angioplasty; ELCA, excimer laser coronary angioplasty.

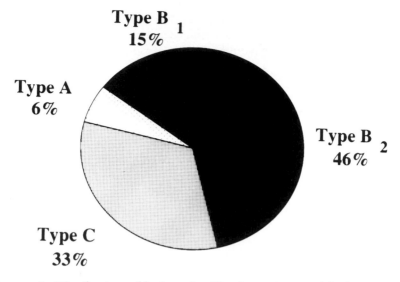

FIGURE 1. *Distribution of lesion classification using modified ACC/AHA criteria.*

TABLE 3	
Specific Lesion Characteristics	
Eccentric lesion	1,365
Calcified	921
Irregular contour	947
Length	
10–20 mm	645
>20 mm	557
Vessel tortuosity	614
Ostial	348
Total occlusion	333
Bifurcation	258
Thrombus present	141
Angulation	
46–90	105
91+	7
Friable graft	60

Total number of adverse lesion descriptors is >1838 because of the presence of more than one adverse characteristic per lesion.

In the entire group, the overall laser success was 86% while the procedural success was 89%. For both laser and procedural success, the rates decreased somewhat, but not statistically significantly with increasing lesion complexity. For type A lesions, procedural success was 92% compared with 88% for type C lesions (Table 4).

TABLE 4

Procedural Outcome

	A	B1	B2	C	Total
Lesions	145	341	1,167	856	2,509
Laser success (%)	92	88	85	86	86
Procedure success (%)	92	91	89	88	89
Complications (%)					
QMI	4.1	1.8	1.4	1.8	1.7
CABG	4.1	6.4	4.1	2.5	3.8
Death	0	1.1	0.7	1.0	0.8
Acute closure	4.0	7.1	5.7	6.7	6.3
Sustained closure	1.0	2.5	3.3	3.3	3.0
Flow-limiting dissection	2.0	4.3	5.2	5.0	4.9
Embolism	0	0	1.2	1.1	1.0
Perforation	3.1	0.7	1.2	1.3	1.2

CABG, coronary artery bypass graft surgery.

Overall, major complication rates were low with Q wave myocardial infarction 1.7%, CABG 3.8%, and death 0.8%. The most common adverse event was acute closure in 6.3%, ranging from 4.0 for type A lesions to 7.1% for B1 lesions and 6.7% for type C lesions. In the majority of cases, the acute closure was transient; overall only 3.0% of patients had persistent occlusion. Perforation rates were highest with type A lesions at 3.1%, perhaps because there was more normal vessel wall impacted by lasing in this group of lesions.

Relation between Lesion Characteristics and Outcome (Table 5)

Specific adverse lesion characteristics were common in the patient cohort undergoing ELCA. There were, however, only relatively small differences in procedural outcomes between any of the specific subsets, ranging from 85% to 92%. Specific lesion characteristics felt to be more optimally treated by laser have been longer lesions: in this experience with lesions from 10–20 mm, the procedural success rate was 92% while for lesions >20 mm, the success rate was 90%. Procedural success rates were less common in calcified lesions ($P<0.001$), chronic total occlusions ($P=0.02$), and lesions with irregular contours ($P<0.001$). Lesions with angiographic thrombus had the lowest success rates (85%); in this group, failure was usually related to sustained occlusion.

TABLE 5

Relationship Between Lesion Characteristics and Outcome

Lesion Characteristic	Proced Succ (%)*	QMI (%)†	Non-QMI (%)	CABG (%)	Death (%)	Sus Occ (%)**
Length						
10–20 mm	92	2.2	2.9	2.6	0.9	2.9
>20 mm	90	2.1	3.1	2.5	1.2	3.3
Angulation						
46–90	86	0	3.8	3.8	1.0	1.0
91+	86	12.5	0	0	0	0
Bifurcation	89	1.2	3.6	4.0	1.2	4.8
Calcification	86	2.5	3.6	4.8	1.3	3.1
Chronic total occlusion	86	0	2.1	1.3	0.9	2.1
Eccentric	88	1.9	3.4	3.9	1.0	3.7
Friable graft	90	0	8.2	0	4.1	2.0
Irregular contour	87	2.0	3.0	3.4	1.1	4.0
Ostial	88	1.4	6.0	4.6	0.9	2.3
Thrombus prior	85	1.5	1.5	3.8	0.8	4.6
Tortuous	88	2.0	3.5	3.3	0.7	4.0
Total occlusion	87	0.3	2.1	1.5	0.6	1.8
Unprot. branch	90	2.2	4.5	5.6	0	5.6

*Procedural success was decreased in lesions with calcification ($P < 0.001$), thrombus prior to procedure ($P = 0.03$), and angulation from 46–90° ($P = 0.04$).
†The incidence of Q-wave myocardial infarction was decreased in chronic total occlusions.
**Rates of sustained occlusion were increased in lesions with side branch involvement ($P = 0.007$) and irregular contour ($P = 0.03$).

Q wave myocardial infarction was more common in patients with calcified lesions ($P=0.02$) and less common in patients with chronic total occlusion ($P=0.05$). No morphologic characteristics strongly predicted non-Q wave myocardial infarction. Occlusion was more common in patients with prior thrombus ($P=0.01$) and less common in patients with prior total occlusion ($P<0.001$). Coronary bypass surgery was less common in patients with moderately long ($P=0.007$), long ($P=0.04$), or totally occluded lesions ($P=0.04$). Finally, death was more common in patients with friable vein grafts ($P=0.01$).

The complication patterns seen varied somewhat depending on the specific lesion subset treated. Friable vein grafts, while they had a procedural success rate of 90%, had a non-Q wave myocardial infarction rate of 8.2% and sustained occlusion of 2.0%, both usually related to distal embolization. The in-hospital mortality was 4.1%. Ostial lesions were also problematic with a 6.0% incidence of non-Q wave myocardial infarction and 4.6% incidence of CABG; death was uncommon (0.9%). Finally, branch vessels remained a problem, although success rates were good at 90%. These lesions still had a slightly increased incidence of sustained occlusion at 4.8% to 5.6%, respectively.

Discussion

A major problem for conventional PTCA has been the inability to predict the acute outcome of balloon inflation on the basis of lesion morphology.[1,3,4] There have been several attempts at categorizing lesion characteristics, most notably the ACC/AHA guidelines that have been modified by Ellis et al[3] to further subcategorize moderate risk type B lesions. This system is based on the concept that increasing lesion complexity will be associated with declining success rates. Ellis et al[3] found that lesion morphology assessed in this manner was the most powerful predictor of procedural outcome in patients with multivessel disease undergoing PTCA. Similar trends have been reported in other series[5,13] although the magnitude of the predictive power has diminished with recent advances in balloon catheter technology.

New therapeutic devices have been developed to avoid the problem of decreasing success rates with increasing lesion complexity. There is limited data on whether this goal has been achieved. Stertzer et al[14] recently reported that the same trend for decreasing success rates with type B and C lesions applies with rotational ablation (Rotablator™, Heart Technology, Bellevue, WA) although specific morphologic subtypes do have an improved outcome. Similar trends have been previously reported for DCA; Ellis et al.[15] documented a substantial decline in success rates from type A lesions (93%) to type B1 lesions (88%) to type B2 lesions (75%). In that experience, the number of type C lesions attempted was too low for meaningful comparison.

In the present multicenter ELCA Registry of 2,509 lesions treated in 2,183 patients, lesion distributions were different than in conventional PTCA series. Only 6% of lesions were type A; B2 lesions were most commonly treated in 46%, while 33% were type C lesions. The differences in lesion subtypes and numbers make comparisons difficult both within this series as well as between ELCA and other devices. In this ELCA series, however, there were no statistically significant differences in laser success rate between the lesion subtypes. Overall, a laser success of 86% was achieved; 92%

for type A, 88% for type B1, 85% for B2, and 86% for type C lesions. This is somewhat different than seen in the recent series of rotational ablation cases in which after rotational ablation, a success rate of 100% was seen with type A lesions, but dropped to 86.9% with type B or C lesions. For this ELCA series, there was also no statistically significant difference in final procedural success rates of 89% with 92% for type A, 91% for B1, 89% for B2, and 88% for type C lesions.

Complications for the entire group were uncommon: 1.7% Q wave myocardial infarction, 3.8% coronary bypass graft surgery, 0.8% death, and 3.0% sustained closure. There was limited variability between lesion subtypes. Of interest, Q wave myocardial infarctions and perforation were more commonly seen with type A lesions being treated. It is possible that in type A lesions there is more normal arterial wall that could be impacted by the laser energy increasing the potential for perforation.[7,16] It is also possible that type A lesions were treated early on in the individual center's experience and represent the learning curve for the procedure. In any case, given the fact that conventional PTCA is so effective for type A lesions, there is very little reason to consider the use of ELCA in this setting. For the other lesion subtypes of B1, B2 and C, complication patterns were very similar. Even in type C lesions, the incidence of sustained acute closure, Q wave infarction and CABG were low at 3.3%, 1.8%, and 2.5%, respectively. There are limited current data on similar lesions treated with conventional PTCA; in the past, type C lesions had definitely decreased success rates and increased complications.

The relation between ACC/AHA type and outcome may not be as definite as the relation between specific lesion morphology and outcome. Moushmoush et al[13] found that the most important predictors of failure in multivessel angioplasty cases were the presence of a chronic total occlusion, a stenosis bend of >90°, and excessive tortuosity. Myler et al[5] found that the presence of thrombus was independently associated with complications whereas the absence of an occlusion >3 months, the absence of an unprotected bifurcation lesion, and a shorter lesion length were all associated with increased success rates on multivariate analysis.

In this ELCA Registry experience, procedural success rates were excellent, irrespective of the specific lesion characteristics. In contrast to PTCA, irrespective of lesion length, success rates were high; 90% for lesions >20 mm versus 92% for lesions from 10–20 mm in length. With conventional dilatation in the past, both of these lesion lengths have been associated with decreased success rates. Bifurcation lesion success rates with ELCA were less and sustained occlusion was increased. In these bifurcation lesions, the laser may damage more normal arterial wall or even the origin of the side branch. A directional laser has been developed for this application that may improve outcome in these patients. As has been true with most other technologies, lesions containing thrombus continue to be associated with decreased success rates and a higher incidence of acute closure which, for the ELCA Registry, were 85% and 4.6%, respectively. Other lesion subsets had good success rates and excellent clinical outcome.

Vein graft lesions continue to be associated with poorer outcome. Although success rates were good, 8.2% of patients had evidence of non-Q wave myocardial infarction, and 2% had sustained occlusion. This is similar to that seen with conventional PTCA and may be less than seen with directional atherectomy. Usually this does not result in adverse clinical sequelae, although it may. In this group of patients, an in-hospital mortality rate of 4.1% was seen, which was far higher than in any other lesion subset. These complications are presumably related to the complex friable nature of the underlying pathophysiology with distal embolization of the material during passage of the catheter.

Follow-up angiography rates have been incomplete with most of the new devices outside of randomized trials. As yet, documentation that restenosis rates will be substantially decreased by any new device with the possible exception of single large stents has not been substantiated; certainly that is true with restenosis after ELCA. During an average follow-up of 6 months, 28% of the patients reported here required another intervention, typically for restenosis.

Limitations

There are limitations to this type of registry study. No core angiography laboratory was used. Instead, the angiograms were interpreted and analyzed at the specific sites for lesion morphology and severity. Core angiographic assessment may have documented specific angiographic subsets of lesions most likely to have adverse outcome although in general, in this study, the success rates were excellent. In addition, this is a clinical patient registry and not a controlled randomized trial. Although trends of success and complication patterns with other technology can be documented, direct comparisons are not valid.

The eventual role of ELCA remains to be determined from randomized trials. It will not supplant conventional dilatation. Ideally, it will be used to treat lesion subsets, B1, B2 and C lesions, which have been documented to have poorer outcome with conventional PTCA. Its role then will be to extend the possibility of catheter-based technology for a larger number of patient subsets with these adverse lesion characteristics to optimize the early outcome.

*Participating Centers

Abbott Northwestern Hospital
Alvarado Hospital Medical Center
Baptist Medical Center of Oklahoma
Cedars-Sinai Medical Center
Carolinas Medical Center
The Christ Hospital
Daniel Freeman Memorial Hospital
Doctors Medical Center
Emory University School of Medicine
Georgetown University Hospital
Goleta Valley Community Hospital
Hillcrest Medical Center
Hoag Memorial Hospital
Massachusetts General Hospital
The Mayo Foundation
Medical College of Virginia
The Mercy Hospital of Pittsburgh
The Methodist Hospital
Miami Heart Institute
Presbyterian Medical Center of Philadelphia

Robert Wood Johnson University Hospital
Rush-Presbyterian-St. Luke's Medical Center
Shands Hospital University of Florida
South Miami Hospital
Saint John's Hospital and Health Center
St. Francis Regional Medical Center
St. Luke's Hospital of Kansas City
St. Luke's Medical Center, Milw
St. Luke's Medical Center, Phoe
St. Vincent Hospital and Health Care Center
Summit Medical Center
The University of Alabama at Birmingham
University of Maryland at Baltimore
Washington Hospital Center
William Beaumont Hospital

References

1. Ryan TJ, Faxon DP, Gunnar RM, et al. Guidelines for percutaneous transluminal coronary angioplasty: a report of the American College of Cardiology/American Heart Association Task Force on Assessment of Diagnostic and Therapeutic Cardiovascular Procedures (Subcommittee of Percutaneous Transluminal Coronary Angioplasty). *Circulation.* 1988;78:486–502.
2. Faxon DP, Holmes DR, Hartzler GO, et al. ABC's of coronary angioplasty: have we simplified it too much? *Cathet Cardiovasc Diagn.* 1992; 25:1–3. Editorial.
3. Ellis SG, Vandormael MG, Cowley MJ, et al. Coronary morphologic and clinical determinants of procedural outcome with angioplasty for multivessel coronary disease. Implications for patient selection. Multivessel Angioplasty Prognosis Study Group. *Circulation.* 1990;82:1193–1202.
4. Kleinman NS, Rodriguez AR, Raizner AE. Interobserver variability in grading of coronary arterial narrowings using the American College of

Cardiology/American Heart Association grading criteria. *Am J Cardiol.* 1992;69:413–415.

5. Myler RK, Shaw RE, Stertzer SH, et al. Lesion morphology and coronary angioplasty. Current experience and analysis. *J Am Coll Cardiol.* 1992;19:1641–1652.

6. Ghazzal ZMB, Hearn JA, Litvack F, et al. Morphological predictors of acute complications after percutaneous excimer laser coronary angioplasty. Results of a comprehensive angiographic analysis: importance of the eccentricity index. *Circulation.* 1992;86:820–827.

7. Bittl JA, Ryan TJ Jr, Keaney JF Jr, et al. Coronary artery perforation during excimer laser coronary angioplasty. *J Am Coll Cardiol.* 1993;21:1158–1165.

8. Cook SL, Eigler NL, Shefer A, et al. Percutaneous excimer laser coronary angioplasty of lesions not ideal for balloon angioplasty. *Circulation.* 1991;84:632–643.

9. Pacala TJ, McDermid IS, Laudenslager JB. Ultranarrow linewidth, magnetically switched, long pulse, xenon chloride laser. *Appl Phys Lett.* 1984;44:658–660.

10. Grundfest WS, Litvack F, Forrester JS, et al. Laser ablation of human atherosclerotic plaque without adjacent tissue injury. *J Am Coll Cardiol.* 1985;5:929–933.

11. Holmes DR Jr, Forrester JS, Litvack F, et al. Chronic total obstruction and short-term outcome: the Excimer Laser Coronary Angioplasty Registry experience. *Mayo Clin Proc.* 1993;68:5–10.

12. Ghazzal ZMB, Leon MB, Shefer A, et al. The novel directional laser catheter: multicenter angiographic core lab analysis. *J Am Coll Cardiol.* 1993;21:288A.

13. Moushmoush B, Kramer B, Hsieh AM, Klein LW. Does the ACC/AHA Task Force grading system predict outcome in multivessel coronary angioplasty? *Cathet Cardiovasc Diagn.* 1992;27:97–106.

14. Stertzer S, Rosenblum J, Shaw RE, et al. Coronary rotational ablation: initial experience in 302 procedures. *J Am Coll Cardiol.* 1993;21:287–296.

15. Ellis SG, DeCesare NB, Pinkerton CA, et al. Relation of stenosis morphology and clinical presentation to the procedural results of directional coronary atherectomy. *Circulation.* 1991;84:644–653.

16. Holmes DR, Reeder GS, Ghazzal ZMB, et al. Coronary perforation after excimer coronary angioplasty: the Excimer Laser Coronary Angioplasty Registry experience. *J Am Coll Cardiol.* 1994;23:330–335.

Chapter 11

Directional Coronary Atherectomy

Michael J. Cowley, MD

Although percutaneous transluminal coronary angioplasty (PTCA) is a highly effective method of coronary revascularization, balloon angioplasty has certain limitations that restrict its wider use. Various new interventional devices have been developed to address the limitations of PTCA. Directional coronary atherectomy (DCA) is a new technique that involves selective plaque removal using a side-cutting catheter system. Coronary atherectomy was first performed in 1986 using prototype catheters. Clinical investigation of DCA was subsequently conducted at a number of clinical sites and results involving single and multicenter experience have been reported.[1-5] Directional coronary atherectomy received FDA premarket approval in 1990, and the technique has since had a rapid increase in clinical usage with an estimated 50,000 procedures performed in the United States in 1993.

Technique

Directional coronary atherectomy is performed in a manner similar to balloon angioplasty. The system uses large (9.5F–11F) guiding catheters with special tip shapes for engaging the coronary arteries. The atherectomy catheters are large (5F–7F diameter) at the distal cylindrical metal housing, which has a 9–10-mm long window, a balloon support member on the opposite side of the window, and a cup-shaped cutter that rotates at 2,000 rpm. The cutter is manually advanced and the excised plaque is trapped in the nosecone collection chamber. Because of the relatively large catheter size and the rigid metal housing, the technique is best suited for proximal lesions in relatively large vessels. Vessels with tortuosity and calcification are less well suited for atherectomy, al-

From Vetrovec GW, Carabello BA, (eds.) *Invasive Cardiology: Current Diagnostic and Therapeutic Issues*. Armonk, NY: Futura Publishing Company, Inc.: © 1996.

though the newer low profile EX catheters are more flexible and have improved access to more distal and tortuous lesions.

Clinical Results

The initial multicenter clinical experience represented more than 1,600 procedures at 24 centers. The multicenter results showed an overall success rate of 85%, with an incidence of major complications of 4.5%.[2] Subsequent reports of the multicenter results and experience from individual centers has shown similar overall results, with success rates ranging from 85% to 95%, and major complication rates of 0.4% to 5% (Table 1).[3-9]

Various predictors of outcome have been identified for success and complications with DCA.[3,5,6,8-10] Presence of calcification was a predictor of lower success rate, as were primary (de novo) lesions and diffuse (>20 mm length) lesions.[3,5] Calcification, diffuse lesions and de novo lesions were also associated with a higher incidence of major complications.[3,5] In several reports, the right coronary artery (RCA) was associated with a lower success rate and higher rate of complications, particularly need for urgent bypass surgery.[3,7,8]

Angiographic restenosis after DCA has been reported in 30% to 58% of patients within 6 months after the procedure.[3,7,11-13] The restenosis rate in the multicenter investigational experience was 42% of 384 lesions (representing a 77% angiographic restudy rate).[3] Restenosis rate in native vessels was 30% for primary lesions and 46% for previously restenotic lesions; similarly, restenosis rate in vein grafts was 31% for primary lesions and 68% for grafts that had previously had restenosis. Fishman[7] reported overall restenosis rate of 32%, with lower restenosis rate (24% versus 39%) when

TABLE 1

Clinical Results with Directional Coronary Atherectomy

	#	Success	Compl	CABG	QMI	Death
Baim[3]	873	85%	4.9%	4.0%	0.9%	0.5%
Hinohara[5]	382	90%	3.4%	3.1%	0.8%	0.3%
Fishman[7]	225	91%	0.4%	0.4%	0%	0%
Cowley[8]	345	95%	4.6%*	3.8%	1.7%	0.3%
Popma[9]	306	95%	2.6%	2.0%	0.3%	0.7%

CABG, urgent coronary artery bypass surgery; Compl, major complication; QMI, Q wave myocardial infarction

* = includes "salvage DCA" procedures for failed angioplasty due to acute vessel closure

postprocedure lumen diameter was >3 mm. Factors associated with a higher rate of restenosis have included diabetes, prior restenosis, lesion length >10 mm, vein graft lesion, smaller vessels (<3 mm diameter), noncalcified lesion, and use of smaller (6F) device.[3,7,11–13]

Specific Clinical Applications of DCA

Eccentric Lesions

Because of the directional cutting capability, eccentric lesions, particularly highly eccentric lesions, are well suited for DCA. These lesions are often not favorable for PTCA or other new interventional devices. Several reports have shown excellent immediate and longer term results with DCA.[5,6] In contrast to balloon angioplasty, the success and complication rates and the final residual percent stenosis were similar for concentric, moderately eccentric, and highly eccentric lesions with DCA.[5] In vessels of suitable size and accessibility with moderately to highly eccentric lesions, DCA has become the interventional procedure of choice. Current clinical indications for DCA are listed in Table 2.

TABLE 2

Current Indications for Directional Coronary Atherectomy

· Eccentric lesions	· Complex lesion morphology
· Proximal LAD	· Thrombus-associated lesions
· Ostial lesions	· Bifurcation lesions
· Vein graft lesions	· Failed/suboptimal PTCA result

LAD, left anterior descending coronary artery; CABG, coronary artery bypass graft surgery

Saphenous Vein Grafts

Directional coronary atherectomy is also well suited for treating focal vein graft (SVG) lesions, which are often eccentric, complex, and friable, and in large caliber vessels without tortuosity or calcification. The multicenter investigational experience of vein graft DCA[14] as well as several individual center reports[13–17] of DCA for vein graft lesions have shown high success and low complication rates. Treatment of vein grafts represents a significant and increasing proportion of interventional procedures, ranging from 15% to 20% or more at many centers. Clinical success rates with SVG DCA have ranged from 85% to more than 95% at various centers, and major complication rates have ranged from 2% to 5% in these reports.[13–17]. Many of the graft lesions treated with DCA were considered to be unsuitable for PTCA due to complex morphology, presence of thrombus, or ostial location. Myocardial infarction occurred in 5% to 6% of patients, with Q wave myocardial infarction in approximately 1% to 2% and non-Q myocardial infarction in approximately 4%. Other complications have included evidence of distal embolization with and without creatine kinase elevation, and vessel perforation. Vessel perforation in vein grafts is often small, localized, and may not be associated with adverse clinical effects due to containment by fibrosis around the graft.[8,16,17] Evidence of embolization (either angiographic or otherwise unexplained creatine kinase-MB elevation) has occurred in about 10% to 15% of procedures. Graft DCA is occasionally performed as a salvage procedure for failed PTCA and may be done in conjunction with thrombolytic therapy.[18] Restenosis rates observed after vein graft DCA have varied widely, ranging from as low as 28% to as high as 65%.[3,5,11–15] Vein graft restenosis after DCA is more common than after native vessel DCA, and restenosis rate is higher for lesions that have had prior restenosis. These associations have also been noted following treatment of vein grafts with balloon angioplasty and with other interventional techniques. Several reports suggest relatively high restenosis rates after vein graft DCA,[5,13,14] however, a recent report by Pomerantz[15] showed a graft restenosis rate of only 28% after DCA. These rates may be lower than seen with balloon angioplasty for similar lesions. Trials such as the CAVEAT II study comparing DCA and angioplasty for vein graft disease should clarify the relative efficacy of DCA for long-term outcome and restenosis.

Thrombus-Associated Lesions

Directional coronary atherectomy is well suited for certain thrombus-containing lesions, which usually have associated underlying complex or ulcerated plaque morphology and are common in patients with unstable angina or recent infarction. In a report by Ellis,[6] DCA was successful in all 35 thrombotic lesions treated and thrombus-containing lesions were a positive multivariate predictor for DCA success. Similarly, at our institution, DCA for thrombus-associated lesions was reported in 42 patients with procedural success achieved in 41 of 42 (98%) and complications occurred in 4.8%.[8] When prominent or extensive thrombus is present, local infusion of a thrombolytic agent such as urokinase may be used prior to catheter intervention. Intracoronary urokinase may also be infused after intervention to treat residual thrombus or embolization. Experience with DCA in conjunction with thrombolytic therapy has been reported,[18] and this combined approach is also effective for totally occluded vein grafts in which patency is restored with prolonged (12–24 hours) urokinase infusion into the graft followed by atherectomy of the complex residual graft lesion. Directional coronary atherectomy appears to be highly effective for focal thrombus-containing lesions in both native vessels and saphenous vein grafts and may be the preferred interventional technique if the target vessel is suitable in size for atherectomy.

Aorto-Ostial Lesions

Ostial lesions have had disappointing results with balloon angioplasty frequently caused by suboptimal dilatation related to elastic recoil and a higher incidence of complications and restenosis.[19] Clinical experience with DCA for aorto-ostial lesions suggests favorable initial results and increasing use for both vein graft and native coronary ostial lesions.[8,20–22] DCA for aorto-ostial lesions is much more difficult than for other lesions due to technical challenges in positioning the atherectomy catheter and the guiding catheter due to angulation and the inability to engage the guiding catheter at the ostium. However, the angiographic results with DCA appear to be significantly better than with PTCA. In a comparison study of final angiographic results with DCA, laser, and balloon angioplasty for aorto-ostial lesions, the final percent stenosis was significantly less with DCA (11%) than with laser (24%) or with balloon angioplasty (35%).[21] Directional coronary atherectomy appears to be highly effective for aorto-ostial lesions of both vein grafts and native vessels. Restenosis rates of aorto-ostial lesions after DCA have not been well characterized, but may be lower than seen with balloon angioplasty for ostial lesions.[20,22]

Directional Coronary Atherectomy for Salvage/Failed PTCA

Directional coronary atherectomy is also effective in achieving improved results in certain situations when balloon angioplasty is unsuccessful or associated with an inadequate or suboptimal result due to elastic recoil or due to localized dissection with occlusive intraluminal intimal flaps and/or acute vessel closure.[8,23–27] The use of "salvage" DCA for unsatisfactory PTCA results has increased in recent experience and multiple reports have shown favorable results (Table 3).[8,23–27]

TABLE 3

DCA for Failed or Suboptimal PTCA Results

	#	Success	CABG	QMI	Death	Perf
Whitlow[23]	67	93%	6.0%	7.4%	4.4%	1.5%
Hofling[24]	40	93%	10.0%	5.0%	0%	0%
Vetter[27]	49	88%	8.9%	4.1%	0%	2.0%
Cowley[8]	36	92%	8.3%	2.8%	0%	2.8%
McCluskey[25]	100	91%	6.0%	6.0%*	2.0%	1.0%

CABG, urgent coronary artery bypass surgery; QMI, Q wave myocardial infarction; Perf, vessel perforation; *, includes Q wave and non-Q MI

Success rates have ranged from 88% to 93% and complication rates have ranged from 6% to 10%. Most of the major complications in these studies occurred in the subgroup with acute vessel closure, and most of the procedure-related myocardial infarctions developed prior to DCA and were not attributable to the atherectomy procedure. Salvage DCA can prevent the need for urgent bypass surgery in selected patients. However, caution is advised because vessel perforation can occur with DCA of a coronary dissection,[8,23,25,27] and extensive, spiral, or deep wall dissections are generally not suitable for DCA. Endoluminal stenting is also effective in treating coronary dissections but currently requires aggressive intravenous and oral anticoagulation, which prolongs hospitalization and is associated with bleeding complications, as well as subacute stent thrombosis in some patients despite anticoagulation.[28] Directional coronary atherectomy is a useful technique for treatment of selected patients with suboptimal/failed PTCA and may be preferable to coronary stenting for certain instances of failed PTCA due to localized dissection, thrombosis, or vessel recoil, because the need for anticoagulation may be avoided.

DCA for Bifurcation Lesions

Directional coronary atherectomy is also effective for treating bifurcation lesions. Although initially considered a relative contraindication because of the inability to protect larger side branches, this approach has actually provided excellent angiographic results without increased complications.[8,29,30] Directional coronary atherectomy of both bifurcation vessels can be done if each is of sufficient size, or DCA of only one of the vessels may allow for better dilatation of the associated branch. The ability to remove plaque material may diminish the incidence of major dissections and suboptimal angiographic results due to plaque shifting at the bifurcation point. Several reports of experience with bifurcation DCA indicate high success and low complication rates for this application.[8,9,29,30]

Randomized Trials of DCA and Coronary Angioplasty

Several randomized clinical trials of DCA and PTCA have recently been completed: the CAVEAT study and the Canadian Coronary Atherectomy Trial (CCAT).[31,32] These studies represent the first randomized comparisons of a new interventional device with balloon angioplasty and provide important clinical information about the use of DCA. The CAVEAT trial enrolled 1,012 patients with primary lesions in native coronary arteries suitable for either technique, and the CCAT trial enrolled 274 patients with proximal LAD lesions suitable for both procedures. Both studies showed higher angiographic and clinical success rates with DCA and lower immediate residual stenosis with DCA than with PTCA. Overall complication rate was higher with DCA than PTCA in the CAVEAT study, primarily due to higher non-Q myocardial infarction and abrupt closure rates with DCA. However, complication rates were not different with DCA and PTCA in the CCAT trial. Angiographic restenosis, the primary end point in each study, was lower with DCA in CAVEAT (50% versus 57%, $P=0.06$), but not in CCAT (46% versus 43%). Subgroup analysis in the CAVEAT study showed significantly lower restenosis rate for proximal LAD lesions with DCA (51%) than with PTCA (63%), $P=0.04$. Clinical status at 6 months showed no difference between DCA and PTCA in either study. Thus plaque removal with DCA resulted in better initial angiographic results, with higher complications and a small reduction in angiographic restenosis in CAVEAT, but the initial better angiographic results did not result in improved clinical outcome at 6-month follow-up. Both studies had surprisingly high restenosis rates for both DCA and PTCA and both studies had substantial residual stenosis after DCA (33% and 25%). Average size of vessels treated in CAVEAT was only 2.77-mm diameter, which was considerably less than the protocol specification of >3.0-mm size. These results demonstrate higher angiographic restenosis rates than encountered in the initial DCA investigational experience or in several single center reports,[3,7,11] as well as showing higher residual stenosis and less initial luminal improvement (acute gain) immediately postintervention. The relation between initial result, vessel size, minimal luminal diameter, and late angiographic outcome has been characterized by Kuntz et al[33] and suggests that the best predictor of restenosis is the immediate postprocedure lumen diameter. The CAVEAT results appear to fit this generalized model of restenosis that they have described. The concept that plaque removal (debulking) provides long-term advantages over plaque remodeling with balloon angioplasty has not been demonstrated in these randomized trials. However, the hypothesis that optimal debulking will provide superior long-term results, which has not yet been tested, will be evaluated in additional clinical trials, such as the BOAT (Balloon versus Optimal Atherectomy Trial) study, which should further clarify the role of DCA in clinical practice.

Summary

Directional coronary atherectomy is a safe and effective coronary interventional therapy that is an alternative to balloon angioplasty for a variety of coronary anatomic and morphologic subsets that are unfavorable for balloon angioplasty. Directional coronary atherectomy is particularly useful for highly eccentric lesions, aorto-ostial lesions, saphenous vein grafts, complex or thrombus-associated lesions, bifurcation lesions, and for treatment of failed or suboptimal PTCA caused by localized dissection or recoil. New, lower profile and more flexible atherectomy catheters have improved results and have allowed treatment of more difficult lesions. Further enhancements such as ultrasound-guided atherectomy are under development and may further improve the utility of this technique. Comparative studies of DCA and balloon angioplasty such as the CAVEAT and CCAT trials have provided important information on the relative advantages and disadvantages of DCA for broad usage and have raised a number of additional questions about optimal debulking versus balloon remodeling that will require further study to help clarify the optimal usage of these techniques.

References

1. Hinohara T, Selmon MR, Robertson GC, et al. Directional atherectomy: new approaches for treatment of obstructive coronary and peripheral vascular disease. *Circulation.* 1990;81(suppl IV):IV-79-IV-91.
2. U.S. Directional Atherectomy Investigator Group: Directional coronary atherectomy: multicenter experience. *Circulation.* 1990;82(suppl IV):IV-71. Abstract.
3. Baim DS, Hinohara T, Holmes D, et al. Results of directional coronary

atherectomy during multicenter pre-approval testing. *Am J Cardiol.* 1993;72:6E–11E.

4. Safian RD, Gelbfish JS, Erny RE, et al. Clinical, angiographic, and histological findings and observations regarding potential mechanisms. *Circulation.* 1990;82:69–79.

5. Hinohara T, Rowe MH, Robertson GC, et al. Effect of lesion characteristics on outcome of directional coronary atherectomy. *J Am Coll Cardiol.* 1991;17:1112–1120.

6. Ellis SG, DeCesare NB, Pinkerton CA, et al. Relation of stenosis morphology and clinical presentation to the procedural results of directional coronary atherectomy. *Circulation.* 1991;84:644–653.

7. Fishman RF, Kuntz RE,Carrozza JP, et al. Long-term results of directional coronary atherectomy: predictors of restenosis. *J Am Coll Cardiol.* 1992;20:1101–1110.

8. Cowley MJ, DiSciascio G. Experience with directional coronary atherectomy since pre-market approval. *Am J Cardiol.* 1993;72:12E–20E.

9. Popma JJ, Mintz GS, Satler LF, et al. Clinical and angiographic outcome after directional coronary atherectomy. *Am J Cardiol.* 1993;72: 55E–64E.

10. Hinohara T, Robertson GC, Selmon MR, et al. Directional coronary atherectomy complications and management. *Cathet Cardiovasc Diagn.* 1993;(suppl 1):61–71.

11. Hinohara TR, Robertson GC, Selmon MR, et al. Restenosis after directional coronary atherectomy. *J Am Coll Cardiol.* 1992;20:623–632.

12. Kuntz RE, Safian RD, Levine MJ, et al. Novel approach to the analysis of restenosis after the use of three new coronary devices. *J Am Coll Cardiol.* 1992;19:1493–1499.

13. Garrett KN, Holmes DR Jr, Bell MR, et al. Results of directional atherectomy of primary atheromatous and restenosis lesions in coronary arteries and saphenous vein grafts. *Am J Cardiol.* 1992;70:449–454.

14. Cowley MJ, Whitlow PL, Baim DS, et al. Directional coronary atherectomy of saphenous vein graft narrowings: multicenter investigational experience. *Am J Cardiol.* 1993;72:30E–34E.

15. Pomerantz RM, Kuntz RE, Carrozza JP, et al. Acute and long-term outcome of narrowed saphenous venous grafts treated by endoluminal stenting and directional atherectomy. *Am J Cardiol.* 1992;70:161–167.

16. DiSciascio G, Cowley MJ, Vetrovec GW, et al. Directional coronary atherectomy of saphenous vein graft lesions unfavorable for balloon angioplasty: results of a single center experience. *Cathet Cardiovasc Diagn.* 1992;26:75. Abstract.

17. Cowley MJ, DiSciascio G. Directional coronary atherectomy for saphenous vein graft disease. *Cathet Cardiovasc Diagn.* 1993;(suppl 1):10–16.

18. Sabri MN, Johnson D, Warner M, Cowley MJ. Intracoronary thrombolysis followed by directional atherectomy: a combined approach for thrombotic vein graft lesions considered unsuitable for angioplasty. *Cathet Cardiovasc Diagn.* 1992;26:15–18.

19. Topol EJ, Ellis SG, Fishman J, et al. Multicenter study of percutaneous transluminal angioplasty for right coronary ostial stenosis. *J Am Coll Cardiol.* 1987;9:1214–1218.

20. Popma JJ, Dick RJL, Haudenschild CC, et al. Atherectomy of right coronary ostial stenoses: initial and long-term results, technical features and histologic findings. *Am J Cardiol.* 1991;67:431–433.

21. Sabri MN, Vetrovec GW, Cowley MJ, et al. Immediate results of non-

balloon devices (directional atherectomy and excimer laser angio-plasty) in aorto-ostial coronary and vein graft lesions. *J Am Coll Cardiol.* 1992;19:263A. Abstract.

22. Kerwin PM, McKeever LS, Marek JC, et al. Directional atherectomy of aorto-ostial stenoses. *Cathet Cardiovasc Diagn.* 1993;(suppl 1):17–25.
23. Whitlow PL, Robertson GC, Rowe MH, et al. Directional coronary atherectomy for failed percutaneous transluminal coronary angio-plasty. *Circulation.* 1990;82(suppl IV):IV-1. Abstract.
24. Hoeffling B, Gonschior P, Simpson L, et al. Efficacy of directional coronary atherectomy in cases unsuitable for percutaneous transluminal coronary angioplasty (PTCA) and after unsuccessful PTCA. *Am Heart J.* 1992;124:341–348.
25. McCluskey ER, Cowley MJ, Whitlow PL: Multicenter clinical experience with rescue atherectomy for failed angioplasty. *Am J Cardiol.* 1993;42E–46E.
26. McKeever LS, Marek JC, Kerwin PM, et al. Bail-out directional atherectomy for abrupt coronary artery occlusion following conventional angioplasty. *Cathet Cardiovasc Diagn.* 1993;(suppl 1):31–36.
27. Vetter JW, Robertson GC, Selmon MR, et al. Use of directional coronary atherectomy for failed PTCA. *Circulation.* 1992;86(suppl I):I-249.
28. Hermann HC, Buchbinder M, Clemen MW, et al. Emergent use of balloon-expandable coronary artery stenting for failed percutaneous transluminal coronary angioplasty. *Circulation.* 1992;86:812–819.
29. Mansour M, Fishman RF, Kuntz RE, et al. Feasibility of directional atherectomy for the treatment of bifurcation lesions. *Coronary Artery Dis.* 1992;3:761–765.
30. Leya FS, Lewis BE, Sumida CW, et al. Modified "kissing" atherectomy procedure with dependable protection of side branches by two-wire technique. *Cath Cardiovasc Diagn.* 1992;27:155–161.$er 31. Topol EJ, Leya F, Pinkerton CA, et al. A comparison of directional atherectomy with coronary angioplasty in patients with coronary artery disease. *N Engl J Med.* 1993;329:221–227.
32. Adelman AG, Cohen EA, Kimball BP, et al. A comparison of directional atherectomy with balloon angioplasty for lesions of the left anterior descending coronary artery. *N Engl J Med* 1993;329:228–233.
33. Kuntz RE, Gibson CM, Nobuyoshi M, Baim DS. A generalized model of restenosis following balloon angioplasty, stenting, and directional atherectomy. *J Am Coll Cardiol.* 1993;21:15–25.

Chapter 12

The Use of Stents in the Treatment of Coronary Artery Disease

Kumar Sridhar, MD and Sheldon Goldberg, MD

The evolution of coronary angioplasty over the last decade has been associated with increasing applications of the technique, including more complex clinical and anatomical scenarios. Gruentzig's initial indications for percutaneous transluminal coronary angioplasty (PTCA) limited its application to single-vessel disease in patients with discrete, concentric lesions, and preserved left ventricular function.[1] With additional operator experience and technological advances, PTCA is now used increasingly for more complex eccentric lesions, often in multiple vessels, or in patients with reduced left ventricular function. Despite these advances, several critical limitations to standard balloon angioplasty are evident. Abrupt vessel closure, restenosis after initially successful procedures, and poor short- and long-term results in saphenous vein bypass grafts remain as problems. Coronary stents were introduced in order to deal with the drawbacks of standard balloon angioplasty. This chapter provides an overview of their role and application in interventional cardiology.

Description of Various Stent Designs

A variety of stent designs have been used in both pre-clinical and clinical study. Several stent types and their features are listed in Table 1. Ideally, metal stents should have a low profile and be flexible in the longitudinal axis, but radially noncompliant. Metal stents should resist corrosion, but also limit thrombogenicity. The overall surface area of the device should be minimized. The device should also be radiopaque to facilitate placement without obscur-

From Vetrovec GW, Carabello BA, (eds.) *Invasive Cardiology: Current Diagnostic and Therapeutic Issues*. Armonk, NY: Futura Publishing Company, Inc.: © 1996.

TABLE 1

Stent	Manufacturer	Expansion	Design	Opacification	Intended Indication
Wallstent	Medivent	Self	Woven-mesh 16 wire filaments 0.08-mm width covering sheath	Fair	Acute or threatened closure restenosis
Gianturco-Roubin	Cook	Balloon	Continuous 0.15cm single strand stainless steel interdigitating loops "clam-shell"	Poor	Acute or threatened closure*
Palmaz-Schatz	Johnson & Johnson	Balloon	2×7 mm rigid tube central 1-mm bridge 0.8-mm thick stainless steel sheath delivery system	Fair	De novo lesions** Suboptimal PTCA** SVG**
Wiktor	Medtronic	Balloon	U-shaped tantalum 127-μm thick	Good	De novo lesions suboptimal PTCA
Cordis	Cordis	Balloon	Single strand sinusoidal helically wrapped tantalum wire 0.005" diameter 7F0.072" can accommodate	Good	De novo lesions suboptimal PTCA
Strecker	Boston Scientific	Balloon	Single filament tantalum 0.07-mm diameter flexible mesh	Good	Suboptimal PTCA de novo lesions

*FDA approved
**potential approval

ing the underlying lesion.[2] The stents most commonly used to date have been the balloon expandable Gianturco-Roubin and Palmaz-Schatz stents, and the self-expanding Wallstent.

The Gianturco-Roubin stent is a balloon expandable device that has been used to treat threatened and abrupt vessel closure (Figure 1). This device has undergone extensive clinical trials for the "bailout" setting, which will be discussed.

The Palmaz-Schatz stent (Figure 2) has a rigid slotted tube design and has been studied in the context of the suboptimal angioplasty result and has been tested in randomized clinical trials, which have addressed restenosis efficacy.

The initially encouraging clinical results reported for the Wallstent[3] were tempered by a report that showed unacceptable rates of delayed stent thrombosis.[4] In that latter study of 105 consecutive patients, thrombosis occurred in 24%, usually within 2 weeks after stent implantation. This resulted in an acute myocardial infarction rate of 14% and a 7.6% mortality rate, but restenosis occurred in only 14%. These early complications made the self-expanding stent fall out of favor. However, the problem of stent thrombosis that occurred with this device may have been related to a variety of factors including variability of operator experience and inconsistent and possibly inadequate anticoagulation regimens.

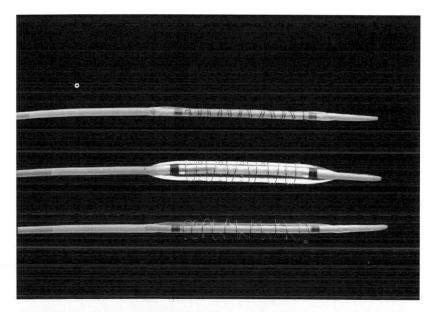

FIGURE 1. *The Gianturco-Roubin Stent.* **Top:** *Mounted, preexpansion.* **Middle:** *Balloon expanded.* **Bottom:** *Postexpansion.*

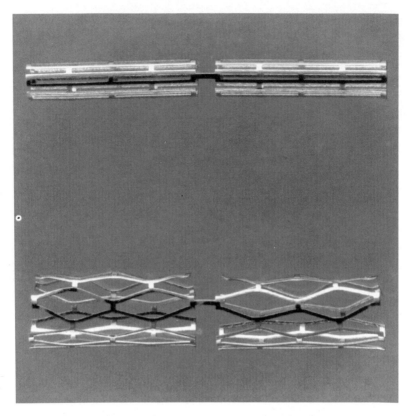

FIGURE 2. *The Palmaz-Schatz stent.* **Top:** *Preexpansion.* **Bottom:** *Expanded.*

Stent Thrombosis and Adjunctive Pharmalogic Regimen

Delayed thrombosis (Figure 3, panels A–E) is the most serious complication of stent placement.[4–8] It occurs an average of 5–6 days after implantation and accounts for the majority of major cardiac complications including death, myocardial infarction, and emergency repeat revascularization (PTCA and cardiopulmonary bypass graft surgery [CABG]). Various angiographic features including small vessel and stent size (<3 mm), the presence of thrombus before and after stent implantation and the persistence of a dissection after stent placement are predictors of thrombosis.[8] Important clinical predictors are recent acute myocardial infarction, presence of unstable angina with significant clot burden and excessively ele-

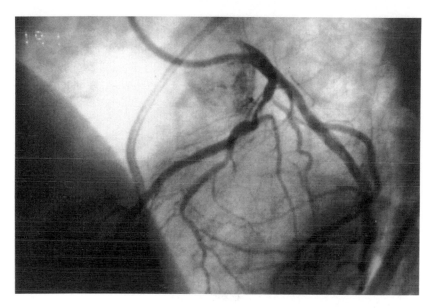

FIGURE 3A. *A 33-year-old male after recent myocardial infarction. Left anterior oblique (LAO) view of left anterior descending (LAD) lesion preintervention.*

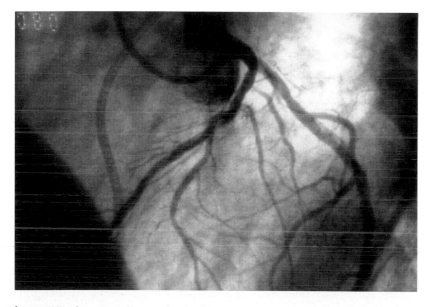

Figure 3B. *Same patient as in A. Postintracoronary stent placement.*

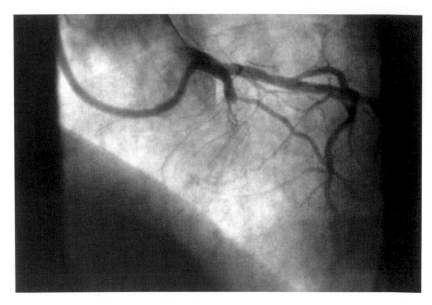

FIGURE 3C. *Same patient as in* **A.** *Delayed thrombosis 2 days after stent placement procedure.*

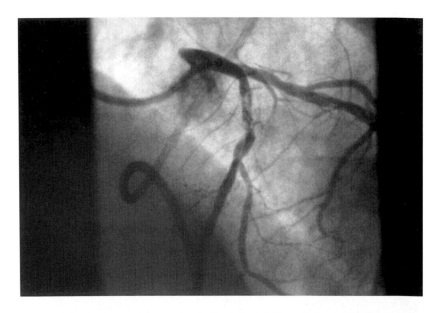

FIGURE 3D. *Same patient as in* **A.** *Residual filling defects after recrossing occlusion.*

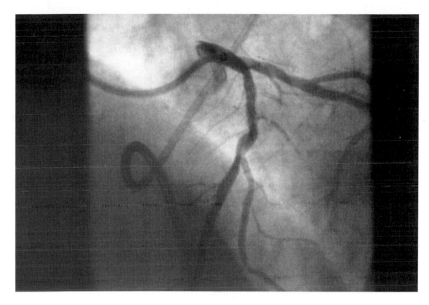

FIGURE 3E. *Same patient as in* **A.** *Final angiogram after intracoronary thrombolysis and multiple balloon inflations. This case illustrates the hazard of stent placement in the peri-infarction period.*

vated platelet counts. In addition, the use of the stent in the bailout setting, ie, for acute or threatened closure, is associated with a markedly increased risk of subsequent thrombosis.[5–7]

In order to decrease the incidence of stent thrombosis, a vigorous and demanding anticoagulation regimen has been used.[8] This consists of pretreatment with aspirin, dipyridamole, and dextran and the institution of warfarin immediately before or just after stent placement. Heparin is given intraprocedurally to achieve an activated clotting time (ACT) >300 seconds. After the procedure, heparin is discontinued and the vascular sheaths are removed on the same day, after the ACT has decreased to <150 seconds. With the dextran infusion still maintained, heparin is reinstituted approximately 6 hours after sheath removal. When the partial thromboplastin time (PTT) is in the desired range, dextran is discontinued. Warfarin and heparin are administered together until the international normalized ration (INR) is 2–3 times control; after this is achieved, heparin is discontinued and warfarin, aspirin, and dipyridamole are given together for 1 month. After 1 month, aspirin is continued indefinitely.

Use of a vigorous anticoagulation regimen has been associated with a reduction in the rate of stent thrombosis.[8] However, the use of such a regimen has been associated with increased bleeding and vascular complications, prolongation of hospital length of stay and additional short term cost.[6,7] The rate of bleeding and vascular complications is roughly doubled compared with conventional balloon angioplasty (approximately 5% to 10%) as is the length of stay after implantation (approximately 3 to 6 days).[6,7] Therefore, these two important limitations of stent implantation, ie, thrombosis and increased bleeding and vascular complications need to be addressed. Strategies to reduce these complications and make the procedure more feasible and applicable are discussed in a subsequent section of this chapter.

Use of the Stent in the Setting of Threatened and Acute Closure

The occurrence of acute closure after routine balloon angioplasty results in a marked increase in major cardiac complications.[9] Acute closure can be expected in 2% to 10% of angioplasty attempts[9] and increases in frequency with increasing lesion complexity[10] and intraprocedural occurrence of a major coronary artery dissection.[11] When vessel closure occurs it is associated with a fivefold increase in mortality rate (1% to 5%) and a 13-fold increase in the rate of myocardial infarction (2% to 27%) in patients undergoing repeat PTCA. When patients undergo emergency CABG for vessel closure, more than 50% sustain an acute myocardial infarction.[9] Various strategies to restore luminal patency including redilation and use of perfusion balloon catheters have been attempted without stable, satisfactory results.[12,13] Accordingly, the metallic intracoronary stents have been studied in an attempt to deal with this dangerous clinical scenario (Figure 4, panels A–C).

A recent study reported on the use of the Gianturco-Roubin stent in 116 consecutive patients whose angioplasty was complicated by threatened or acute closure.[7] These patients had significant balloon-induced dissections that were associated with lumen compromise and/or a decrease in perfusion that did not respond to repeated balloon inflations. The coronary stent was successfully placed in 103 patients (89%). The placement of stents resulted in resolution of angina and electrocardiographic changes in 84% of patients. Nine patients developed stent thrombosis (8.6%) during the initial hospitalization, with six having repeat PTCA. While urgent CABG was performed in 29 patients, 9 of these patients had CABG mandated by protocol requirement, and 9 additional patients with good angiographic and clinical results after stent place-

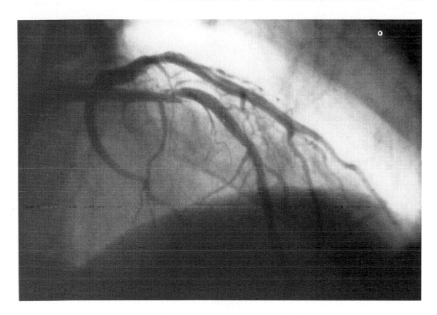

FIGURE 4. *A 65-year-old male post-PTCA to high-grade LAD lesion. **A:** Right anterior oblique (RAO) projection of LAD lesion with residual stenosis and intraluminal flap.*

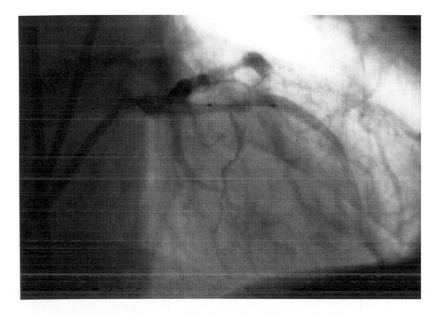

FIGURE 4. ***B:** RAO projection of stent placement with markers spanning lesion.*

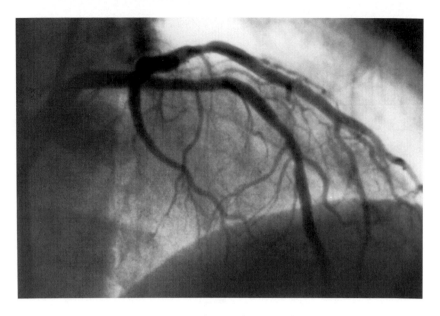

FIGURE 4. C: *Final angiogram of LAD lesion after Palmaz-Schatz stent placement.*

ment underwent CABG because of the large amount of myo-cardium supplied by the stented artery. Long-term clinical follow-up (mean 14 months) showed a 3% incidence of death and 2% rate of late myocardial infarction. Sixteen percent of patients had re-peat PTCA and 15% late CABG. Angiographic restenosis occurred in 53% of patients eligible for follow-up study. Overall, event-free survival (death, CABG, Q wave myocardial infarction and PTCA) was 39%. In a similar population, a matched case control study was performed in 61 patients treated with the Gianturco-Roubin stent for threatened (28 patients) or abrupt closure (33 patients) and compared to 61 patients treated with conventional methods in an 18-month period prior to stent availability.[13] The placement of stents was associated with superior immediate results such as residual diameter stenosis (26% versus 49%, $P<0.001$), an increased chance of restoration of TIMI-3 flow (97% versus 72%, $P<0.001$), and a reduced need for emergency bypass surgery (4.9% versus 18%, $P=0.02$). Despite these findings, there was no difference in the overall rate of Q wave myocardial infarction (32% and 20%); importantly, the rate of Q wave myocardial infarction in patients treated early after vessel closure (<45 minutes) was only 3.9%. Fur-thermore, in-hospital mortality was identical in both groups

(3.3%). Long-term follow-up at a mean of 6.3 months showed that freedom from late death, myocardial infarction, coronary artery bypass or PTCA was not different between the two groups (75% versus 81%, P=NS).

A large multicenter study was recently reported using the Gianturco-Roubin stent in acute or threatened closure involving 518 patients.[6] The majority of patients (69%) had threatened closure. The stent was successfully deployed in 95% of patients with angiographic improvement in stenosis severity from 63% to 15% after stent deployment. The in-hospital incidence of death (2.2%), myocardial infarction (5.5%), and CABG (4.3%) was very low for this population. However, the incidence of subacute thrombosis (8.7%) and the requirement of blood transfusions (17%) remain cause for concern. Late complications during the 6-month follow-up period included death in 7 patients (1.4%) and CABG in 34 patients (6.9%).

In a separate study, 56 patients who underwent emergency unplanned stenting with the Palmaz-Schatz device, were evaluated.[5] The population consisted of a group of 23 patients who had a suboptimal PTCA result, another group of 15 patients who had evidence of impending closure, and a third group with frank acute occlusion (18 patients). The short-term and 30-day results of coronary stent implantation were described with respect to major cardiac complications including death, myocardial infarction, and the requirement for CABG surgery. While successful stent implantation was achieved in 98% of the patients, the success rate fell to only 71% at 1 month, due primarily to stent thrombosis and associated complications. Major cardiac events occurred in 29% of 56 patients within the 30-day period. Long-term follow-up showed that angiographic restenosis occurred in 23% of 35 eligible patients. Overall long-term success, excluding patients who died, had CABG, myocardial infarction, or restenosis was 57%.

When taken together, these studies show that stent placement is effective in solving the immediate problem of threatened or acute closure in the majority of patients; however, subacute thrombosis continues to be a significant problem in the bailout setting; this results in reclosure, reinfarction, death or the need for repeat intervention.

Stents for Restenosis

Two recently completed randomized studies compared the efficacy of elective stent implantation with balloon angioplasty. In the Stent Restenosis Study (STRESS Trial), 407 patients with discrete (<15 mm) de novo lesions in relatively large (>3 mm) epicardial coronary arteries were randomly assigned to either elective stent placement or elective angioplasty with availability of the stent for failed angioplasty procedures.[14] The primary end point of the trial was angiographic restenosis, defined as ≥50% residual stenosis at 6-month angiographic restudy. Ischemia-driven target lesion revascularization and clinical event rates were secondary end points of the trial. Patients in both groups had identical baseline stenosis severity (75%) and similar minimal lumen diameters (0.78 versus 0.76 mm). There was significantly greater acute gain in patients assigned to stent placement (1.72 versus 1.23 mm, $P<0.001$). This resulted in a greater postprocedure lumen diameter (2.49 versus 1.99, $P<0.001$) and less residual diameter stenosis (19% versus 35%, $P<0.001$). The greater initial gain was due to the scaffolding effect of the device as stent placement was associated with less intimal disruption and reduced elastic recoil. At 6-month follow-up, there was greater late loss in the stented lesions (0.74 versus 0.38 mm $P<0.001$), but the cumulative frequency curve showed a persistent difference at 6-month follow-up (Figure 5). The final minimal lumen diameter was significantly greater in the stent group (1.74 versus 1.56 mm, $P=0.007$). This translated into a reduction in angiographic restenosis from 42% in the PTCA group to 31% in the

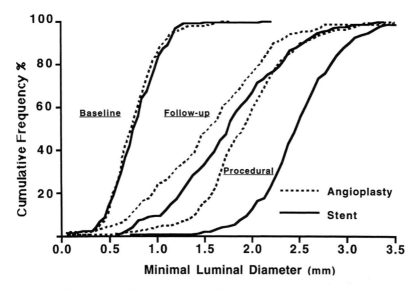

FIGURE 5. *Cumulative frequency distribution as a function of minimal lumen diameter. (Copyright* New England Journal of Medicine. *331:499, 1994. Reprinted with permission.)*

stent group by intention-to-treat analysis. Therefore, patients randomly assigned to stent implantation had a relative reduction in restenosis frequency of 25%.

Subacute closure occurred in 3.4% of patients assigned to stent placement and 1.4% of patients assigned to angioplasty (P=NS). Delayed closures occurred 5±3 days after implantation and were due to stent thrombosis in 7 patients in the stent group and 3 patients in the PTCA group who received bailout stenting for failed angioplasty. Bleeding and vascular complications were higher in stented patients (7.3% versus 4.9%, P=0.14) as was the length of stay after the procedure (5.8 versus 2.8 days, P<0.001).

A composite clinical end point analysis that included death, myocardial infarction, and the need for repeat revascularization showed no difference at 6 months between the stent and angioplasty groups. However, the need for ischemia-driven target lesion revascularization was less in patients assigned to stent implantation (Figure 6).

In the Belgium and Netherlands Stent Trial (BENESTENT), 520 patients were similarly randomized to either stent implantation or angioplasty.[15] Angiographic restenosis was reduced in the patients treated with stent as compared with the PTCA arm (22% versus 32%, P<0.002), a relative reduction of 33%. Late event-free survival was also greater in the stent group (79% versus 67%, rela-

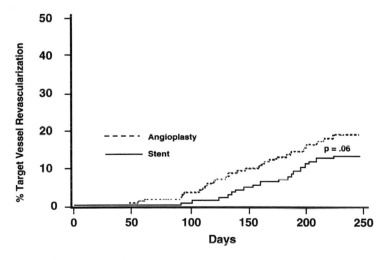

FIGURE 6. *Target vessel revascularization percentage as a function of days postprocedure. A trend toward reduced requirement for vessel revascularization was seen in the stent arm. (Copyright New England Journal of Medicine. 331:500, 1994. Reprinted with permission.)*

tive risk 0.63, 0.47–0.84) and target lesion revascularization was reduced by 40% in the stent group. Again, bleeding and vascular complications occurred more frequently in the stent group (14.6% versus 2.4%, *P*<0.0001).

The combined results of these trials indicate that stent implantation reduced angiographic restenosis and late repeat intervention, but at the cost of increased bleeding complications and prolonged initial hospitalization.

Stent for Saphenous Vein Bypass Graft Stenosis

Previous reports have indicated high restenosis and event rates in patients who undergo angioplasty of saphenous vein graft lesions.[16,17] A recent study assessed the long-term clinical and angiographic outcome of patients electively treated with Palmaz-Schatz stents in saphenous vein graft stenoses.[18] One hundred and ninety-eight patients had single stent placement in 209 saphenous vein bypass graft lesions. Coronary angiography was performed at baseline after stent implantation and 6 months later. Restenosis, defined as ≥50% diameter narrowing, was assessed at the 6-month follow-up period. In addition, clinical end points were analyzed for 1 year in all patients. These end points included death, nonfatal infarction, and the need for repeat intervention. Stent implantation was successful in 99% of patients with only one case of stent thrombosis. Restenosis occurred in 33% of restudied lesions. Importantly, de novo lesions had a lower restenosis rate as compared to lesions that had prior angioplasty (21% versus 47%, *P*<0.001). The overall mortality rate at 1 year was 9%, with myocardial infarction developing in 6% of patients. Coronary bypass surgery was used in 11% and repeat PTCA in 12% of patients. Repeat target lesion revascularization was more common in patients who had undergone prior angioplasty of the stented lesion compared with the de novo lesion group (35% versus 10%, *P*<0.001). The 1-year event-free survival was 70% for the entire group. However, 82% of the patients with de novo lesions remained event-free at 1 year compared to only 55% of patients who had prior angioplasty procedures (*P*<0.001). Conclusions from this initial nonrandomized study suggested that use of the Palmaz-Schatz stent for the treatment of saphenous vein graft lesions was associated with high primary success and a low rate of subacute thrombosis. The incidence of angiographic restenosis and clinical event rates in the de novo group was encouraging and compares favorably with other published data.[19] Future randomized trials to address the usefulness of stents in patient populations with previous bypass surgery are underway.

Future Trends in Coronary Stent Implantation

As has been discussed, coronary stents have shown encouraging results in treating the major limitations of standard balloon angioplasty, ie, acute closure, restenosis, and saphenous vein graft stenoses. However, as with most new technologies, drawbacks have become evident. In the case of coronary stents, these problems include subacute thrombosis and peripheral vascular complications.

Subacute thrombosis remains the most serious limitation to coronary stent placement, especially in the failed angioplasty or bailout setting. The use of a more intense anticoagulation protocol has lowered the incidence of delayed thrombosis, but with more bleeding complications. Improvements in the pharmacologic prevention of thrombosis, including better antithrombotic and antiplatelet agents, as well as direct delivery of such agents through "coated" stents, may prove advantageous. Furthermore, improved deployment techniques using intracoronary ultrasound may allow for improved assessment of stent-vessel contact and strut expansion, thereby decreasing the potential for thrombus formation at the lesion site.[20] Preliminary work has shown that when the Palmaz-Schatz stent struts are fully expanded, the incidence of stent thrombosis decreases, even when anticoagulation with warfarin is omitted.

Vascular access site complications also pose a major impediment to stent placement. Recent studies employing pneumatic vascular compression devices or collagenous vascular sealents have shown promise in reducing its incidence.[21]

Restenotic lesions are poorly served by standard balloon angioplasty. Randomized trials to assess the efficacy of coronary stents in this subset of patients are ongoing. In de novo lesions, the greater late loss observed in the stent arm of randomized trials suggests that smooth muscle cell proliferation is greater in stent patients. Therefore, future studies utilizing locally delivered antiproliferative compounds may reduce restenosis further.

Stent placement is a relatively new technique for myocardial revascularization that provides an optimal angiographic result and a large smooth lumen. The device effectively seals intimal flaps and decreases elastic recoil, thereby acting as an intravascular scaffold. These effects make it a useful tool for treating dissections post balloon angioplasty. Furthermore, the large initial lumen is associated with a reduction in angiographic restenosis at 6-month follow-up. The major limitations of coronary stent placement are being addressed in ongoing clinical trials. If these limitations can be overcome, then the use of stents may become the preferred therapy in selected patients with coronary artery disease.

References

1. Gruentzig AR, Senning A, Siegenthaler WE. Nonoperative dilatation of coronary artery stenoses. *N Engl J Med.* 1979;301:61–68.
2. Wong SC, Schatz RA. Developmental background and design. In: Herrmann HC, Hirshfeld JS, eds. *Clinical Use of the Palmaz-Schatz Intracoronary Stent.* Mount Kisco, NY: Futura Publishing Company; 1993.
3. Sigwart U, Puel J, Mirkovitch VS, et al. Intravascular stents to prevent occlusion and restenosis after transluminal angioplasty. *N Engl J Med.* 1987;316:701–706.
4. Serruys PW, Strauss BH, Beatt KJ, et al. Angiographic follow-up after placement of a self expanding coronary artery stent. *N Engl J Med.* 1991;324:13–17.
5. Hermann HC, Buchbinder M, Clemen MW, et al. Emergent use of balloon-expandable coronary artery stenting for failed percutaneous transluminal coronary angioplasty. *Circulation.* 1992;86:812–819.
6. George BS, Voorhees WD, Roubin GS, et al. Multicenter investigation of coronary artery stenting to treat acute or threatened closure after percutaneous transluminal coronary angioplasty: clinical and angiographic outcomes. *J Am Coll Cardiol.* 1993;22:135–143.
7. Hearn JA, King SB, Douglas JS, et al. Clinical and angiographic outcomes after coronary stenting for acute or threatened closure after percutaneous transluminal coronary angioplasty: initial results with a balloon-expandable, stainless steel design. *Circulation.* 1993;88:2086–2096.
8. Schatz RA, Baim DS, Leon MB, et al. Clinical experience with the Palmaz-Schatz coronary stent. Initial results of a multicenter study. *Circulation.* 1991;83:148–161.
9. Detre KM, Holmes DR, Holubkov R, et al. Incidence and consequences of periprocedural occlusion. The 1985–86 National Heart, Lung and Blood Institute percutaneous transluminal coronary angioplasty registry. *Circulation.* 1990;82:739–750.
10. Ellis SG, Roubin GS, King SB, et al. Angiographic and clinical predictors of acute closure after native vessel coronary angioplasty. *Circulation.* 1988;77:372–379.
11. Bredlau CE, Roubin GS, King SB, et al. In hospital morbidity and mortality in patients undergoing elective coronary angioplasty. *Circulation.* 1985;72:1044–1052.
12. Foley JB, Sridhar K, Dawdy J, et al. Pros and cons of perfusion balloons in failed angioplasty. *Cathet Cardiovasc Diagn.* 1994;31:264–269.
13. Lincoff AM, Topol EJ, Chapekis AT, et al. Intracoronary stenting compared with conventional therapy for abrupt vessel closure complicating coronary angioplasty: a matched case-control study. *J Am Coll Cardiol.* 1993;21:866–875.

14. Fischman DL, Leon MP, Baim D, et al. A randomized comparison of coronary stent placement and balloon angioplasty in the treatment of coronary artery disease. *N Engl J Med.* 1994;331:496–501.
15. Serruys PW, de Jaegen P, Kiemeniej F, et al. A comparison of balloon expandable stent implantation with balloon angioplasty in patients with coronary artery disease. *N Engl J Med.* 1994;331:489–495.
16. Reeves F, Bonan R, Cote G, et al. Long-term angiographic follow-up after angioplasty of venous coronary bypass grafts. *Am Heart J.* 1991; 122:620–627.
17. Cote G, Myler R, Stertzer S, et al. Percutaneous transluminal angioplasty of stenotic coronary bypass grafts: 5 years' experience. *J Am Coll Cardiol.* 1987;9:8–17.
18. Fenton SH, Fischman DL, Savage MP, et al. Long-term clinical and angiographic outcome after implantation of balloon-expandable stents in saphenous vein grafts. *Am J Cardiol.* 1994,74.1187–1191.
19. Carozza J, Kuntz R, Levine MJ, et al. Angiographic and clinical outcome of intracoronary stenting: immediate and long term results for a large single center experience. *J Am Coll Cardiol.* 1992;20:328–337.
20. Nakamura S, Columbo A, Gaglione A, et al. Intracoronary ultrasound observations during stent implantation. *Circulation.* 1994;89:2026–2034.
21. Sridhar K, Porter D, Gupta B, et al. Peripheral vascular complications after coronary stenting: incidence and management. *Cathet Cardiovasc Diagn.* 1994;32:98. Abstract.

Chapter 13

Thermal Angioplasty

Ezra Deutsch, MD

There are a number of problems that impact on the initial success and also limit the long-term effectiveness of percutaneous transluminal coronary angioplasty (PTCA). The remodeling of coronary artery stenoses by PTCA in humans is achieved by the application of radial compressive forces to the atherosclerotic arterial wall. There is mechanical compression of atheroma and concurrent splitting or fracture of noncompliant, calcified aspects of obstructive plaque. The more compliant components of the arterial wall are stretched.[1] There is exposure of subendothelial surfaces and thrombus formation at the dilatation site that may evolve to threatened or even acute closure of the dilated vessel. Histologic analysis of atherosclerotic arteries immediately after balloon dilatation in animal and necropsy specimens reveals endothelial denudation, linear and spiral tears in the intimal surface that often extend into the media, and subintimal hemorrhage and thrombus formation at the angioplasty site.[2,3] Dissection is observed angiographically in up to 30% of cases.[4] The presence of intimal flaps and thrombus formation postangioplasty in humans has been confirmed by angioscopy.[5]

Restenosis after successful PTCA occurs with an observed incidence ranging from 30% to 50%,[6] and is the primary limitation of the procedure. Certain angiographic, morphologic predictors of restenosis after PTCA have been described, and imply that the cost of arterial remodeling in eccentric, severe stenoses (minimum luminal diameter [MLD] < 0.5 mm) is reflected in an increased incidence of restenosis.[7,8] Thus, the localized barotrauma that occurs during arterial recanalization in balloon angioplasty causes the conditions that predispose to these short- and long-term complications.

Many of the short- and long-term reparative processes that oc-

From Vetrovec GW, Carabello BA, (eds.) *Invasive Cardiology: Current Diagnostic and Therapeutic Issues.* Armonk, NY: Futura Publishing Company, Inc.: © 1996.

cur in response to angioplasty-induced barotrauma are likely to contribute to the restenosis process. Endothelial denudation results in the loss of endothelial antithrombotic function,[9] including diminished synthesis of platelet binding inhibitors and an impaired ability for endogenous thrombolysis due to reduced plasmin generation. The depth of arterial injury caused by experimental angioplasty has been directly correlated to the magnitude of local platelet adherence.[9] Platelet adhesion to exposed subendothelial matrix proteins including collagen, elastin, and medial smooth muscle is followed by degranulation and aggregation, the recruitment of additional platelets, and thrombus formation. Sufficient thrombus burden at the site of angioplasty may result in acute closure of the vessel.[10]

After angioplasty there is also loss of endothelial vasodilator effectors such as endothelium-dependent relaxing factor. Endothelial denudation may promote production of endothelin, which is a powerful vasoconstrictor.[9] Platelet degranulation results in the release of potent vasoconstrictors such as thromboxane A2 and serotonin.[11] The balance of vasoconstrictor and vasodilator forces are unfavorably shifted toward vasoconstriction after angioplasty. This phenomenon may predispose to turbulent flow, a propensity to increased thrombus formation at the angioplasty site, and thus, a greater likelihood of acute thrombotic closure and subsequent restenosis. Tissue factor released from injured cells activates the contact system of thrombosis, resulting in thrombin generation and thrombus formation.[12]

Platelet-derived growth factor and transforming growth factor-b are also released at the angioplasty site by aggregating platelets, are chemotactic for the local recruitment of inflammatory cells, and serve as mitogenic stimuli for subsequent medial smooth muscle cell proliferation.[13] Thrombin also stimulates smooth muscle cell proliferation in a receptor-mediated fashion.[14] Direct injury to medial smooth muscle may also provoke a fibroproliferative response.[15] Histologic examination of angioplasty sites in experimental models and in human necropsy studies consistently reveal intimal hyperplasia or thickening, irrespective of whether there is angiographic evidence of restenosis.[16,17] The extent to which neointimal hyperplasia occurs may thus be dependent on the degree of arterial damage that occurs as a result of the remodeling process during PTCA. Restenosis lesions are typically concentric, suggesting that the process of renarrowing due to neointimal hyperplasia involves the entire dilated segment in a circumferential fashion.[8]

Rationale of Thermal Angioplasty

The concept of applying thermal energy during angioplasty evolved from observations that the principal complications of PTCA—acute closure, whether due to significant dissection and/or thrombus formation, and restenosis, the result of neointimal hyperplasia—could be effectively treated by the simultaneous application of heat (at 85°C to 120°C) and pressure during angioplasty.[18] The geometry of the disrupted tissue planes at the luminal surface post-PTCA produces zones of separated flow that serve as substrate for ongoing platelet aggregation and microthrombus formation.[18] Welding of these dissected tissue planes should provide a smooth, nonthrombogenic lumen with restoration of laminar flow. Elastic recoil following balloon dilatation has been described.[18,19] Thus, the residual lumen post-PTCA is typically less than the desired end point, in part related to the viscoelastic properties of the arterial wall. Thermal angioplasty abolishes elastic recoil after PTCA,[20] likely the result of straightening of elastic fibers[21–23] and medial smooth muscle cell damage.[21] Inhibition of smooth muscle cell proliferation by direct damage to the cells during the initial thermal angioplasty might also impede the restenosis process. Current research in thermal angioplasty includes the concept of local drug delivery facilitated by heating.[24] A description of the different thermal angioplasty devices is outlined in Table 1.

Table 1

Laser balloon angioplasty (LBA)	85 to 125°C (in vitro) Nd:Yag optic fiber Thermal fusion of dissected tissue layers Dessication of thrombus Disruption of connective tissue at higher temperatures
Microwave angioplasty	85°C Guide wire is microwave antenna Thermal injury to media
Physiologically controlled Low-stress angioplasty (PLOSA)	60°C Radiofrequency energy source Facilitated remodeling of Plaque Minimal arterial barotrauma

Laser Balloon Angioplasty

Laser balloon angioplasty (LBA) is a thermal angioplasty technique that permits the heating of vascular tissue during angioplasty using laser energy. Conceptually, LBA was designed to address the problems of acute thrombotic closure and restenosis by achieving two primary effects on dilated tissue. Thermal energy would fuse the disrupted tissue elements and reappose the separated tissue planes, leaving a smooth, relatively nonthrombogenic surface. Dessication of thrombus would occur as well, reducing the potential for acute thrombotic complications and the release of growth factors that contribute to neointimal hyperplasia. The second effect of LBA would be the reduction of elastic recoil by a direct thermal effect on the elastic fibrils in the arterial wall. A larger lumen would be achieved, preserving laminar flow through the dilated segment.[18]

The LBA Catheter and Laser Delivery System

The LBA system consists of a modified PTCA catheter and a laser source.[22] A three-lumen catheter with a polyethylene teraphthalate balloon contains a central lumen to accommodate the guide wire, a second lumen for balloon inflation, and a third lumen that houses a 100-mm silica fiberoptic that terminates in a spiral-shaped specialized diffusing tip. The diffusing tip allows for even distribution of laser energy over the length and circumference of the balloon. Laser transmission efficiency is optimized by inflating the balloon with a 50% solution of metrizamide in deuterium oxide, rather than water.[25] The laser source is a 50-W continuous wave neodymium:yttrium-aluminium-garnet (Nd:YAG) laser that delivers laser radiation in the near infrared spectrum at 1,060 nm. In the coronary protocol, laser doses of 205 to 380 J are delivered in a stepwise decremental dose format over 25 seconds in the following fashion: 25 W for 5 seconds, 15 W for 5 seconds, and 12 W for 10 seconds (for a 3-mm diameter, 20-mm length balloon catheter). These doses achieve tissue temperatures of 90°C to 110°C in vitro.[25] In humans, an additional 30–40 seconds of balloon inflation is required as the balloon temperature cools to body temperature.

Experimental Studies

Thermal welding of separated tissue planes by LBA was initially evaluated in segments of cadaveric human atherosclerotic aortae.[26] A thermal sealing effect of separated medial and adventitial layers could be achieved, and there was a linear correlation between the thermal weld strength and the peak adventitial temperature achieved using laser energy input. Welding did not occur at tissue temperatures below 80°C, but was reliably achieved at temperatures above 95°C. There was a direct correlation between the peak tissue temperature achieved and the depth of thermal penetration into the arterial wall. Temperatures over 120°C penetrated 2 mm into the arterial wall, whereas the depth of penetration when temperatures <100°C were applied averaged 1 mm.[26] Tissue temperatures above 140°C produced charring and tissue perforation. The duration of laser exposure required to weld tissue ranged between 10–20 seconds. Simultaneous tissue pressure up to 2 atm was an additional requirement to achieve tissue welding. No additional benefit was derived from pressures above this value.

The effects of LBA on elastic recoil have been studied in a rabbit iliac artery and canine coronary angioplasty models.[22,23] The acute response to overstretching of a 2.1-mm rabbit iliac artery to 2.8 mm by balloon angioplasty was recoil of the vessel to 2.2 mm. However, arteries treated with LBA using a 2.8-mm LBA catheter maintained lumenal diameters of 2.4–2.6 mm. This increase in arterial diameter was maintained at 1 month in those animals treated with laser energy doses that achieve temperatures of 80°C–100°C in vitro. In contrast, with higher doses of laser energy, these acute gains were not maintained long term, paralleled by histologic evidence of medial fibrosis and adventitial injury. LBA performed in the left circumflex coronary artery of normal dogs produced acute gains in luminal diameter that exceeded those observed in control arteries subjected to balloon angioplasty. Although those arteries treated with balloon angioplasty demonstrated significant vasoconstriction in response to intracoronary ergonovine, there was no evidence of vasoconstriction in the LBA-treated segments. A typical constrictive response was observed in the untreated areas adjacent to the LBA-treated segment. This vascular response persisted up to 1 month after treatment. Angiographically, the LBA-treated segments had the appearance of a "biologic stent."[23] Histologic analysis revealed straightening of elastic fibrils limited to those areas in direct contact with the LBA balloon.[23] Thus, LBA results in larger luminal diameters than those achieved with balloon angioplasty. Acute and late elastic recoil is minimized, in parallel with the finding that vasoconstriction is inhibited in the region of thermal angioplasty. These observations correlated with the histologic observation that there is straightening of elastic fibers in the treated arterial segments.

One other important experimental study demonstrated that arterial dissections and perforations could be sealed by LBA application.[27] Atherosclerotic rabbits were subjected to iliac artery angioplasty with oversized balloons, producing severe dissections and perforations. LBA was then performed, with angiographic evidence for sealing of dissections and perforations. Angiography performed at 4 months confirmed long-term patency in the majority of animals. Thus, thermal welding of dissected arterial tissue planes in an atherosclerotic model is feasible in vivo.

Human Clinical Trials

The initial phase I clinical trial was performed in 15 patients in whom LBA was applied after conventional angioplasty. In addition to demonstrating safety and efficacy, the aim of this study was to determine whether LBA could further improve luminal diameter and arterial geometry at the site of balloon dilatation. All patients had lesions treated with a 3.0-mm PTCA balloon followed by a 3.0-mm LBA application. A 20-second decremental laser dose was applied, with laser energy delivered that produced temperatures of 90°C–110°C in vitro. In this small series of patients, MLD increased from a mean of 2.17 ± 0.71 mm post-PTCA to 2.61 ± 0.26 mm after LBA ($P < 0.05$), as measured by quantitative coronary angiography. Repeat angiography performed at 24 hours and 1 month revealed no change in MLD, confirming the absence of arterial recoil after thermal angioplasty.

A multicenter registry was established to evaluate the short- and long-term effects of LBA as an adjunct to arterial remodeling in patients undergoing PTCA.[28] Fifty-five patients who underwent PTCA of a discrete coronary stenosis with an appropriately sized 3.0-mm balloon catheter were then treated with LBA. One to three 20-second doses of laser energy (250 to 420 J) were delivered in a decremental stepwise fashion. No adverse effects of LBA on the arterial lumen were observed in any patient. The initial MLD increased from 0.67 ± 0.25 mm to 1.73 ± 0.57 mm 10 minutes after PTCA. A significant increase in MLD to a mean diameter of 2.27 ± 0.33 mm was achieved after LBA, as determined by quantitative angiographic analysis. Follow-up angiography performed 24 hours and 1 month after the procedure revealed a stable MLD of 2.27 ± 0.39 mm and 2.39 ± 0.35 mm, respectively. The mean reference diameter of 3.00 ± 0.34 mm was unchanged post-PTCA and post-LBA.

The overall restenosis rate at 6-month angiographic follow-up was 51%. However, two specific variables identified patient populations with an increased probability of restenosis. Patients who had previously undergone conventional PTCA of the treated coronary segment (restenosis lesions) had a significantly higher incidence of restenosis of 67%, as compared with a 46% renarrowing in patients with de novo lesions. In addition, patients who received higher laser doses (380 to 450 J) had an increased incidence of restenosis (67% vs. 36% for doses of 250 to 320 J). In those patients with de novo lesions treated with a lower dose of laser energy, the restenosis rate was only 29%. Importantly, those patients who had an unsuccessful PTCA procedure due to angiographic evidence of a significant coronary dissection (n=8) or acute closure due to thrombus (n=3), a successful angiographic and clinical result was achieved after LBA treatment. The severity of the dissection was moderately reduced in 4 patients and significantly reduced in the other 4 patients.[28]

In a subsequent study, 10 patients were treated urgently with LBA after acute failure of PTCA due to abrupt closure or severe dissection unresponsive to prolonged inflations with a conventional or perfusion balloon catheter.[25] Again, only a 3-mm diameter, 20-mm long LBA catheter was available. Seven of 10 patients were successfully treated with this LBA device. Complete sealing of dissection was achieved in 3 patients, and stabilization of the dissection occurred in 3 additional patients. In 1 patient, dessicated thrombus was present on the LBA catheter after successful treatment. Normal (TIMI grade 3) antegrade flow and resolution of ischemic symptoms was observed in these 7 patients. Mean MLD was 2.31±0.47 mm post-LBA, corresponding to a residual stenosis of 19%±14%. One such patient is illustrated in Figure 1. Failure of LBA in the remaining 3 patients occurred due to an inability to seal the dissection due to its excessive length (60 mm in 2 patients) or a mismatch in the size of the 3.0-mm LBA catheter and the vessel lumen. Although restenosis subsequently occurred in 5 of the 7 patients successfully treated, the need for emergent coronary artery bypass graft (CABG) surgery was obviated in this high-risk cohort. Directional atherectomy was subsequently performed in 3 patients for restenosis after LBA. Histologic analysis of tissue obtained in these patients revealed intimal hyperplasia identical to that found in patients with restenosis after conventional angioplasty.

One novel application of LBA may be in the deployment of local pharmacologic therapy at the angioplasty site using LBA.[24] In this approach, the goal of LBA is to deploy a bioprotective material to reduce or eliminate the thrombogenic potential of the injured arterial surface at the site of angioplasty. Given the release of mitogenic

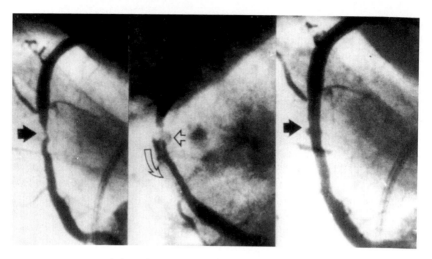

FIGURE 1. *Successful sealing of a coronary dissection by laser balloon angioplasty.* **Left panel:** *significant stenosis in the midportion of a right coronary artery (dark arrow).* **Middle panel:** *spiral dissection after PTCA, extending distal to the site of the initial lesion (open arrows).* **Right panel:** *welding of dissected tissue planes successfully performed with laser balloon angioplasty. The arterial lumen is now widely patent (dark arrow). Figure provided courtesy of Gregg Reis, MD.*

growth factors from adherent thrombus, and the potential to apply drugs that might reduce the proliferative response to PTCA, the concept of thermally-mediated local drug delivery is an attractive one. Preliminary experiments in canine carotid and superficial femoral arteries in vivo have demonstrated that albumin microspheres containing heparin can be adhered to the site of arterial angioplasty injury using LBA. Fluorescence microscopy confirmed the presence of microspheres at the angioplasty site. No evidence for thrombus formation at the angioplasty site was seen 24 hours after angioplasty injury and subsequent LBA/microsphere treatment, even in the absence of systemic anticoagulation, suggesting a local heparin effect.[24] This technique has the promise of deploying a bioprotective material to the angioplasty site, which might permit specific targeting of antithrombotic and antiproliferative drug therapies.

Microwave Balloon Angioplasty

Microwave balloon angioplasty (MBA) was developed as an alternative form of thermal angioplasty that could provide carefully regulated delivery of thermal energy using a small and relatively inexpensive microwave generator. Goals similar to laser balloon angioplasty have been described for this device.[29] The microwave system consists of a microwave generator that emits microwave energy at a frequency of 2,450 MHz, coupled to a cable 0.023 inches in diameter. The cable terminates in an antenna that is inserted into a modified conventional angioplasty balloon catheter. When the cable is fully advanced, the antenna is positioned in the middle of the balloon. Microwave energy is transmitted through the medium in the balloon to surrounding tissue. Heating of tissue occurs primarily, and not as the result of heating of balloon contents with conduction to the arterial wall in contact with the inflated balloon.[29]

Initial range-finding studies in normal rabbit iliac arteries demonstrated a direct correlation between the extent of medial injury and the peak temperature attained in a range of 50°C–100°C. When temperatures above 80°C were applied, there was late histologic evidence of a loss of cellularity in the media and replacement by fibrous elements.[29] Thus, there was the potential for selective thermal injury to the media, with the hope of a reduction in neointimal hyperplasia. Comparison of MBA at 85°C and conventional angioplasty in atherosclerotic rabbit iliac arteries revealed a significant increase in MLD in MBA-treated segments compared with conventional angioplasty. There was evidence for less thrombus at the angioplasty site in the MBA-treated vessels. A trend toward a persistent larger arterial lumen was observed at 4 weeks.[29] In an atherosclerotic rabbit model of coronary dissection, MBA was effective in sealing dissections and perforations at temperatures ranging from 70°C–100°C.[30] There is presently no clinical experience in humans for the treatment of peripheral or coronary stenoses.

PLOSA

Physiologically controlled low-stress angioplasty (PLOSA) is a technique based on the premise that the application of heat at 60°C and a minimal balloon distending pressure during angioplasty would permit arterial remodeling with less intimal disruption than is observed with conventional angioplasty. Phase change of the cholesterol ester components of atherosclerotic plaque might occur utilizing thermal energy at these temperatures in vivo. The "softened" plaque could subsequently be dilated at lower inflation pressures. Thus, in PLOSA, the angioplasty component of arterial remodeling would be achieved with "low-stress" inflation pressures. A reduction in the extent of arterial barotrauma that occurs during conventional PTCA would theoretically minimize the extent of intimal damage and dissection, paralleled by a diminished likelihood of acute thrombotic closure and subsequent neointimal hyperplasia.

The hypothesis on which PLOSA is based is the observation that the lipid component of human atheroma comprises as much as 30% to 65% of the total dry weight[31] and is thus the major constituent of the atherosclerotic plaque. The development of arterial atheroma in humans begins in early childhood. Fatty streaks are seen in the intimal surface of the arterial wall, and are the result of cellular cholesterol uptake in excess of excretion. Cholesterol is solubilized to form cholesterol esters, which coalesce to form droplets that are typically seen as foam cells. Over time, there is nucleation of cholesterol to form inert crystals, paralleled by cell necrosis and plaque formation. Atherosclerotic plaques are thus stratified. The most rigid cholesterol crystals comprise the base of the plaque, and the softer, more recently deposited cholesterol esters (cholesteryl oleate, linoleate, and palmitate) are found on the luminal aspect of the intima.[31]

The distribution of lipids in the arterial wall is divided between three major populations: phospholipid, free cholesterol, and cholesterol esters. The lipid content of normal intima is approximately 5% of cell constituents. In infancy, >70% of this lipid is in the form of phospholipid; <3% are cholesterol esters. However, a significant cholesterol ester phase is seen by age 10, and by 50 years of age, 50% of lipid in normal intima are cholesterol esters. In contrast to normal intima, atherosclerotic intima may be composed of as much as 30% to 65% lipid.[31] As the plaque develops, there is a shift from a phospholipid-rich to a cholesterol ester-rich state. This is demonstrated clinically by the age-related increase in low-density lipoprotein-like lipids.

These three classes of lipid have marked differences in their thermal properties in vitro. Both phospholipid and cholesterol monohydrate have melting points of 85°C. In contrast, cholesterol esters exhibit a complex thermal behavior. Cholesteryl oleate melts from a crystal to a liquid at 51°C. On cooling, first a cholesteric state forms at 47.5°C, followed by a stable smectic state below 42°C. Cholesteryl linoleate melts from crystal to liquid at 42°C. Cholesteryl palmitate does not melt to a liquid state until 83.5°C.[24] Furthermore, it is likely that the higher melting point cholesterols soften before melting, perhaps at temperatures under 85°C. These physiochemical properties may thus permit thermal remodeling of atherosclerotic plaque in the temperature range of 50°C to 60°C.

The PLOSA System

The PLOSA System™ (Boston Scientific Corporation, Water-town, MA) consists of a modified conventional angioplasty balloon catheter and a control unit. Two platinum electrodes are mounted on the catheter shaft inside the balloon, and are attached to the control unit by wires. A radiofrequency potential is applied at 650 kHz across these resistive elements. As current flows between the electrodes, heat is generated by resistive power loss in the fluid inside the balloon (typically a 50/50 mixture of 0.9 M NaCl and ionic contrast). This heat is in turn transmitted to the arterial wall by conduction. No radiofrequency energy passes through tissue; it is confined to the balloon. The temperature of the fluid is selectable by the operator and is accurate to within ±2°C. A temperature sensor mounted on the catheter shaft inside the balloon is in direct contact with the balloon fluid and is connected to a feedback system in the control unit. This thermistor provides continuous temperature monitoring to the control unit, which instantaneously regulates radiofrequency input, thus preventing temperature overshoot. Uniform heating of the balloon to 60°C, as confirmed by thermal map profiles, is achieved within seconds. Cooling of the saline/contrast mixture inside the balloon to 37°C occurs after cessation of radiofrequency energy input. Data from our laboratory has demonstrated that only those areas of the arterial wall in direct contact with the PLOSA balloon will be heated.

One striking difference between PLOSA and other devices that utilize thermal energy to treat obstructive coronary stenoses is the relatively low temperature of 60°C used during PLOSA. Thermal ablation of atherosclerotic plaque, initially thought to be a beneficial effect of laser therapy (temperature range 100°C–400°C), produces a charred endothelial surface that may result in vascular spasm and resultant thrombosis.[32,33] The incidence of restenosis has not been diminished by laser therapy, either as independent therapy or in conjunction with balloon angioplasty.[1,32,33] Laser balloon angioplasty (applied temperature estimated at 85°C–120°C, inflation pressures of 6–10 atm) also has a high restenosis rate when applied as either primary or adjunctive therapy.[28] One explanation for the significant incidence of restenosis with these devices is that thermal injury, with attendant cell necrosis, occurs at these temperatures. In contrast, only minimal medial cell injury was observed after PLOSA at 60°C in an in vivo porcine coronary artery angioplasty model.[21] It is interesting to note that the extent of cell damage in this model was significantly increased when PLOSA was performed at 70°C. One distinct advantage of the PLOSA system is the use of radiofrequency energy as the source of thermal output. The magnitude of energy output can be closely regulated, permitting tight control of the applied temperature. Early studies using prototype bipolar radiofrequency balloon angioplasty catheters with electrodes on the balloon surface demonstrated that thermal "molding" of postmortem human atherosclerotic arterial segments could be successfully performed, and that larger luminal diameters were achieved, with no evidence of subsequent elastic recoil.[34] These authors demonstrated that thermal energy was applied only to that segment of artery in contact with the balloon system. However, there was histologic evidence of medial myocyte damage with this system. A major concern in the design of the initial radiofrequency system with surface electrodes was the inability to have precise control of the applied temperature. Thus, the PLOSA system was modified such that two radiofrequency electrodes were mounted on the catheter shaft inside the balloon. Radiofrequency energy applied between these electrodes is confined to the balloon and results in heating of the contrast/saline mixture inside the balloon. Thermal energy reaches the arterial wall by thermal conduction. A thermistor is also mounted on the catheter shaft inside the balloon. The balloon temperature in the present system can be regulated by a control unit to within 1°C.

Experimental Studies

Proof of Principle: In Vitro Cadaver Atherosclerotic Iliac Artery Studies

The initial evaluation of the PLOSA system was performed in freshly excised cadaver atherosclerotic human iliac arteries. Range-finding experiments with this experimental system demonstrated that 60°C and 2 atm were optimal temperature and pressure settings necessary to achieve stenosis reduction utilizing a single 60-second treatment. Heating commenced in parallel with inflation of the balloon, so as to avoid any isolated "angioplasty effect." Lower temperatures (40°C–50°C) required inflation pressures of 6 atm to reduce the initial stenoses, and were associated with an equivalent incidence of dissection to PTCA, as assessed by postprocedure angioscopy. There was no additional improvement in angiographic or angioscopic outcomes at temperatures above 60°C when compared with the 60°C treatments at 2 atm.

In this model, PLOSA resulted in improved stenosis reduction, a lower incidence of dissection, and a significant reduction in the extent of intimal disruption compared with conventional angio-plasty.[35] On morphometric analysis of histologic arterial cross sections, only 4.6%±2.6% of the intimal surface was damaged after PLOSA, which contrasts sharply with the 29.3%±10.4% observed after conventional angioplasty. These effects are not the result of balloon inflation at a lower pressure, as the incidence of dissection and the extent of intimal disruption in a cohort of segments dilated at low pressure and 37°C was significantly higher than that observed in the PLOSA group.

Effects of PLOSA on Arterial Elastic Properties

Further insight into the mechanism of PLOSA comes from studies examining the effect of simultaneous application of heat at 60°C and a minimal distending pressure on the elastic properties of intact porcine iliac vessels.[36] Progressive inflation of a conventional angioplasty balloon in an appropriately sized, freshly excised porcine common iliac artery generates a pressure-volume curve that describes the compliance of the arterial segment. Inflation of a PLOSA balloon at 60°C in the contralateral paired arterial segment resulted in a rightward shift of this pressure-volume curve, even at a minimal balloon volume. Thus, the compliance of the artery is increased when subjected to heating at 60°C and progressive inflation of the PLOSA balloon. Histologic straightening of elastic fibers was observed in PLOSA treated segments, in parallel with this alteration in arterial compliance. These alterations in arterial compliance, likely the result of combined thermal-pressure effects on elastic fibers, may have important effects on arterial remodeling in humans.

Time Course of Transmural Arterial Heating

To gain further insight into the mechanism of PLOSA, we examined the time course of transmural heating and the relation between arterial wall thickness and temperature gradients in normal and atherosclerotic rabbits[37] in vivo. Three thermistors were placed on the adventitial surface of the infrarenal aorta in a radial pattern, and the wires externalized. PLOSA was performed at 60°C, 1 atm for 60 seconds with the balloon centered at the level of the thermistors. Balloon and adventitial aortic temperatures were continuously monitored during the inflation sequence. The time for the adventitial surface to reach 50°C and the lag in adventitial heating from the onset of thermal input were also examined. Animals were then killed, and histologic analysis of these aortic segments was performed. The heating profiles of normal and atherosclerotic aorta are quite different. Higher peak temperatures, immediate and rapid transmural heating were observed in normal rabbits, in the setting of significantly less intimal-medial thickness than the atherosclerotic animals. Heating profiles for atherosclerotic animals were further separated into two cohorts based on a peak adventitial temperature >55°C. The group of thermistors where higher peak temperatures were achieved again had a minimal lag in adventitial heating and a more rapid heating profile. However, intimal-medial thickness in this group was significantly greater than in aorta where thermistors recorded a peak adventitial temperature <55°C. Thus heat transfer during PLOSA is rapid in atherosclerotic arteries, and is amplified in areas of larger plaque thickness. Thermal energy may thus be focused to the area of greatest plaque burden in PLOSA. This observation suggests that plaque and the surrounding media and adventitia are a rapid conductor of heat in this model. The eccentric nature of atherosclerotic plaque may also account for the rapid heat transfer, as more surface area of the plaque is in direct contact with the balloon surface, and thus receives augmented thermal input.

Preservation of Arterial Vasoreactivity

The effects of balloon angioplasty on coronary arterial vasoreactivity in humans are well known.[19] There is persistent vasoconstriction that may in part be due to the uniform endothelial denudation in those areas of the coronary artery in direct contact with the balloon surface. This results in the loss of synthesis of endogenous vasodilators such as endothelium-dependent relaxing factor and prostacyclin. In addition, stretching and tearing of medial smooth muscle fibers results in progressive coronary vasoconstriction postangioplasty, both at the site of the dilatation and in the distal vessel. This phenomenon can be reversed with intracoronary nitroglycerin, and is thought to occur due to direct balloon injury to medial smooth muscle. As PLOSA is performed at significantly lower inflation pressures, the attendant reduction in arterial barotrauma might result in preservation of endothelium and smooth muscle architecture and thus in preserved vascular responsiveness. In addition, the effect of heating at 60°C on arterial vasoreactivity is not known.

To assess the effect of PLOSA on arterial vasoreactivity, the vasomotor responses of arterial rings of atherosclerotic rabbit abdomi-

nal aorta subjected to either PLOSA, conventional balloon angioplasty, or no intervention were evaluated.[38] Contraction and relaxation responses to norepinephrine and nitroglycerin were similar in
the three groups, and paralleled the responses of normal (nonatherosclerotic) aortic rings. However, methacholine-induced vasorelax-
ation was observed only in normal rings and in atherosclerotic rings
treated with PLOSA. The vasodilator response to methacholine in this
model requires intact endothelium, and implies that endothelial function is preserved after PLOSA but not after conventional angioplasty.
The response of nonintervened atherosclerotic rings to methacholine
is blunted in comparison to the nonatherosclerotic, nonintervened
controls. The recovery of a vasodilator response to methacholine after PLOSA raises the issue of whether there is a beneficial effect of
heat on vascular responsiveness in this model.

In Vivo Atherosclerotic Rabbit Studies

The short- and long-term effects of PLOSA were directly compared with conventional angioplasty in the atherosclerotic rabbit.
In the acute and long-term animals, angiographic and histologic
outcomes after arterial remodeling using the PLOSA system were
significantly better than after conventional balloon angioplasty.
There was a marked increase in the extent of arterial barotrauma
seen on histologic sections from the angioplasty group as compared with the PLOSA group. A mean of 82.2% of the intimal surface was damaged after balloon angioplasty, as compared with only
35.5% damage of the intimal circumference after PLOSA. The minimal extent of arterial barotrauma after PLOSA contrasts the difference in mechanisms of plaque reduction between PLOSA and
balloon angioplasty. Thus PLOSA is a better method of initial arterial remodeling in this model.[39] The long-term outcomes in this
atherosclerotic model reflect the observations made in those animals studied acutely.[40] The cross-sectional area of neointima (in
mm^2), a measure of neoimtimal hyperplasia, defined as the region
of arterial wall from the endothelial surface at the lumen to the luminal margin of the media, was significantly less in PLOSA-treated
segments than in paired arteries treated with conventional angioplasty. This finding was consistent in the animals studied either at
30 days or at 60 days. A larger cross-sectional luminal area, measured from histologic sections, was also observed in the 30- and 60-
day PLOSA groups compared with angioplasty controls.
Quantitative analysis of follow-up angiograms at 30 and 60 days
demonstrated a significant increase in the MLD in the PLOSA

group at 30 days compared with the angioplasty cohort, with a trend to significance at 60 days. Thus, neointimal hyperplasia is significantly reduced after PLOSA compared with balloon angioplasty. Angiographic restenosis is significantly less at 30 days, with a trend to significance at 60 days, in parallel with a larger lumen in the PLOSA group. These data show that the less traumatic mechanism of arterial remodeling in PLOSA impacts favorably on the incidence of restenosis in this model, and suggests that PLOSA may offer similar benefits in humans.

Clinical Experience

Phase I Human Coronary Trial

Study Design

The initial human coronary cases were performed in Europe and Canada prior to the onset of the United States Phase I clinical trial. The inflation protocol was designed in such a fashion as to derive a maximal benefit from the application of thermal energy at 60°C to "soften" the atherosclerotic plaque such that only a minimum distensile force (applied by the balloon) would be required to remodel the coronary stenosis. The PLOSA balloon is made of a unique blend of polyethylene tetraphalate, and exhibits minimal compliance, achieving nominal size at 1 atm, with less than a 2% increase in size at 5 atm. This design minimizes the potential for any isolated angioplasty effect. Exact sizing of the balloon to the arterial diameter of the stenosed segment is thus necessary to achieve optimal stenosis reduction. These first cases demonstrated that PLOSA was a safe and effective percutaneous technique of remodeling atherosclerotic coronary stenoses. One critical observation was that a significant time period (approximately 1 second of cooling for each second of heating) was required for the saline/contrast mixture inside the balloon to cool from 60°C to 42°C prior to deflation after each PLOSA treatment. The inflation sequence for the United States Phase I protocol is outlined in Table 2. The first inflation is limited to a peak pressure of 2 atm. A peak pressure of 5 atm can be used during the second inflation in an effort to provide additional dilating force without overexpansion of those aspects of the balloon unopposed by obstructive plaque. After two inflations, the operator may elect to upsize the balloon by 0.25 mm in diameter. Indeed, if straightening of elastic

TABLE 2

PLOSA Human Coronary Protocol

infl#	balloon:artery ratio	peak pressure	max infl time
1	1:1	2 atm	90 sec
2	1:1	5 atm	90 sec
3	>1:1	2 atm	90 sec
4	>1:1	5 atm	90 sec

Inflations 2 and 4 may be repeated multiple times at the investigator's discretion. An angiographic end point of < 20% residual stenosis is desired.

fibers occurs after the initial inflations, a larger balloon may be required to achieve complete remodeling of the stenosed coronary segment. A residual stenosis of <20% is the desired end point.

The phase I protocol permits treatment of a single lesion with PLOSA. Patients with de novo lesions or lesions that have restenosed after previous treatment with conventional angioplasty are considered eligible for participation in this protocol. Angiographic inclusion criteria require greater than a 70% stenosis in a vessel 2.5 to 3.5 mm in diameter, and lesions must be <20 mm in length. Patients suffering an acute myocardial infarction or who have received thrombolytic therapy <1 week prior to intervention are excluded from this study, as are patients with severe left ventricular dysfunction (LVEF <35%). Patients who are pacemaker-dependent (permanent or temporary) are also ineligible for this protocol. Other angiographic criteria that preclude consideration for this study are an unprotected left main stenosis >50%, 100% occluded lesions, and the presence of either intracoronary thrombus or a severely calcified lesion.

Seventy-two patients comprise the human coronary experience.[41] Forty-six patients had an isolated coronary stenosis, 22 had two-vessel disease, and 5 had three-vessel disease. Mean left ventricular ejection fraction (LVEF) was 63%. Anginal symptoms were present in 90%, and 30% of patients with angina were unstable (Canadian Cardiovascular Society Class IV) at the time of the procedure. Two patients had clinical evidence of congestive heart failure. Twenty-nine patients had a documented prior myocardial infarction. Risk factors for coronary artery disease include a family history of premature coronary artery disease in 52%, tobacco abuse in 72%, hyperlipidemia in 59%, hypertension in 36%, and diabetes in 14%. All patients were treated with aspirin, 60% were treated with β-receptor blocking agents, and 70% received calcium channel antagonists. Seventy-three stenoses (52 de novo, 20 restenotic) were treated with PLOSA, with the following distribution of stenosis locations: 37 LAD, 22 RCA, 12 LCFX, and two saphenous vein bypass graft stenoses. Fifty lesions were type B, 20 were type A, and two were type C morphology (American College of Cardiology/ American Heart Association typology). All patients received 325 mg of aspirin the morning of the procedure. All oral and intravenous cardiac medications were continued for each patient. Anticoagulation with intravenous heparin was achieved after insertion of arterial and venous femoral cannulas. Additional heparin was administered as needed throughout the case in order to maintain an activated clotting time >350 seconds. All patients described typical anginal chest discomfort during PLOSA inflations, and in addition, a number of patients described a sensation of "heat" in parallel with temperatures over 55°C. An angiographic success was achieved in 93% of patients. A mean initial stenosis of 80.6%±1.5% (mean±SEM) was reduced to 30.8%±1.7%. Mean MLD increased from 0.57±0.04 mm preprocedure to 2.06±0.06 mm 5 minutes after PLOSA, with no evidence of elastic recoil at 15 minutes (MLD 2.01±0.06 mm). Localized dissection at the PLOSA site occurred in 11 patients (15%). Adjunctive PTCA was performed in 6 patients. In 2 cases, PTCA was utilized in an effort to further improve the arterial lumen at the site of the stenosis. In 2 patients a perfusion balloon catheter was used to treat a dissection after PLOSA. In one case a low-pressure inflation was performed with a conventional PTCA balloon to break up arterial thrombus at the PLOSA site. There was one instance of abrupt closure of the treated vessel that occurred after premature deflation of the PLOSA balloon at 60°C. This patient required emergent CABG surgery.[41]

In each case, arterial remodeling was achieved at a significantly lower inflation pressure than would be expected with conventional balloon angioplasty (mean 3.85±0.12 atm). Longer inflation times were required, accounted for in part by 30- to 90-second periods as the device cooled to 42°C prior to deflation, after individual heating inflations of 55 to 90 seconds. Total heating time ranged from 55 to 480 seconds (mean 190 seconds). A mean of 3.5±1.5 inflations were performed. A mean of 1.3±0.4 balloons were used per case.[37] The typical angiographic appearance of an arterial segment after treatment with PLOSA is a smooth, tubular lumen that resembles the shape of the fully inflated balloon. Intracoronary ultrasound reveals a minimum of intimal disruption and a smooth, circular lumen. Representative cases are presented in Figures 2 and 3.

To compare the procedural variables and angiographic outcomes of PLOSA to PTCA directly, we performed a retrospective, case-matched control study of 20 human coronary lesions treated with PLOSA as sole therapy with 35 randomly selected lesions matched for lesion location and arterial location that were treated with PTCA.[42] Angiograms were analyzed at a core laboratory using a computer-based edge detection system. Stenosis reduction was achieved with significantly lower inflation pressures after PLOSA than with conventional angioplasty. Although longer inflation periods were required during PLOSA, the number of inflations per case was similar in the two groups. Initial lesion severity, as measured by percent stenosis and MLD, was similar in the PLOSA and PTCA cohorts. However, the residual stenosis postprocedure was significantly less after PLOSA, paralleled by a significantly greater MLD in the PLOSA group. These procedural variables and angiographic outcomes are outlined in Table 3.

Arterial recoil is a commonly observed phenomenon after PTCA. Straightening of elastic fibers has been observed after PLOSA in experimental models.[21] Utilizing the PLOSA and case-matched control PTCA cohort described above, quantitative analysis of angiograms performed 5 and 15 minutes after the final inflation in each case revealed no change in the MLD in the PLOSA group. However, MLD declined 0.25 mm 15 minutes after PTCA, representing an 18% loss of the acute gain. Thus, a greater initial improvement in MLD and the absence of elastic recoil are observed after PLOSA in comparison with PTCA.[42]

One further insight into the mechanism of PLOSA comes from analysis of changes in lesion eccentricity. To compare the coronary arterial remodeling that occurs with PLOSA and conventional PTCA, the eccentricity of the vessel wall at the site of stenosis was assessed from pre- and post-intervention angiograms using a computer-based edge detection system. Changes in the morphology of each side of the vessel wall were separately assessed based on changes in the standard deviation of the radius of curvature (SDC) averaged across the stenotic zone. An eccentricity index was generated from a ratio of the SDCs of the opposing vessel walls. This technique permits evaluation of lesion eccentricity independent of the course of the arterial segment in space. Lesion eccentricity was similar in the PLOSA and case-matched groups pre-intervention. However, lesions were significantly less eccentric after PLOSA. The more diseased arterial wall (evidenced by the greatest SDC pre-intervention) changed significantly more toward paralleling the midline with PLOSA than with PTCA. These data suggest that the mechanism of stenosis reduction is different in PLOSA than in

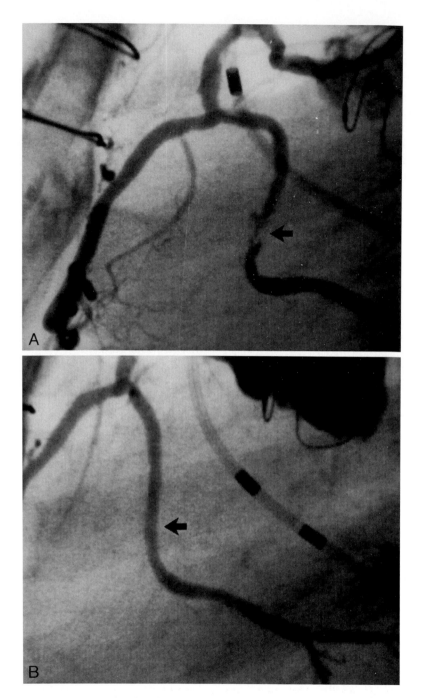

FIGURE 2. *PLOSA of a distal right coronary artery stenosis. An initial 90% stenosis (MLD 0.3 mm, arrow) in the distal right coronary artery is depicted in panel* **A.** *The angiographic appearance is that of an ulcerated, ruptured plaque.* **B:** *This lesion was reduced to a 7% narrowing after two inflations with a 3.25-mm PLOSA balloon (MLD 2.82 mm, arrow).*

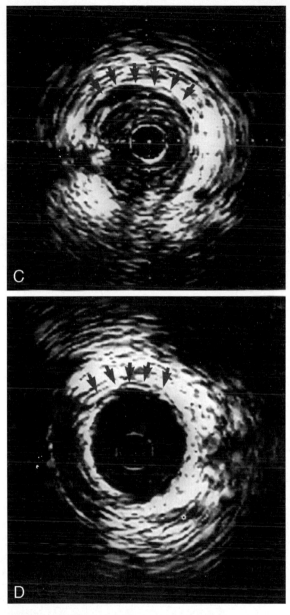

FIGURE 2. (continued). *C: Intracoronary ultrasound of the lesion pre-PLOSA. There is a large plaque burden and a spontaneous dissection superiorly (arrows).* **D:** *Intracoronary ultrasound of the same lesion after PLOSA. There is a smooth, circular lumen. The dissection plane has been sealed (arrows).*

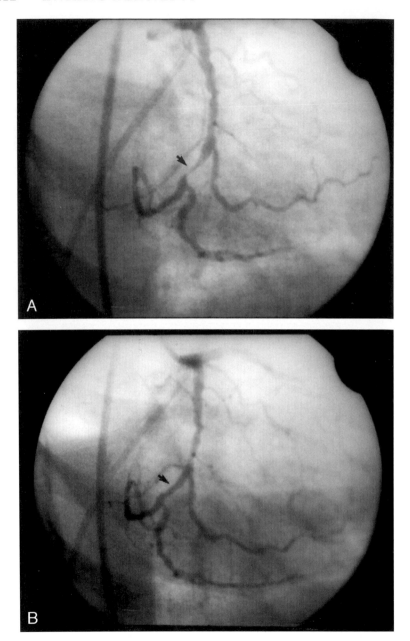

FIGURE 3. *PLOSA of a left circumflex artery stenosis. An initial 75% stenosis (MLD 0.7 mm, arrow) in the distal left circumflex artery is depicted in **A. B:** This lesion was reduced to an 18% narrowing after three inflations with a 2.75-mm PLOSA balloon (MLD 2.06 mm, arrow). An angiogram at 6 months revealed further improvement in the remodeled PLOSA site (MLD 2.27 mm, arrow). A new lesion is seen in the proximal vessel.*

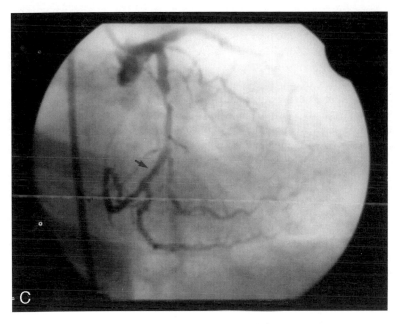

FIGURE 3. *(continued)*

TABLE 3

PLOSA vs Conventional Angioplasty:Procedural Variables and Angiographic Outcomes

	PTCA	PLOSA	*P* value
Peak Pressure (ATM)	8.2±.32	3.7±.22	0.0001
# of Inflations	3.5±.25	2.8±.25	ns
Total Inflation Time (sec)	224±24	402±44	0.0003
% Diameter Stenosis pre	80±1.8	85±1.5	0.04
% Diameter Stenosis post	31±2.0	24±1.9	0.03
Minimum Luminal Diameter pre	0.62±.06	0.49±.05	ns
Minimum Luminal Diameter 5 min post	2.04±.07	2.41±.11	0.005
Minimum Luminal Diameter 15 min post	1.79+.07	2.37±.11	0.0001

PTCA. PLOSA results in more concentric dilatation with facilitated remodeling of regions with greater plaque burden.[43]

Treatment of Suboptimal PTCA Due to Acute Arterial Recoil

Suboptimal dilatation complicating PTCA may occur as the result of elastic recoil. Based on the observations that PLOSA results in straightening of elastic fibers in experimental models and that there is no acute recoil of dilated segments after PLOSA in humans, the inclusion criteria for PLOSA were expanded to permit acute PLOSA treatment of patients who have a suboptimal result after conventional angioplasty due to recoil at the dilatation site. Eight patients have been treated with PLOSA for this indication. Five lesions were de novo and three were restenotic. Three lesions were in the LAD, four in the left circumflex, and there was one RCA stenosis. During conventional PTCA, 4.9 ± 0.4 inflations were performed to a peak of 11.5 ± 1.1 atm with at least 1:1 balloon:artery sizing. In each case, at least two inflations were performed where the PTCA balloon was fully expanded. PLOSA was then performed using a balloon of comparable size to the largest PTCA balloon. An average of 3.6 PLOSA inflations were performed, with a mean total heating time of 281 ± 69 seconds at a peak of 4.0 ± 0.4 atm. MLD increased from 0.76 ± 0.13 mm pre-PTCA to 1.1 ± 0.10 mm post-PTCA, with a further increase to 1.67 ± 0.11 mm post-PLOSA ($P=0.01$). This corresponded to a reduction in residual percent stenosis from $59.0\% \pm 4.1\%$ post-PTCA to $35.6\% \pm 5.6\%$ after PLOSA treatment. Thus the application of thermal energy appears to have beneficial effects on the elastic properties of coronary vasculature in this setting.

Summary

The application of heat at 60°C and a minimal distending pressure distinguishes PLOSA from other percutaneous forms of coronary remodeling. The magnitude of the initial gain achieved after PLOSA is significantly greater than that observed after PTCA. It has recently been proposed that greater acute gains in coronary MLD are associated with a reduced incidence of subsequent restenosis.[44] In PLOSA, the large increase in MLD is achieved at lower inflation pressures than are typically required with either conventional angioplasty or other balloon facilitated coronary remodeling techniques. Experimental studies with PLOSA demonstrate that the application of heat and only a minimal inflation pressure minimizes the extent of barotrauma and permits a significant degree of functional preservation of vascular endothelium. The effects of PLOSA on arterial recoil are likely the direct result of thermal energy on the elastic elements of the arterial wall. Ongoing examination of long-term outcomes after PLOSA will broaden our understanding of the thermal behavior and subsequent responses of atherosclerotic coronary vasculature. Future studies, including concurrent intraluminal imaging and thermal-mediated drug delivery, may further optimize this technique for better short- and long-term outcomes.

References

1. Waller BF. "Crackers, breakers, stretchers, drillers, scrapers, shavers, burners, welders and melters"—the future treatment of athersclerotic coronary disease? A clinical-morphologic assessment. *J Am Coll Cardiol.* 1989;13:969–987.969–987.
2. Faxon DP, Weber VJ, Haudenschild C, Gottsman SB, McGovern WA, Ryan TJ. Acute effects of transluminal angioplasty in three experimental models of atherosclerosis. *Arteriosclerosis.* 1982;2:125–133.
3. Block PC, Baughman KL, Pasternak RC, Fallon JT. Transluminal angioplasty: correlation of morphologic and angiographic findings in an experimental model. *Circulation.* 1980;61:778–785.
4. Matthews BJ, Ewels CJ, Kent KM. Coronary dissection: a predictor of restenosis? *Am Heart J.* 1988;115:547–554.
5. Ramee SR, White CJ, Collins TJ, Mesa JE, Murgo JP. Percutaneous angioscopy during coronary angioplasty using a steerable microangioscope. *J Am Coll Cardiol.* 1991;17:100–105.
6. Hirshfeld JW Jr, Schwartz JS, Jugo RS, et al. Restenosis after coronary angioplasty: a multivariate model to relate lesion and procedure variables to restenosis. *J Am Coll Cardiol.* 1991;18:647–656.
7. Deutsch E, Hirshfeld JW Jr, Pepine CJ, Bove AA. Analysis of initial lesion characteristics and arterial remodelling six months after angioplasty in a stable population. *J Am Coll Cardiol.* 1992;19:258A.
8. Deutsch E, Gerber RS, Martin JL, Burke JA, Combs WG, Bove AA. Initial lesion eccentricity predicts restenosis after successful coronary angioplasty. *J Am Coll Cardiol.* 1993;21:89A.
9. Chesebro JH, Lam YHT, Badimon L, Fuster V. Restenosis after arterial angioplasty: a hemorrheologic response to injury. *Am J Cardiol.* 1987;60:10B–16B.
10. Lucas MA, Deutsch E, Hirshfeld JW, Barnathan ES, Laskey WK. Influence of heparin therapy on PTCA outcome in patients with coronary thrombus. *Am J Cardiol.* 1990;65:179–182.
11. Fuster V, Badimon L, Cohen M, Ambrose J, Badimon JJ, Chesebro JH. Insights into the pathogenesis of acute ischemic syndromes. *Circulation.* 1988;77:1213–1220.
12. Wilcox JN. Thrombin and other potential mechanisms underlying restenosis. *Circulation.* 1991;84:432–434.
13. Ross R. The pathogenesis of atherosclerosis: an update. *N Engl J Med.* 1986;314:488–500.
14. McNamara CA, Sarembock IJ, Gimple LW, Fenton JW III, Coughlin SR, Owens GK. Thrombin stimulates proliferation of cultured rat aortic smooth muscle cells by a proteolytically activated receptor. *J Clin Invest.* 1993;91:94–98.
15. Liu MW, Roubin GS, King SB. Restenosis after coronary angioplasty: potential biologic determinants and role of intimal hyperplasia. *Circulation.* 1989;79:1374–1387.
16. Austen GE, Ratliff NH, Hollman J, Tabei S, Phillips DF.Intimal proliferation of smooth muscle cells as an explanation for recurrent coro-

nary artery stenosis after percutaneous transluminal coronary angioplasty. *J Am Coll Cardiol.* 1985;6:369–375.
17. Giraldo AA, Esposo OM, Meis JM. Intmial hyperplasia as a cause of
   restenosis after percutaneous transluminal coronary angioplasty. *Arch
   Pathol Lab Med.* 1985;109:173–175.
18. Spears JR. Percutaneous transluminal coronary angioplasty restenosis: potential prevention with laser balloon angioplasty. *Am J Cardiol.*
   1987;60:61B–64B.
19. Fischell TA, Derby G, Tse TM, Stadius ML. Coronary artery vasoconstriction routinely occurs after percutaneous tranluminal coronary angioplasty. *Circulation.* 1988;78:1323–1334.
20. O'Neill BJ, Title LM, Makowski S, et al. Absence of early recoil after
   successful physiologic low stress angioplasty. *Circulation.* 1993;88:I-
   150.
21. Fram DB, Aretz TA, Fisher JP, et al. In vivo radiofrequency balloon angioplasty of porcine coronary arteries: histologic effects and safety.
   J Am Coll Cardiol. 1992;19:217A.
22. Jenkins RD, Sinclair IN, Leonard BM, Sandor T, Schoen FJ, Spears RJ.
   Laser balloon angioplasty vs. balloon angioplasty in normal rabbit iliac arteries. *Lasers Surg Med.* 1989;9:237–247.
23. Sinclair IN, Jenkins RD, James LM, et al. Effect of laser balloon angioplasty on normal dog coronary arteries in vivo. *J Am Coll Cardiol.*
   1988;11(suppl):108A.
24. Spears JR, Kundu SK, McMath LP. Laser balloon angioplasty: potential for reduction of the thrombogenicity of the injured arterial wall
   and for local application of bioprotective materials. *J Am Coll Cardiol.*
   1991;17:179B–188B.
25. Reis GJ, Pomerantz RM, Jenkins RD, et al. Laser balloon angioplasty:
   clinical, angiographic and histologic results. *J Am Coll Cardiol.* 1991;
   18:193–202.
26. Jenkins RD, Sinclair IN, Anand RK, Kalil AG Jr, Schoen FJ, Spears JR.
   Laser balloon angioplasty: factors affecting plaque—arterial wall thermal "weld" strength. *Lasers Surg Med.* 1988;8:30–39.
27. Jenkins RD, Sinclair IN, McCall PE, Schoen FJ, Spears JR. Thermal
   sealing of arterial dissections and perforations in atherosclerotic rabbits with laser balloon angioplasty. *Lasers Life Sci.* 1989;3:13–30.
28. Spears JR, Reyes VP, Wynne J, et al. Percutaneous coronary laser balloon angioplasty: initial results of a multicenter experience. *J Am Coll
   Cardiol.* 1990;16:293–303.
29. Walinsky P, Rosen A, Martinez-Hernandez A, Smith DL, Nardone DO,
   Brevette B. Microwave balloon angioplasty. *J Invasive Cardiol.* 1991;3:
   152–156.
30. Landau C, Currier JW, Haudenschild CC, Heyman D, Minihan AC,
   Faxon DF. Microwave balloon angioplasty to treat arterial dissections
   in an atherosclerotic rabbit model. *J Am Coll Cardiol.* 1991;17:234A.
31. Small DM. Progression and regression of atherosclerotic lesions: insights from lipid physical biochemistry. *Arteriosclerosis.* 1988;8:103–
   129.
32. Forrester JS, Litvak F, Grundfest W. Vaporization of atheroma in man:
   the role of lasers in the era of balloon angioplasty. *Int J Cardiol.* 1988;
   20:1–7.
33. Sanborn TA. Laser angioplasty. What has been learned from experimental and clinical trials? *Circulation.* 1988;78:769–774.

34. Lee BI, Becker GJ, Waller BF, et al. Thermal compression and molding of atherosclerotic vascular tissue with use of radiofrequency energy: implications for radiofrequency balloon angioplasty. *J Am Coll Cardiol.* 1989;13:1167–1175.

35. Deutsch E, Martin JL, Budjak R, et al. Low stress angioplasty at 60°C: attenuated arterial barotrauma. *Circulation.* 1990;82(suppl III):72.

36. Mitchel JF, Fram DB, Fisher JP, et al. Low grade (60°C) heating increases vascular compliance during balloon angioplasty. *Circulation.* 1991;84(suppl II):300.

37. Deutsch E, Martin JL, Budjak R, Bove AA. Timecourse of transmural heating during low stress angioplasty at 60°C in the atherosclerotic rabbit: preferential heating of plaque. *Cathet Cardiovasc Diagn.* 1992; 22:75.

38. Morley D, Zhang XY, Budjak R, Martin JL, Bove AA, Deutsch E. Preservation of arterial vasoreactivity following low stress angioplasty at 60°C in the atherosclerotic rabbit. *Circulation.* 1991;84-II:299.

39. Deutsch E, Morley D, Martin JL, Budjak R, Bove AA. Conventional angioplasty vs low stress angioplasty at 60°C in the atherosclerotic rabbit iliac artery: angiographic and histologic outcomes and platelet deposition. *Circulation.* 1991;84:II-299.

40. Deutsch E, Martin JL, Budjak R, Goldman BI, Bove AA. Low stress angioplasty at 60°C in the atherosclerotic rabbit results in reduced neointimal hyperplasia. *Circulation.* 1992;86:I-185.

41. Deutsch E, Martin JL, Makowski S, O'Neill BJ, McKay RG. Acute and chronic outcomes after physiologic low stress angioplasty (PLOSA) of de novo coronary stenoses:results of the phase I trial. *Circulation.* 1993;88:I-646.

42. O'Neill BJ, McKay RG, Martin JL, et al. Physiologic low stress angioplasty at 60°C: comparison to matched controls undergoing conventional coronary angioplasty. *Circulation.* 1992;86:I-457.

43. Martin JL, Deutsch E, McKay RG, et al. Coronary remodelling with low stress angioplasty at 60°C vs conventional angioplasty in man: analysis of changes in plaque eccentricity. *J Am Coll Cardiol.* In press.

44. Kuntz RE, Baim DS. Defining coronary restenosis: newer clinical and angiographic paradigms. *Circulation.* 1993;88:1310–1323.

Chapter 14

High-Speed Rotational Coronary Atherectomy

Andrew I. MacIsaac, MBBS and
Patrick L. Whitlow, MD

Percutaneous transluminal coronary angioplasty (PTCA) was first introduced by Andreas Gruentzig to treat discrete, proximal coronary artery lesions.[1,2] The technique rapidly became widely accepted,[3,4] but its limitations soon became apparent. The major limitations of balloon angioplasty are threefold. First, in 1% to 2% of cases the target lesion cannot be dilated[5]; second, acute coronary closure complicates 4% to 5% of cases[6-8]; and third, restenosis develops in 30% to 50% of treated lesions.[9-12] The incidence of procedure failure and short-term complications increase with the complexity of the target lesion. Lesions that are long, ostial, calcified, thrombus containing, angulated or chronic total occlusions have the highest complication rates.[13] Restenosis is related to a number of factors, including the minimal luminal diameter achieved by the intervention.[14] The residual stenosis after angioplasty is often on the order of 30%,[15] and recent data suggest less residual stenosis and reduced restenosis with new interventional devices.[16]

These limitations of balloon angioplasty led to the development of the Rotablator™ (Heart Technology Inc., Redmond, WA). The use of a high-speed, diamond-coated burr to ablate coronary atherosclerosis has proven effective in treating complex lesions, and potentially may limit restenosis. It has become a valuable addition to the percutaneous treatments of advanced coronary atherosclerosis. This chapter describes the equipment, technique, indications for and results of high-speed rotational atherectomy using the Rotablator.

From Vetrovec GW, Carabello BA, (eds.) *Invasive Cardiology: Current Diagnostic and Therapeutic Issues.* Armonk, NY: Futura Publishing Company, Inc.: © 1996.

Mode of Action

Percutaneous high-speed rotational atherectomy was originally developed by David Auth to debulk atheromatous plaque while minimizing injury to disease-free arterial regions. The Rotablator consists of an elliptical metal burr that is coated with diamond chips. This burr rotates at 200,000 revolutions per minute (rpm) abrading atherosclerotic lesions while preserving normal regions. Such differential cutting is possible because of the elastic nature of the normal arterial wall and the more rigid, inflexible nature of diseased arterial segments. As the high-speed cutting burr passes down a diseased artery, it displaces the normal segments and abrades rigid lesions encroaching into the vessel lumen. This results in the selective removal of atheromatous plaque, leaving a polished smooth surface (Figure 1). Histological studies of focal lesions in atherosclerotic rabbit iliac arteries have shown that the Rotablator denudes endothelium, leaving a smooth intimal surface without injuring the arterial media (Figure 2).[17] These findings have also been confirmed in cadaver studies.[18] In vivo studies using three-dimensional reconstructions of intravascular images after high-speed rotational atherectomy have also shown a cylindrical smooth lumen, especially in heavily calcified lesions.[19] Angioscopy after Rotablator has demonstrated significantly fewer plaque fractures and smoother residual lesions than seen after balloon angioplasty.[20]

The Rotablator abrades atheromatous plaque into particles <5 μm in diameter. The small size of these particles enables them to traverse the microvasculature and to be eventually taken up by the reticulo-endothelial system.[21] This particulate debris could theoretically impair flow through the distal capillary bed, especially if particle size was increased or blood viscosity altered. However, this is normally not the case. Positron emission tomography has demonstrated a significant improvement in myocardial perfusion defects after uncomplicated rotational atherectomy.[22] Studies of left ventricular wall motion after rotational atherectomy have also demonstrated normal myocardial contraction in segments supplied by vessels treated with the Rotablator.[23,24] However, reduced distal flow has been reported after rotational atherectomy and described as the "slow reflow" phenomenon. Slow reflow has been reported to occur in 1.8% to 9.5% of cases,[25,26] and to be complicated by Q wave myocardial infarction in 9% and non-Q wave myocardial infarction in 33% of cases.[25] It is most likely to occur when there is a large plaque burden and where distal run-off is limited. Multivariate analysis has shown that the incidence of slow reflow is highest

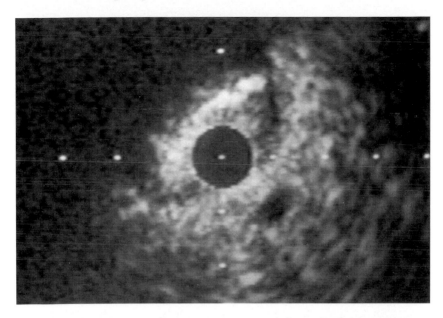

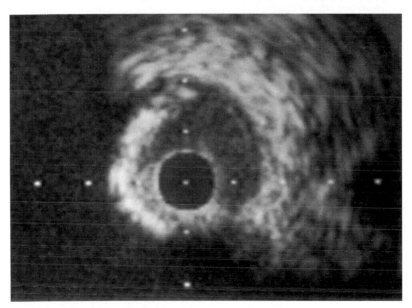

Figure 1. *Intravascular ultrasounds demonstrating differential cutting by the Rotablator.* **Top:** *before high-speed rotational atherectomy, an eccentric calcified lesion is present on the left of the vessel lumen.* **Bottom:** *after rotational atherectomy the luminal area is greatly increased, but the normal intimal (right side of lumen) is preserved. (Ultrasounds courtesy of Dr. S. Nissan.)*

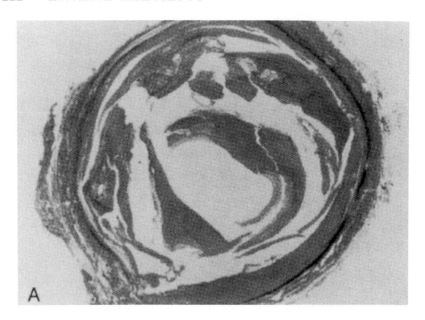

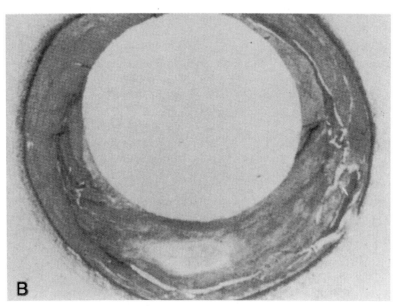

Figure 2. *Arterial cross sections.* **A:** *After balloon angioplasty showing a fractured plaque with multiple intimal and medial tears.* **B:** *After high-speed rotational atherectomy with no significant residual plaque and a smooth lumen. (Reproduced with permission from Reference 31.)*

if myocardial infarction had occurred in the territory supplied by the target lesion within 2 weeks, in patients with a history of hypertension, in long lesions, and after prolonged total burr activation time.[25] It may be due to either plugging of the distal capillary bed by microparticulate debris, arteriolar spasm, or microcavitation. Microcavitation or the formation of minute bubbles within blood at the tip of the Rotablator burr at speed >20,000 rpm has been demonstrated in vitro, but its clinical significance is uncertain.[27]

Equipment and Procedure

The Rotablator unit consists of an elliptical burr coated with diamond chips (Figure 3), connected by a flexible drive shaft to a gas driven turbine. The drive shaft is covered by a 4F Teflon sheath that is continuously flushed with saline to minimize friction around the drive shaft. The gas turbine is driven by compressed nitrogen. A console unit that is activated by a foot pedal controls the rate of gas delivery to the turbine. A fiberoptic cable connects the turbine and console enabling the speed of burr rotation to be measured and displayed. The burr tracks over a specialized 0.009-inch stainless steel guide wire that has a 0.017-mm radiopaque tip.

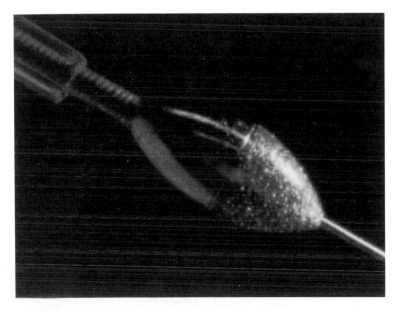

Figure 3. *Diamond chip coated elliptical Rotablator burr. (Reproduced with permission from Reference 31.)*

Procedure

The size of the guiding catheter depends on the size of the burr to be used. Burrs are manufactured in quarter millimeter gradations between and including 1.25 mm and 2.5 mm. Burrs <2.0 mm pass through an 8F guide; the 2.0 mm and 2.25 mm burrs require a 9F guide; and a 10F system is required for the 2.5-mm burr (Table 1). The diameter of the largest burr to be used should not exceed 80% of the vessel diameter.[28] If the target is a de novo lesion >5 mm in length, the initial burr size should be the 1.75 mm burr or smaller to minimize the initial volume of microparticulate debris. The burr size can then be increased; the second burr should not have a diameter 0.5 mm greater than the first. A larger initial burr can be used for short or restenotic lesions, but except in unusual circumstances, the 2.5-mm burr should not be used first as it may produce an excessive amount of debris.

Bradycardia is common if the vessel supplying the atrioventricular node is treated, therefore, a pacing wire should be placed prior to the treatment of a lesion in a dominant right or dominant circumflex coronary artery. Likewise, if a dominant right or circumflex artery is occluded and the target artery supplies collaterals to the atrioventricular node, a pacemaker should also be placed. After the administration of intravenous heparin and the selection of the appropriate size guiding catheter, the lesion is crossed using a bare wire technique. The "C" flexible wire is used in most cases but a stiffer "A" wire is available. These wires are not as maneuverable as usual PTCA guide wires. Occasionally a complex lesion may need to be crossed with a conventional guide wire, and then the wire exchanged for a 0.009-inch wire through a catheter. It is essential that the guide wire is placed with the radiopaque tip distal

TABLE 1

Recommended Guide Catheter Sizes for Use with the Rotablator

Rotablator Burr Size	Internal Diameter	Minimum Guide Size
1.25 mm	0.059″	8F
1.50 mm	0.069″	8F
1.75 mm	0.078″	8F
2.00 mm	0.088″	9F
2.15 mm	0.092″	9F
2.25 mm	0.097″	10F
2.50 mm	0.107″	10F

to the intended site of treatment, as the Rotablator will not advance over this distal guide wire segment.

The burr and turbine unit are then loaded onto the guide wire. The turbine is connected to the console and to high-pressure flush. With the flush running, the burr is tested before it is advanced into the guiding catheter. The flow of gas to the turbine is set so that the burr rotates at 200,000 rpm. The burr is advanced into a disease-free arterial segment proximal to the lesion and activated. The burr is then advanced using the sliding control knob on the turbine unit. A pecking motion with very gradual advancement of the burr is recommended to minimize the size and rate of production of debris. The speed of rotation is constantly monitored and should not drop below 160,000–175,000 rpm. The burr should be activated for no more than 40–60 seconds per run. Once the burr has crossed the lesion an additional "polishing" run is made, and the burr is withdrawn. Subsequently, a larger burr or adjunctive balloon angioplasty can be performed until a residual stenosis of less than 30% is achieved. The optimal balance between high-speed rotational atherectomy and adjunctive PTCA has not been determined. Multiple burrs have been used on the premise that maximal tissue debulking will limit restenosis. Conversely, the use of a single undersized burr may alter the target lesion's characteristics sufficiently to facilitate safer PTCA. Nino et al.[29] studied the effect of rotational atherectomy on the results of adjunctive balloon angioplasty. In 103 lesions treated by balloon angioplasty alone, the ratio of the minimal luminal diameter obtained to the diameter of the largest balloon used was 0.71 ± 0.11. In 32 lesions treated with rotational atherectomy, the ratio of the minimal luminal diameter to the diameter of the adjunctive balloon was significantly at $>0.86 \pm 0.16$ ($P<0.001$). Adjunctive PTCA is often required when the final burr artery ratio is <70%; however, even when larger burrs are used, adjunctive balloon angioplasty often optimizes the acute gain in lesion diameter, minimizing the residual stenosis.

Results

Angiographic and Procedural Success

Early experience with the Rotablator demonstrated that adjunctive PTCA was often necessary to achieve a satisfactory result. Teirstein et al.[30] reported results in 42 patients who were considered suboptimal candidates for balloon angioplasty. Most of these patients had diffuse coronary artery disease, defined as lesions >10 mm in length. The Rotablator was used as a stand-alone procedure, therefore no adjunctive balloon angioplasty was performed. Procedural success was obtained in 92% of lesions <10 mm in length, but only in 70% of longer lesions.

More recently, data from the United States Coronary Rotary Ablation Multicenter Registry[31,32] and the European Registry[23] have been reported. This United States registry contains data on 1,042 patients and 1,688 treated lesions from fourteen United States centers. Adjunctive PTCA was used as necessary to achieve the optimum result. The mean age of patients treated with the Rotablator was 62.4 years and 75% were male. Almost 50% had stable angina, while 39% had Canadian Class III or IV angina. The target lesion was in the left anterior descending in 49% of lesions, 29% were located in the right coronary artery, 18% in the circumflex, and 3% in the left main trunk. Multivessel coronary artery disease was present in 64% of these patients. Seventy percent of the lesions were de novo and 30% restenotic. Calcification was present in 42% of lesions, 25% of lesions involved a bifurcation, and 25% were located in tortuous vessels.

As shown in Table 2, 94.5% of lesions were successfully treated, with success defined as a reduction in lesion percent stenosis to <50% without death, Q wave myocardial infarction, or urgent coronary artery bypass surgery. Success was more likely in restenotic lesions (96.8%) than de novo lesions (93.6%, $P=0.0002$).

TABLE 2

Coronary Rotary Ablation Multicenter Registry Data

Number of Procedures	1,403
Number of Lesions	1,688
Males/Females	1,042/361
Mean Age	62.4
Overall Success	1,602 (95%)
Success by Lesion Location	
RCA	96%
LAD	93%
Circ	98%
Left Main Trunk	96%
Success by Lesion Type	
Type A	97%
Type B	96%
Type C	93%

RCA, right coronary artery; LAD, left anterior descending artery; Circ, circumflex artery; MI, circ infarction; CABG, coronary artery bypass grafting. (*Modified with permission from Reference 31.*)

Success rates were 96.0% in American Heart Association/American College of Cardiology type A lesions, 95.5% in type B lesions, 93% in type C lesions (P=0.0001, C vs. other). Success was more frequent in lesions that were <10 mm in length (94.9% vs. 93.0%, P=0.043). The presence of calcification did not reduce the success rate of the Rotablator in the 2,161 procedures in which a single lesion was treated (Table 3), despite the more frequent complex nature of these calcified lesions.[33,34] Death occurred in 0.9% of patients, Q wave myocardial infarction in 0.9%, and urgent coronary artery bypass grafting in 2.3%. In addition, 4.4% had a non-Q wave myocardial infarction.

The European registry contains data on 129 patients.[23] Over 50% of the patients had either severe exertional angina (53% Canadian Class III) or rest pain (10% Canadian Class IV). Forty-eight percent of the lesions were American Heart Association/American College of Cardiology Class A, 36% Class B, and 16% Class C. The success rate was 86% with 31% of the patients requiring balloon angioplasty because of an initially inadequate result. The mean percent stenosis decreased from 73±12% to 42±13%. There were no deaths, 1.3% of patients required urgent coronary bypass surgery, and 2.3% had a Q wave myocardial infarction.

In the Cleveland Clinic experience[26] with 153 patients and 164 lesions, the procedural success rate was 92%. Complication rates were similar to those in the multicenter registry. In-hospital death occurred in 1.3% of patients, Q wave myocardial infarction in 1.3%, emergency coronary artery bypass surgery in 2%, and 5.3% of patients had a non-Q wave myocardial infarction. At the Washington Hospital Center, angiographic failure, defined as a residual stenosis >50% by quantitative angiography, occurred in 3.3% of lesions treated, and procedural failure (angiographic failure or death, Q wave myocardial infarction or urgent coronary artery bypass surgery) in 4.9% of cases. Both angiographic and procedural

TABLE 3

Procedural Outcome of Calcified and Noncalcified Lesions

Lesions	Success	Death	CABG	Q wave MI
Calcified	1,106 (94%)	14 (1.3%)	24 (2.2%)	6 (0.6%)
Noncalcified	1,031 (95%)	5 (0.5%)	26 (2.4%)	5 (0.5%)
P	ns	0.04	ns	ns

Success = <50% residual stenosis without major complication. CABG, coronary artery bypass surgery; MI, myocardial infarction.

failures were more common in angulated lesions with proximal tortuosity. High success rates were achieved even in complex lesions, with 94.8% in calcified lesions, 94.1% in eccentric lesions, 94.7% in lesions greater than 10 mm, 94.7% in de novo lesions, and 90.6% in lesions with >45° angulation.[35]

Bertrand et al.[31] reported the results of rotational atherectomy as assessed by quantitative angiography. In 47 patients treated by Rotablator alone, the mean burr to artery ratio was 0.70 ± 0.17. The diameter of the lesion as a percentage of the reference vessel diameter fell significantly from 72%±10% to 40%±13%. In 30 patients treated with Rotablator and adjunctive PTCA, the lesion diameter was reduced from 74%±9.2% to 30%±9.8%.

Recoil

Lesions treated with high-speed rotational atherectomy have less recoil than those treated primarily with PTCA. These data need to be interpreted with caution, as the Rotablator often causes arterial spasm that may reduce both vessel and lesion diameters. However, Safian et al.[36] reported that the lumen produced by the Rotablator is equal to 91% of the burr diameter, with only 9% of the burr diameter "lost" due to recoil or spasm. Gilmore et al.[37] reported significantly less recoil 24 hours after rotablation than occurred after balloon angioplasty (0% vs. 57%, $P<0.001$).[37]. This lack of lesion recoil after rotational atherectomy has been confirmed by other investigators.[31]

Complications

Coronary artery dissection and perforation have been reported after rotational atherectomy. Data from the multicenter registry showed that dissection was reported in 13% of treated lesions, 73% of which were caused by the passage of the burr and the remainder were visible only after adjunctive balloon angioplasty.[38] Dissection is seen more frequently in tortuous, eccentric and longer lesions and resulted in acute closure in 14% of dissections (1.8% of all treated lesions).[38] Acute closure is relatively infrequent after rotational atherectomy; the reported incidence ranges from 1.4% to 7.8%.[23,26,38,39] It is more frequent in hinge lesions and long lesions and is seen less frequently when lesions are treated with a small burr first.[39] Coronary perforation has been reported in 1.4% of treated lesions; of five patients reported by Ellis et al.[25] three required urgent bypass surgery, and two died. Perforation was more frequent in lesions located on a bend (odds ratio=4.0, $P=0.039$).

Restenosis

Restenosis rates have varied between series from 25% to 40%. These are similar to the restenosis rates reported with balloon angioplasty. Five hundred and forty-six of the patients in the United States Multicenter Rotary Ablation Registry have had angiographic follow-up.[31] Restenosis, defined as a recurrent lesion >50% diameter narrowing, occurred in 43% of patients. The restenosis rate in lesions treated with the Rotablator alone was 40%. When adjunctive balloon angioplasty was used, the restenosis rate was 46%. In the European experience, angiographic follow-up was reported from 57.3% of patients at a mean of 4.6 months.[23] The restenosis rate was 37.8%, 46% in those who had Rotablator alone, and 29.7% in those who had adjunctive balloon angioplasty. The restenosis rate for de novo lesions appears to be lower (27.8%) than for restenotic lesion (32.5%).[40]

Indications for Rotational Atherectomy

The indications for rotational atherectomy include discrete complex lesions, especially those that are calcified, ostial, or cannot be dilated. The complications of rotational atherectomy are higher for diffuse, angulated lesions or those in patients with recent myocardial infarction. Data from the United States Multicenter Registry on the use of rotational atherectomy show that success is more likely in restenotic lesions (96.8%) than de novo lesions (93.6%, $P=0.0002$), and in lesions ≤ 10 mm in length (94.9% vs. 93.0%, $P=0.043$).[32] The presence of tortuosity, eccentricity, calcification, bifurcation lesion and stenosis >90% were not predictive of outcome. Successful use of the Rotablator in chronic occlusions has been reported in a small number of patients,[41] but its role in this situation has not been established. Similarly, although one report indicates that saphenous vein graft lesions can be successfully treated with rotational atherectomy, restenosis occurred in eight of the nine patients reported,[42] and the risk of embolization from diseased vein grafts is likely to be excessive.

Calcified Lesion

We recently reported data from 2,161 procedures on 1,078 calcified and 1,083 noncalcified lesions.[33] The patients with calcified lessons had a mean age of 65.9 years that was significantly older than the group with noncalcified lesions whose mean age was 60.5

years (*P* = 0.001). The calcified lesions were located in tortuous vessels more frequently (27% vs. 22%, *P* = 0.02), were more often eccentric (75% vs. 64%, *P* = 0.0001), were longer (32% vs. 27%, ≥ 10 mm in length, *P* = 0.01), more frequently ACC/AHA type C (26% vs. 11%, *P* = 0.0001) and located in the left anterior descending coronary artery more frequently (51% vs. 44%, *P* = 0.001). The procedural outcome of these patients is shown in Table 3. There was no difference in procedural success between the two groups. Complication rates were similar, but more patients with calcified lesions died following the procedure (1.3% vs. 0.5%, *P* = 0.04). Leon et al.[43] also reported on the use of the Rotablator to treat calcified lesions. The success rate of rotational atherectomy as a stand-alone procedure was 82% in the 220 calcified lesions and 86% in the 275 noncalcified lesions. After adjuctive balloon angioplasty, the success rate for both groups was 95%. Intravascular ultrasound has also demonstrated that the Rotablator effectively removes calcified lesions (Figure 4, panels A–E).[19] Because of these high success rates, rotational atherectomy has become the treatment of choice for heavily calcified lesions.

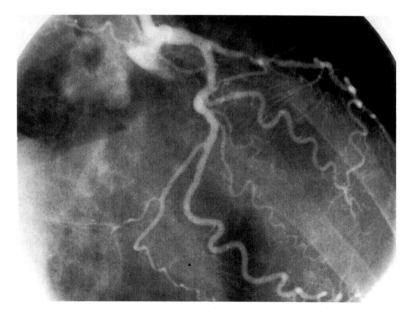

Figure 4. *A complex irregular lesion in the proximal left anterior descending coronary artery (**A**). Intravascular ultrasound from within the lesion. Note the heavy calcification*

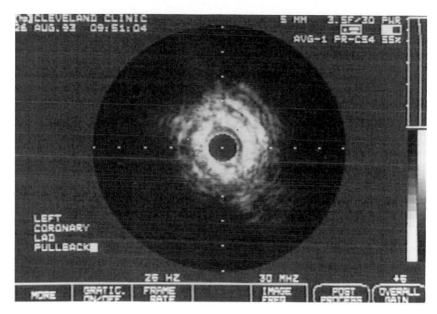

FIGURE 4B. *Stand-alone rotational atherectomy using a 1.75-mm burr.*

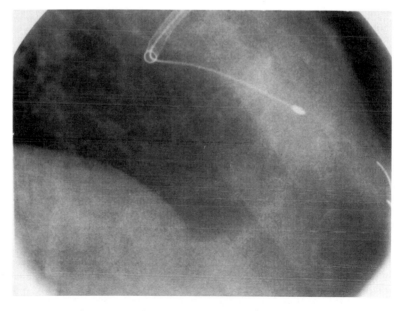

FIGURE 4C. *Subsequent further rotational atherectomy was performed with a 2.25-mm burr. Target lesion postrotational atherectomy.*

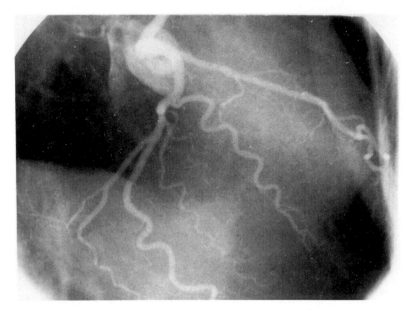

FIGURE 4D. *Intravascular ultrasound from lesion site following Rotablator demonstrating the removal of calcium.*

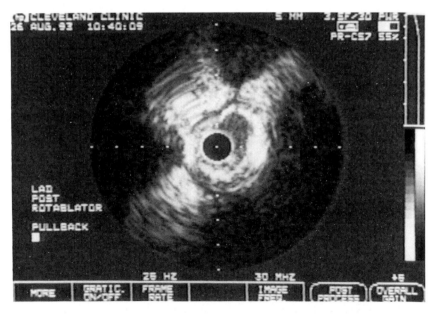

FIGURE 4E. *(Ultrasounds courtesy of Dr. S. Nissan.)*

Ostial Lesions

Percutaneous balloon angioplasty has lower success rates and high restenosis rates for ostial lesions. Goudreau et al.[44] reported a 97% success rate in the 31 ostial lesions they treated with rotational atherectomy. Complication rates were low, and the acute angiographic result was not influenced by lesion morphology. Kent et al.[45] reported the registry data on 147 ostial lesions treated with rotational atherectomy. Procedural success was achieved in 93% of lesions, coronary artery bypass surgery was required in 3.4%, 2.1% died and none had a Q wave myocardial infarction. Angiographic restenosis occurred in 47% of the patients. These results compare well to those of percutaneous balloon angioplasty, which has been reported to have a success rate of 75% to 88% in ostial lesions with a 13% major complication rate.[15,46,47] The Rotablator is highly effective in treating ostial lesions, especially when they are calcified.

Complex Lesions

The Rotablator has a high success rate in complex lesions. In order to assess the influence of multiple angiographic risk factors on procedural success, we analyzed data on 874 lesions.[34] The angiographic risk factors considered were lesion calcification, lesion eccentricity, lesion length >10 mm, stenosis severity, the presence of a bifurcation within the lesion, and proximal vessel tortuosity. The overall success rate was 95%. Individually, these angiographic risk factors did not reduce the success rate. Furthermore, success was not reduced by increasing lesion complexity. When no angiographic risk factor was present, the success rate was 96%, with one factor it was 95%, two factors 95%, and three factors 97% (P=NS). These data suggest that the presence of one or more angiographic risk factor does not reduce procedural success, and that use of the Rotablator should be considered in complex lesions.

Undilatable Lesions

Brogan et al[48] reported their experience with rotational atherectomy in a group of patients in whom percutaneous transluminal balloon angioplasty had been unsuccessful. Rotational atherectomy was used in 41 patients in whom balloon angioplasty was unsuccessful because of either lesion rigidity (inability to dilate), inability to cross the lesion with a balloon or elastic recoil. The percent diameter stenosis was reduced from a mean of 72%±14% to 41%±16% with the Rotablator. In 20% of lesions a significant (>50%) lesion remained after high-speed rotational atherectomy, but after adjunctive PTCA, the angiographic success rate was 49 of 50 lesions (98%). Procedural success was obtained in 90% of cases. One patient died of left ventricular failure and two required urgent coronary artery bypass surgery because of acute vessel closure. Restenosis occurred in 35% of the patients who had follow-up angiography, and 24% of the group developed recurrent symptoms. Therefore, rotational atherectomy enables the treatment of selected lesions that previously were not amenable to percutaneous interventions.

Summary

Rotational coronary atherectomy with the Rotablator provides a means to ablate coronary artery lesions, leaving a polished smooth residual lesion. The effectiveness and safety of the Rotablator has been proven by numerous studies. Indications for the use of the Rotablator include discrete lesions, especially those that are calcified, ostial or complex. It must be used with caution however, as complications can occur, especially in long, angulated lesions.

The Rotablator has widened the indications and improved the success of percutaneous coronary interventions. However, in the absence of randomized trials, its benefit over conventional therapy has not been definitively proven, except in cases of PTCA failure. Several issues remain to be resolved, in particular the correct balance between the degree of high-speed rotational atherectomy required prior to adjunctive balloon angioplasty, and the long-term effectiveness of adjunctive PTCA versus stand-alone rotational atherectomy. These issues and the exact role of high-speed rotational atherectomy will be established by a series of clinical trials that are planned for the near future.

Acknowledgments

The authors would like to thank Dr. Maree Barnes and Kathryn Brock for their editorial assistance, and Paula Shalling and Brian Keough for preparing the figures.

References

1. Gruentzig AR. Transluminal dilatation of coronary artery stenoses. *Lancet.* 1978;1:268.
2. Gruentzig AR, Senning A, Siegenthaler WE. Nonoperative dilatation of coronary artery stenoses. Percutaneous transluminal coronary angioplasty. *N Engl J Med.* 1979;301:61–68.

3. Stack RS. Impact of new technology on interventional cardiology. *J Interven Cardiol.* 1992;5:51–56.
4. Weintraub WS, Jones EL, King SB, et al. Changing use of coronary angioplasty and coronary artery bypass surgery in the treatment of chronic coronary artery disease. *Am J Cardiol.* 1990;65:183–188.
5. Kahn JK, Hartzler GO. Frequency and cause of failure with contemporary balloon angioplasty and implications for new technology. *Am J Cardiol.* 1990;66:858–860.
6. Ellis SE, Roubin GS, King SB. Angiographic and clinical predictors of acute closure after native coronary vessel angioplasty. *Circulation.* 1988;77:372–379.
7. Cowley MJ, Dorros G, Kelsey SF, et al. Acute coronary events associated with percutaneous transluminal coronary angioplasty. *Am J Cardiol.* 1984;53:112C 116C.
8. Bredlau CE, Roubin GS, Leimgruber P, et al. In-hospital morbidity in patients undergoing elective coronary angioplasty. *Circulation.* 1985;72:1044–1052.
9. Levine S, Ewels CJ, Rosing DR, et al. Coronary angioplasty: Clinical and angiographic follow up. *Am J Cardiol.* 1985;55:673–676.
10. Holmes DR, Vliestra RE, Smith HC, et al. Restenosis after percutaneous transluminal coronary angioplasty: a report from the National Heart, Lung and Blood Institute. *Am J Cardiol.* 1984;53:77C–81C.
11. Nobuyoshi M, Kimura T, Nosaka H, et al. Restenosis after successful percutaneous coronary angioplasty: serial angiographic follow up of 299 patients. *J Am Coll Cardiol.* 1988;12:616–623.
12. Beatts KJ, Serruys PW, Hugenholtz PG. Restenosis after coronary angioplasty: new standards for clinical studies. *J Am Coll Cardiol.* 1990;15:491–498.
13. Ellis SG, Vandormael MG, Cowley MJ, et al. Coronary morphologic and clinical determinants of procedural outcome with angioplasty for multivessel disease. Implications for patient selection. *Circulation.* 1990;82:1193–1202.
14. Kuntz RE, Hinohara T, Safian RD, Selmon MR, Simpson JB, Baim DS. Restenosis after directional coronary atherectomy. Effects of luminal diameter and deep wall excision. *Circulation.* 1992;86:1394–1399.
15. Topol EJ, Leya F, Pinkerton CA, et al. A comparison of directional atherectomy with coronary angioplasty in patients with coronary artery disease. The CAVEAT Study Group. *N Engl J Med.* 1993;329:221–227.
16. Carrozza JP, Kuntz RE, Levine MJ, et al. Angiographic and clinical outcome of intracoronary stenting: immediate and long term results from a large single-center experience. *J Am Coll Cardiol.* 1992;20:328–337.
17. Hansen DD, Auth DC, Vrako R, et al. Rotational atherectomy in atherosclerotic rabbit iliac arteries. *Am Heart J.* 1988;115:160–165.
18. Ahn SS, Arca MJ, Marcus JR, et al. Histological and morphological effects of rotational atherectomy on human cadaver arteries. *Ann Vasc Surg* 1990;4:563–569.
19. Mintz GS, Potkin BN, Keren G, et al. Intravascular ultrasound evaluation of the effect of rotational atherectomy in obstructive atherosclerotic coronary artery disease. *Circulation.* 1992;86:1383–1393.
20. Bass TA, Gilmore PS, White CJ, et al. Surface luminal characteristics following coronary rotational atherectomy (PTCRA) vs. balloon angioplasty (PTCA): angioscopic, ultrasound and angiographic evaluation. *J Am Coll Cardiol.* 1993;21:444A. Abstract.

21. Ahn SS, Auth D, Marcus DR, et al. Removal of focal atheromatous lesions by angioscopically guided high speed rotary atherectomy. *J Vasc Surg.* 1988;7:292–300.
22. Sherman CT, Bruken R, Chan A, Krivokapich J, Buchbinder M. Myocardial perfusion and segmental wall motion after coronary rotational atherectomy. *Circulation.* 1992;86:I-652. Abstract.
23. Bertrand ME, Lablanche JM, Leroy F, et al. Percutaneous Transluminal coronary rotary ablation with Rotablator (European Experience). *Am J Cardiol.* 1992;69:470–474.
24. O'Neill WW. Mechanical rotational atherectomy. *Am J Cardiol.* 1992; 69:12F–18F.
25. Ellis SE, Franco I, Satler LF, Whitlow PL. Slow reflow and coronary perforation after Rotablator therapy—Incidence; clinical, angiographic and procedural predictors. *Circulation.* 1992;86:I-652. Abstract.
26. Villa AE, Whitlow PL. Rotational coronary atherectomy. In: Topol EJ, ed. *Textbook of Interventional Cardiology.* Philadelphia: W.B. Saunders; 1993:135–146.
27. Zotz R, Stahr P, Erbel R, et al. Analysis of high frequency rotational angioplast induced echo contrast. *Cathet Cardiovasc Diagn.* 1991;22: 137–144.
28. Fajadet J, Doucet S, Caillard J, et al. Coronary rotational ablation in complex lesions: clinical, angiographic and procedural predictors of success and complications. *Circulation.* 1992;86:I-511. Abstract.
29. Nino CL, Freed M, Blankenship L, et al. Procedural cost and benefits of new interventional devices. *J Am Coll Cardiol.* 1993;21(2):78A.
30. Teirstein PS, Warth DC, Haq N, et al. High speed rotational coronary atherectomy for patients with diffuse coronary artery disease. *J Am Coll Cardiol.* 1991;18:1694–1701.
31. Bertrand ME, Bauters C, Lablance JM. Percutaneous coronary rotational angioplasty with the Rotablator. In: Topol EJ, ed. *Textbook of Interventional Cardiology.* 2nd ed. Philadelphia: W.B.Saunders; 1993: 659–667.
32. MacIsaac AI, Whitlow PL, Cowley MJ, Buchbinder M. Angiographic predictors of outcome of coronary rotational atherectomy from the completed multicenter registry. *J Am Coll Cardiol.* 1994;23:353A.
33. MacIsaac AI, Whitlow PL, Cowley MJ, Buchbinder M. Coronary rotational atherectomy for calcified and non calcified lesions: final registry report. *J Am Coll Cardiol.* 1994;23:285A.
34. Whitlow PL, Buchbinder M, Kent K, Kipperman R, Bass T, Cleman M. Coronary rotational atherectomy: angiographic risk and their relationship to success/complications. *J Am Coll Cardiol.* 1992;19:334A.
35. Popma JJ, Satler LF, Pichard AD, et al. Clinical and angiographic predictors of procedural outcome after rotational coronary atherectomy in complex lesions. *J Am Coll Cardiol.* 1993;21:228A. Abstract.
36. Safian RD, Niazi KA, Strzelecki M, et al. Detailed angiographic analysis of high-speed mechanical rotational atherectomy in human coronary arteries. *Circulation.* 1993;88:961–968.
37. Gilmore PS, Bass TA, Conetta DA, et al. Coronary intravascular ultrasound delineation of elastic recoil following balloon angioplasty and absence of recoil following rotational atherectomy. *Circulation.* 1992;86:I-331. Abstract.
38. Satler LF, Warth D. Dissection after high speed rotational atherec-

tomy: frequency, predictive factors and clinical consequences. *Circulation*. 1992;86:I-785. Abstract.

39. Ellis SE, Popma JJ, Raymond RR, Whitlow PL. Abrupt coronary occlusion after Rotablator therapy—Incidence; clinical, angiographic and procedural predictors. *Circulation*. 1992;86:I-652. Abstract.

40. Rosenblum J, Zipkin RE, Myler RK, Murphy MC, Hansell HN. Restenosis after successful rotational ablation. *Circulation*. 1992;86:I-653. Abstract.

41. Warth D, Cowley M. Percutaneous transluminal coronary rotational ablation of total coronary occlusions. *Circulation*. 1992;86:I-781.

42. Bass TA, Gilmore PS, Buchbinder M, Cleman MW, Stertzer SH. Coronary rotational atherectomy (PTCRA) in patients with prior coronary revascularization: a registry report. *Circulation*. 1992;86:I-653.

43. Leon MB, Kent KM, Pichard AD, et al. Percutaneous transluminal rotational angioplasty of calcified lesions. *Circulation*. 1992;84:II-84.

44. Goudreau E, Cowley MJ, DiSciascio G, deBottis D, Vetrovec GW, Sabri N. Rotational atherectomy for aorto-ostial and branch ostial lesion. *J Am Coll Cardiol*. 1993;21:31A.

45. Kent KM, Stertzer S, Bass T, et al. High speed rotational ablation in patients with ostial lesions. *Circulation*. 1992;86:I-512.

46. Bedotto JB, McConahay DR, Rutherford BD, et al. Balloon angioplasty of aorto-ostial coronary stenoses revisited. *Circulation*. 1991;84:II-251. Abstract.

47. Mathias DW, Fishman JM, Lange HW, et al. Frequency of success and complications of coronary angioplasty of a stenosis at the ostium of a branch. *Am J Cardiol*. 1991;67:491–495.

48. Brogan WC, Popma JJ, Pichard AD, et al. Rotational coronary atherectomy after unsuccessful coronary balloon angioplasty. *Am J Cardiol*. 1993;71:794–798.

Chapter 15

Ultrasound Angioplasty

Robert J. Siegel, MD, Wolfgang Steffen, MD,
Julian Gunn, MD, Michael C. Fishbein, MD,
and David C. Cumberland, MD

Catheter-Delivered Ultrasound Ablation Angioplasty

Therapeutic intravascular ultrasound is markedly different from intravascular ultrasound imaging as lower frequencies (of nonionizing mechanical energy, namely 19–30 kHz) are used for therapeutic ultrasound compared to those (10–40 MHz) used in diagnostic intravascular imaging.

Using a 20-kHz system, probe tip oscillations of 20–110 μm at a rate of 20,000 cycles per second or 1.2 million times per minutes are produced causing mechanical ablation characteristics not seen with the high-frequency megahertz diagnostic intravascular imaging catheters. The effects of therapeutic ultrasound on tissue are thought to be due to: 1) mechanical pulverization; 2) the formation of intracellular microcurrents; 3) thermal warming; and 4) cavitation.

In hard arterial plaques, those that are calcified or densely fibrotic, the mechanism of therapeutic ultrasonic angioplasty is primarily mechanical, resulting from the rapid (approximately 20,000 cycles per second or greater) movement of the titanium ball-tipped probe impacting on the rigid, immobile segments of the arterial wall. Normal compliant portions of blood vessels are not significantly damaged due to the small amplitude (20–110 μm) of motion of the probe, as the vessel wall tends to move out of the way of the vibrating probe tip. This process can be likened to an orthopedic cast-cutting device that cuts through the rigid immobile plaster

From Vetrovec GW, Carabello BA, (eds.) *Invasive Cardiology: Current Diagnostic and Therapeutic Issues.* Armonk, NY: Futura Publishing Company, Inc.: © 1996.

cast without harming the normal (elastic) underlying skin that moves away from the cutter's teeth.[1] The longitudinal and transverse oscillation of the probe tip (20,000 cycles per second), as well as nonlinear interactions of sound waves contribute to the mechanical alterations induced by catheter-delivered high-intensity, low-frequency ultrasound. Sinusoidal ultrasonic waves have been shown to propagate in the direction of the probe as force is generated within the medium. As the speed of sound increases with pressure, the pressure maxima of the wave travels faster than the pressure minima, resulting in a distortion of the ultrasonic pressure waveform. This generates harmonics, with a pressure component that is thought to cause tissue alterations.[2]

High-intensity ultrasound exerts nonthermal cellular effects independent of the presence of standing ultrasonic waves. These effects are considered to be caused by acoustic streaming and cavitation.[3] Acoustic streaming, defined as the unidirectional movement in an acoustic pressure field, results from the radiation pressure that is produced when an ultrasound wave travels through a compressible medium such as cell suspensions or tissue. High-velocity gradients, located at boundaries within the acoustic field, induce intense short stresses that can, if sufficiently high, impact on cells and adjacent membranes.[4]

Heating of tissues may result from dissipation of the ultrasound probe's mechanical energy. Thermal effects can be avoided with the use of an irrigation solution to cool the ultrasound probe. Without irrigation, however, we have generated probe temperatures with continuous wave energy in excess of 75°C.[5,6] Thermal energy at this temperature may either facilitate therapeutic tissue ablation or cause tissue damage. However, we believe thermal effects should be avoided to prevent undesired tissue damage. Therefore, we infuse saline during activation of the probe. When 10 mL/min of irrigation fluid is applied during ultrasound activation of the coronary probe, the temperature, as assessed with a thermocouple, rises <2°C in the arterial wall when using the coronary ultrasound catheter (Baxter Edwards, Irvine, CA).

Cavitation is the formation of microbubbles in tissues or fluids in response to the alternating pressure fields induced by an acoustic field. Ultrasound dissolution of thrombi is thought to be primarily due to stable and unstable cavitation, defined as the generation and subsequent collapse of vapor-filled cavities (bubbles) in tissues, fluids, or cells.[7,8] These cavitation nuclei are thought to result from the consolidation of gas dissolved in the medium or tissue. Cavitation during pulsed or continuous wave ultrasound produces effects when bubbles formed at the probe tip implode.

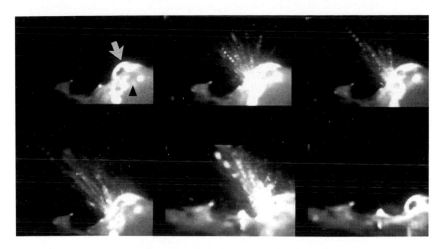

FIGURE 1. *High-speed filming at 1,500 frames per second reveals ultrasound effect on an in vitro clot. The **middle top panel** shows initial activation of ultrasound energy. The clot is liquified in milliseconds. In the **top left panel** the white arrow identifies probe tip and an arrowhead identifies the clot. The time sequence goes left to right along top panel, and then followed by bottom panel left to right.*

Such implosions generate several atmospheres of pressure. Maximal cavitation occurs at the interface of materials with differing acoustic impedance. The asymmetric collapse of these bubbles close to a tissue boundary results in the generation of high-speed cavitation microjets. As shown in Figure 1 using high-speed filming at 1,500 frames per second, we have found support for cavitation being the primary mechanism of ultrasound clot dissolution as microbubbles form and implode at the probe tip. The collapse of these bubbles results in intense shear stresses that are thought to mediate important aspects of the effects of ultrasound energy on thrombus and possibly on plaque as well.

Plaque Ablation In Vitro

Since 1965 there have been 12 in vitro studies[9–20] that have shown that catheter-delivered ultrasound ablates human atherosclerotic plaques and can recanalize calcific atherosclerotic occlusions (Figure 2). In more than 1,000 human arteries, ultrasound effectively ablated and/or recanalized occluded vessels. Despite varied experimental designs, ultrasound power outputs ranging from

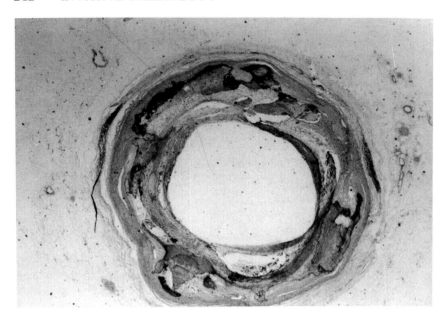

FIGURE 2. *Histologic arterial cross section from the occluded calcific and atherosclerotic coronary artery recanalized by ultrasound ablation shows a smooth lumenal surface.*

20 to 250 W, and ultrasonic frequencies ranging from 19.5 to 30 kHz, investigators were able to demonstrate plaque ablation.

Effects on the Arterial Wall

Catheter-delivered ultrasound increases the distensibility of postmortem in vitro calcific atherosclerotic human arteries.[21] Figure 3 demonstrates that intra-arterial pressure-volume curves are altered after exposure to ultrasound. The left curve shows the pressure-volume relationship before ultrasound exposure; the right curve illustrates the change in the pressure-volume relationship after 2 minutes of ultrasound ablation. This rightward shift in the pressure curve is indicative of increased arterial distensibility after ultrasound application. This change in vessel distensibility could result clinically in the facilitation of balloon dilatation of calcific or "balloon dilation resistant" lesions.

Figure 4 illustrates findings from an in vitro study of perfusion mounted rabbit aortas by Fischell et al.[22] They found that ultrasound induced vasodilation, and that it was independent of the

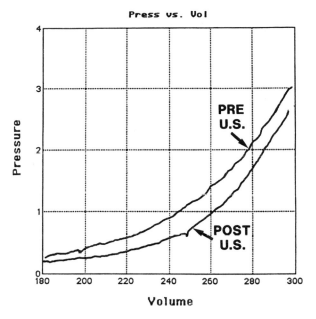

FIGURE 3. *Effect of ultrasound on compliance of atherosclerotic artery. Pressure-volume curves obtained prior to (left curve) and immediately after application of ultrasound energy (right curve) to calcific atherosclerotic arteries. The right ward shift is indicative of increased arterial distensibility after ultrasound exposure (Reproduced with permission from Siegel RJ, Cumberland DC, Crew JR. Ultrasound recanalization of diseased arteries. In: The Surgical Clinics of North America. Ahn S, Seeger J, eds. Philadelphia, PA: W.B. Saunders Co.; 1992.)*

presence or absence of arterial endothelium.[22] As demonstrated by electron microscopy and by the ability of vessels to reconstrict after ultrasound, vasodilation was not due to arterial damage. Importantly, vasodilation occurs with the same amount of ultrasound energy used to ablate diseased coronary arteries in a clinical setting.

In Vivo Animal Studies

Plaque Ablation

Prior to clinical testing, we studied two different animal models of arterial occlusion for evaluation of ultrasound plaque abla-

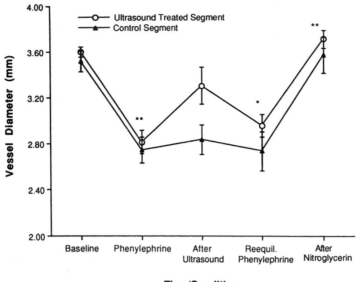

FIGURE 4. *Effects of ultrasound energy on arterial relaxation. Rabbit aortas after precontraction with phenylephrine show ultrasound dose dependent (watts), vasodilation; the aortas are also able to reconstrict in response to reexposure to phenylephrine, and again vasodilate after exposure to nitroglycerin. (Reproduced with permission from Reference 22.)*

tion. Figure 5A shows a long, subtotal, superficial femoral artery stenosis with extensive collateral circulation. This fibrocellular lesion was induced in the dog's femoral artery several months previously.[1] After ultrasound recanalization (Figure 5B), the artery appears more widely patent and the collateral vessels are no longer present. Histology (Figure 5C) reveals a smooth residual lesion that is eccentric, but without thermal damage or blast injury. In our cases of canine fibrocellular occlusions and stenoses, there was a reduction from 93%±13% to 40%±14% after passage of the ultrasound probe.[6]

The other model we have used[5] consists of occluded human atherosclerotic arteries that were implanted into dog arteries (aorta, carotid, iliac). The occluded xenografts were guide wire resistant as well as impassable to the nonactivated ultrasound probe (excluding the Dotter effect when ultrasound recanalization was performed). In this study using this xenograft model the ultrasound probe recanalized obstructions of up to 7 cm in length in an average of 3.2 minutes. There were no ultrasound-related vessel perfo-

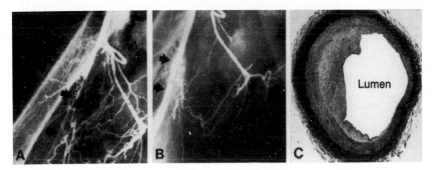

FIGURE 5. *Recanalization of chronic canine fibrocellular, femoral arterial occlusion.* **A.** *Prior to ultrasound angioplasty a long and severely narrowed right femoral artery is seen with extensive collateral vessels.* **B.** *After ultrasound angioplasty, the lumen appears wider and the collateral vessels have disappeared on the angiogram.* **C.** *A histologic section from a cross section of femoral artery exposed to ultrasound angioplasty demonstrates a mild residual fibrous eccentric stenosis without arterial damage. (Hematoxylin and eosin stain) (Reproduced with permission from Reference 1.)*

rations. Ultrasound alone resulted in an occlusion decrease to a 62% residual stenosis; subsequent balloon angioplasty further reduced it to 29%±13%. No evidence of ultrasound-induced vasospasm, thrombosis, or arterial dissection was found by angiography. Histology revealed occasional deposition of platelets and fibrin at the site of recanalization, but no other significant histologic abnormalities, including thermal damage.[5]

Freeman[23] and Gal[24] tested ultrasound angioplasty in Yucatan microswine with fibrous atherosclerotic lesions. These atherosclerotic lesions in Yucatan microswine consist principally of collagen with minimal calcium or lipid. Their catheter-delivered ultrasound probe recanalized high-grade porcine arterial stenoses or occlusions without ultrasound-associated vascular trauma or perforation. In Freeman's study the residual stenoses ranged from 20% to 30% after the use of ultrasound recanalization in subtotal occlusions.[23] The findings from our canine studies and the work in porcine models by Freeman and Gal on over 40 vessels (femoral and iliac arteries) demonstrate that stenoses are reduced and occlusions recanalized with catheter-delivered, high-intensity, low-frequency ultrasound. Neither significant particle embolization or ultrasound-mediated perforation were found to be problematic in the studies of these animal models.

All interventional devices that ablate or disrupt plaque such as laser,[25] high-speed rotational atherectomy (Rotablator™, Heart Technology, Inc., Redmond, WA),[26] Kensey catheter,[27] as well as ultrasound generate particulate debris. Lane[10] and Dobrinski[12] have reported particulates <5 μm. Monteverde et al[15] have measured particulates of up to 110 ± 30 μm. In using a peripheral ultrasound ablation device with probe tip oscillations of 50 ± 25 μm, we found 95% of particulates measured <25 μm. However, when using a coronary device with a probe tip applitude of 15–30 μm, 99% of the particulates measured <10 μm. The differences in the reported particle sizes could be a result of using different ultrasound ablation systems, as well as using different methods to analyze those particulates. After injecting the effluent from recanalized calcific coronary arterial segments measuring 1–3 cm long into the left coronary artery of three dogs in vivo, we found no evidence of myocardial ischemia or injury by ECG, no emboli by selective coronary arteriography, no wall motion by left ventriculography or myocardial necrosis histologic studies. Current data indicate the particulates generated by ultrasound plaque ablation are similar in size to those particulates that have been reported for lasers and the high-speed rotational ablation catheter (Rotablator).

Thrombus Dissolution

In our initial series of in vitro studies of ultrasound for thrombus dissolution, we found that it was rapid and effective. The particulate size was largely <10 μm, and was not affected by the addition of streptokinase.[28] Hong (from our laboratory) demonstrated that ultrasound lysis did not produce a significant increase in D-dimer. These findings indicate that the fibrinolytic system is not activated during ultrasound clot dissolution.[28] Further, clot age did not affect the rate of disruption by ultrasound. Using a more powerful ultrasound probe system, we found that a power output of 23 W (102 μm peak-to-peak probe tip displacement) disrupted 1 g of thrombus in <15 seconds.[29] Of the particles measured using this system 99% were <10 μm in size. Marzelle and co-workers used ultrasound ablation and tissue plasminogen activator (TPA), and showed that this combination was synergistic in the dissolution of "chronic" collagen-containing thrombi.[30] Hartnell has recently described a prototype coronary ablation system (1.6 mm overall diameter) that in vitro has demonstrated effective thrombus dissolution.[31] Similarly, in our laboratory, we have been testing a 160-cm long 5F over-the-wire coronary ultrasound ablation probe (Baxter Edwards, Irvine, CA).[32] To study the efficacy of this monorail coronary ultrasound probe in dissolving clots, we exposed 1-, 2-, and 4-hour old human blood clots to catheter-delivered ultrasound for 1 to 3 minutes. We have exposed more than 200 clots in vitro with the coronary ultrasound ablation device. Using this ultrasound system, clots are dissolved at a rate of 100–200 mg/min. We have found that there is little difference in the dissolution rate if the probe is in a straight or bent configuration. Further, the irrigation of 10 mL/min routinely used with this device, does not cause clot dissolution in and of itself, but the irrigation does serve as a potent amplifier of ultrasound clot lysis—presumably by augmenting cavitation. Our in vitro data then document that this prototype monorail coronary ultrasound probe effectively dissolves clots in vitro.

In Vivo Animal Studies

Thrombus Dissolution

Initial studies on "ultrasound thrombolysis" were performed in 1975 by Trubestein, Stumpff, and colleagues.[33,34] They were able to disrupt and aspirate femoral arterial and venous thrombi in an in vivo canine model with a hollow 2-mm diameter metal probe. Rosenschein and co-workers studied catheter-delivered ultrasound thrombus disruption in a series of canine femoral arteries[14] and found that with occlusive and nonocclusive thrombi, the mean stenosis fell from 98% to 18% after ultrasound. Ariani et al.[29] from our laboratory also showed in an angiographic and angioscopic study of 21 canine femoral arteries that ultrasound dissolves arterial thrombi. High-intensity (25 W), low-frequency (20 kHz) ultrasound dissolved all thrombi in <4 minutes. Angioscopy studies revealed that ultrasound probe activation causes clot disruption. As shown in Figure 6, histologic studies of the femoral arteries after ultrasound recanalization revealed no intimal disruption, thermal or cavitational injury, occlusive distal embolization, or perforation. Recent work by Steffen et al. from our laboratory has shown the feasibility of in vivo thrombus dissolution in a series of canine coronary arteries. We have been able to demonstrate ultrasound recanalization of acute thrombotic coronary occlusions.[35] These findings suggest that this method could serve as an alternative or adjunct to systemic thrombolysis for myocardial infarction or other thrombus-mediated acute coronary ischemic syndromes.

The in vitro and in vivo animal studies on catheter-delivered ultrasound thrombus dissolution indicate that this method is effec-

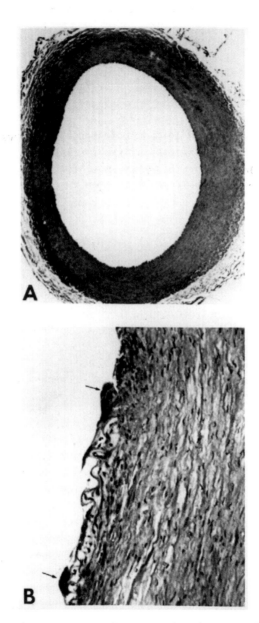

FIGURE 6. *Histologic section of a recanalized previously thrombosed artery. The arterial lumen is widely patent and free of thrombus. (Hematoxylin and Eosin stain; original magnification × 20). (Reproduced with permission from Reference 29.)*

tive, results in small particulate debris, is associated with minimal intimal damage, and is relatively rapid for thrombus dissolution.

Clinical Ultrasound Ablation System

We have utilized a low-frequency ultrasound system composed of an ultrasound generator, piezoelectric transducer, flexible metal waveguide and catheter (Baxter Edwards, Irvine, CA) (Figure 7). The system features include a 19.5 kHz operational frequency with a 50% duty cycle operating at 30 m/sec on and 30 m/sec off. Power activation is controlled by a foot or hand switch. Infusion of heparinized saline or crystalloid (10 mL/min for coronary and 25 mL/min for peripheral arteries) is used for adequate cooling of the waveguide inside the catheter body. The ultrasound energy is due to the alternate excitation of the piezoelectric crystals inside the transducer with positive and negative sine wave voltage. This results in expansion and contraction of the crystals proportionate to the applied voltage. The mechanical displacement generated from the crystals is amplified by an acoustical horn attached to the piezoelectric crystals. This system generates a longitudinal wave of energy (a compressional wave) that is then imparted to the waveguide, (ultrasound wire probe). Along the waveguide there are nodal points and antinodal points. The nodal points are areas within the metal where the molecules are stationary but are under maximum stress. The antinodal points are areas where the molecules show maximum displacement but minimum stress. The system is designed so that the antinodes occur at the transducer horn tip and the waveguide tip, in order to produce maximal tip displacement.

The ultrasound transducer containing the piezoelectric elements and the acoustic horn is hand-held during the ultrasound ablation procedure. This transducer is an amplifier that transmits the sound waves from piezoceramic crystals to the wire (titanium) probe. The range of power output at the acoustic horn using the current Baxter system is up to 25 W, depending on the setting used.

Clinical Cases

Peripheral Arterial Studies

We have used percutaneous ultrasound angioplasty to treat 50 peripheral arterial lesions in 45 patients.[36] The clinical indication

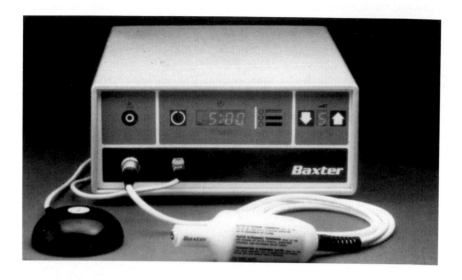

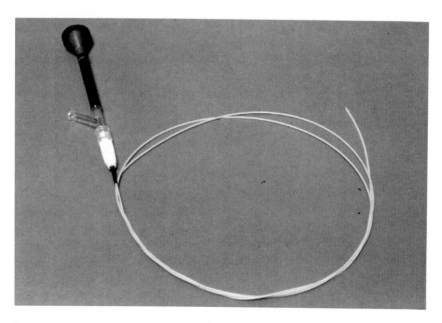

FIGURE 7. Top. *Baxter-Edwards Ultrasound Ablation System with power generator, transducer, and foot pedal.* **Bottom.** *Coronary of ultrasound probe used in initial clinical coronary trials.*

for peripheral arterial ultrasound angioplasty was disabling or worsening claudication of <100 m or resting limb ischemia manifested by lower extremity ulceration or gangrene. There were 35 arterial occlusions and 15 stenoses: 40 superficial femoral arterial lesions; 7 popliteal lesions; and 3 tibial-peroneal lesions. The minimum length of the 35 total arterial occlusions was 6.2±5.7 cm with a range in length from 0.5–28 cm. Radiographic calcification was present in one third of the lesions. Thirty of the 35 total occlusions were recanalized with the ultrasound probe. We failed to recanalize 5 lesions using the ultrasound catheter, as well as a number of different guide wire manipulations. Seven lesions were treated with stand-alone ultrasound angioplasty and the remainder received adjunctive balloon angioplasty. The baseline angiographic percent stenosis fell from 94% to 55% after ultrasound and to 12% after balloon angioplasty.

In the course of this study we changed from a non–over-the-wire probe to an over-the-wire system. The mean residual stenosis after ultrasound in cases undergoing subsequent balloon angioplasty was similar for both systems (62% vs. 56%, P=NS). However, after balloon angioplasty of the over-the-wire cases, the mean residual stenosis was 0% compared to 13.0%±7.1% for the non–over-the-wire cases (P<0.001). There were no differences in lesion length or percent stenosis before or after initial ultrasound treatment. The only apparent significant difference between the two groups of lesions was the duration of exposure of the arterial wall to ultrasound energy. With the over-the-wire system, arterial lesions were exposed to ultrasound energy for 1 min/cm of lesion length compared to <15 sec/cm of ultrasound energy for the straight, non–over-the-wire probe. The previously described in vitro studies using pressure-volume curves demonstrated that the distensibility of calcific atherosclerotic arteries increases after exposure to high-intensity low-frequency ultrasound. We believe that the significant difference in residual stenosis between the non–over-the-wire and over-the-wire probes is due to longer ultrasound exposure with the over-the-wire probe with secondary enhancement of arterial distensibility, which facilitated dilatation by adjunctive balloon angioplasty.

In our series of 50 peripheral arterial lesions, there was no evidence of distal embolization, acute reocclusion within the first 24 hours, or vasospasm. The recanalization rate (86%) is similar to that reported by investigators using other methods of accessing total femoropopliteal occlusions, such as laser angioplasty,[37,38] Kensey catheter,[39] or standard guide wire manipulation.[40–42] Because of differences in study design, population, and lesion type, and the relatively small number of cases used with any of the three ultrasound probe catheter designs, it is difficult to compare this technology to others for primary recanalization. Experimental in vitro, animal, and intraoperative studies, suggest that this method may result in a superior recanalization rate over guide wire techniques.[5,6,12,14,16] However, the precise role of the ultrasound ablation catheter system in guide wire resistant lesions needs to be determined.

Based on the 50 lesions treated, the safety profile of this technique appears comparable to other recanalization devices. However, early prototypes of this device were stiff with limited steerability. As a consequence, during advancement of the stiff probes (0.030-inch wire probe) at an oblique angle in occluded vessels, four mechanical perforations occurred as did four arterial dissections. None of these complications had significant clinical sequelae. No other clinical complications were identified. Importantly, no embolization was detected, no patient required surgical intervention, and no transducer or generator malfunctions were identified. While early probe designs were stiff and difficult to guide, the current system is more flexible and tracks over a guide wire. With the over-the-wire system, there have been no perforations, dissections, or other complications identified.

Our findings are compatible with the three other clinical series that have been reported. Rosenschein[43] also demonstrated the effectiveness of ultrasound angioplasty in an intraoperative study. In addition to recanalization of all seven occlusions studied, this study found that particulate size generated during ultrasound recanalization was small (89%±6% <30 μm). An intraoperative study by Drobinski and colleagues[44] evaluated ultrasound angioplasty in peripheral arteries. They angioscopically documented rapid thrombus dissolution by catheter-delivered ultrasound in 4 of 5 patients. Monteverde and co-workers[45] have used percutaneous peripheral ultrasound angioplasty to treat 50 lesions, with an 80% recanalization rate for total occlusions. They also had no evidence of distal emboli, but did have a 5% perforation rate with a non–over-the-wire system. In Monteverde's study, of the 23 patients treated by ultrasound alone, the restenosis rate was 12% at 1 year. Their findings along with the 20% clinical restenosis rate (not angiographic) found in our patients is lower than that reported with the use of other devices for peripheral vascular occlusions.

In summary, the clinical experience in treating peripheral arterial lesions[36,43–46] indicates that peripheral ultrasound angioplasty is feasible and safe. The clinical results consistent with the experimental in vitro and animal studies clearly demonstrate that catheter-delivered ultrasound is relatively atraumatic to the normal arterial wall, causes localized vasodilation, appears to enhance arterial distensibility, and debulks arterial lesions by plaque ablation and/or thrombus dissolution, and did generate detectable emboli in the patient group studied (82% arterial occlusions).

Preliminary Clinical Coronary Studies

Between January and March, 1993 we initiated a trial of percutaneous coronary ultrasound angioplasty in 19 patients.[20] The ultrasound probe system (Baxter-Edwards, Healthcare Corporation, Bentley Laboratories, Europe B.V., Uden, The Netherlands) that we used was a 4.6F catheter ensheathing a titanium wire probe that transmits the ultrasound energy. The ultrasound coronary catheter, or monorail design, is 160 cm long, has a 1.7-mm ball tip, a distal lumen that is flushed with heparinized saline at a rate of 10 mL/min to prevent heating of the probe during activation of ultrasound, and a lumen for an 0.014- or 0.018-inch coronary guide wire. This catheter is passable through an 8F guide catheter. The power output at the transducer was 16–20 W in a pulsed mode with a 50% duty cycle of 30 msec.

The 19 patients undergoing coronary ultrasound angioplasty were all symptomatic on medications and had obstructive single vessel coronary artery disease. Three of the patients had unstable angina. There were coronary lesions in the proximal or mid left anterior descending coronary artery (n=8) and in the midportion of the right coronary artery (n=11). The diameter stenosis for the group was 80%±12%. The average lesion length was 18 mm (range 4–7 mm). The minimal lumen diameter was 0.6±0.3 mm and the reference vessel diameters ranged from 2.5–3.5 mm. By ACC/AHA criteria, there were 6 type A, 10 type B, and 3 type C lesions.[47] The catheter-delivered ultrasound energy was applied for an average of 439 (range 138–890) seconds.

Our procedure for performing coronary ultrasound angioplasty is similar to that for standard coronary balloon angioplasty. We place an 8F introducer sheath in the patient's femoral artery and administer 10,000 units of heparin intravenously. Standard 8F guiding catheters are used for ultrasound and adjunctive balloon angioplasty. For standardization purposes, angiograms are done after 200 μg of intracoronary nitroglycerin at baseline, after ultrasound exposure, and after balloon angioplasty. The smallest luminal diameter within the stenosis, as well as a normal reference segment, were measured using a Philips digital quantitative angiographic system.

Adjunctive balloon angioplasty was performed on all patients. Eighteen of 19 patients were studied by repeat coronary arteriography 18–24 hours after the angioplasty procedure to reevaluate the acute results. Patients were discharged 24 hours after angiography on 75 mg of aspirin daily in addition to their standard medications.

Coronary ultrasound angioplasty reduced the stenosis in 17 of 19 coronary lesions treated. The percent reduction in the stenoses for the group was 20% from 80%±12% to 60%±18% ($P<0.0001$) and the mean (±SD) minimum lumen diameter (MLD) increased from 0.6±0.3mm to 1.1±0.5 ($P<0.001$) after application of catheter-delivered ultrasound energy. As shown in Figures 8 and 9, the residual lumenal contours appeared angiographically smooth with no clefts or haziness visible and there was brisk arterial run-off.

In one patient there was a guiding catheter-induced dissection of a right coronary artery after use of the ultrasound catheter. In this case, balloon dilatation failed to restore arterial patency, but there were no clinical sequelae. All the other 18 patients underwent successful adjunctive balloon angioplasty, with the final mean residual stenosis being 26%±11% ($P<0.001$) and the MLD increasing to 2.4±0.5 mm ($P<0.001$).

Potential complications were carefully monitored. There was no evidence of ultrasound-induced emboli, arterial dissection, perforation, vasospasm, abrupt closure, or bradyarrhythmias. There was no chest pain or significant electrocardiographic ST-T wave changes or rhythm disturbances associated with the intracoronary ultrasound angioplasty. In these studies, all patients were premedicated with intracoronary nitroglycerin. Subsequent ultrasound did not result in coronary vasodilation for the patients as a group but there was one case in which the coronary ultrasound probe reversed vasospasm after 30 seconds of exposure. This case had been unresponsive to 700 μg of intracoronary nitroglycerin.

During adjunctive balloon angioplasty after clinical coronary ultrasound angioplasty, it was noted that the mean balloon pressures to achieve full inflation, ie, the yield pressure of the underlying lesion, were relatively low at 2.7 (range 1–5.5) atmospheres. These findings are also consistent with our in vitro[21] and initial clinical observations in treating peripheral arteries.[46] Specifically, we noted that after ultrasound application, there was only a slight "waist" or deformation of the inflated balloon, suggesting that the arterial compliance or resistance of the lesions to pressure had

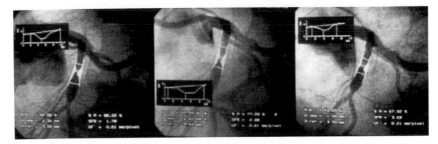

FIGURE 8. *Angiogram of left anterior descending coronary artery at base-line (**left**), after ultrasound (**middle**), and after adjunctive balloon angio-plasty (**right panel**)*

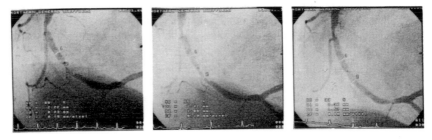

FIGURE 9. *Angiogram of right coronary artery at baseline (**left**), after ul-trasound (**middle**), and after adjunctive balloon angioplasty (**right panel**).*

been decreased.[46] There are three clinically significant implications of this ultrasound effect: first, the "nondilatable", balloon-resistant lesion may become amendable to balloon dilation after ultrasound ablation; second, dilation at a lower pressure may reduce the risk of acute dissection; and third, if the barotrauma of high balloon in-flation pressures potentiates the problem of restenosis, a method that reduces the requisite balloon inflation pressure might have a favorable impact on the long-term results of coronary balloon an-gioplasty.

At 24 hours of follow-up, all patients were free of chest pain and there was no ECG or cardiac enzyme evidence of myocardial damage in any patient. Repeat angiograms done 18–24 hours after coronary ultrasound angioplasty showed lumenal patency of all but one artery, a previously occluded left anterior descending. This artery silently reoccluded without pain, ECG, or creatine phospho-kinase changes. Subsequent repeat balloon angioplasty at 24 hours opened this vessel. For the remaining 17 patients, the mean MLD of 2.4 mm did not change on the 24-hour angiogram, but the arterial stenosis increased slightly from 26%±11% to 32%±11% in the same period (*P*<0.02).

Current limitations of the coronary ultrasound ablation device include the following: 1) only one probe tip size is presently available; 2) the size of the lumen generated is restricted by the probe tip size; 3) increased power output may be needed to augment plaque ablation; and 4) limited flexibility restricts application of ultrasound energy to the major epicardial coronary vessels. We believe that the use of larger probe tips as well as increasing the ultrasound power output to augment plaque ablation may result in more plaque ablation and a larger lumen size.

The findings of the experimental and clinical studies to date indicate that ultrasound angioplasty may have clinical utility as a device for: 1) facilitation of balloon angioplasty by lesion debulking and altering arterial distensibility; 2) the possible benefit of vasodilation during angioplasty; 3) the possible recanalization of complete occlusions; and 4) disruption of intra-arterial clot. Additional clinical studies will need to be performed in peripheral and coronary arteries to assess the potential benefits on the acute and long-term outcome of this new technique and to compare its outcomes with that of balloon angioplasty and other interventional technologies.

Acknowledgments

The authors acknowledge the numerous contributions made by Clare Wales, RN, Theresa De Bell, RN, and Martha Hibbitt.

References

1. Siegel RJ, Fishbein MC, Forrester J, et al. Ultrasound plaque ablation: a new method for recanalization of partially or totally occluded arteries. *Circulation.* 1988;78:1443–1448.
2. Miller DL. A review of the ultrasonic bioeffect of microsonation, gas-body activation, and related cavitation like phenomena. *Ultrasound Med Biol.* 1987;13:443–470.
3. Dyson M. Nonthermal cellular effects of ultrasound. *Br J Cancer.* 1982; 45:165–171.
4. Kerr CI, Gregory DW, Chan KK, et al. Ultrasound-induced damage of veins in pig ears as revealed by scanning electron microscopy. *Ultrasound Med & Biol.* 1989;15:45–52.
5. Siegel RJ, Don Michael TA, Fishbein MC, et al. In vivo ultrasound arterial recanalization of atherosclerotic total occlusions. *J Am Coll Cardiol.* 1990;15:345–351.

6. Siegel RJ, Ariani M, Forrester JS, et al. Cardiovascular applications of therapeutic ultrasound. *J Invasive Cardiol.* 1989;1:219–229.

7. Miller DL, Williams AR. Bubble cycling as the explanation of the promotion of ultrasonic cavitation in a rotating tube exposure system. *Ultrasound Med & Biol.* 1989;15:641–648.

8. Miller DL, Thomas RM, Williams AR. Mechanisms for hemolysis by ultrasonic cavitation in the rotating exposure system. *Ultrasound Med & Biol.* 1991;17:171–178.

9. Anschuetz R, Bernard HR. Ultrasonic irradiation and atherosclerosis. *Surgery.* 1965;57:549–553.

10. Lane WZ, Minot HD. Ultrasonic coronary endarterectomy. *Ann Thoracic Surg.* 1965;6:693–696.

11. Marracini P, Orsini E, Pelosi G, Landini L. Low frequency ultrasound energy for selective dissolution of atherosclerotic plaque. *Circulation.* 1988;81:235. Abstract.

12. Drobinski G, Kremer D. Elaboration d'un systeme a ultrasons pour desobstruction des artere coronaire. *Arch Mal Coeur.* 1989;82:377–380.

13. Ernst A, Schenk E, Woodlok T. Feasibility of high intensity ultrasound recnalization of human coronary arteries. *J Am Coll Cardiol.* 1990;15:104. Abstract.

14. Rosenschein U, Bernstein JJ, DiSegni E, et al. Experimental ultrasonic angioplasty. Disruption of atherosclerotic plaques and thrombi in vitro and arterial recanalization in vivo. *J Am Coll Cardiol.* 1990;15:711–717.

15. Monteverde C, Velez M, Liata R, et al. Angioplastia coronaria transluminal por ultrasonido. *Arch Inst Cardiol Mex.* 1990;60:27–38.

16. Ernst A, Schenk BA, Graccwski SM. Ability of high-intensity ultrasound to ablate human atherosclerotic plaques and minimize debris size. *Am J Cardiol.* 1991;68:242–246.

17. Muller-Leise CR, Schmitz-Rode T, Boehm N, et al. US-angioplasty: experimental in vitro penetration of fibrous and calcified atherosclerotic plaque. *Radiol Soc North Am.* 1991;181:170. Abstract.

18. Strunk H, Weber W, Steffen W, et al. Percutaneous sonographic angioplasty. Initial experimental results. *Rofo: Fortschritte auf dem Gebiete der Roentgenstrahlen und der neuen Bildgebenden Verfahren.* 1992;156:33–36.

19. Ernst A, Shenk EA, Woodlock TJ, et al. Feasibility of recanalization of human coronary arteries using high intensity ultrasound. *Am J Cardiol.* 1994;73:126–132.

20. Siegel RJ, Gunn J, Ahsan A, et al. Use of therapeutic ultrasound in percutaneous coronary angioplasty: Experimental in vitro studies and initial clinical experience. *Circulation.* 1994;89:1587–1593.

21. Demer LL, Ariani M, Siegel RJ. High intensity ultrasound increases distensibility of calcific atherosclerotic arteries. *J Am Coll Cardiol.* 1991;1:1259–1262.

22. Fischell TA, Abbas MA, Grant GW, Siegel RJ. Ultrasonic energy—effects on vascular function and integrity. *Circulation.* 1991;84:1783 1795.

23. Freeman I, Isner J, Gal D, et al. Ultrasonic angioplasty using a flexible wire probe. *J Am Coll Cardiol.* 1989;13. Abstract.

24. Gal DV, Monteverde C, Hogan J, et al. In vivo assessment of ultrasound angioplasty of fibrotic total occlusions. *Circulation.* 1991;84:1679. Abstract.

25. Labs JD, Merillat JC, Williams GM. Analysis of solid phase debris from laser angioplasty: potential risk of atheroembolism. *J Vasc Surg.* 1988; 7:326–335.
26. Friedman HZ, Elliot MA, Gottlieb GJ, O'Neill WW. Mechanical rotary atherectomy: the effects of microparticle embolization on myocardial blood flow and function. *J Interventional Cardiol.* 1989;2:77–83.
27. Weibull H, Lundqvist B, Falt K, Spangen L, Feith F, Bergqvist D. Perioperative arterial recanalization with Kensey dynamic angioplasty. *Eur J Surg.* 1991;157:385–387.
28. Hong AS, Chae JS, Dubin SB, Lee S, Fishbein MC, Siegel RJ. Ultrasonic clot disruption: an in vitro study. *Am Heart J.* 1990;120:418–422.
29. Ariani M, Fishbein MC, Siegel RJ. Dissolution of peripheral arterial thrombi by ultrasound. *Circulation.* 1991;84:1680–1688.
30. Marzelle J, Combe S, Mnoushehr M, et al. Catheter delivered ultrasound dissolves organized thrombi resistant to tissue plasminogen activator (tPA). *Circulation.* 1991;84:468. Abstract.
31. Hartnell GG, Saxton JM, Friedl SE, Abela GS. Rapid ablation of fresh thrombus by a new ultrasonic device—in vitro assessment. *J Am Coll Cardiol.* 1992;19:108. Abstract.
32. Siegel RJ, Nita H, Steffen W, Fishbein MC, Passafaro J. Development of a flexible over-the-wire ultrasound coronary ablation catheter. *Circulation.* 1992;86:I-457.
33. Trubestein G, Engel C, Etzel P, Sobbe A, Cremer A, Stumpff U. Thrombolysis by ultrasound. *Clin Sci Mol Med.* 1976;51:697s–698s.
34. Trubestein G. Entfernung intravasaler Thromben durch Ultraschall. *Fortschr Med.* 1978;14:755–760.
35. Steffen W, Luo H, Nita H, et al. Catheter delivered therapeutic ultrasound recanalizes thrombotically occluded canine coronary arteries. *J Am Coll Cardiol.* 1993;21:338A.
36. Siegel RJ, Gaines P, Crew J, Cumberland D. Clinical results of percutaneous ultrasound angioplasty. *J Am Coll Cardiol.* 1993;22:460–468.
37. Sanborn TA, Cumberland DC, Greenfield AJ, Welsh CL, Guben JK. Percutaneous laser thermal angioplasty. Initial results and 1-year follow-up in 129 femoropopliteal lesions. *Radiology.* 1988;168:121–125.
38. Arlart IP, Gerlach A, Grass HG. Laser-assisted balloon angioplasty in complete femoropopliteal occlusions: preliminary results. *Cardiovasc Intervent Radiol.* 1991;14:233–237.
39. Triller J, Do D, Maddern G, Mahler F. Femoropopliteal artery occlusion: clinical experience with the Kensey catheter. *Radiology.* 1992;182:257–261.
40. Gallino A, Mahler F, Probst P, Nachbur B. Percutaneous angioplasty of the arteries of the lower limbs: a 5-year follow-up. *Circulation.* 1984; 70:619–623.
41. Zeitler E, Richter EI, Roth FJ, Schoop W. Results of percutaneous transluminal angioplasty. *Radiology.* 1983;146:57–60.
42. Capek P, McLean GK, Berkowitz HD. Femoropopliteal angioplasty: factors influencing long-term success. *Circulation.* 1991;83(suppl I):I-70-I-80.
43. Rosenschein U, Rozenszajn LA, Kraus L, et al. Ultrasonic angioplasty in totally occluded arteries. *Circulation.* 1991;83:1976–1986.
44. Drobinski G, Brisset D, Phillipe F, et al. Effects of ultrasound energy on peripheral arterial total occlusions: initial angiographic and angioscopic results. *J Intervent Cardiol.* In press.

45. Monteverde C, Velez M, Jaurequi R, Garcia R, Guillermo N. An-giosonoplasty: Percutaneous intravascular plaque ablation with ultra-sound. Late results in peripheral arteries. *Circulation.* 1991;84:69. Abstract.
46. Siegel RJ, Cumberland DC, Myler RK, Don Michael TA. Percutaneous ultrasonic angioplasty—initial clinical experience. *Lancet.* 1989;9:772–774.
47. Ryan TJ, Klocke FJ, Reynolds WA. Clinical competence in percuta-neous transluminal coronary angioplasty. *J Am Coll Cardiol.* 1990;15: 1469–1474.

Chapter 16

Lesion-based Device Choices:
Defining the Niches

Michael A. Kutcher, MD
and Gustavo A. Solis, MD

As detailed in previous chapters, there is a vast array of new technology with which to perform percutaneous transluminal coronary angioplasty (PTCA). This chapter is written from a clinical perspective and addresses the question that many of the readers of this book face on a daily basis—which, if any, of the new angioplasty devices should the interventional cardiologist use to provide the most effective form of revascularization for the individual patient? This chapter offers a lesion-based format to define specific niches where new technology may be considered.

Background

Over the past 10 years, there has been an improvement in coronary balloon angioplasty technology. Success has remained at a high level with relatively low risk despite the expansion of PTCA into increasingly complex settings. Any new device must at least match or improve upon the current standards of PTCA[1] that include an incidence of: 90%–95% success rate; 5%–7% dissection; 3%–4% myocardial infarction; 2%–3% emergency cardiopulmonary bypass graftin (CABG); 0.5%–1% mortality; and 35%–40% late restenosis.

For the present and future, the foremost challenges to coronary angioplasty are:

The authors would like to acknowledge the support of the Wuliger Angioplasty Research Fund in the preparation of this manuscript.

From Vetrovec GW, Carabello BA, (eds.) *Invasive Cardiology: Current Diagnostic and Therapeutic Issues*. Armonk, NY: Futura Publishing Company, Inc.: © 1996.

1. **Expand indications:** to treat cases that cannot be effectively performed with balloon dilatation.[2]
2. **Eliminate emergency surgery:** to reduce the necessity for surgical intervention to resolve failed angioplasty.
3. **Reduce restenosis:** to lower the recurrence rate and allow angioplasty to be a better long-term solution to coronary atherosclerotic heart disease.

New Technology

Part of the appeal of new devices has been the promise that they may be more comprehensive catheter-based revascularization alternatives than balloon dilatation. Specifically, new technology may result in actual plaque removal, a larger residual lumen, less chance of dissection, reduction of elastic recoil, less proliferative response, and the capability to address cases unsuitable for balloon dilatation.

The major device categories of atherectomy, lasers, and stents that have undergone investigational evaluation are listed in Table 1. The first new technology device approved by the Food and Drug Administration (FDA) in September, 1990 was directional coronary atherectomy (DCA), Simpson AtheroCath® (Devices for Vascular Intervention, Redwood City, CA). DCA uses a balloon centered cutting cylinder that permits intraluminal excision and extraction of atheroma. The Rotablator® (Heart Technologies, Bellevue, WA) uses a high-speed rotational burr to ablate plaque into small particles. The Transluminal Extraction Catheter (TEC®) system (Inter-

---

·TABLE 1

New Technology in Coronary Angioplasty
Recent and Current Devices

Atherectomy	Laser	Stents	Diagnostic
DCA	Laser probe	Wallstent	ICUS
Rotablator	Lastac	Gianturco-Roubin	Angioscope
TEC	LBA	Palmaz-Schatz	
	ELCA	Wiktor	
	PELCA	Strecker	
	Holmium		

DCA, directional coronary atherectomy; TEC, transluminal extraction catheter; LBA, laser balloon angioplasty; ELCA, excimer laser coronary angioplasty; PELCA, percutaneous excimer laser coronary angioplasty; ICUS, intracoronary ultrasound.

Ventional Technologies, San Diego, CA) is a high-speed rotational cutting catheter with the capability to suction debris out of the artery. The Rotablator and TEC device were approved for general use by the FDA in 1993.

The field of lasers has been littered with high hopes, false starts, and failures. Laser devices that have undergone initial investigational trials, but never proceeded to more expanded studies or to FDA approval and are now defunct include the Laser Probe® (Trimedyne, Santa Ana, CA), the LASTAC® (GV Medical, Minneapolis, MN), and the Spears (LBA) Laser Balloon Angioplasty® (USCI, Billerica, MA).

The Excimer Laser Coronary Angioplasty (ELCA®) system (Advanced Interventional Systems, Irvine, CA) was approved by the FDA in January, 1992. Within the same year, the FDA approved the Percutaneous Excimer Laser Coronary Angioplasty (PELCA®) system (Spectronetics, Colorado Springs, CO). As of 1994, AIS and Spectronetics have merged into one excimer laser company. In this chapter, the designation ELCA will refer to both the AIS system and the Spectronetics system unless otherwise specified. A Holmium laser system (Eclipse®, Palo Alto, CA) is currently undergoing investigational study, but has not yet been approved by the FDA.

A variety of intracoronary stents have undergone clinical investigation. The Wallstent® (Medinvent SA, Lausanne, Switzerland) was the first intracoronary stent to undergo clinical trials in Europe. However, due to a high thrombosis and restenosis rate there are no plans for this stent to be released in the United States. The Gianturco-Roubin or Flex-Stent® (Cook Inc., Bloomington, IN) was approved by the FDA in June, 1993 for use in acute or threatened closure after coronary angioplasty. The Palmaz-Schatz® Stent (Johnson & Johnson Interventional Systems, Warren, NJ) received FDA approval in 1994 for use in preventing restenosis in selected coronary arteries. In addition, there are nonsponsored protocols utilizing biliary stents in old saphenous vein grafts. Current multicenter investigational trials are underway with the Wiktor® Stent (Medtronics, San Diego, CA), and the Strecker® Stent (Boston Scientific, Watertown, MA). Other stent designs, bioabsorbable stents, and temporary retrievable devices are also being investigated, but are several years away from clinical approval.

The evolution of intracoronary ultrasound (phased array or mechanical) has allowed actual in vivo quantitative assessment of lesions prior to and after intervention. Intracoronary angioscopy shows great promise in the qualitative identification of lesions. These two diagnostic modalities may be used to more precisely define lesion subsets for new technology.

The specifics of each new device have been thoroughly discussed in other chapters in this book. This chapter centers on the
FDA approved or soon-to-be approved devices and their application
in subsets of patients requiring coronary angioplasty.

Assessment of New Technology

There are four phases of development for the clinical assessment of new devices in coronary angioplasty. The first phase consists of the initial device evolution in one or two centers. The
second phase involves open label multicenter trials where indications are clarified and safety and efficacy are assessed by an industry sponsored open registry. Once the device has fulfilled stringent
criteria set up by the FDA it receives approval for general use. Prior
to using new technology, interventional cardiologists must attend
an official training workshop to be certified to use the new device.
The last phase involves the continuation of a postmarket approval
open registry and randomized comparative trials of the new technology.[2]

Since 1990, The National Heart, Lung, and Blood Institute has
sponsored the New Approaches to Coronary Intervention (NACI)
Registry to monitor the continuing impact of new technology in
high-volume clinical centers. A recent publication from this registry summarizing the major technologies of atherectomy, lasers,
and stents reported a 66.5% device success rate and a 75.5% incidence of adjunctive balloon angioplasty for an overall 92.2% lesion
success rate.[3] Major complications consisted of an incidence of
1.6% mortality, 1.3% Q wave myocardial infarction, and 1.7%
emergency surgery. General procedure success without a major
complication was achieved in 90.8% of patients.

Since new devices usually require higher caliber catheters and
sheaths, there are specific unique vascular complications that may
occur. In a recent comparative study by Popma et al,[4] a 14% incidence of significant complications of hematoma, vascular repair, or
retroperitoneal bleed occurred in an intracoronary stent group. The
TEC group had a major vascular complication rate of 12.5%. Standard balloon angioplasty had only a 3.2% incidence with the DCA,
Rotablator, and ELCA groups averaging rates of 2.5%–4.7%.

In this era of health care reform, it will be increasingly important to monitor the cost of new technology. Cohen et al[5] reported
that procedural costs between DCA and coronary balloon angioplasty were similar and involved a 2.3–2.6-day hospital stay. Intracoronary stent patients averaged a 5.5-day stay with significantly

higher procedural and total costs, which reflects the necessity for a high-intensity anticoagulation prophylaxis against thrombosis. Future evaluation and assessment of the cost of new technology should also consider the likelihood that adjunctive coronary balloon angioplasty will be required in the majority of cases.

In general, it may be said that in open registry assessment, new devices have had similar success and risks comparable to balloon angioplasty. However, the restenosis rates have not been appreciably reduced. Thus, the current question exists: where does new technology fit into the scheme of catheter-based coronary revascularization?

Challenges to Angioplasty

A starting point is to go back to the basic challenges to coronary angioplasty and logically assess each challenge from the vantage point of new technology.

Expand Indications

The ACC/AHA criteria for type A, type B, and type C lesions are well-accepted definitions of lesion morphology that correlate with the success and risks of PTCA.[6] Under these criteria, type A lesions are minimally complex with the following characteristics: discrete length <10 mm, concentric, readily accessible, nonangulated segment <45° smooth contour, little or no calcification, less than totally occlusive, nonostial in location, no major side branch involvement, and/or with absence of thrombus. Extensive clinical experience with type A lesions has indicated balloon angioplasty success rates of 95% or greater with significant complication rates of 1.2% or less.[7] Thus, in view of the absence of a lower restenosis rate with new technology, there are few indications where new devices would have an edge over conventional balloon angioplasty in type A lesions.

Type B lesions, however, represent moderately complex subsets that include characteristics of tubular shape with length 10–20 mm, eccentricity, moderate tortuosity of proximal segment, moderate angulated segments >45° or <90° irregular contour, moderate or heavy calcification, total occlusions <3 months old, ostial in location, bifurcation lesions, and/or some thrombus present. Ellis et al[8] have further subdivided this group into type B1 and type B2, with the former having one characteristic and the latter having two or more characteristics of type B lesions. In this study, type B1 stenoses had an 84% success and 4% complication rate, type B2 a 76% success and 10% complication rate with balloon angioplasty. In particular, eccentric stenoses and increasing degrees of calcification increase the risk of acute occlusion with balloon dilatation. Although Topol[9] has reported success rates of 85% with balloon dilatation of ostial lesions, the complications and long-term restenosis rate of >50% limit the application of PTCA in this group.

Type C or severely complex lesions have the highest complication rate and least chance of success with balloon angioplasty. Ellis[8] reported a 61% success rate with a 21% complication rate in this subgroup. Characteristics of type C lesions include diffuse length >20 mm, excessive tortuosity of proximal segments, extremely angulated segments >90°, total occlusions >3 months old, inability to protect major side branches, and/or old degenerated vein grafts with friable lesions. Diffuse lesions >20 mm continue to have a lower incidence of success and a higher chance of dissection with balloon angioplasty. Although balloon dilatation of chronic total occlusions has an acceptable complication rate, the success rate is low and the long-term restenosis rate of >50% is prohibitively high.[10] The most disturbing subgroup of type C lesions are the degenerative vein grafts, particularly grafts >5 years old with friable lesions. These have been notoriously difficult to successfully treat and maintain long-term patency with balloon angioplasty.[11]

New technology may have a particular application in these high-risk subsets of type B and type C lesions that uniformly do poorly with standard balloon angioplasty. Considering the challenge of angioplasty to expand indications, one may divide lesion subsets into those indicated on Table 2. In addition, the restenotic plaque itself may be a sub-subset of these lesion types. Table 3 outlines the lesion subsets and new device options. The following discussion reviews the experience and justification for new technology in these subsets.

TABLE 2

Expand Indications
Lesion Subsets

- Chronic total occlusion
- Significant calcium
- Ostial
- Eccentric
- Long >20 mm
- Old bypass grafts

TABLE 3

Lesion-Based Device Choices

| | Total Occlusion | Calcium | Ostial | Eccentric | Long | Old Bypass Grafts |
	TO	**CA**	**OS**	**ECC**	**LONG**	**SVG**
TO	ELCA DCA	ELCA	ELCA DCA	DCA	ELCA	TEC STENT
CA	ELCA	ROTA ELCA	ROTA ELCA	ROTA DELCA	ELCA	ELCA ROTA STENT
OS	ELCA DCA	ROTA ELCA	DCA ROTA ELCA	DCA	ELCA	DCA ELCA STENT
ECC	DCA	ROTA DELCA	DCA	DCA	DCA DELCA	DCA STENT
LONG	ELCA	ELCA	ELCA	DCA DELCA	ELCA	TEC STENT
SVG	TEC STENT	ELCA ROTA STENT	DCA ELCA STENT	DCA STENT	TEC STENT	STENT

DCA, directional coronary atherectomy; DELCA, directional excimer laser coronary angioplasty; ELCA, excimer laser coronary angioplasty; ROTA, Rotablator; STENT, intracoronary stent; TEC, transluminal extraction catheter.

An algorithm of lesion subsets and new device options. The shaded blocks represent an uncomplicated lesion subset. After each subgroup and its potential, sub-subsets may be done by either vertical or horizontal movement within the table. Of the six major lesion types, there are 36 blocks with inherent redundancy, but 21 distinctive niches of complex morphology. Each lesion subset may also need adjunctive balloon angioplasty, multiple devices, and/or stenting to achieve the most optimal final lumen diameter.

Chronic Total Occlusion

The two major problems associated with chronic total occlusion are obtaining access across the occlusion and debulking the totally obstructive lesion to improve initial success and reduce the long-term restenosis rate. If attempts to cross the occlusion are unsuccessful, the options are limited. Both the Laser Probe and the Lastec systems are defunct. Recently, investigational use of an 0.018-inch diameter excimer laser wire has been reported to have a success rate of 62% in a small group of patients with total occlusion.[12] In Europe, an 85% success rate has been reported utilizing

a low-speed rotational wire.[13] Both of these investigational devices
are flawed by an inherent danger of perforation.

Special steering wires may be helpful in crossing chronic total
occlusions. Meier[14] has reported success rates >65% with the Mag-
num® wire (Schneider, Europe), which has a 0.21-inch shaft with a
1-mm olive-type tip. In the United States, the Glidewire® (Mansfield, Boston Scientific, Watertown, MA) with a 0.014- or 0.016-inch
diameter, a nitinol shaft with hydrophilic coating, and an angled
tip may have an advantage over conventional steering wires.

Once crossed with a steering wire, pure chronic total occlusions may be successfully debulked with ELCA.[15] Depending on
vessel size, DCA has also been reported to be successful in reducing
plaque load, particularly if the lesion is eccentric.[16] When chronic
total occlusion is associated with calcification and/or long length,
ELCA may be the more appropriate choice. Total occlusion of the
ostia may be treated with either ELCA or DCA. Chronic total occlusions of bypass grafts are a particularly difficult subset that
could conceivably be treated with TEC or stenting.

Significant Calcium

Clinical experience with the Rotablator has indicated a 90%
or greater success rate with few complications in debriding inelas-
tic or calcified vessels.[17] Recent studies using sequential intravascular ultrasound imaging have shown that high-speed rotational
atherectomy causes luminal enlargement by selective ablation of
hard calcified atherosclerotic plaque with little tissue disruption.[18]
Thus, in most subsets of calcified stenoses the Rotablator may be
the technology of choice. ECLA may be a better option to vaporize
calcific deposits with less distal debris in total occlusions or long
diffuse calcified stenoses.[19] A directional ELCA system (DELCA) is
currently under investigation to address eccentric calcified lesions.[20]

Ostial Lesions

Pure ostial lesions may be effectively treated by a variety of devices, depending on the morphology subsets. DCA has been successfully used when the vessel is large and/or eccentric.[21] With
greater degrees of calcification, ostial lesions may be best treated
with rotational atherectomy.[22] Eigler et al[23] have recently reported
the safety and effectiveness of ELCA in aorto-ostial lesions of the
right coronary and saphenous vein grafts.

Eccentric Stenoses

Pure eccentric stenoses are probably most effectively treated with DCA because of the capability of spatially and selectively eliminating plaque with this system.[21] Braden et al[24] have documented with pre- and postintracoronary ultrasound imaging that actual plaque removal is the predominant mechanism in DCA compared to a mere stretching effect with balloon angioplasty. The DELCA system may have promise in eccentric calcified lesions or eccentric long lesions, but experience with this system is still in investigational trials.[20]

Long (>20 mm) Stenoses

ELCA has been demonstrated clinically to be effective in long stenoses (>20 mm).[25] Although the Rotablator system has been used to some benefit in diffuse lesions,[26] the concern of distal embolization of small particulate matter may limit the use of this device.

Old Bypass Grafts

Old saphenous vein graft body lesions continue to pose a major impediment for PTCA and new technology. Recently, a 39.2% device success and an 84% procedural success rate without complications has been reported with the TEC system in saphenous vein grafts.[27] However, the mortality and morbidity of TEC in this group continues to be high, which is a reflection of the diffuse and friable disease in these old grafts. Depending on other subsets of eccentricity, calcification, ostial location, eccentricity, or total occlusion, other technology may be tried. The greatest promise for the successful long-term treatment of old graft body lesions may be in the de novo placement of the Palmaz-Schatz stent.[28] Because vein grafts tend to be large, oversize stents may provide a better mechanism for long-term patency with less chance of acute thrombosis. At present, stents may be considered in old bypass grafts any time either new technology results in suboptimal results or if acute or threatened closure is present.

Eliminate Emergency Surgery

The second major challenge to coronary angioplasty is the elimination of the incidence of emergency surgery. Perhaps the necessity of standby surgery may not be totally eliminated, however, the mortality and morbidity inherent in emergency surgery for failed angioplasty may be reduced by more effective plaque reduction by the new technology.

The widespread experience and success with intracoronary stenting to stabilize extensive dissection, threatened occlusion, and abrupt closure has been documented by trials using the Gianturco-Roubin stent.[29,30] Experience with the Palmaz-Schatz stent in bail-out situations has been accumulating[31] and may in the future be an acceptable indication for the use of this device.

Figure 1 is a proposed schema for the thought process of dealing with threatened occlusion or abrupt closure. Emphasis should be placed on the morphology and etiology of the lesion as the lesion-based device choices outlined in Table 3 may be of help to abort a threatened or abrupt occlusion. For example, DCA has been shown to be effective in eliminating ulcerative flaps and/or dissection lines.[32] ELCA and the Rotablator have been successful in hard noncompressible lesions, but if dissection has occurred, they are contraindicated due to the high incidence of perforation and/or extension of dissection.

Prolonged autoperfusion with a balloon catheter would also be an appropriate first step of action to try to stabilize the threatened occlusion.[33] If either autoperfusion or lesion-based device choices are unsuccessful, the options would then be to proceed with intracoronary stenting using the FDA approved Gianturco-Roubin stent, or in the future, the Palmaz-Schatz stent. Emergency CABG

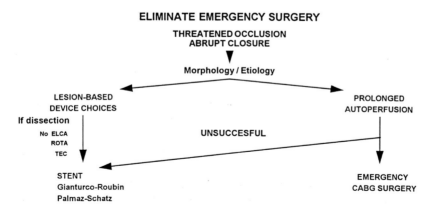

FIGURE 1. *Strategy to eliminate the need for emergency bypass surgery when threatened occlusion or abrupt closure complicate coronary angioplasty. ELCA, excimer laser coronary angioplasty; ROTA, rotational atherectomy (Rotablator); TEC, transluminal extraction catheter.*

surgery would be another consideration if extensive dissection or multivessel disease were present. The long-term safety and efficacy of stents compared to emergency surgery is still controversial and needs to be further assessed.[34]

Reduce Restenosis

The initial hope that new technology would reduce restenosis has been tempered by the reality that no new device has significantly reduced restenosis in open label trials.[17,19,21] However, the recent advent of randomized trials pitting new technology against conventional balloon angioplasty has reopened the promise of technology as a means to reduce restenosis.

The Coronary Angioplasty Versus Excisional Atherectomy Trial (CAVEAT) and the Canadian Coronary Atherectomy Trial (CCAT) were the first randomized studies to compare a new technology, in this case DCA, against standard balloon angioplasty.[35,36] Although restenosis was not significantly reduced with DCA in either study, these trials set the standard for future comparisons.

The recent observations by Baim et al[37] emphasize that initial luminal gain, late luminal loss, and net luminal gain are important parameters to reduce restenosis. With additional experience, new improvements in technology, and the concept of a large but safe luminal gain, future comparisons of DCA or other devices with balloon angioplasty may have a more favorable impact on restenosis.

The Stent Restenosis Study (STRESS) and the Belgium Netherlands Stent Trial (BENESTENT) initially reported at the 1993 American Heart Association Scientific Sessions indicated a reduced restenosis rate with Palmaz-Schatz stenting of large de novo native coronary lesions compared with coronary balloon angioplasty.[38,39] These reports were confirmed by peer-reviewed publications in 1994. In the STRESS study, the 6-month restenosis rate as defined by >50% diameter stenosis was 42% compared with 32% in the stent group.[40] In the BENESTENT trial, the restenosis rate was 32% compared with 22% in the stent group.[41] These studies seem to reaffirm the concept of "bigger is better" or that the largest residual lumen possible after an intervention may be the best mechanical chance of reducing restenosis. However, this initial enthusiasm must be tempered against the inherent vascular and bleeding complications as a result of heavy anticoagulation to prevent stent thrombosis. Perhaps newer generations of stent surface coatings and regimens of less intesive systemic anticoagulation will reduce this morbidity. Finally, the aplicability of stents to smaller more tortuous vessels and the long-term effects of permanent implantation must be assessed before stents can be categorically recommended to reduce restenosis.

The future of randomized trials comparing new technology with standard balloon angioplasty is exciting. The CAVEAT II trial will compare DCA with balloon angioplasty in saphenous vein grafts. Comparative trials of ELCA versus PTCA, ELCA versus Rotablator, and other multiple combinations of comparative new technology are underway. For the present, however, until the results of randomized trials are available, the application of new technology rests with the art and science of the clinician to deal with the individual patient.

Approach to Individual Patient

Table 4 outlines an overall thought process that may be used to assess an individual patient in deciding the best choice of catheter revascularization therapy. It should be emphasized that in spite of all the excitement of new technology, 80% of coronary angioplasty procedures are still best done with balloon dilatation, and even in the 20% of cases treated with new technology, adjunctive balloon angioplasty will be required in the majority of cases.

TABLE 4

Approach to the Individual Patient
Lesion-based Device Choices
What is the Justification for New Technology
Over Balloon Angioplasty in this Case?

Definite Considerations
  · unable to cross
  · unable to dilate
  · abrupt occlusion
Possible Considerations
  · better success?
  · less complications?
  · larger post precedural lumen?
  · less elastic recoil?
  · less restenosis?
  · more cost effective?
    in hospital
    long term

Summary

New technology is best poised to expand the indications of angioplasty in the problematic subsets of chronic total occlusion, calcified lesions, ostial stenoses, eccentric morphology, long lesions, or old friable bypass grafts. Because balloon angioplasty is less optimal in these situations, lesion-based subsets provide an appropriate entry point for new technology.

There is promise that intracoronary stenting may reduce the indications for emergency CABG surgery. However, there always will be a subset, hopefully increasingly small, that will ultimately require surgery for failed angioplasty.

Finally, there is still a possibility that technology may reduce restenosis. As more clinical experience with new devices occurs in the lesion-based subsets, the additional information from intracoronary ultrasound and angioscopy may translate to a better understanding of the mechanical aspects of optimal luminal diameter. Randomized trials comparing new technology are essential to assess the safety and effectiveness of devices to reduce restenosis. Realistically, however, some combination of technology and pharmacologic applications will probably be the key to resolve the restenosis problem.

In summary, this chapter offers suggestions as to where new technology may best be used in the clinical arena based on lesion specifics. However, there is an ongoing evolution of technology and recommendations made today may change in the future depending on additional experience and new data.

Acknowledgment

The authors would like to thank Ms. Peggy Gordon for her expert secretarial assistance and Drs. Bill Little and Greg Braden for their review and suggestions in the preparation of this chapter.

References

1. Holmes D, Myler R, Kent K, et al. National Heart, Lung, and Blood Institute Percutaneous Transluminal Coronary Angioplasty Registry as a standard for comparison of new devices. *Circulation.* 1991;84:1828–1830.
2. Participants in the National Heart, Lung, and Blood Institute Conference on the Evaluation of Emerging Coronary Revascularization Technologies: evaluation of emerging technologies for coronary revascularization. *Circulation.* 1992;85:357–361.

3. Baim DS, Kent KM, King SB III, et al. Evaluating new devices: acute (in-hospital) results from the New Approaches to Coronary Intervention Registry. *Circulation.* 1994;89:471–481.
4. Popma JJ, Satler LF, Pichard AD, et al. Vascular complications after balloon and new device angioplasty. *Circulation.* 1993;88:1569–1578.
5. Cohen DC, Ho K, Carrozza J, et al. Analyzing charges and costs for elective coronary revascularization—a comparison of conventional angioplasty, atherectomy, stenting, and bypass surgery. *J Am Coll Cardiol.* 1993;22:1052–1059.
6. Ryan TJ, Bauman WB, Kennedy JW, et al. Guidelines for percutaneous transluminal coronary angioplasty. A report of the ACC/AHA Task Force on Assessment of Diagnostic and Therapeutic Cardiovascular Procedures (Committee on PTCA).*J Am Coll Cardiol.* 1993;22:2033–2054.
7. Myler RK, Shaw RE, Stertzer SH, et al. Lesion morphology and coronary angioplasty: current experience and analysis. *J Am Coll Cardiol.* 1992;19:1641–1652.
8. Ellis S, Vandormael M, Cowley M, et al. Coronary morphologic and clinical determinants of procedural outcome with angioplasty for multivessel coronary artery disease. Implications for patient selection. *Circulation.* 1990;82:1193–1202.
9. Topol E. Multicenter study of percutaneous transluminal angioplasty for right coronary artery ostial stenoses. *J Am Coll Cardiol.* 1987;9:1214–1218.
10. Ivanhoe RJ, Weintraub WS, Douglas JS, et al. Percutaneous transluminal coronary angioplasty of chronic total occlusions. *Circulation.* 1992;85:106–115.
11. Douglas JS. Percutaneous intervention in patients with prior coronary bypass surgery. In: Topol EJ, ed. *Textbook of Interventional Cardiology.* Philadelphia, PA: WB Saunders Co.; 1994:339–354.
12. Sanborn TA, Spokojny AM, Bergruan GW, et al. A 0.018" excimer laser guidewire to recanalize chronic total occlusions and guide conventional angioplasty catheters. *Circulation.* 1993;88:I-504.
13. Kaltenbach M, Hartmann A, Vallbracht C. Procedural results and patient selection in recanalization of chronic coronary occlusions by low speed rotational angioplasty. *Eur Heart J.* 1993;14:826–830.
14. Meier B, Carlier M, Finci L, et al. Magnum wire for balloon recanalization of chronic total coronary occlusions. *Am J Cardiol.* 1989;64:148–154.
15. Werner G, Buchwald C, Voth E, et al. Recanalization of chronic total coronary arterial occlusions by percutaneous excimer-laser and laser-assisted angioplasty. *Am J Cardiol.* 1990;66:1445–1450.
16. Dick RJL, Haudenschild CC, Popma JJ, et al. Directional atherectomy for total coronary occlusions. *Coronary Artery Dis.* 1991;2:189–199.
17. Ellis SG, Popma JJ, Buchbinder M, et al. Relation of clinical presentation, stenosis morphology, and operator technique to the procedural results of rotational atherectomy and rotational atherectomy-facilitated angioplasty. *Circulation.* 1994;89:882–891.
18. Kovach JA, Mintz GS, Pichard AD, et al. Sequential intravascular ultrasound characterization of the mechanisms of rotational atherectomy and adjunct balloon angioplasty. *J Am Coll Cardiol.* 1993;22:1024–1032.
19. Litvack F, Eigler N, Margolis J, et al. Percutaneous excimer laser coro-

nary angioplasty: results in the first consecutive 3,000 patients. *J Am Coll Cardiol.* 1994;23:323–329.

20. Leon MB, Henson KD, Javier SP, et al. Early results with directional laser angioplasty in unfavorable coronary lesions. *Circulation.* 1993;88:I-23.

21. Ellis S, De Cesare N, Pinkerton C, et al. Relation of stenosis morphology and clinical presentation to the procedural results of directional coronary atherectomy. *Circulation.* 1991;84:644–653.

22. Popma J, Brogan W, Pichard A, et al. Rotational coronary atherectomy of ostial stenoses. *Am J Cardiol.* 1993;71:436–438.

23. Eigler NL, Weinstock B, Souglas JS, et al. Excimer laser coronary angioplasty of aorto-ostial stenoses. *Circulation.* 1993;88(part 1):2049–2057.

24. Braden GA, Herrington DM, Downes TR, et al. Qualitative and quantitative contrasts in the mechanisms of lumen enlargement by coronary balloon angioplasty and directional coronary atherectomy. *J Am Coll Cardiol.* 1994;23:40–48.

25. Cook SL, Eigler NL, Shefer A, et al. Percutaneous excimer laser coronary angioplasty of lesions not ideal for balloon angioplasty. *Circulation.* 1991;84:632–643.

26. Teirstein PS, Warth DC, Haq N, et al. High speed rotational coronary atherectomy for patients with diffuse coronary artery disease. *J Am Coll Cardiol.* 1991;18:1694.

27. Safian RD, Grines CL, May MA, et al. Clinical and angiographic results of transluminal extraction coronary atherectomy in saphenous vein bypass grafts. *Circulation.* 1994;89:302–312.

28. Strumpf RK, Mehta SS, Ponder R, et al. Palmaz-Schatz stent implantation in stenosed saphenous vein grafts: clinical and angiographic follow-up. *Am Heart J.* 1992;5:1329–1336.

29. Roubin GS, Cannon AD, Agrawal SK, et al. Intracoronary stenting for acute and threatened closure complicating percutaneous transluminal coronary angioplasty. *Circulation.* 1992;85:916–927.

30. Hearn JA, King SB, Douglas JS, et al. Clinical and angiographic outcomes after coronary artery stenting for acute or threatened closure after percutaneous transluminal coronary angioplasty. *Circulation.* 1993;88:2086–2096.

31. Maiello L, Colombo A, Gianrossi R, et al. Coronary stenting for treatment of acute or threatened closure following dissection after coronary balloon angioplasty. *Am Heart J.* 1993; 125:1570–1575.

32. McKeever LS, Marek JC, Kerwin PM, et al. Bail-out directional atherectomy for abrupt coronary artery occlusion following conventional angioplasty. *Cathet Cardiovasc Diagn.* 1993;(Suppl 1):31–36.

33. Van Lierde JM, Glazier JJ, Stammen FJ, et al. Use of an autoperfusion catheter in the treatment of acute refractory vessel closure after coronary balloon angioplasty: immediate and six month follow up results. *Br Heart J.* 1992;68:51–54.

34. Lincoff AM, Topol EJ, Chapekis AT, et al. Intracoronary stenting compared with conventional therapy for abrupt vessel closure complicating coronary angioplasty: a matched case-control study. *J Am Coll Cardiol.* 1993;21:866–875.

35. Topol EJ, Leya F, Pinkerton C, et al. A comparison of directional atherectomy with coronary angioplasty in patients with coronary artery disease. *N Engl J Med.* 1993;329:221–227.

36. Adelman AG, Cohen EA, Kimball BP, et al. A comparison of directional

atherectomy with balloon angioplasty for lesions of the left anterior descending coronary artery. *N Engl J Med.* 1993;329:228–233.

37. Kuntz RE, Gibson CM, Nobuyoshi M, et al. Generalized model of restenosis after conventional balloon angioplasty, stenting and directional atherectomy. *J Am Coll Cardiol.* 1993;21:15–25.

38. Schatz RA, Penn IM, Baim DS, et al. STent RESTenosis Study STRESS): analysis of in-hospital results. *Circulation.* 1993;88:I-594.

39. Serruys PW, Macaya C, de Jaegers P, et al. Interim analysis of the BENESTENT trial. *Circulation.* 1993;88:I-594.

40. Fischman DL, Leon MB, Baim DS, et al. A randomized comparison of coronary stent placement and balloon angioplasty in the treatment of coronary artery disease. *N Engl J Med.* 1994;331:496–501.

41. Serruys PW, de Jaegere P, Kiemeneij F, et al. A comparison of balloon-expandable-stent implantation with balloon angioplasty in patients with coronary artery disease. *N Engl J Med.* 1994;331:489–495.

Chapter 17

The Pathology of Restenosis

*Jeffrey M. Isner, MD, Marianne Kearney, BS,
J. Geoffrey Pickering, MD, PhD,
Guy Leclerc, MD, Sigrid Nikol, MD,
and Lawrence Weir, PhD*

For many years, the use of human tissues as an alternative or even supplementary source of clues to the basis for restenosis was precluded by access. The advent of directional atherectomy[1] solved this dilemma by providing tissues in a form that is sufficiently intact to perform light microscopic analyses from human patients in vivo at the peak of their clinical course. The fact that the freshly obtained specimen may be immediately snap-frozen or otherwise fixed preserves the opportunity to study such tissues by contemporary analytic techniques. This chapter outlines certain features of restenosis that have been recognized in such studies of human atherectomy specimens, and discusses the implications that these findings may have for future therapeutic approaches.

Light Microscopic Findings

Light microscopic features of atherectomy specimens retrieved from the peripheral and coronary arteries of patients undergoing percutaneous revascularization have been characterized by several laboratories and, in general, have proved to be remarkably similar. In particular, studies of specimens excised in vivo[2-6] have confirmed observations made in reports of patients studied at necropsy[7-19] suggesting that primary and restenosis lesions could often be distin-

Supported in part by Grants (HL40518, HL02824 [JMI] and AR40580 [LW]) from the National Heart, Lung, and Blood Institute, NIH, Bethesda, MD.

From Vetrovec GW, Carabello BA, (eds.) *Invasive Cardiology: Current Diagnostic and Therapeutic Issues.* Armonk, NY: Futura Publishing Company, Inc.: © 1996.

guished from each other on the basis of certain light microscopic findings (Figures 1 and 2). Primary lesions appear typically hypocellular, consisting predominantly of well-organized collagen and ambiguous ground substance. In contrast, restenosis lesions typically include a focus of hypercellularity; cells within these foci have phe-

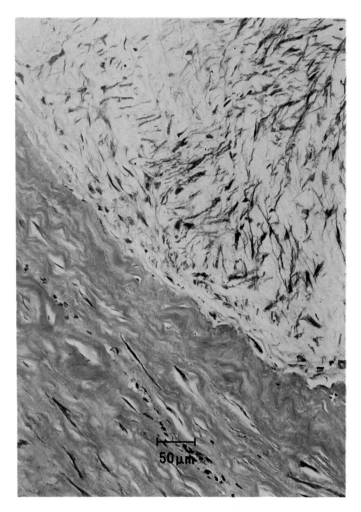

FIGURE 1. *Classic light microscopic bilayer appearance of restenosis specimen obtained by directional atherectomy. "Restenosis focus" includes: **A:** hypercellularity in which cells have phenotypic characteristics of proliferative vascular smooth muscle cells; and **b** loose extracellular matrix with distinctive light hue. Underlying primary atherosclerotic plaque is hypocellular, and extracellular matrix, consisting predominantly of ambiguous ground substance and collagen, has a more compact appearance and darker hue. (Elastic-tissue trichrome).*

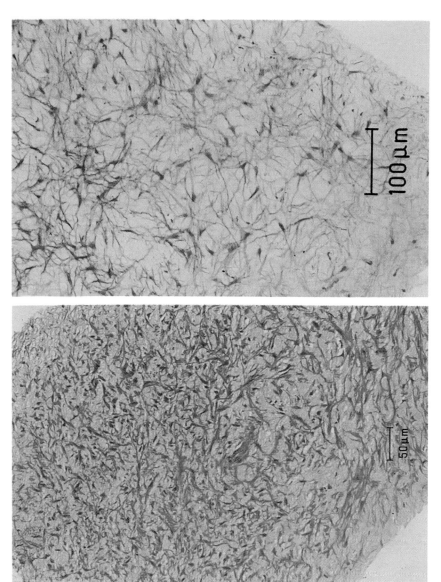

FIGURE 2. *Atherectomy specimens retrieved from restenosis lesions demonstrating variable relation between cell density and extracellular matrix. Hypercellularity predominates in specimen shown on **left** (hematoxylin and eosin); specimen on **right** (elastic-tissue/trichrome) is hypercellular, but includes proportionately more matrix.*

notypic characteristics of proliferative vascular smooth muscle cells, and the matrix surrounding these cells typically has a distinctly lighter hue and less compact appearance than the matrix of primary or adjacent plaque. These contrasting findings between primary and restenosis lesions are perhaps best illustrated in a group of 18 patients studied in our laboratory[20] in whom directional atherectomy had been performed as the primary intervention, and again at the time that the patient returned with restenosis. Thus, these 18 patients offered a unique opportunity to study the same lesion site in the same artery of the same patient at two different points in time. Light microscopic examination documented distinctive features, including hypercellular foci consisting of proliferative vascular smooth muscle cells surrounded by a loose neomatrix, in 13 of 18 (72%) cases. In 5 patients, neither the primary nor the restenosis specimen demonstrated such a "restenosis focus." A similar restenosis focus has been observed in 165 (65%) of 253 restenosis specimens retrieved by directional atherectomy in our laboratory.

The fact that the lesion illustrated in Figure 1 is not a universal feature of restenosis lesions should not be surprising. There are at least four factors that may contribute to this observation. First, this is almost certainly the best evidence that the phenomenon that we call "restenosis" lumps together several disorders, each with its own pathogenesis, ie, restenosis is multifactorial. Second, this observation underscores the heterogeneous nature of not only primary atherosclerosis, but retenosis as well. Third, there may well be previously unappreciated differences between the pathology of lesions that develop in the lower extremity versus the coronary versus the carotid arterial circulations. Restenosis foci were observed more frequently, for example, in 37 of 42 (88%) peripheral arterial specimens versus 20 of 27 vein graft specimens (74%) versus 108 of 184 coronary specimens (59%). Fourth, it must be assumed that some degree of sampling error is inherent in the atherectomy procedure itself.

Finally, it must also be acknowledged that this lesion is not specific for restenosis. Among 425 primary specimens examined in our laboratory as part of the CAVEAT investigation, a similar lesion was observed in 31 (7%) primary specimens.[21] Whether this finding in primary lesions identifies accelerated lesion development in a patient with unstable angina, denotes a population of "activated" smooth muscle cells poised to proliferate, or is simply a coincidental finding, remains to be determined.

Evidence of Activated Smooth Muscle Cells

Isoforms of nonmuscle myosin have been shown to be differentially expressed during development and in different animal tissues.[22] Changes in nonmuscle myosin/smooth muscle myosin content have also been demonstrated in atherosclerotic rabbits.[23] Proliferation of vascular smooth muscle cells, considered to play an important role in the development of atherosclerotic and restenotic lesions, is associated with a major shift in myosin isoform distribution.[24] From these observations, it has been suggested that nonmuscle myosin may be required for smooth muscle cell proliferation by virtue of its involvement in cytokinesis, cell migration, and secretion.

Therefore, we investigated the distribution of nonmuscle myosin heavy chain (NMMHC) at the mRNA level using in situ hybridization. This technique is particularly valuable for analysis of atherectomy specimens because it can be performed on the very small amounts of tissue that are typically retrieved by this technique, particularly from the coronary arteries. Northern blot analysis typically requires at least 10 μg of total RNA and nuclease analysis requires even more (40 μg is recommended). The amount of RNA that we have been able to obtain from a specimen is typically less than this: previous analysis of 78 coronary and 72 peripheral atherectomy specimens performed in our laboratory using quantitative polumerase chain reaction (PCR) yielded median values of 1.97 and 7.58 μg of total RNA respectively (L. Weir, unpublished data).

Moreover, in situ hybridization provides information regarding the localization of mRNA. In the case of specimens obtained from atherosclerotic arteries, one can thus localize expression of mRNA to neointima, as well as media and adventitia when present, and potentially cell types as well. Analysis of pathologic vascular segments by in situ hybridization is complicated by certain features indigenous to atherosclerotic neointima. Because cryopreservation of tissues performed in preparation for in situ hybridization typically results in disruption of cellular cytoarchitecture, it is often difficult to determine with certainty that silver grains are exclusively localized within cytoplasmic boundaries as opposed to the extracellular matrix. This issue is particularly problematic in heterogeneous tissues, such as atherosclerotic plaque, in which cell density is greatly variable, and in which extensive and "sticky" extracellular matrix may exacerbate nonspecific adherence of silver grains.[25] Fortuitously, a generally consistent feature of in situ hybridization of atherosclerotic plaque is that mRNA expression appears clustered around cell nuclei.[26-32] This clustering is never seen with control sense probes. Accordingly, we have used the convention adopted by previous investigators in which positive hybridization is determined by the finding of silver grain clusters in relation to the cell nuclei.[28,33-35] This interpretation is supported by previous work[36-38] indicating that the mRNA for certain proteins may be preferentially limited to a perinuclear site, particularly in the case of mRNA encoding for proteins that govern cellular functions such as cell division.

It must be recognized that the finding in the autoradiograph of silver grains clustered about the nucleus does not imply that the mRNA to which the radiolabeled probe has hybridized is necessarily intranuclear. Studies performed in our Laboratory using confocal microscopy have illustrated the manner in which silver grains are essentially restricted to a superficial layer of the tissue section (Figure 3); serial scans recorded at 0.9-μm intervals into the tissue section indicate that few silver grains can be recognized at a depth of $\geq 2\mu$m below the surface of the section. The three-dimensional geometry of the cell allows emissions from radiolabeled probes that have hybridized to mRNA transcripts near and/or above the nucleus to cause developed silver grains in the superficial layer of emulsion to appear intranuclear (Figure 4).

We have also taken advantage of the juxtanuclear location of exposed silver grains, and the fact that cell nuclei, as opposed to cytoplasmic boundaries, are readily identified even in cryopreserved sections of atherosclerotic plaque, to perform semiquantitative analysis of the autoradiographs generated by in situ hybridization (Figure 5). The strength of the hybridization signal may be gauged by manual counting of the juxtanuclear silver grains to define an area for comparison between different tissue types with variable cell densities. Applying this approach to analysis of primary and restenosis specimens obtained by directional atherectomy, we observed that mRNA for the IIB isoform of NMMHC was present in greater abundance among restenotic versus primary vascular stenoses.[26] Further prospective investigation of a pilot group of patients undergoing directional atherectomy for primary stenoses suggested that elevated levels of NMMHC-IIB mRNA in primary lesions correlated with the subsequent development of restenosis.[32]

The amount of protein within a given atherectomy specimen is of course not necessarily reflected by the amount of mRNA present; translational regulation and differential stability of mRNA and protein may contribute to such potential discrepancy. Accordingly, investigation of the differential distribution of nonmuscle myosin isoforms was subsequently extended to the protein level using isoform-specific antibodies to perform Western blot and immunohistochemistry analyses for NMMHC-IIB and a related, but separately encoded isoform, NMMHC-IIA.[39] Previously published studies have shown that NMMHC-IIB and NMMHC-IIA are differentially expressed in a tissue-specific manner.[22,24,40] Among atherectomy

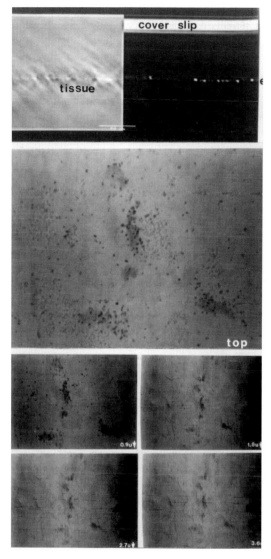

FIGURE 3. *Distribution of silver grains, studied by confocal microscopy, after in situ hybridization of retenosis specimen with antisense probe to nonmuscle myosin heavy chain IIB (NMMHC-IIB).* **Top:** *three-dimensional reconstruction of 9-μm thick optical sections of tissue specimen shown here in profile: exposed silver grains (emulsion, e) are limited to superficial aspect of tissue section.* **Middle:** *top-most optical section shows perinuclear distribution of silver grains, indicating positive hybridization to mRNA for NMMHC-IIB. Subsequent optical sections, photographed at 0.9, 1.8, 2.7, and 3.6 μm deep into tissue block demonstrate that few grains can be identified more than 2 μm into block.*

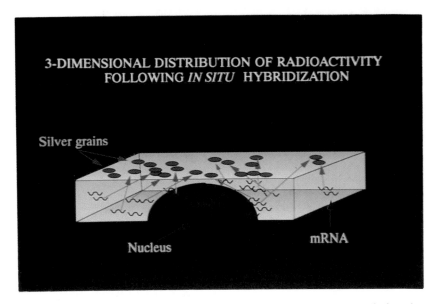

3-DIMENSIONAL DISTRIBUTION OF RADIOACTIVITY FOLLOWING *IN SITU* HYBRIDIZATION

Silver grains

Nucleus

mRNA

FIGURE 4. *Schematic correlate to Figure 3. Three-dimensional distribution of radioactivity after in situ hybridization. Radiolabeled antisense probes hybridize to mRNA. Randomly oriented emissions from hybridized probes result in exposure of silver grains in superficial layer of the section, including silver grains located above and around nucleus.*

specimens from primary and restenotic lesions, mRNA and protein for NMMHC-IIA were present to an equivalent degree in all types of tissues specimens. In contrast, NMMHC-IIB mRNA levels were again significantly greater in restenotic versus primary atherosclerotic lesions. This difference was even more apparent at the protein level: while NMMHC-IIB was consistently observed in restenotic specimens, it was undetectable in primary lesions. Particularly intriguing was the observation that the contractile ring, in dividing cells in culture, stained positively with the antibody against NMMHC-IIB. These results suggest that NMMHC-IIA is constitutively expressed, whereas NMMHC-IIB is potentially involved in cell division, including vascular restenosis.

Analysis of Cellular Proliferation

Beyond the factors responsible for smooth muscle cell proliferation in restenotic lesions, the extent to which such proliferation continues to be ongoing at the time of percutaneous revasculariza-

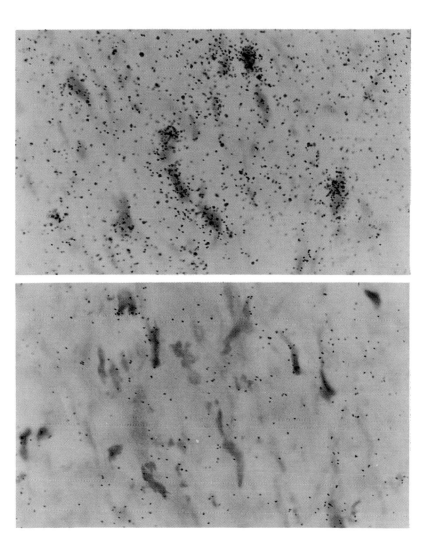

FIGURE 5. Photomicrographs of sense (**left**) and antisense (**right**) treated sections of restenosis lesion studied by in situ hybridization for nonmuscle myosin heavy chain IIB (NMMHC-IIB). **Left panel** shows paucity of silver grains; **right panel**, with prominent clustering of silver grains, denotes strong hybridization signal. (Hematoxylin and eosin). (Reproduced with permission from Reference 62.)

tion is of fundamental and practical significance. Many of the novel treatment strategies designed to prevent recurrent episodes of restenosis are predicated on local delivery of drugs or novel biologicals known to interfere with cell proliferation. To determine the degree of cell proliferation in symptom-producing vascular lesions, we examined the expression of the proliferating cell nuclear antigen (PCNA) in primary and restenotic atherosclerotic lesions retrieved by directional atherectomy. PCNA is an essential cofactor for DNA polymerase delta and its presence in the cell is considered to be a specific indication that the cell is replicating. Gordon and coworkers[41] had previously used anti-PCNA immunostaining to quantify proliferation in the coronary arteries of hearts explanted from patients undergoing cardiac transplantation. In that patient population, some 3 of 14 atherosclerotic lesions displayed no evidence of proliferation and the overall proportion of PCNA-positive cells was relatively low (mean = 0.85%).

In contrast, immunohistochemical analyses applied in our laboratory to atherectomy specimens retrieved from actively symptomatic patients disclosed that 5 of 7 primary and 8 of 8 restenotic lesions contained proliferating cells[31] (Figure 6). The mean rate of proliferation (percent of PCNA-positive cells) was higher in restenotic (15.2%±13.6%) than in primary (3.6%±3.5%) lesions. Proliferating cells were detected as late as 1 year after angioplasty. To verify these obsevations, a parallel series of 22 additional lesions was studied using as a wholly independent technique, in situ hy-

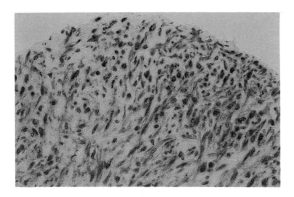

FIGURE 6. *Light photomicrograph of restenotic lesion double-labeled with antibodies to proliferating cell nuclear antigen (PCNA) and smooth muscle alpha actin. Reaction product for PCNA is localized to nucleus of cell; double immunostaining for HHF-35 indicates that PCNA-positive cell is vascular smooth muscle cell.*

bridization. Among the 22 plaques analyzed by in situ hybridization, 7 of 11 primary and 11 of 11 restenotic lesions contained PCNA-positive cells. The mean rate of proliferation was $7.2\% \pm 10.8\%$ in primary lesions and $20.6\% \pm 18.2\%$ in restenotic lesions ($P<0.05$).

These findings thus suggest that in patients referred for percutaneous revascularization, some lesions may be indolent, but many have a detectable proliferative component. It is likely that the more advanced atherosclerotic lesions from patients studied initially by Gordon et al[41] with end-stage cardiac disease undergoing cardiac transplantation are correspondingly more quiescent than lesions retrieved by directional atherectomy from patients with active symptoms of myocardial ischemia. Indeed, subseqent analysis[42] of vascular lesions developing in arteriovenous fistulas created for hemodialysis of patients with renal insufficiency disclosed PCNA indices similar to those cited above for restenosis lesions.

Several caveats concerning the methodology used to apply immunohistochemical identification of PCNA in human atherectomy specimens merit specific comment. First, previous investigators have underscored the critical impact which the fixative selected for tissue preservation may have on accessability of PCNA antigen to antibody detection.[43,44] Formalin fixation in particular may severely attenuate the antigenicity of PCNA. In fact, even formalin that has been introduced into the automatic tissue processor after the first morning run may be sufficient to blunt the degree of PCNA immunostaining apparent on specimens processed during subsequent runs through the same processor. In contrast, methanol appears to optimally preserve PCNA antigenicity. Consistent with experience reported previously by others, we have observed that duration of fixation is equally important and thus routinely preserve specimens designated for PCNA immunostaining overnight in methanol preservative. Implicit in these remarks is the routine use of control tissues such as tonsil or gut.

Second, the fundamental distinction between PCNA and other indices of cell proliferation must be recognized. Radiolabeled thymidine and the thymidine analog, bromodeoxyuridine (BrdU), for example, are frequently used to assess cellular proliferation in autoradiographs and immunohistochemical studies, respectively. Cells exposed to either of these agents are labeled when these agents are incorporated into the DNA of dividing cells during DNA synthesis; ie, thymidine and BrdU are S-phase specific indices of cell proliferation. Expression of PCNA, in contrast, is not limited to S-phase, but occurs during the G1 and G2 components of the growth cycle as well. Therefore, for any given population of cells that are PCNA-positive, only a fraction of those cells will have been labeled during DNA synthesis, and only this fraction will be labeled by incorporation of thymidine and/or BrdU. Studies that index the intensity of PCNA immunostaining according to an S-phase specific marker such as BrdU[45] will predictably result in a far lower index of cell proliferation; this is simply a consequence of the fact that the small fraction of PCNA-positive cells in S phase will be counted, while the much larger number of PCNA-positive cells in other phases of the growth cycle will not be included.

This distinction is perhaps best illustrated in the results of studies that have used similar techniques to evaluate the proliferative activity of neoplastic lesions. Studies of bronchogenic carcinoma and Hodgkin's lymphoma[46,47], for example, have disclosed proliferative indices of up to 40% using S-phase specific indices such as BrdU; analyses of cell proliferation observed in tissues from these same neoplastic lesions, however, typically disclosed PCNA indices of 50% to 100%. The latter are clearly and quite substantially in excess of PCNA indices observed in our atherectomy data, as would be expected for malignant lesions versus the "benign" lesion of vascular restenosis.

Ex Vivo Studies of Cell Proliferation

Additional evidence supporting the proliferative nature of restenosis versus primary lesions is derived from studies of vascular smooth muscle cells grown in cultures of explanted fragments of human atherectomy specimens. A traditional method of evaluating growth properties of cultured cells is to generate growth curves by serially counting subcultured cells at various intervals after seeding. While characterizing the proliferative profile of the cells, the cell counting approach typically necessitates multiple subcultivation to obtain sufficient cells for analysis. It is well recognized that the growth characteristics of cells in primary culture will change with time due to the selection of cell clones with the greatest capacity to proliferate. Furthermore, the low initial cell yield from atherectomy material may preclude this as a routine form of analysis. Dartsch and coworkers,[48] for example, found that growth curves could not be generated for cells derived from 14 of 19 primary lesions studied because of insufficient cell yield.

Therefore, we examined the behavior of smooth muscle cells growing directly out of intact explants of tissue specimens retrieved by directional atherectomy.[49] From a practical standpoint, our experience and that of others,[48,50] has shown that initiating cell growth from atherectomy tissues by explant outgrowth is more successful than by enzymatic dispersion of cells within the plaque. Furthermore, cell migration and proliferation underlie the phenomona of cellular outgrowth from vascular explants and, although quantifying outgrowth kinetics does not discern the relative role of each, it provides a straightforward means of assessing the combined effect of these important cellular events shortly after the tissue has been placed in the ex vivo environment.

Use of the explant outgrowth technique provided a highly successful means of cultivating smooth muscle cells from a variety of human plaque types and demonstrated that the outgrowth kinetics of these cells are indeed dependent on the type of the lesion. Among 41 lesions retrieved by directional atherectomy, in only 1 did none of the explant fragments result in an outgrowth of smooth muscle cells. The mean proportion of explant fragments yielding outgrowth, per lesion, was 69%±4%. This varied according to the nature of the lesion. Specifically, the prevalence of outgrowth from restenotic lesions (81%±3%) was greater than that obtained from primary lesions (56%±6%, $P<0.001$).

The time-course of initiation of smooth muscle cell outgrowth also varied among the different types of lesions. Initiation of outgrowth proceeded most rapidly among explants derived from restenotic lesions and was half-maximal by 5.9±0.6 days; this was significantly earlier than that of primary lesions (8.7±0.4 days, $P<0.001$). Serial outgrowth values for the peripheral artery lesions (primary and restenotic) yielding outgrowth are depicted in Figure 7. Initiation of outgrowth was clearly more immediate in the restenotic lesions: by 5 days, smooth muscle cell outgrowth had begun among 32%±4% of the explants from restenotic lesions versus 9%±5% of explants from primary lesions ($P<0.001$). Statistically significant differences between the groups persisted throughout the outgrowth period.

The rate of accumulation of cells around the explant was also substantially higher in tissue from restenotic lesions than from primary plaque. Twenty-one days after half-maximal outgrowth was attained, the total number of cells per adherent explant was 2,791±631 for restenotic tissue and 653±144 for primary tissue ($P<0.01$). The 5-day outgrowth of smooth muscle cells from a primary and restenotic lesion is illustrated in Figure 8. Outgrowth, while present from the primary and restenotic lesions, was considerably more abundant from the restenotic specimen.

The specimens evaluated by this ex vivo approach were obtained from a variety of locations and likely reflect a spectrum of morphologic features and stages of development. Nevertheless, ex-

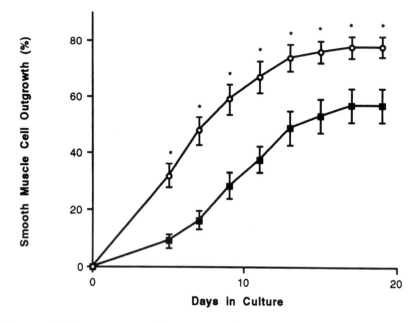

FIGURE 7. *Time course of initiation of smooth muscle cell outgrowth from explants of primary atherosclerotic (closed squares) and restenosis lesions (open circles) retreived by directional atherectomy from peripheral arteries. The initiation of outgrowth was considerably more prompt in the restenosis lesions. (Reproduced with permission from Reference 48.)*

plants of primary and restenotic lesions gave rise to smooth muscle cell outgrowth indicating that smooth muscle cells were a component of each plaque type; this finding is consistent with the studies from our laboratory cited above regarding cell proliferation in primary and restenotic lesions obtained by directional atherectomy. As expected, outgrowth from heavily calcified lesions was frequently scant and in one case unsuccessful. The reliable (>80%) outgrowth of smooth muscle cells from explants of restenotic tissue, as well as the onset of outgrowth and rate at which the outgrowing cells accumulated around the explants of restenotic lesions is consistent with the prominence of smooth muscle cells in these lesions.

The difference between the rates at which outgrowing cells accumulated around the explant of restenotic versus primary lesions (approximately four times higher for cells originating from restenotic than from primary lesions) may be partly accounted for by differences in the initial number of cells within the respective ex-

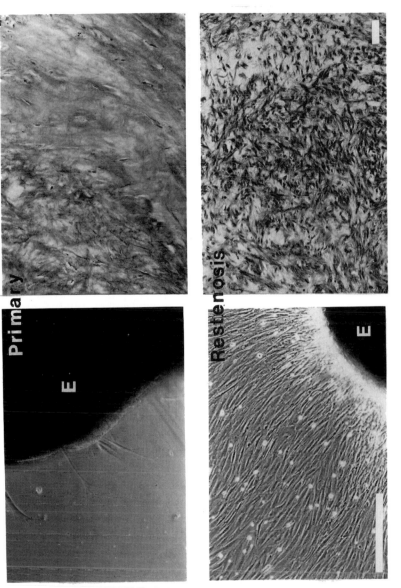

FIGURE 8. *Five-day cell outgrowth from a peripheral artery primary lesion (**top row**) and a peripheral artery restenotic lesion (**bottom row**). Light photomicrograph of a section from the respective lesions is shown on the right (elastic/trichrome). Cell outgrowth from the primary lesion is at a very early stage. The corresponding histologic features demonstrate the paucity of cells within this lesion. In contrast, a dense population of cells has already accumulated around the restenotic tissue; the lesion itself was highly cellular. E, explant. White bar at bottom left 250 μm; white bar at bottom right = 50 μm.*

plants. When cells were subcultured and seeded at identical densities, however, thymidine incorporation was found to be significantly (1.3-fold) higher in cells originating from restenotic lesions. This is consistent with the observation by Dartsch and coworkers[48] that cells derived from restenotic tissue have shorter doubling times than those from primary lesions. These findings imply that there are intrinsic differences in the growth behavior of smooth muscle cells derived from primary and restenotic tissue, independent of initial cell number. We speculate that one reason for the difference in outgrowth kinetics may be the different phenotypic states of smooth muscle cells within the various lesions. Thus the prompt egress of smooth muscle cells from explants of restenotic tissue[50] may reflect the prominence of preexisting, so-called synthetic-state smooth muscle cells that are in effect "primed" for outgrowth in vitro. Conversely, the delayed onset of outgrowth from explants of primary lesions may reflect the existence of smooth muscle cells that are predominantly nonproliferating or slowly proliferating. Electron microscopic studies of primary lesions of peripheral arteries have demonstrated a mixed population of smooth muscle cells, some of which have abundant contractile elements, while others have ultrastructural features more typical of so-called synthetic-state cells.[51] The variability in outgrowth kinetics among primary lesions may reflect this heterogeneity in smooth muscle cell phenotypes.

The Extracellular Matrix

Although vascular smooth muscle cell proliferation and the resulting hypercellular nature of the fibroproliferative tissue have been the focus of most studies of restenosis, it is the extracellular matrix that in fact accounts for the bulk volume of these lesions. Previous investigations have outlined certain pathways through which deposition of extracellular proteoglycans are regulated.[52] Moreover, it is now established that these constituents of the extracellular matrix may serve as important modulators of cell proliferation, as well as feedback regulators of growth factors governing their synthesis. While experiments performed in animals have demonstrated that intimal hyperplasia resulting from balloon injury incorporates proteoglycans and collagen, however, little is known regarding the distribution of proteoglycan and collagen subtypes in human, particularly restenosis, tissues.

To further characterize the extracellular matrix of restenotic tissues, in collaboration with Thomas Wight from the University of

Washington, we studied the codistribution of two proteoglycans, biglycan and decorin, known to be differentially modulated during extracellular matrix elaboration; both may be part of a natural feedback mechanism that regulates the biological activity of transforming growth factor-β (TGF-β). Extracellular deposits of biglycan were found to be characteristic of the loose, rich extracellular matrix comprising the restenosis focus.[53] Examination of serial sections revealed that biglycan staining was intimately related to the intensity of collagen type I and III staining in the same areas. Staining for decorin was limited to weak staining intensity in the more compact transition zone between loose extracellular matrix and dense connective tissue typical of advanced lesions composed of hypocellular fibrous plaque.

We[29,30] and others[54] have previously shown that expression of TGF-β is increased in restenotic lesions retrieved from human coronary and peripheral arteries. Others have shown that when TGF-β1 is used to stimulate cultures of human fibroblasts or primate vascular smooth muscle cells, biglycan expression is upregulated, whereas decorin expression is unaffected or even reduced.[55,56] In vivo studies carried out in experimental models of pulmonary[57] and hepatic[58] fibrosis have demonstrated that TGF-β and biglycan are upregulated during early stages of fibrosis; decorin, in contrast, was found only during the chronic stages of fibrosis. Furthermore, biglycan and decorin can bind and neutralize the effect of TGF-β; systemic adminsitration of decorin, in fact, has been shown to inhibit TGF-β-mediated production of extracellular matrix in a rat model of glomerulonephritis.[59] It is therefore possible that proteoglycans such as decorin and biglycan are part of a natural feedback mechanism that regulates the biologic activity of TGF-β. This may be relevant to neointimal extracellular matrix formation, given the documented expression of TGF-β in human primary and, to an even greater extent, restenosis lesions cited above. These preliminary findings thus illustrate the complex interplay between cellular proliferation and extracellular matrix constituents in regulating development of the restenosis lesion; and at the same time implicitly illustrate the potential for modifying lesion formation postrevascularization by strategies designed to interfere with growth factors and/or their subject molecules.

Microscopic Angiogenesis

Folkman and colleagues[60] have pioneered the concept that antagonism of the neovascular substrate that nourishes developing neoplasms constitutes a potential treatment strategy for a variety of oncologic disorders. An intriguing analog in vascular biology was suggested by the demonstration in selected necropsy specimens of vasa vasora extending from the adventitia into the thickened intima of atherosclerotic segments of human coronary arteries.[61] Interference with this microvascular network represents a theoretical means of inhibiting the development of restenosis and/or primary atherosclerosis. To investigate further the extent and potential role of microangiogenesis in lesions obtained from live patients, we studied specimens obtained consecutively by directional atherectomy from 94 patients, 62 (66%) of whom were undergoing primary revascularization, and 32 (34%) were patients with restenosis. Sections from each specimen were examined by standard light microscopy and immunostaining using Ulex Europaeus I, an endothelial-cell specific lectin, to identify endothelium of microangiogenic foci (Figure 9). Among the 62 primary lesions, microvessels (2–30, mean = 8.6) were identified in 17 (32%). Of the 32 restenosis lesions, microvessels (2–32, mean = 9.2) were observed in 11 (34%); in 5 of these 11 cases, the microvessels were localized to the hypocellular, fibrous (primary) portion of the specimen. Light microscopic examination was performed to assess the pres-

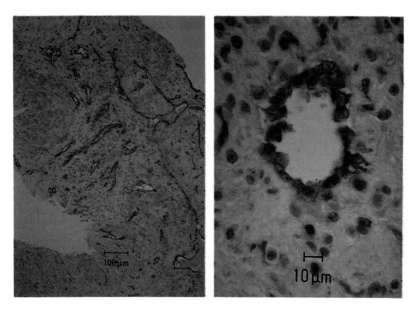

FIGURE 9. *Identification of neovascularity in primary lesion (low power, left; higher power, right) retrieved by directional atherectomy. Ulex stain identifies endothelium of neovascular network.*

ence of adventitia, media, calcific deposits, foam cells, cholesterol clefts and foam cells; none of these features was found to be related to the degree of neovascularization. These preliminary analyses thus confirm that microangiogenesis is a feature of primary and restenotic lesions in human atherosclerosis, and therefore a potential target for therapies designed to prevent luminal arterial narrowing, although such neovascularity is observed within the restenosis focus less often than in the primary atherosclerotic component of the tissue specimen.

Future Studies

Access to human lesions by virtue of directional atherectomy will continue to provide a unique opportunity to study the vascular pathology of patients, and thereby complement a variety of laboratory experiments, including those performed in live animals. The heterogeneous nature of luminal arterial narrowing, whether primary or restenotic, will remain a persistent challenge for those attempting to identify unifying concepts of pathogenesis. Such heterogeneity, however, must not be ignored, since the varied faces of this complex disorder are almost certain to contain the very clues required to segregate its multiple etiologies and thereby develop effective prevention and treatment strategies.

References

1. Simpson JB, Selmon MR, Robertson GC, et al. Transluminal atherectomy for occlusive peripheral vascular disease. *Am J Cardiol*. 1988;61: 96G–101G.
2. Garratt KN, Edwards WD, Kaufmann UP, et al. Differential histopathology of primary atherosclerotic and restenotic lesions in coronary arteries and saphenous vein bypass grafts: analysis of tissue obtained from 73 patients by directional atherectomy. *J Am Coll Cardiol*. 1991;17:442–448.
3. Johnson DE, Hinohara T, Selmon MR, et al. Primary peripheral arterial stenoses and restenoses excised by transluminal atherectomy: a histopathologic study. *J Am Coll Cardiol*. 1990;15:419–425.
4. Safian RD, Galbfish JS, Erny RE, et al. Coronary atherectomy: clinical, angiographic, and histological findings and observations regarding potential mechanisms. *Circulation*. 1990;82:69–79.
5. Schwarcz TH, Yates GN, Ghobrial M, et al. Pathologic characteristics of recurrent carotid artery stenosis. *J Vasc Surg*. 1987;5:280–288.
6. Strauss BH, Umans VA, vanSuylen R-J, et al. Directional atherectomy for treatment of restenosis within coronary stents: clinical, angiographic and histologic results. *J Am Coll Cardiol*. 1992;20:1465–1473.
7. Austin GE, Ratliff NB, Hollman J, et al. Intimal proliferation of smooth muscle as an explanation for recurrent coronary artery stenosis after

percutaneous transluminal coronary angioplasty. *J Am Coll Cardiol.* 1985;6:369–375.

8. Bruneval P, Guermoprez JL, Perrier P, et al. Coronary artery restenosis following transluminal coronary angioplasty. *Arch Path Lab Med.* 1986;110:1186–1187.

9. Essed CE, Van Den Brand M, Becker AE. Transluminal coronary angioplasty and early restenosis. Fibrocellular occlusion after wall laceration. *Br Heart J.* 1983;49:393–396.

10. Farb A, Virmani R, Atkinson JB, et al. Plaque morphology and pathologic changes in arteries from patients dying after coronary balloon angioplasty. *J Am Coll Cardiol.* 1990;16:1421–1429.

11. Garratt KN, Edwards W, Vlietstra RE, et al. Coronary morphology after percutaneous directional coronary atherectomy in humans: autopsy analysis of three patients. *J Am Coll Cardiol.* 1990;16:1432–1436.

12. Forrester JS, Fishbein M, Helfant R, et al. A paradigm for restenosis based on cell biology: clues for the development of new preventive therapies. *J Am Coll Cardiol.* 1991;17:758–769.

13. Giraldo AA, Esposo OM, Meis JM. Intimal hyperplasia as a cause of restenosis after percutaneous transluminal coronary angioplasty. *Arch Path Lab Med.* 1985;109:173–175.

14. Gravanis MB, Roubin GS. Histopathologic phenomena at the site of percutaneous transluminal coronary angioplasty: the problem of restenosis. *Hum Path.* 1989;20:477–485.

15. Kohchi K, Takebayashi S, Block PC, et al. Aterial changes after percutaneous transluminal coronary angioplasty: results at autopsy. *J Am Coll Cardiol.* 1987;10:592–599.

16. Mittal V, Karl EM, Atkinson JB, et al. Early and late morphologic changes after transluminal balloon angioplasty of the iliac arteries. *Am J Cardiol.* 1986;58:182–184.

17. Nobuyoshi M, Kimura T, Ohishi H, et al. Restenosis after percutaneous transluminal coronary angioplasty: pathologic observations in 20 patients. *J Am Coll Cardiol.* 1991;17:433–439.

18. Ueda M, Becker AE, Fujimoto T. Pathological changes induced by repeated percutaneous transluminal coronary angioplasty. *Br Heart J.* 1987;58:635–643.

19. Waller BF, Pinkerton CA, Orr CM, et al. Beyond angioplasty: 1. Remodeling and removing. *Practical Cardiol.* 1990;16:70–86.

20. Isner JM, Kearney M, Bortman S, et al. Sequential biopsy of human atheromata in vivo: longitudinal analysis of atheromatous coronary arterial wall in 11 patients treated for primary and restenosis lesions by directional atherectomy. *J Am Coll Cardiol.* 1993;21:74A. Abstract.

21. Isner JM, Kearney M, Berdan LG, et al. Core pathology lab findings in 425 patients undergoing directional atherectomy for a primary coronary artery stenosis and relationship to subsequent outcome: the CAVEAT study. *J Am Coll Cardiol.* 1993;21:380A. Abstract.

22. Murakami N, Trenkner E, Elzinger M. Changes in expression of nonmuscle myosin heavy chain isoforms during muscle and nonmuscle tissue development. *Dev Biol.* 1993;157:19–27.

23. Kuro-o M, Nagai R, Nakahara K-I, et al. cDNA cloning of a myosin heavy chain isoform in embryonic smooth muscle and its expression during vascular development and in arteriosclerosis. *J Biol Chem.* 1991;266:3768–3777.

24. Kawamoto S, Adelstein RS. Chicken nonmuscle myosin heavy chains: differential expression of two mRNAs and evidence for two different polypeptides. *J Cell Biol.* 1991;112:917–925.

25. Grabb ID, Hughes SS, Hicks DG, et al. Nonradioactive in situ hybridization using digoxigenin-labeled oligonucleotides. *Am J Pathol.* 1992;141:579–589.

26. Leclerc G, Isner JM, Kearney M, et al. Evidence implicating nonmuscle myosin in restenosis: use of in situ hybridization to analyze human vascular lesions obtained by directional atherectomy. *Circulation.* 1992;85:543–553.

27. Lindner V, Reidy MA. Expression of basic fibroblast growth factor and its receptor by smooth muscle cells and endothelium in injured rat arteries. *Circ Res.* 1993;73:589–595.

28. Nelken NA, Soifer SJ, O'Keefe J, et al. Thrombin receptor expression in normal and atherosclerotic human arteries. *J Clin Invest.* 1992;90:1614–1621.

29. Nikol S, Isner JM, Pickering JG, et al. Expression of transforming growth factor-b1 is increased in human vascular restenosis lesions. *J Clin Invest.* 1992;90:1582–1592.

30. Nikol S, Weir L, Sullivan A, et al. Persistent increased expression of the transforming growth factor-b1 gene in human vascular restenosis. *Cardiovasc Path.* 1994;3:57–64.

31. Pickering JG, Weir L, Jekanowski J, et al. Proliferative activity in peripheral and coronary atherosclerotic plaque among patients undergoing percutaneous revascularization. *J Clin Invest.* 1993;91:1469–1480.

32. Simons M, Leclerc G, Safian RD, et al. Relation between activated smooth muscle cells in coronary artery lesions and restenosis after atherectomy. *N Engl J Med.* 1993;328:608–613.

33. Brown LF, Yeo K-T, Berse B, et al. Expression of vascular permeability factor (vascular endotehlial growth factor) by epidermal keratinocytes during wound healing. *J Exp Med.* 1992;176:1375–1379.

34. Hoefler H, Childers H, Montminy MR, et al. In situ hybridization methods for the detection of somatostatin mRNA in tissue sections using antisense RNA probes. *Histochemistry.* 1986;18:597–604.

35. Long AA, Mueller J, Andre-Schwartz J, et al. High-specificity in situ hybridization. Methods and applications. *Diag Mol Path.* 1992;1:45–47.

36. Lawrence JB, Singer RH, Marselle LM. Highly localized tracks of specific transcripts within interphase nuclei visualized by in situ hybridization. *Cell.* 1989;57:493–502.

37. Lawrence JB, Singer RH. Intracellular localization of messenger RNAs for cytoskeletal proteins. *Cell.* 1986;45:407–415.

38. Xing Y, Johnson CV, Dobner PR, et al. Higher level organization of individual gene transcription and RNA splicing. *Science.* 1993;259:1326–1336.

39. Nikol S, Weir L, Kearney M, et al. Nonmuscle myosin: two isoforms with different functions in vascular restenosis. *J Am Coll Cardiol.* 1992;19:166A. Abstract.

40. Katsuragawa Y, Yanagisawa A, Inour A, et al. Two distinct nonmuscle myosin-heavy-chain mRNAs are differentially expressed in various chicken tissues. *Eur J Biochem.* 1989;184:611–616.

41. Gordon D, Reidy MA, Benditt EP, et al. Cell proliferation in human coronary arteries. *Proc Natl Acad Sci USA.* 1990;87:4600–4604.

42. Rekhter M, Ferguson SN, Gordon D. Cell proliferation in human arte-riovenous fistulas used for hemodialysis. *Arterioscler Thromb.* 1993;13: 609–617.

43. Gelb AB, Kamel OW, LeBrun DP, et al. Estimation of tumor growth fractions in archival formalin-fixed, paraffin-embedded tissues using two anti-PCNA/cyclin monoclonal antibodies. *Am J Pathol.* 1992;141: 1453–1458.

44. Kreipe H, Alm P, Olsson H, et al. Prognostic significance of formalin-resistant nuclear proliferation antigen in mammary carcinomas as de-termined by the monoclonal antibody Ki-S1. *Am J Pathol.* 1993;142: 651–657.

45. O'Brien ER, Alpers CE, Stewart DK, et al. Proliferation in primary and restenotic coronary atherectomy tissue: implications for antiprolifera-tive therapy. *Circ Res.* 1993;73:223–231.

46. Fontanini G, Pingitore R, Bigini D, et al. Growth fraction in non-small cell lung cancer estimated by proliferating cell nuclear antigen and comparison with Ki-67 labeling and DNA flow cytometry data. *Am J Pathol.* 1992;141:1285–1290.

47. Klemi PJ, Alanen K, Jalkanen S, et al. Proliferating cell nuclear antigen (PCNA) as a prognostic factor in non-Hodgkin's lymphoma. *Br J Can-cer.* 1992;66:739–743.

48. Dartsch PC, Voisard R, Bauriedel G, et al. Growth characteristics and cytoskeletal organization of cultured smooth muscle cells from human primary stenosing and restenosing lesions. *Arteriosclerosis.* 1990;10: 62–75.

49. Pickering JG, Weir L, Rosenfield K, et al. Smooth muscle cell out-growth from human atherosclerotic plaque: implications for the as-sessment of lesion biology. *J Am Coll Cardiol.* 1992;20:1430–1439.

50. Bauriedel G, Windstetter U, DeMaio SJ, et al. Migratory activity of hu-man smooth muscle cells cultivated from coronary and peripheral pri-mary and restenotic lesions removed by percutaneous atherectomy. *Circulation.* 1992;85:554–564.

51. Ross R, Wight TN, Strandness E, et al. Human atherosclerosis I. Cell constitution and characteristics of advanced lesions of the superficial femoral artery. *Am J Pathol.* 1984;114:79–93.

52. Hay ED. *Cell Biology of Extracellular Matrix Second Edition.* New York, NY: Plenum Press; 1991.

53. Riessen R, Isner JM, Blessing E, et al. Regional differences in the dis-tribution of the proteoglycans biglycan and decorin in the extracellu-lar matrix of atherosclerotic and restenotic human coronary arteries. *Am J Pathol.* 1994;144:962–974.

54. Rakugi H, Gibbons G, Wang D, et al. Expression of transforming growth factor beta 1 in human atherectomy specimens from primary and restenotic coronary artery lesions. *J Am Coll Cardiol.* 1992;19: 329A. Abstract.

55. Kahari VM, Larjava H, Uitto J. Differential regulation of extracellular matrix proteoglycan (PG) gene expression. *J Biol Chem.* 1991;266: 10608–10615.

56. Schonherr E, Jarvelainen HT, Kinsella MG, et al. Platelet derived growth factor and transforming growth factor-b1 differentially affect the synthesis of biglycan and decorin by monkey arterial smooth mus-cle cells. Differential regulation of extracellular matrix proteoglycan (PG) gene expression. *Arterioscler Thromb.* 1993;13:1026–1036.

57. Westergreen-Thorsson G, Hernnas J, Sarnstrand B, et al. Altered expression of small proteoglycans, collagen, and transforming growth factor-b1 in developing bleomycin-induced pulmonary fibrosis in rats. *J Clin Invest.* 1993;92:632–637.
58. Krull NB, Zimmermann T, Gressner AM. Spatial and temporal patterns of gene expression for the proteoglycans biglycan and decorin and for transforming growth factor-b1 revealed by in situ hybridization during experimentally induced liver fibrosis in the rat. *Hepatology.* 1993;18:581–589.
59. Border WA, Noble NA, Yamamoto T, et al. Natural inhibitor of transforming growth factor-b protects against scarring in experimental kidney disease. *Nature.* 1992;360:361–364.
60. Folkman J. Tumor angiogenesis: therapeutic implications. *N Engl J Med.* 1971;285:1182–1186.
61. Barger AC, Beeuwkes R, Lainey LL, et al. Hypothesis: vasa vasorum and neovascularization of human coronary arteries. *N Engl J Med.* 1984;310:175–177.
62. Leclerc G, Pickering JG, Weir L, et al. Percutaneous gene therapy for cardiovascular disease. In: Topol E, ed. *Interventional Cardiology.* Philadelphia, PA: W.B. Saunders; 1993:1019–1029.

Chapter 18

Restenosis:
Pathophysiology and Rational
Approches to Interventions.
Theseus and Minotaur?

*George Sopko, MD, MPH
and Peter Libby, MD*

The treatment of coronary heart disease (CHD), which is the leading cause of mortality in the United States, has progressed significantly over the past several decades with new approaches emerging and becoming an accepted form of therapy. Coronary revascularization by percutaneous transluminal coronary angioplasty (PTCA) can provide relief of symptoms and/or ischemia in patients with CHD by reducing luminal obstruction and improving coronary flow. Since the first PTCA done in 1977, there has been a rapid increase in the number of PTCAs performed with over 360,000 done in 1992, surpassing 309,000 coronary bypass graft surgeries (CABG).[1] Despite significant improvements in device technology, the high rate of restenosis remains the major limitation of PTCA and other percutaneous revascularization techniques. It has been reported to range from 12% to nearly 60% and peaking 1–3 months after successful dilation.[2,3] Conceptually, restenosis represents a specialized, time-limited excessive form of healing to localized injury, perhaps a form of "endovascular keloid formation".

Because intimal hyperplasia has been consistently observed in patients after PTCA, whether or not restenosis occurred, it would appear that this narrowing is closely related to the healing process that follows injury induced by arterial dilatation. Although laboratory investigations have led to a number of important observations,

From Vetrovec GW, Carabello BA, (eds.) *Invasive Cardiology: Current Diagnostic and Therapeutic Issues*. Armonk, NY: Futura Publishing Company, Inc.: © 1996.

understanding restenosis is hampered by the many gaps in knowledge of the biologic determinants of the healing process. Thus, the design of experimental approaches to unravel the pathophysiology of restenosis remains a considerable challenge.

The National Heart, Lung and Blood Institute (NHLBI) has and continues to play a significant role in advancing our understanding of this complex problem. One of the important missions of the NHLBI is to foster innovative research to facilitate the understanding of disease mechanism(s), to develop effective treatments and prevention strategies for significant public health problems, and to improve and enhance the quality of life. Many advances in diagnosis, treatment, and prevention of CHD have been made and a steady decrease in CHD mortality has been observed. However, many important issues remain to be resolved. Over the past decade the NHLBI has supported research projects directly and indirectly related to restenosis. Among the first to collect and report data on PTCA systematically, the NHLBI funded PTCA Registry (I and II) provided a comprehensive report on the success and complications of PTCA at that time, becoming a standard for comparison.[4] It became clear that there was a significant need to foster research to investigate mechanisms of restenosis after angioplasty, so that a rational approach for modulation of the repair process and ultimately for prevention of this complication of angioplasty can be developed. As a result an NHLBI initiative (RFA NIH 91-HL-02-H) was released in November 1990. The objective of the initiative was to encourage multidisciplinary research directed at the elucidation of fundamental mechanisms of the humoral, cellular and other responses responsible for restenosis. The NHLBI funded the five most meritorious. The following is a brief review of some of the complexities of restenosis, many of which have been addressed with NHLBI support.

Clinical Risk Factors

Several risk factors for restenosis have been identified. It is most likely to occur in patients over 60 years of age, diabetics, smokers, and those with class IV angina.[4] Recently, lipoprotein(a) (Lp(a)) and low levels of HDL cholesterol have been also implicated.[5-10] The angiographic correlates of restenosis include significant residual stenosis after dilation, lesion eccentricity, lesion length over 10 mm, calcification, proximal lesion location and major intimal/medial dissection. Mechanical factors, such as oversized balloon and high inflation pressures have also been implicated.[11-14]

Other variables include: a magnitude of vessel stretch with subsequent damage to deeper layers of the vessel wall and the extent of vessel wall changes resulting from plaque formation and rupture. Despite various strategies targeted to relieve obstruction, such as bulk removal via atherectomy, laser ablation, or rotoblade, the rate of restenosis remains high.[3] Recent studies using stents have shown significant reduction in restenosis by angiography defined by percent residual stenosis at follow-up.[15] However, this benefit appears consequent to an improved immediate result rather than reduced luminal encroachment over time.[16,17] Furthermore, the effect of prolonged intravenous heparin administration in relation to reduction in restenosis with stents is unknown.

The Empiric Therapies

Given the importance of the problem of restenosis, a number of pharmacologic agents that empirically were thought to have the potential to prevent restenosis have been tested. Although heparin and prostaglandin inhibitors reduce the incidence of early (acute) post-PTCA thrombotic occlusion, late restenosis has not been prevented.[18] This lack of effectiveness of heparin was surprising because the drug has multiple effects, including direct inhibition of smooth muscle cell proliferation and migration in vitro and in vivo.[19,20] In animals, low molecular weight heparin reduced the proliferative response to injury, including stent implantation.[21-24] Based on studies in vitro showing some growth inhibiting effects and recognizing that vessel constriction facilitates thrombosis as well as influencing remodeling of the vessel wall, calcium channel blockers are conceptually very appealing. Most of the studies showed that these agents either have not successfully reduced restenosis or at best had only marginal benefit.[25-27] However, recent meta-analysis of five randomized clinical trials suggests a benefit with the use of these drugs.[28] Many other agents including lovastatin, a HMG-CoA reductase agent, high-dose steroid therapy, antiplatelet agents, and various anticoagulants have been tried and have not been shown to prevent restenosis.[29-33] Administration of an antibody directed against the platelet adhesive glycoprotein IIb/IIIa reduces the incidence of acute events post-PTCA, but has not yet been shown to reduce restenosis.[34] It is likely that many phenomena contribute to the observed clinical failure of agents with promising in vitro results. Some of this disparity may relate to many factors. The lack of therapeutic effect may be related to the conventionally dosed therapies not producing adequate levels to inhibit the restenosis.[35-37] Many of these therapies focused on modulation of vessel tone and partly on abolishing thrombosis rather than on mechanism(s) of specific cell function such as proliferation, migration, matrix production, and their inhibition. A search for effective agents continues.

Pathobiology

It is well appreciated that PTCA results in unavoidable vessel wall injury. Disruption of endothelial and vessel wall structure triggers molecular and cellular responses that in some patients lead to restenosis. There are similarities between the atherosclerotic process and restenosis; however, time course and specific features are unique to restenosis.[38] Briefly, the histology of restenosis specimens obtained by atherectomy reveals an abundance of what appear to be smooth muscle cells with a substantial amount of extracellular matrix, particularly proteoglycan and collagens.[39-41] The current opinion is that these cells are predominantly smooth muscle cells, perhaps phenotypically modulated compared to normal medial smooth muscle cells.[42-43] However, other cells may be involved.[44] Cells propagated from restenotic lesions show lower sensitivity to growth inhibition by heparin suggesting aberrant growth cell regulation.[45] However, selection artifacts and responses to in vitro conditions hamper the extrapolation of such cell culture results to the in vivo situations. Intimal thickening is a complex process involving endothelial and vascular smooth muscle cells, platelets, growth factors, immune responses and the multiple consequences of disruption of an atherosclerotic plaque. A number of proposed mechanisms are reviewed.

Humoral and Vascular Interaction

Interaction between vascular (endothelium) and blood elements (platelets, neutrophils, RBC) plays a significant role in the initiation and in the determination of the severity of response to the injury. Endothelial cells receive and process signals from the endovascular (luminal) space and regulate underlying specific responses of smooth muscle cells.[46] The intact endothelium is the only biologic nonthrombogenic surface. The antithrombotic defense mechanisms of endothelial cells include endothelial-derived relaxing factor (EDRF), eicosanoids (in particular prostacyclin), binding of heparin, thrombomodulin (which allows activation of protein C, a potent anticoagulant), and smooth muscle cell and endothelial cell production of heparan sulfate proteoglycans, which inhibit smooth muscle cell proliferation.[47,48] EDRF is a potent vasodilator with properties similar to nitric oxide (NO) while inhibiting platelet adhesion and adhesion.[49] Endothelium actively regulates vascular tone and response to various physical and hormonal stimuli through releasing vasodilating substances, chiefly EDRF, prostacyclin, adenosine di- and triphosphate or vasoconstricting factors, such as endothelin, thromboxane A2, superoxide anion, and endothelium-derived constricting factor.[50,51] This vasoactive function of endothelium is disturbed, with impaired EDRF-dependent responses observed, in vascular injury, atherosclerosis, and hypertension.[52,53] The issue of endothelial-related relaxation being dependent on formation of NO, which in turn affects intimal hyperplasia, has been raised. For example, administration of L-arginine, a precursor of NO, inhibited intimal hyperplasia by 39%.[54]

The injury initiates a complex interaction between endothelium and blood components with activation and release of specific factors, including calcium, serotonin, LDL particles, oxygen free radicals, mitogens, and chemoattractants.[55] Activated blood elements (ie, platelets and leukocytes) produce intermediates, which are then converted to new products. This allows the use of precursors and intermediates from different cells to form new metabolites with completely new functions. This phenomenon is known as "transcellular metabolism." It also provides for cell-to-cell communication. It is therefore reasonable to postulate that transcellular metabolism between endothelial cells, smooth muscle cells, neutrophils, platelets, and erythrocytes form a critical linkage in determining pathophysiologic events of restenosis as a result of vascular injury.

Mitogens and Smooth Muscle Cell Transformation

Neointimal thickening is assumed to require "phenotypic transformation" of smooth muscle cells from the normal "contractile" state, characterized by the presence of myosin and a lack of response to mitogens, to a modulated, so-called "synthetic" state noted in young growing cells, which is sensitive to mitogens and to growth stimuli.[56] Increased expression of the B isoform of nonmuscle myosin heavy chain was increased in human restenosis lesions.[57] This transformation correlates with the ability to assemble extracellular matrix components and promote cell division, and with hypersensitivity to vasoconstrictors. Serotonin, released from platelets, and also a neurotransmitter, exhibits vasoconstricting as well as mitogenic and chemotactic (for smooth muscle cells) effects.[58] However, results from recent randomized clinical trials showed that ketanserin, a serotonin S2-receptor antagonist inhibiting mitogenesis, platelet activation, vasoconstriction did not reduce restenosis.[59] The shift in phenotype between neointimal smooth muscle cells and normal medial smooth muscle cells may be triggered by mediators released or activated during injury, or may reflect amplification of a population of phenotypically distinct intimal smooth muscle cell precursors; or most likely a combination of these events. Intimal smooth muscle cells display many distinct characteristics such as production of a PDGF-like mitogen and expressing of PDGF A-chain MRNA.[60] The expression of the PDGF-A gene and the PDGF α and β receptor mRNA favor modulation of smooth muscle cells phenotype.[61] The data suggest that PDGF may also induce endogenous PDGF formation. Neointimal rat smooth muscle cells can proliferate independently of extracellular PDGF and exogenous growth factors.[62,63] It has been speculated that endogenous PDGF-like mitogen(s) and transforming growth factor (TGF-β-1) produced by regenerating smooth muscle cells may stimulate cell proliferation acting intracellularly without extracellular release. Angiotensin II and TGF-β-1 increase expression of PDGF-A mRNA and PDGF-like mitogens.[64–66] Vascular injury induces tissue angiotensin converting enzyme (ACE) expression with increased angiotensin II promoting smooth muscle cell proliferation in vitro.[67,68] ACE inhibition prevents intima formation in rats and inhibits injury-induced intimal hyperplasia.[69,70] However, in humans treatment with ACE inhibitor did not reduce restenosis.[71,72] Leukotrienes LTB4, LTC4, LTD4 stimulate phenotypic, induce smooth muscle cell DNA synthesis and facilitate a proliferative response to mitogens.[73] Conversely, prostaglandins PGE1, PGE2, and PGI2 inhibit smooth muscle cell growth.

However, prostaglandin inhibitors have not affected restenosis clinically.[18] Because in vascular injury there appears to be an upregulation of the mitogens, attention has been turned toward chemotherapeutic agents such as colchicine, vincristine, methotrexate, and actinomycin-D in hopes of thwarting the hyperproliferative response.[74–76] One of the important questions that remain is to what extent the replication of smooth muscle cells so characteristic after injury to animal arteries applies to human restenosis.[77,78]

Coagulation Cascade

One of the original hypotheses regarding the pathogenesis of restenosis is that thrombin generation and platelets are key elements. Acute thrombosis plays a significant role in the multifaceted hypercellular response to injury by angioplasty. Exposure of subendothelilal space or lesional tissue factor to blood elements leads to rapid thrombus formation. Fibrin and fibronectin facilitate the attachment and migration of smooth muscle cells. In experimental injury, thrombin activity remains elevated for several weeks.[79] Thrombin is thought to have direct and indirect mitogenic effects.[80–84] It can activate growth-related gene expression in smooth muscle cells and then evoke production of other growth factors. Compared with thrombin receptor expression only in the endothelial layer of normal vessel segments, the receptor was widely expressed in regions rich in smooth muscle cells and macrophages.[85] Plasminogen activators facilitate smooth muscle cell migration and proliferation. Injury and partial loss of endothelium secondary to angioplasty may facilitate smooth muscle cell migration and proliferation. This may be also due to loss of endothelial-derived heparin sulfate and TGF-β1, which can inhibit smooth muscle cell activity as well as due to loss of anticoagulant effect due to vessel injury.

There is a need to establish a time course for and measure the quantity of cell proliferation, thrombus formation, thrombin generation, and growth factor gene expression after human angioplasty injury. Various strategies targeting platelet adhesion, cohesion, and release after vascular injury are being tested. These include administration of a monoclonal antibody to platelet glycoprotein Gp-IIb/IIIa to inhibit platelet adhesion. This latter therapy reduces the acute thrombotic events post-PTCA, but as yet there is no evidence that this treatment actually inhibits restenosis.[34] Other innovative specific thrombin inhibitors are also being studied. It will be important to assess the effectiveness of thrombin inhibition at the site of injury and correlate that with smooth muscle cell growth responses. Restoration of endothelial confluence by attaching autologous cultured endothelial cells to sites of mechanical denudation to interrupt vascular lesion formation has also been proposed. We may also ask whether mesothelial cells (or any other suitable cell) could be used as a therapeutic substitute for endothelial cell. Factor Xa, another important coagulation factor is another (in vitro) mitogen for smooth muscle cells. Specific inhibition with recombinant antistasin (RATS) or tick anticoagulant (rTAP) reduced angiographic restenosis with lesser cross-sectional narrowing in hypercholesteremic rabbits.[86]

Fibrinolytic System

The plasminogen activator system plays a key role in the control of fibrinolysis by converting plasminogen to the active enzyme plasmin.[87] In addition to fibrinolysis, plasmin has been implicated in other cellular events, such as vascular wound repair, particularly cell migration through the extracellular matrix and the stimulation of cell replication. Plasminogen activators are expressed during cell migration and tissue remodeling. Plasminogen activators and their inhibitors comprise an extracellular system involved in proteolytic and antiproteolytic activities regulating matrix turnover. This class of fibrinolytic molecules that also facilitate the movement of cells through the tissue barriers and extracellular matrix, while plasminogen activator inhibitor type 1 (PAI-1) may inhibit this process. Activated plasminogen yielding plasmin amplifies the proteolytic activity of cells producing plasminogen activators.[88] Plasmin can also activate latent forms of certain growth factors, such as TGF-β1.[89] The final effect is determined by the complex interaction and balance of various (growth) factors. For example, although TGF-β1 and bFGF increase endothelial PA-1 and urokinase (u-PA) mRNA and synthesis, TGF-β1 facilitates antiproteolysis while bFGF enhances proteolysis.[90] It is also possible that growth factor inactivation could result from activity of the proteolytic plasminogen/plasmin system. In vascular injury models, increased expression of u-PA and tissue plasminogen (t-PA) tissue activators in temporal association with vascular smooth muscle cell proliferation and migration have been observed. t-PA produced by endothelial cells is likely to limit inappropriate clot formation. Minimal information exists about plasminogen activator receptor regulation in smooth muscle cells. It is also appreciated that plasminogens play an important role in vessel wall homeostasis but there is virtually no information available on alterations post-PTCA. Low levels of circulating plasminogen activator (rapid) inhibitor (PAI-1) were observed in patients with restenosis.[10] Many important questions need to be resolved. What is the interaction of t-PA (or u-PA) with endothelial cell surface receptors, and those growth factors, cytokines and pharmacological compounds that might regulate the plasminogen activators and their respective cell surface receptors? How is expression of plasminogen activators, their receptors and matrix-degrading proteases regulated by growth factors and cytokines on vascular cells in vitro? Will blocking (for example, by antisense oligonucleotides) of the synthesis of PAI-1 or u-PA affect smooth muscle cell proliferation, migration and invasion?

Leeches have been used for over a century for their anti-inflammatory effects. Hirudin has been isolated from the salivary gland of the European common leech. Recombinant hirudin differs from the natural compound by an absence of sulfated tyrosine group in position 63.[91] Hirudin can block thrombin at the thrombin-fibrinogen recognition site, the thrombin-fibrinogen binding site, and the thrombin-platelet activation site. Because of its effect of blocking thrombin activation of fibrinogen and retarding platelet aggregation, hirudin has also been used primarily for clot lysis.[92,93] Recent provocative findings indicate that early administration of recombinant hirudin also inhibits restenosis after experimental angioplasty in rabbits.[94,95] The mechanisms by which thrombin may promote neointimal thickening following PTCA and how recombinant hirudin results in a lower restenosis rate need to be examined. Related questions include: Does hirudin block smooth muscle cell migration and/or proliferation and does it influence the type and distribution of cells in these lesions including endothelial regrowth and smooth muscle cell distribution and the "phenotype"? What is thrombin's ability to act as a mitogen for endothelial and smooth muscle cells and its ability to elicit the production of or potentiate the effects of other growth factors and cytokines?

Growth Factors

Platelets release multiple growth factors such as PDGF, TGF-β1, serotonin, and thromboxane A2. Thromboxane A2 is a potent platelet aggregator and may facilitate smooth muscle cell proliferation. However, a clinical trial with thromboxane A2-receptor inhibitor did not prevent restenosis.[96] With the injury healing process there is an up-regulation of serotonin (primarily coupled to phospholipase C) that in turn makes the site more sensitive to vasoconstrictors and growth factors. Besides its release from platelets, PDGF is also produced by endothelial and smooth muscle cells. PDGF can stimulate smooth muscle cell migration and exhibit chemotactic activity for smooth muscle cells, leukocytes, and fibroblasts attracting them to the subendothelial space.[97–99] Through this "paracrine" action PDGF mediates subendothelial tissue reactivity and responses. At the site of smooth muscle cell proliferation resulting from injury, PDGF-receptor β expression is increased.[100] Trapidil, a PDGF antagonist, has been shown to have antiproliferative properties and can reduce restenosis.[101,102]

Basic fibroblast growth factors (bFGF), members of the heparin-binding growth factor family, are potent mitogens stimulating angiogenesis and regulating components of extracellular matrix, possibly in an autocrine manner.[103] Excellent in vivo evidence supports a causal role for bFGF released from injured intimal smooth muscle cells in signaling the "first wave" of medial smooth muscle cell proliferation in the rat carotid artery after balloon injury.[104-107] As with other growth factors in injury, there is an increased expression of FGF receptors in this situation. Recently, efforts directed at using FGF to target proliferating cells have used chimeric molecules with different activities combining them synthetically. Chimeric molecules of TGF-α and acidic FGF, targeted to receptors on smooth muscle cells, were bound to *Pseudomonas exotoxin* fragments (PE40) to achieve cytolysis of rapidly proliferating smooth muscle cells.[108] This strategy takes advantage of receptor-bound complexes and endocytosis to deliver the toxin.

Another substance likely to play a significant role in the injury healing process is insulin-like growth factor (IGF-I). An omnipresent polypeptide, structurally similar to insulin, it is necessary for cells in order to go through the cell division cycle. Its production by smooth muscle cells is increased with (endothelial) injury while the number of receptors is markedly decreased. Recently, significantly higher concentrations of IGF-I were noted in the smooth muscle cells of the modulated versus the contractile phenotype.[109] It has been suggested that IGF-I may play a role in allowing cells to continue to grow after induction by PDGF.[110] Compared to PDGF-BB, IGF-I is a weaker mitogen, but with a potent stimulation of directed migration of smooth muscle cells.[111] Somatostatin, a polypeptide, inhibits cellular proliferation and secretion of other peptides and hormones. Somatostatin analogs, octreotide and angiopeptin, inhibited IGF-I and bFGF-induced human coronary smooth muscle cell proliferation.[109] In animals, angiopeptin has been shown to inhibit smooth muscle cell proliferation.[112,113] However, in humans, subcutaneous administration twice a day did not prevent restenosis.[114] TGF-β1 is released from platelets, and belongs to a superfamily of regulatory cytokines that play a role in the injury healing process beginning with chemotaxis for macrophages and monocytes and induction of angiogenesis. The repair activity includes synthesis and assembly of new extracellular matrix.[115] As a part of tissue repair TGF-β1 can induce its own production, thus potentially initiating a vicious and chronic cycle leading to restenosis.[116,117] Compared to normal and atherosclerotic tissues, expression of TGF-β1 mRNA was highest in restenosis tissues.[118] However, TGF-β1 also inhibits endothelial cells via oxygen-dependent (pro-oxidant) effect and can be a mitogen. The antiproliferative effects on endothelial cells are early and late, with the latter being reversible.[119] The precise role of medial versus neointimal smooth muscle cells and TGF-β1 in "final" regulation leading to restenosis remains to be clarified. TGF is one of the most potent stimuli known for interstitial collagen production by smooth muscle cells. As most of the volume of the restenotic lesion consists of matrix rather than cells, this function of TGF may be as important as any effects on smooth muscle cell proliferation. Therapies using anti-TGF-β1 inhibitors are being studied.

It appears that activation of various endovascular "stressors" can induce new growth promoting signaling pathways, such as phospholipase C and protein kinase C activation. Protein kinase C is a multifunctional calcium and phospholipid-dependent serine/threonine kinase system important in regulating the number of cellular surface receptors.[120] Growth factors alter transduction and expression of early response genes which then alter cellular function that may promote neointima formation.[121] For example, angiotensin II, PDGF, and (α) thrombin induce c-*fos* proto-oncogene in smooth muscle cells.[64,122–123] The c-*fos* and c-*jun* protein complex appears to be important for cell proliferation.[124] The KC gene appears also easily inducible by the above factors. JE gene product protein is induced by PDGF and vessel injury.[125] JE encodes the rodent homolog of the human monocyte chemoattractant protein MCP-1, a monocyte and smooth muscle cell attractant. KC encodes a neutrophil chemoattractant. In contrast to KC, c-*fos* and c-*myc*, is inhibited by glucocorticoids. It is possible that KC and JE recruit neutrophils and monocytes to the site of injury with JE stimulating smooth muscle cell migration. Neuropeptides, such as substance P and K can also spur DNA synthesis and smooth muscle cell proliferation.[126] The expression of c-*myc* gene is needed for maximal activity.[127] Many factors have potent proliferative properties, however, the proliferative effects are also counteracted by antiproliferative effects. Angiotensin II, a powerful vasoconstrictor, modulates smooth muscle cell growth and hypertrophy that is accompanied by elevated levels of mRNA proto-oncogenes, c-*fos*, c-*myc*, and c-*jun*, and increased expression of PDGF, an autocrine growth factor.[128] It also evokes an antiproliferative response mediated by the protein kinase C pathway leading to an expression of TGF-β1.[129] The net effect of these simultaneous bifunctional responses is likely to be the production of cellular hypertrophy rather than hyperplasia at least in rat aortic smooth muscle cells.[130] Endothelin, another potent vasoconstrictor binds specifically to smooth muscle cells and stimulates expression of the proto-oncogenes c-*myc* and c-*fos*. Under some circumstances endothelin may induce DNA synthesis.[131,132]

Lipids and Oxidized Lipid Products

Another central hypothesis regarding restenosis is that immediately after PTCA, oxidants and lipid oxidation products act as direct stimuli of smooth muscle cell proliferation adding to the effects of other growth factors present, such as bFGF or PDGF. Oxidized LDL particles are thought to recruit leukocytes and facilitate their adhesion to endothelium with oxidant-producing inflammatory leukocytes accompanying platelets into the injury site.[133] The response shortly thereafter includes smooth muscle cell proliferation that ceases in a matter of weeks and is accompanied by hypertrophy and enhanced connective tissue synthesis. Conversion of LDL to oxidized LDL is done by endothelial cells, smooth muscle cells, monocytes and macrophages. Oxidized LDL is cytotoxic, interferes with endothelium-dependent relaxation, and augments agonist-induced vasoconstriction.[134,135] The inhibitory effect of oxidized LDL on endothelium appears to be caused by direct interaction between NO and oxidized LDL inactivating EDRF.[136] It is also hypothesized that these lipid oxidation products suppress the production of TGF-β1, which has strong inhibitory effects on smooth muscle proliferation and that the inhibitory action of the TGF-β1 ultimately signals the end of the proliferatory response to PTCA and is responsible for the enhancement of connective tissue synthesis. In a swine model of restenosis treatment with probucol, an antioxidant and lipid lowering agent significantly reduced neointimal formation after balloon injury.[137] Preliminary results suggest that lipoprotein Lp(a) lowering by LDL-apheresis can reduce restenosis rate.[138] The question here is whether lipid and cytokine/growth factors can explain the restenotic response to PTCA in individuals with atherosclerosis.

Immunologic and Inflammatory Mechanism(s)

A novel hypothesis has been put forth that immunologic and inflammatory mechanisms involve monokine release from tissue macrophages that initiate and perpetuate a restenosis "cascade."[139] Acute local thrombosis and/or mechanical injury triggers initial cytokine gene expression by macrophages and smooth muscle cells. This acute generation of cytokines evokes a secondary growth factor and cytokine response establishing a positive, self-stimulatory, autocrine and paracrine feedback loop that amplifies and sustains smooth muscle cell proliferation over time. This multistage schema would account for the lag between injury and restenosis, and failure of chronic antithrombotic therapy to eliminate the process.

There are many questions to be answered. What is the effect of angioplasty injury to an atheromatous plaque on endogenous mononuclear phagocytes as judged by local expression of cytokines? Is there delayed (more than 24 hours) and continuing (1–28 days) local expression of endogenous cytokine and growth factor genes after angioplasty injury leading to ongoing smooth muscle cell proliferation and matrix production. Can hirudin or analogous peptides to inhibit thrombin and cytokine antagonists modulate the initiation of propagation of the proliferative responses following angioplasty? Do lesions initially richer in macrophages have a greater potential to develop restenosis? An endothelial injury evokes leukocyte adhesion. It is thought that monocytes play an important role in vascular repair. Agents able to inhibit injury-induced monocyte adhesion such as heparin and antibody to monocyte chemotactic protein JE have been shown to decrease intimal proliferation.[140,141] The role of autoimmunity in restenosis has been also proposed. Elevated anticardiolipin antibodies are frequently seen in patients with lupus with propensity toward arterial thrombosis. Patients with restenosis had more often elevated levels of IgM-anticardiolipin antibodies.[142]

Fish oil-derived φ-3 fatty acids exhibit many effects potentially beneficial for the cardiovascular system. They are rapidly taken up by platelets, leukocytes and endothelial cells affecting their function. Fish oil-derived φ-3 fatty acids are thought to affect leukocyte-endothelial interaction by inhibition of leukotriene biosynthesis.[143,144] However, non-prostanoid pathways also exist. Leukotriene B4 is a potent factor mediating leukocyte adhesion and trans-endothelial migration. It has been also shown that leukotriene B4 up-regulates surface leukocyte adherence receptors.[145] Furthermore, leukotrienes LTB4, LTC4, LTD4, and LTE4 can accelerate phenotypic conversion of smooth muscle cells.[146] Peptidoleukotrienes and lipoxin A4 are released into a lumen during angioplasty and interestingly, their appearance is enhanced by aspirin.[147] In animals, fish oil administration prevented oxidized LDL-mediated leukocyte recruitment and endothelial adhesion.[148] Early studies on restenosis in humans showed promising results. Relatively large amounts of φ-3 fatty acids given shortly before angioplasty and continued for at least 3 months afterwards have been shown to reduce the frequency of restenosis.[149,150] However, other studies failed to detect beneficial effect with sufficient power being limited by small sample sizes.[151,152] Recent meta-analysis of trials suggested dose-dependent benefits of φ-3 fatty acids.[153] A large multicenter study funded by NHLBI is in progress to clarify issues regarding safety and efficacy of fish oils in restenosis.

Genetic Manipulation

Conceptually, mechanical injury of the endothelium by angioplasty may result in down-regulation of some growth-inhibiting mechanisms and up-regulation of growth factors facilitating smooth muscle cell proliferation and migration. The interferons, such as interferon-gamma (IFN-g) produced by T lymphocytes in the atherosclerotic lesion, can exhibit antiproliferative effects and inhibit collagen synthesis. It has been speculated that neointimal smooth muscle cell proliferation could be a result of local inhibition by gamma interferon and promotion by TGF-β1.[154–157] Expression of nuclear proto-oncogenes (c-*myb*, c-*fos*, and c-*myc*) a group of phosphoproteins linked to cellular proliferation, has been observed following mitogenic stimulation and after balloon injury to vessel wall in vitro.[158–160] Proto-oncogenes are thought to represent a common final path of mitogenic signals either as direct transcriptional activators or as gene regulators at post- transcriptional levels.[161] This common path represents an attractive target for therapeutic interventions. One of the important oncogenes is p53, a tumor suppressor oncogene.

p53 has been extensively studied and its mutations have been implicated in many malignancies. Conceptually, it is possible to view atherosclerotic lesions to some extent as benign smooth muscle cells tumors. p53 is a part of the system overviewing cell cycle function and division and plays an important role in DNA damage control.[162–164] Recent provocative findings from NHLBI suggest that in a substantial proportion of patients, angioplasty-induced injury activates latent cytomegalovirus, which in turn inactivates p53 protein in smooth muscle cells. With no longer (tumor) suppressor activity present, the smooth muscle cells can replicate more easily and lead to restenosis.[165] Thus, agents restoring p53 integrity or antiviral agents could represent alternative strategies to combat restenosis.

In animals, gene transfer, gene knockout, or manipulation of gene expression offers experimental tools and novel avenues of therapy in the control of restenosis.[166,167] The artery can be directly transfected using retroviral or adenoviral infection or liposome-mediated transfection. Both endothelial and smooth muscle cells can express transferred genes.[167] With antisense techniques, short segments of synthetic DNA complement and bind segments of native messenger RNA, translation or transcription is blocked ("a transient neutralization of gene expression") leading to a specific protein synthesis decrease. Administration of antisense oligomers directed against c-*myc* or c-*myc* mRNA inhibit human smooth muscle cell proliferation in vitro.[168,169] Conceptually, this approach offers an opportunity to target selectively proliferating cells and modulate their activity although many issues regarding selectivity and practicality remain unresolved. In a rat model c-*myc* mRNA peaks after 2 hours of a balloon injury. Antisense c-*myc* oligodeoxynucleotide reduced peak of c-*myc* expression and smooth muscle cell proliferation.[170] Ability to inhibit human smooth muscle cell growth with c-*myc* antisense oligonucleotides and neointimal formation (by adventitial delivery) with c-*myb* in vivo has been reported.[168-172] Human adenoviruses are able to infect many cells including vascular endothelium, offering an opportunity to specifically target smooth muscle cells. Recently, a successful transfer of a recombinant adenoviral vector expressing cell regulatory gene was made.[173 176] Also recently, adenovirus was used to deliver the thymidine kinase (tk) gene into the damaged smooth muscle cells making the cells more sensitive to ganciclovir in a pig model. The treated animals had 50% to 90% less arterial wall thickening than controls.[177] Similar findings have been observed in carotid vessels of rats treated with tk gene and ganciclovir.

However, many issues need to be addressed. These include a choice of the "optimal" gene, gene expression activity limited to a specific cell type, bioavailability and therapeutic efficacy of gene transfer strategy, selection of the best method of delivery, and application and long-term safety in humans.[178] Current animal models also used injured but nondiseased vessels in testing these strategies. One of the attractive features of gene therapy is that it can also be targeted directly to the site of angioplasty by the infusion catheters, leading to a rapid though transient transgene (local) expression.[179] Compared to other therapeutic strategies gene transfer can be targeted locally providing high levels of antiproliferative products without side effects accompanying systemic administration. The duration and concentration or "dose" of this mode of therapy could be tailored to correspond to the optimal course necessary to inhibit smooth muscle cell proliferation; if this process is indeed a sensibly therapeutic target in humans. What then needs to be determined is whether an endothelial lesion can be transfected and whether transfected cells can secrete antiproliferative proteins sufficient to inhibit the neoproliferation.

Extracellular Matrix

Extracellular matrix contains among other components proteoglycans, interstitial collagen, and fibronectin. It binds and acts as a reservoir of growth factors responsible for cellular proliferation (bFGF, TGF-β1-). Through cell surface receptors, smooth muscle cells interact with extracellular matrix proteins, influencing the intimal cytoskeleton. Integrins, one class of transmembrane cellular surface receptors, have extracellular and cytoplasmic domains. The extracellular component interacts with extracellular matrix, while the intracellular component interacts with cytoskeletal proteins, such as vinculin, talin, or α-actinin. Integrins provide a linkage, and mediate interaction, between the extracellular matrix and cells, potentially modifying cell behavior and migration. Remodelling of extracellular matrix by proteinases from vascular cells could lead to release of growth factors.[180] Migration of cells requires release of the cells from the cytoskeleton matrix. This may require interaction among various extracellular matrix proteins and stored growth factors.[181] Induction of specific proteinases can lead to initiation and perpetuation of degradation of extracellular matrix. For example, urokinase could release bFGF that then could initiate cellular proliferation.[182] Thus, remodeling may involve induction of proteolytic enzymes and their respective inhibitors. For example, activated TGF-β1 can stimulate PAI-1 and subsequently inhibit plasmin-dependant activation of TGF-β1.[183] Therefore the interaction among various components of extracellular matrix and growth factors may influence the direction and magnitude of cellular migration and proliferation. Thus, the extracellular matrix is important in lesion formation.[184]

One of the problems of therapy has been that in view of the large number of growth factors and receptors, it has been difficult to inhibit smooth muscle cells with antibodies or other antagonists directed at them. As proliferating smooth muscle cells express more bFGF receptors than nonproliferating smooth muscle cells, the alternative approach would be to selectively obliterate the proliferating subpopulation of smooth muscle cells.[185] However, there are problems with this strategy. Antibodies to specific growth factors are being counteracted by neutralizing antibodies on repeat exposure, limiting its effect to the initial decrease of smooth muscle cell migration from media to intima. There is also a problem with a penetration of the endothelial barrier. With recent advances in molecular technology, fragments or "small" antibodies capable of crossing capillaries have been produced together with other small molecules designed to achieve specific characteristics.

Summary

The dominant effect of angioplasty is intimal injury, accompanied by varying degrees of thrombosis and subsequent tissue healing by a hyperplastic response. Substantial amounts of (nonfederal) monies have been spent on multiple drug strategies, mostly empiric ones, with no significant success. Many endogenous substances with endocrine or autocrine properties such as endothelin, TGF-β-1, PDGF, FGF, LDL, glucocorticoids, insulin-like growth factor-1, angiotensin II, epinephrine, and norepinephrine may play a significant role in smooth muscle cell growth and migration. They can act as mitogens or factors facilitating a hyperplastic response. We need to learn not only about agents' inhibitory effects on smooth muscle proliferation, but also about their effect on endothelium. Because all attempts to halt the restenotic process have concentrated on suppressing the activity of vascular smooth muscle cells and since those attempts are unsuccessful in humans, we might ask the question "are we targeting the wrong cell or process?" It is clear that healing after angioplasty injury involves complex biologic mechanisms that ultimately regulate the development of prothrombotic and proliferative activities facilitated by vascular and blood elements, and native tissue antithrombotic defenses. Understanding these mechanisms and interactions is critical to the development of more rational interventions to combat restenosis, subsequently reducing the morbidity and cost associated with repeated revascularization by percutaneous techniques. As in the myth of Theseus and Minotaur, we must not get lost in the labyrinth in our quest to slay the beast.

References

1. National Hospital Discharge Survey, NCHS, 1992.
2. Liu MW, Roubin GS, King SB. Restenosis after coronary angioplasty: potential biologic determinants and role of intimal hyperplasia. *Circulation.* 1989;79:1374–1387.
3. Topol EJ, Leya F, Pinkerton CA, et al. A comparison of directional atherectomy with coronary angioplasty in a patients with coronary artery disease. The CAVEAT Study Group. *N Engl J Med.* 1993;329:221–227.
4. Kent K, Mullin SM, Passamani ER. Proceedings of the National Heart, Lung, and Blood Institute Workshop on the Outcome of Percutaneous Transluminal Angioplasty. *Am J Cardiol.* 1984;53:1c–146c.
5. Hearn JA, Donohue BC, Ba'albaki H, et al. Usefulness of serum lipoprotein(a) as a predictor of restenosis after percutaneous transluminal angioplasty. *Am J Cardiol.* 1992;69:736–739.
6. Donohue B, Lasorda D, Barker E, et al. Lp(a) correlates with restenosis after PTCA. *J Am Coll Cardiol.* 1993;21:33A.
7. Desmarais RL, Ayers CR, Gimple LW, et al. Serum lipoprotein(a) levels as a risk for restenosis after coronary angioplasty. *Circulation.* 1993 (suppl);88:I-272A.
8. Grainger DJ, Kirschenlohr IIL, Metcalfe JC, et al. Proliferation of human smooth muscle cells promoted by lipoprotein(a). *Science.* 1993; 260:1655–1658.

9. Cooke T, Shean R, Foley D, et al. Lipoprotein(a) in restenosis after percutaneous transluminal coronary angioplasty and coronary artery disease. *Circulation.* 1994;89:1593–1598.
10. Shah PK, Amin J. Low high density lipoprotein level is associated with increased restenosis rate after coronary angioplasty. *Circulation.* 1992; 85:1279–1285.
11. Holmes DR, Vlietstra RE, Smith HC, et al. Restenosis after percutaneous transluminal coronary angioplasty (PTCA): a report from the PTCA registry of the National Heart, Lung, and Blood Institute. *Am J Cardiol.* 1984;53:77C–81C.
12. Mabin TA, Holmes DR, Smith HC, et al. Follow-up clinical results in patients undergoing percutaneous transluminal coronary angioplasty. *Circulation.* 1985;71:754–760.
13. Roubin GS, Douglas JS Jr, King SB III, et al. Influence of balloon size on initial success, acute complications, and restenosis after percutaneous transluminal coronary angioplasty. A prospective randomized study. *Circulation.* 1988;78:555–565.
14. Rensing BJ, Hermans WR, Vos J, et al, on behalf of the Coronary Artery Restenosis Prevention on Repeated Thromboxane Antagonism (CARPORT): Luminal narrowing after percutaneous transluminal coronary angioplasty. A study of clinical, procedural, and lesional factors related to long-term angiographic outcome. *Circulation.* 1993;88: 975–985.
15. Larrazet FS, Dupouy PJ, Rande JLD, et al. Angioscopy after laser and balloon coronary angioplasty. *J Am Coll Cardiol.* 1994;23:1321–1326.
16. Serruys PW, Jaegere PDK, Kilmeney P, et al, for a BENESTENT Study. A comparison of balloon-expandable-stent implantation with balloon angioplasty in patients with coronary artery disease. *N Engl J Med.* 1994;331:489–495.
17. Fischman DL, Leon MB, Baim DS, et al, for the Stent Restenosis Study Investigation. *N Engl J Med.* 1994;331:496–501.
18. Gershlick AH, Spriggins D, Davies SW, et al. Failure of eprostenol (prostacyclin, PGI2) to inhibit platelet aggregation and to prevent restenosis after coronary angioplasty: results of a randomized placebo controlled trial. *Br Heart J.* 1994;71:7–15.
19. Lindner V, Olson NE, Clowes AW, Reidy MA. Inhibition of smooth muscle cell proliferation in injured rat arteries. *J Clin Invest.* 1992;90:2044–2049.
20. Kenagy RD, Nikkari ST, Welgus HG, Clowes AW. Heparin inhibits the induction of three metalloproteinases (stromelysin, 92-kD gelatinase, and collagenase) in primate arterial smooth muscle cells. *J Clin Invest.* 1987;93:1987–1993.
21. Hanke H, Oberhoff M, Hanke S, et al. Inhibition of cellular proliferation after experimental balloon angioplasty by low-molecular-weight heparin. *Circulation.* 1992;85:1548–1556.
22. Buchwald AB, Unterberg C, Nebendahl K, et al. Low-molecular-weight heparin reduces neointimal proliferation after coronary stent implantation in hypercholesteremic minipigs. *Circulation.* 1992;86:531–537.
23. Currier JW, Pow TK, Haudenschild CC, et al. Low molecular weight heparin (enoxaparin) reduces restenosis after iliac angioplasty in the hypercholesteremic rabbit. *J Am Coll Cardiol.* 1991;17(suppl B):118B–125B.

24. Faxon DP, Spiro TE, Minor S, et al. Low molecular weight heparin in prevention of restenosis after angioplasty. Results of Enoxaparin Restenosis (ERA) Trial. *Circulation.* 1994;90:908–914.
25. Corcos T, David PR, Bal PG, et al. Failure of diltiazem to prevent restenosis after percutaneous transluminal coronary angioplasty. *Am Heart J.* 1985;109:926–931.
26. Whitworth HB, Roubin GS, Hollman J, et al. Effect of nifedipine on recurrent stenosis after percutaneous transluminal coronary angioplasty. *J Am Coll Cardiol.* 1986;8:1271–1276.
27. Hoberg E, Dietz R, Frees U, et al. Verapamil treatment after coronary angioplasty in patients at high risk of recurrent stenosis. *Br Heart J.* 1994;71:254–260.
28. Hilegass WB, Ohman EM, Leimberger JD, Califf RM. Meta-analysis of randomized trials of calcium antagonists to reduce restenosis after coronary angioplasty. *Am J Cardiol.* 1994;73:835–839.
29. Lovastatin Restenosis Trial Study Group. Lovastatin restenosis trial: final results. *Circulation.* 1993;88(suppl):I-506A.
30. Schwartz L, Bourassa MG, Lesperance J, et al. Aspirin and dipyridamole in the prevention of restenosis after percutaneous transluminal coronary angioplasty. *N Engl J Med.* 1988;318:1714–1719.
31. Thornton MA, Gruentzig AR, Hollman J, et al. Coumadin and aspirin in prevention of recurrence after transluminal coronary angioplasty: a randomized study. *Circulation.* 1984;69:721–727.
32. Pepine CJ, Hirschfeld JW, Macdonald RG, et al. A controlled trial of corticosteroids to prevent restenosis after coronary angioplasty. *Circulation.* 1990;81:1753–1761.
33. Serruys PW, Rutsch W, Heyndrickx GR, et al. Prevention of restenosis after percutaneous transluminal coronary angioplasty with thromboxane A2-receptor blockade. A randomized, double-blind, placebo-controlled trial. *Circulation.* 1991;84:1568–1580.
34. The EPIC Investigators. Use of a monoclonal antibody directed against the platelet glycoprotein IIb/IIIa receptor in high-risk coronary angioplasty. *N Engl J Med.* 1994;330:956–961.
35. Singh JP, Rothfuss KJ, Wiernicki TR, et al. Dipyridamole directly inhibits vascular smooth muscle cell proliferation in vitro and in vivo: implications in the treatment of restenosis after angioplasty. *J Am Coll Cardiol.* 1994;23:665–671.
36. Edelman ER, Karnowsky MJ. Contrasting effects of the intermittent and continuous administration of heparin in experimental restenosis. *Circulation.* 1994;89:770–776.
37. Rogers C, Karnovsky MJ, Edelman ER. Inhibition of experimental neointimal hyperplasia and thrombosis depends on the type of vascular injury and the site of drug administration. *Circulation.* 1993;88:1215–1221.
38. Gravanis MB, Roubin GS. Histopathologic phenomena at the site of percutaneous transluminal coronary angioplasty: The problem of restenosis. *Hum Pathol.* 1989;20:477–485.
39. Safian RD, Gelbfish JS, Erny RD, et al. Coronary atherectomy: clinical, angiographic, and histologic findings and observations regarding potential mechanisms. *Circulation.* 1990;82:69–79.
40. Garratt KN, Holmes DR, Bell MR Jr, et al. Differences between primary atheromatous and restenosis lesions and influence of subintimal tissue resection. *J Am Coll Cardiol.* 1991;17:442–448.

41. Garratt KN, Edwards WD, Kaufmann UP, et al. Differential histopathology of primary atherosclerotic and restenotic lesions from coronary arteries and saphenous vein bypass grafts in tissue obtained from 73 patients by percutaneous atherectomy. *J Am Coll Cardiol.* 1990;16:1665–1671.
42. Hofling B, Welsch U, Heimerl J, et al. Analysis of atherectomy specimens. *Am J Cardiol.* 1993;72:96E–107E.
43. Waller BF, Johnson DE, Schnitt SJ, et al. Histologic analysis of directional coronary atherectomy samples. A review of findings and their clinical relevance. *Am J Cardiol.* 1993;72:80E–87E.
44. Wilcox JN, Scott N, Lumsden AB, et al. Onset of cell proliferation and growth factor expression after clinical angioplasty of primate vascular lesions. *Circulation.* 1993;88(suppl):I-469A.
45. Chan P, Patel M, Betteridge L, et al. Abnormal growth regulation of vascular smooth muscle cells by heparin in patients with restenosis. *Lancet.* 1993;341:341–342.
46. Daniel TO, Ives HE. Endothelial control of vascular function. *News Physiol Sci.* 1989;4:139–142.
47. Castellot JJ Jr, Favreau LV, Karnovsky MJ, Rosenberg RD. Inhibition of vascular smooth muscle cell growth by endothelial cell-derived heparin: possible role of platelet endoglycosidase. *J Biol Chem.* 1982;257: 11256–11260.
48. Fritze LMS, Reilly CF, Rosenberg RDA. Antiproliferative heparan sulfate species produced by post confluent smooth muscle cells. *J Cell Biol.* 1985;100:1041–1049.
49. Furchgott RF, Zawadzki JV. Obligatory role of endothelial cells in the relaxation of arterial smooth muscle by acetylcholine. *Nature (Lond).* 1980;288:373–376.
50. Marshall JJ, Kontos HA. Endothelium-derived relaxing factors: a perspective from in vivo data. *Hypertension.* 1990;16:371–386.
51. Dubin D, Pratt RE, Cooke JP, Dzau VJ. Endothelin, a potent vasoconstrictor, is a vascular smooth muscle mitogen. *J Vasc Med Biol.* 1989;1: 150–154.
52. Healy B. Endothelial cell dysfunction: an emerging endocrinopathy linked to coronary disease. *J Am Coll Cardiol.* 1990;16:357–358.
53. Luscher TF, Yang Z, Diedrich D, Buhler FR. Endothelium derived vasoactive substances: potential role in hypertension, atherosclerosis and vascular occlusion. *J Cardiovasc Pharmacol.* 1989;14(suppl 6):S63–S69.
54. McNamara DB, Ignarro LJ, Akers DL. L-Arginine inhibits balloon catheter-induced intimal hyperplasia without improving neoendothelial-dependent acetylcholine-induced relaxation. *Circulation.* 1993; 88(suppl):I-371A.
55. Hoshi H, Kan M, Chen J-K, McKeehan WL. Comparative endocrinology- paracrinology-autocrinology of human adult large vessel endothelial and smooth muscle cells. *In Vitro Cell Dev Biol.* 1988;24: 309–319.
56. Hedin U, Bottger BA, Forsberg D, et al. Diverse effects of fibronectin and laminin on phenotypic properties of cultured arterial smooth muscle cells. *J Cell Biol.* 1988;107:307–319.
57. Simons M, Leclerc G, Safian RD, et al. Relation between activated smooth-muscle cells in coronary artery lesions and restenosis. *N Engl J Med.* 1993;328:608–613.

58. Nemecek GM, Coughlin SR, Handley DA, Moskowitz MA. Stimulation of aortic smooth muscle cells mitogenesis by serotonin. *Proc Natl Acad Sci.* 1986;83:674–678.
59. Serruys PW, Klein W, Tijssen JP, et al. Evaluation of ketanserin in the prevention of restenosis after percutaneous transluminal coronary angioplasty. A multicenter randomized double-blind placebo-controlled trial. *Circulation.* 1993;88:1588–1601.
60. Libby P, Warner SJC, Salomon RN, Birinyi LK. Production of platelet-derived growth factor-like mitogen by smooth muscle cells from human atheroma. *N Engl J Med.* 1988;318:1493–1498.
61. Sjolund, Hedin U, Sejersen T, et al. Arterial smooth muscle cells express platelet derived growth factor (PDGF) A chain mRNA, secrete a PDGF-like mitogen, and bind exogenous PDGF in a phenotype- and growth state dependent manner. *J Cell Biol.* 1988;106:403–413.
62. Schwartz SM, Foy L, Bowen-Pope DF, Ross R. Derivation and properties of platelet-derived growth factor-independent rat smooth muscle cells. *Am J Pathol.* 1990;136:1417–1428.
63. Walker LN, Bowen-Pope DF, Ross R, Reidy MA. Production of platelet-derived growth factor-like molecules by cultured arterial smooth muscle cells accompanies proliferation after arterial injury. *Proc Natl Acad Sci USA.* 1986;83:7311–7315.
64. Naftilan AJ, Pratt RE, Dzau VJ. Induction of platelet-derived growth factor A-chain and c-*myc* gene expressions by angiotensin II in cultured rat vascular smooth muscle cell cells. *J Clin Invest.* 1989;83:1419–1424.
65. Bobik A, Grinpukel S, Little PG, et al. Angiotensin II and noradrenaline increase PDGF-BB receptors and potentiate PDGF-BB stimulated DNA synthesis in vascular smooth muscle. *Biochem Biophys Res Commun.* 1990;166:580–588.
66. Majack RA, Majesky MW, Goodman LV. Role of PDGF-A expression in the control of vascular smooth muscle cell growth by transforming growth factor-beta. *J Cell Biol.* 1990;111:239–247.
67. Rakugi H, Kim DK, Krieger JE, et al. Induction of angiotensin converting enzyme in the neointima after vascular injury. Possible role in restenosis. *J Clin Invest.* 1994;93:339–346.
68. Powell JS, Clozel JP, Muller PK, et al. Inhibitors of angiotensin-converting enzyme prevent myointimal proliferation after vascular injury. *Science.* 1989;245:186–188.
69. Clozel JP, Muller RK, Roux S, et al. Influence of the status of the renin-angiotensin system on the effect of cilazapril on neointima formation after vascular injury in rats. *Circulation.* 1993;88:1222–1227.
70. Powell JS, Muller RK, Baumgartner HR. Suppression of the vascular response to injury: the role of angiotensin-converting enzyme inhibitors. *J Am Coll Cardiol.* 1991;17(supplB):137–142B.
71. Desmet W, Vrolix M, De Scheerder I, et al. Angiotensin-converting enzyme inhibition with fosinopril sodium in the prevention of restenosis after coronary angioplasty. *Circulation.* 1994;89:385–392.
72. Does the new angiotensin converting enzyme inhibitor cilazapril prevent restenosis after percutaneous transluminal angioplasty? Results of the MERCATOR study: a multicenter randomized, double-blind placebo-controlled trial. *Circulation.* 1992;86:100–110.
73. Palmberg L, Claesson HE, Thyberg J. Leukotrienes stimulate initiation of DNA synthesis in cultured arterial smooth muscle cells. *J Cell Sci.* 1987;88:151–159.

74. O'Keefe JH Jr, McCallister BD, Bateman TM, et al. Ineffectiveness of colchicine for the prevention of restenosis after coronary angioplasty. *J Am Coll Cardiol.* 1992;19:1597–1600.
75. Freed MS, Safian MA, Safian RD, et al. An intensive poly-pharmaceutical approach to the prevention of restenosis: the mevacor, ACE inhibitor, colchicine (BIG-MAC) pilot trial. *J Am Coll Cardiol.* 1993; 21:33A.
76. Muller DW, Topol EJ, Abrams GD, et al. Intramural methotrexate therapy for the prevention of neointimal thickening after balloon angioplasty. *J Am Coll Cardiol.* 1992;20:460–466.
77. O'Brien ER, Alpers CE, Stewart DK, et al. Proliferation in primary and restenotic coronary atherectomy tissue. Implications for antiproliferative therapy. *Circ Res.* 1993;73:223–231.
78. Pickering JG, Weir L, Jekanowski J, et al. Proliferative activity in peripheral and coronary atherosclerotic plaque among patients undergoing percutaneous revascularization. *J Clin Invest.* 1993;91:1469–1480.
79. Hatton MSW, Moar SL, Richardson M. Deendothelialization in vivo initiates a thrombogenic reaction at the rabbit aorta surface. Correlation of uptake of fibrinogen and antithrombin III with thrombin generation by the exposed endothelium. *Am J Pathol.* 1989;135:499–508.
80. McNamara CAI, Sarembock IJ, Gimple LW, et al. Thrombin stimulates proliferation of cultured rat aortic smooth muscle cells by a proteolytically activated receptor. *J Clin Invest.* 1993;91:94–98.
81. Carney DH, Mann R, Redin WR, et al. Enhancement of incisional wound healing and neovascularization in normal rats by thrombin and synthetic thrombin receptor-activating peptides. *J Clin Invest.* 1992;89: 1469–1477.
82. Bar-Shavit R, Benezra M, Eldor A, et al. Thrombin immobilized to extracellular matrix is a potent mitogen for vascular smooth muscle cells: nonenzymatic mode of action. *Cell Regul.* 1990;1:453–463.
83. Stouffer GA, Sarembock IJ, McNamara CA, et al. Thrombin-induced mitogenesis of vascular smooth muscle cells is partially mediated by autocrine production of platelet-derived growth factor-AA. *Am J Physiol.* 1993;265:C806–C811.
84. Bachhuber BG, Sarembock IJ, McNamara CA, et al. Thrombin-induced proliferation of cultured vascular smooth muscle cells requires prolonged exposure to thrombin. *Circulation.* 1993;88(suppl):I-468A.
85. Nelken NA, Soifer SJ, O'Keefe J, et al. Thrombin receptor expression in normal and atherosclerotic human arteries. *J Clin Invest.* 1992;90: 1614–1621.
86. Ragosta M, Gimple LW, Gertz SD, et al. Specific factor Xa inhibition reduces restenosis after balloon angioplasty of atherosclerotic femoral arteries in rabbits. *Circulation.* 1994;89:1262–1271.
87. Vassalli J-D, Sappino A-P, Belin D. The plasminogen activator/plasmin system. *J Clin Invest.* 1991;88:1067–1072.
88. Andrade-Gordon P, Strickland S. Interaction of heparin with plasminogen activators and plasminogen: effects on the activation of plasminogen. *Biochemistry.* 1986;25:4033–4040.
89. Rifkin DB, Moscatelli D, Bizik J, et al. Growth factor control of extracellular proteolysis. *Cell Diff Dev.* 1990;32:313–318.
90. Pepper MS, Belin D, Montesano R, et al. Transforming growth factor-beta 1 modulates basic fibroblast growth factor-induced proteolytic

and angiogenic properties of endothelial cells in vitro. *J Cell Biol.* 1990;111:743–755.

91. Markwardt F. Pharmacology of hirudin: one hundred years after the first report of the anticoagulant agent in medicinal leeches. *Biomed Biochem Acta.* 1985;44:1007–1013.

92. Heras M, Chesebro JH, Webster MWI, et al. Hirudin, heparin and placebo during deep arterial injury in the pig: the in vivo role of thrombin in platelet-mediated thrombosis. *Circulation.* 1990;82:1476–1484.

93. Cannon CP, Maraganore JM, Loscalzo J, et al. Anticoagulant effects of Hirulog, a novel thrombin inhibitor, in patients with coronary artery disease. *Am J Cardiol.* 1993;71:778–782.

94. Sarembock I, Gertz SD, Gimple LW, et al. Effectiveness of recombinant desulphatohirudin in reducing restenosis after balloon angioplasty of atherosclerotic femoral arteries in rabbits. *Circulation.* 1991;84:232–243.

95. McCoy K, Gimple LW, Gertz SD, et al. Effectiveness of hirulog in reducing restenosis after balloon angioplasty of atherosclerotic femoral arteries in rabbits. *Circulation.* 1993;88(suppl):I-338A.

96. Serruys PW, Rutsch W, Heyndrickx GR, et al. Prevention of restenosis after percutaneous transluminal coronary angioplasty with thrombaxane A2-receptor blockade. A randomized, double blind, placebo controlled trial. *Circulation.* 1991;84:1568–1580.

97. Jawien A, Bowen-Pope DF, Lindner V, et al. Platelet-derived growth factor promotes smooth muscle migration and intimal thickening in a rat model of balloon angioplasty. *J Clin Invest.* 1992;89:507–511.

98. Ross R, Raines EW, Bowen-Pope DF. The biology of platelet-derived growth factor. *Cell.* 1986;46:155–169.

99. Thyberg J, Hedin U, Sjolund M, et al. Regulation of differentiated properties and proliferation of arterial smooth muscle cells. *Arteriosclerosis.* 1990;10:966–990.

100. Majevsky MW, Lindner V, Twardzik DR, et al. Production of transforming growth factor beta-1 during repair of arterial injury. *J Clin Invest.* 1991;88:904–910.

101. Liu MW, Roubin GS, Robinson KA, et al. Trapidil in preventing restenosis after balloon angioplasty in atherosclerotic rabbit. *Circulation.* 1990;81:1089–1093.

102. Okamoto S, Inden M, Setsuda M, et al. Effect of trapidil (triazolopyrimidine), a platelet-derived growth factor antagonist, in preventing restenosis after percutaneous transluminal coronary angioplasty. *Am Heart J.* 1992;123:1439–1444.

103. Winkles JA, Friesel R, Alberts GF, et al. Elevated expression of basic fibroblast growth factor in an immortalized rabbit smooth muscle cell line. *Am J Pathol.* 1993;143:518–527.

104. Lindner V, Reidy MA, Fingerle J. Regrowth of arterial endothelium. Denudation with minimal trauma leads to complete cell regrowth. *Lab Invest.* 1989;61:556–563.

105. Lindner V, Majack RA, Reidy MA. Basic fibroblast growth factor stimulates endothelial regrowth and proliferation in denuded arteries. *J Clin Invest.* 1990;85:2004–2008.

106. Lindner V, Lappi DA, Baird A, et al. Role of basic fibroblast growth factor in vascular lesion formation. *Circ Res.* 1991;68:106–113.

107. Lindner V, Reidy MA. Proliferation of smooth muscle cells after vascular injury is inhibited by an antibody against basic fibroblast growth factor. *Proc Natl Acad Sci USA.* 1991;88:3739–3743.
108. Epstein SE, Siegall CB, Biro S, et al. Cytotoxic effects of a recombinant chimeric toxin on rapidly proliferating vascular smooth muscle cells. *Circulation.* 1991;84:778–787.
109. Grant MB, Wargovich TJ, Ellis EA, et al. Localization of insulin-like growth factor I and inhibition of coronary smooth muscle cell growth by somatostatin analogues in human coronary smooth muscle cells. A potential treatment for restenosis. *Circulation.* 1994;89:1511–1517.
110. Khorsani MJ, Fagin JA, Giannella-Neto D, et al. Regulation of insulin-like growth factor-I and its receptor in rat aorta after balloon denudation. Evidence for local bioactivity. *J Clin Invest.* 1992;90:1926–1931.
111. Bornfeldt KE, Raines EW, Nakano T, et al. Insulin-like growth factor-I and platelet-derived growth factor-BB induce directed migration of human arterial smooth muscle cells via signaling pathways that are distinct from those of proliferation. *J Clin Invest.* 1994;93:1266–1274.
112. Lundergan C, Foegh ML, Vargas R, et al. Inhibition of myointimal proliferation of the rat carotid artery by the peptides, angiopeptin and BIM 23034. *Atherosclerosis.* 1989;80:49–55.
113. Santoian ED, Schneider JE, Gravanis MB, et al. Angiopeptin inhibits intimal hyperplasia after angioplasty in porcine coronary arteries. *Circulation.* 1993;88:11–14.
114. Kent KM, Williams DO, Cassagneau B, et al. Double blind controlled trial of the effect of angiopeptin on coronary restenosis following balloon angioplasty. *Circulation.* 1993;88(suppl):I-506A.
115. Pettinen RP, Kobayashi S, Bernstein P. Transforming growth factor-beta increases mRNA for matrix proteins both in the presence and in the absence of changes in mRNA stability. *Natl Acad Sci USA.* 1988;85:1105–1108.
116. Border WA, Ruoslahti E. Transforming growth factor-beta in disease: the dark side of tissue repair. *J Clin Invest.* 1992;90:1–7.
117. van Obberghen-Schilling E, Roche NS, Flanders KC, et al. Transforming growth factor-beta1 positively regulates its own expression in normal and transformed cells. *J Biol Chem.* 1988;263:7741–7746.
118. Nikol S, Isner JM, Pickering JG, et al. Expression of transforming growth factor-beta 1 is increased in human vascular restenosis lesions. *J Clin Invest.* 1992;90:1582–1592.
119. Das SK, White AC, Fanburg BL. Modulation of transforming growth factor-beta1 antiproliferative effects on endothelial cells by cysteine, cystine, and N-acetylcysteine. *J Clin Invest.* 1992;90:1649–1656.
120. Nishizuka Y. The molecular heterogeneity of protein kinase C and its implication for cellular regulation. *Nature (Lond).* 1988;334:661–665.
121. Miano EP, Ehsani N, Palmer H, Libby P. Cytokines positively and negatively regulate interstitial collagen gene expression in human vascular smooth muscle cells. *Arteriosclerosis.* 1991;11:1223–1230.
122. Poon M, Marmur JD, Rosenfield C-L, et al. The KC gene is induced in vivo by vascular injury and in smooth muscle culture by growth factors. *Circulation.* 1990;82(suppl):III-208A.
123. Naftilan AJ, Pratt RE, Dzau VJ. Angiotensin II induces c-fos expression in smooth muscle via transcriptional control. *Hypertension.* 1989;13:706–711.

124. Miller AD, Curran T, Verma IM. C-fos protein can induce cellular transformation: A novel mechanism of activation of cellular oncogene. *Cell.* 1984;35:51–60.
125. Marmur JD, Friedrich VL, Rossikhina M, et al. The JE gene encodes a smooth muscle chemotactic factor that is induced by vascular injury. *Circulation.* 1990;82(suppl):III-698.
126. Nilsson J, von Euler AAM, Dalsgaard C-J. Stimulation of connective tissue cell growth by substance P and substance K. *Nature.* 1985; 315:61–63.
127. Nilsson J, Sejersen T, Hultgardh-Nilsson A, Dalsgaard C-J. DNA synthesis induced by the neuropeptide substance K correlates to the level of myc-gene transcripts. *Biochem Biophys Res Commun.* 1986;137: 167–174.
128. Daemen MJAP, Lombardi DM, Bosman FT, Schwartz SM. Angiotensin II induces smooth muscle cell proliferation in the normal and injured rat arterial wall. *Circ Res.* 1991;68:450–456.
129. Gibons GH, Pratt RE, Dzau VJ. Vascular smooth muscle cell hypertrophy vs. hyperplasia: Autocrine transforming growth factor-beta expression determines growth response to angiotensin II. *J Clin Invest.* 1992;90:456–461.
130. Gibons GH, Pratt RE, Dzau VJ. Angiotensin II is a bifunctional modulator of vascular smooth muscle cell growth: interaction with basic fibroblast growth factor. *Hypertension.* 1989;14:358A.
131. Bobik A, Grooms A, Millar JA, et al. Growth factor activity of endothelin on vascular smooth muscle. *Am J Physiol.* 1990;258:C408–C415.
132. Hirata Y, Takagi Y, Fukuda Y, Marumo F. Endothelin is a potent mitogen for rat vascular smooth muscle cells. *Atherosclerosis.* 1989; 78:225–228.
133. Quinn MT, Parthasarathy S, Fong LG, Steinberg D. Oxidatively modified low density lipoprotcins: a potential role in recruitment and retention of monocyte/macrophages during atherogenesis. *Proc Natl Acad Sci USA.* 1987;84:2995–2998.
134. Simon BC, Cunningham LD, Cohen RA. Oxidized low density lipoproteins cause contraction and inhibit endothelium-dependent relaxation in pig coronary artery. *J Clin Invest.* 1990;86:75–79.
135. Berliner JA, Territo MC, Sevanian A, et al. Minimally modified low density lipo-protein stimulate monocyte endothelial interactions. *J Clin Invest.* 1990;85:1260–1266.
136. Chin JH, Azhar S, Hoffman BB. Inactivation of endothelial derived relaxing factor by oxidized lipoproteins. *J Clin Invest.* 1992;89:10–18.
137. Schneider JE, Berk BC, Gravanis MB, et al. Probucol decreases neointimal formation in a swine model of coronary artery balloon injury. A possible role for antioxidants in restenosis. *Circulation.* 1993;88:628–637.
138. Daida H, Yamaguchi H, Yokoi H, et al. Prevention of restenosis after percutaneous coronary angioplasty by LDL-apheresis: LDL-apheresis Angioplasty Restenosis Trial (LART). *J Am Coll Cardiol.* 1993;21:34A.
139. Libby P, Schwartz D, Brogi E, et al. A cascade model for restenosis. A special case of atherosclerosis progression. *Circulation.* 1992;86: 47–52.
140. Rogers C, Karnovsky MJ, Edelman ER. Heparin's inhibition of monocyte adhesion to experimentally injured arteries matches its antiproliferative effects. *Circulation.* 1993;88(suppl):I-370A.

141. Guzman LA, Whitlow PL, Beall CJ, Kolattakudy P. Monocyte chemotactic protein antibody inhibits restenosis in the rabbit atherosclerotic model. *Circulation.* 1993;88(suppl):I-371A.
142. Eber B, Schumaker M, Auer-Grumbach P, et al. Increased IgM-anticardiolipin antibodies in patients with restenosis after percutaneous transluminal coronary angioplasty. *Am J Cardiol.* 1992;69:1255–1258.
143. Lee TH, Hoover RL, Williams JD, et al. Effect of dietary enrichment with eicosapentoic and docohexaenoic acids on in vitro neutrophil and monocyte leukotriene generation and neutrophil function. *N Engl J Med.* 1985;312:1217–1224.
144. Endres S, Ghorbani R, Kelley VE, et al. The effect of dietary supplementation with omega-3 polyunsaturated fatty acids on the synthesis of interleukin-1 and tumor necrosis factor by mononuclear cells. *N Engl J Med.* 1989;320:265–271.
145. Lindstrom P, Lerner R, Palmblad J, Patarroyo M. Rapid adhesive responses of endothelial cells and of neutrophils induced by leukotriene B4 are mediated by leukocytic adhesion protein CD18. *Scand J Immunol.* 1990;31:737–744.
146. Palmberg L, Claesson H-E, Thyberg J. Effects of leukotrienes on phenotypic properties and growth of arterial smooth muscle cells. *J Cell Sci.* 1989;93:403–408.
147. Brezinski DA, Nesto RW, Serhan CN. Angioplasty triggers intracoronary leukotrienes and lipoxin A4. Impact of aspirin therapy. *Circulation.* 1992;86:56–63.
148. Lehr H-A, Hubner C, Finckh B, et al. Dietary fish oil reduces leukocyte/endothelium interaction following systemic administration of oxidatively modified low density lipoprotein. *Circulation.* 1991;84:1725–1731.
149. Dehmer GJ, Popman JJ, van den Berg EK, et al. Reduction in the rate of early restenosis after coronary angioplasty by a diet supplemented with n-3 fatty acids. *N Engl J Med.* 1988;319:733–740.
150. Bairati I, Roy L, Meyer F. Double-blind, randomized, controlled trial of fish oil supplements in prevention of recurrence of stenosis after coronary angioplasty. *Circulation.* 1992;85:950–956.
151. Reis GJ, Boucher TM, Sipperly ME, Silverman DI. Randomized trial of fish oil for prevention of restenosis after coronary angioplasty. *Lancet.* 1989;2:177–181.
152. Grigg LE, Kay TWH, Valentine PA, et al. Determinants of restenosis and lack of effect on the incidence of effect of dietary supplementation with eicosapentoic acid on the incidence of coronary artery restenosis after angioplasty. *J Am Coll Cardiol.* 1989;13:665–672.
153. Gapinski JP, VanRuiswyk JV, Heudebert GR, Schectman GS. Preventing restenosis with fish oils following coronary angioplasty. A meta-analysis. *Arch Intern Med.* 1993;153:1595–1601.
154. Heyns AP, Eldor A, Vlodavsky I, et al. The antiproliferative effect of interferon and the mitogenic activity of growth factors are independent cell cycle events. *Exp Cell Res.* 1985;161:297–306.
155. Hansson GK, Johansson L, Holm J, et al. Gamma-interferon regulates vascular smooth muscle proliferation and Ia antigen expression in vivo and in vitro. *Circ Res.* 1988;63:712–719.
156. Amento EP, Ehsani N, Palmer H, Libby P. Cytokines and growth factors positively and negatively regulate interstitial collagen gene ex-

pression in human vascular smooth muscle cells. *Arteriosclerosis.* 1991;11:1223–1230.

157. Hansson GK, Holm J. Interferon-gamma inhibits arterial stenosis after injury. *Circulation.* 1991;84:1266–1272.

158. Kindy MS, Sonenshein GE. Regulation of oncogene expression in cultured aortic smooth muscle cells. *J Biol Chem.* 1986;261:12856–12868.

159. Brown KE, Kindy MS, Sonenshein GE. Expression of the c-myb proto-oncogene in bovine vascular smooth muscle cells. *J Biol Chem.* 1992;267:4625–4630.

160. Miano Jm, Tota RR, Vlasic N, et al. Early proto-oncogene expression in rat aortic smooth muscle cells following endothelial removal. *Am J Pathol.* 1990;137:761–765.

161. Prendergast GC, Cole MD. Posttranscriptional regulation of cellular gene expression by the c-*myc* oncogene. *Mol Cell Biol.* 1989;9:124–134.

162. Friend S. P53: a glimpse at the puppet behind the shadow play. *Science.* 1994;265:334–335.

163. Cho Y, Gorina S, Jeffrey PD, Pavletich NP. Crystal structure of a p53 tumor suppressor-DNA complex: Understanding tumorigenic mutations. *Science.* 1994;265:346–355.

164. Clore GM, Omichinski JG, Sakaguchi K, et al. High-resolution structure of the oligomerization domain of p53 by multidimensional NMR. *Science.* 1994; 265:386–391.

165. Speir E, Modali R, Huang E-S, et al. Potential role of human cytomegalovirus and p53 interaction in coronary restenosis. *Science.* 1994;265:391–394.

166. Lim CS, Chapman GD, Gammon RS, et al. Direct in vivo gene transfer into the coronary and peripheral vasculature of the intact dog. *Circulation.* 1991;83:2007–2011.

167. Nabel EG, Plautz G, Nabel GJ. Site-specific gene expression in vivo by direct gene transfer into the arterial wall. *Science.* 1990;249:1285–1288.

168. Shi Y, Hutchinson HG, Hall DJ, Zalewski A. Down-regulation of c-*myc* expression by antisense oligonucleotides inhibits proliferation of human smooth muscle cells. *Circulation.* 1993;88:1190–1195.

169. Simons M, Rosenberg RD. Antisense nonmuscle myosin heavy chain and c-myb oligonucleotides suppress smooth muscle cell proliferation in vitro. *Circ Res.* 1992;70:835–843.

170. Bennett MR, Anglin S, McEwan JR, et al. Inhibition of vascular smooth muscle cell proliferation in vitro and in vivo by c-*myc* antisense oligodeoxynucleotides. *J Clin Invest.* 1994;93:820–828.

171. Simons M, Edelman ER, DeKeyser J-L, et al. Antisense c-myb oligonucleotides inhibit intimal arterial smooth muscle cell accumulation in vivo. *Nature.* 1992;359:67–80.

172. Speir E, Epstein SE. Inhibition of smooth muscle cell proliferation by antisense oligonucleotide targeting the messenger RNA encoding proliferating cell nuclear antigen. *Circulation.* 1992;86:538–547.

173. Lee SW, Trapnell BC, Rade JJ, et al. Adenoviral-mediated gene transfer into rat carotid artery. *Circulation.* 1993;88(suppl):I-371A.

174. March KL, Bauriedel G, Trapnell BC. Gene therapy to block restenosis following percutaneous transluminal coronary angioplasty: feasibility of strategies to target smooth muscle cells using adenoviral vectors. *Circulation.* 1993;88(suppl):I-371A.

175. Morishita R, Gibbons GH, Ellison KE, et al. A viral-mediated antisense oligonucleotide delivery system to prevent restenosis. *Circulation*. 1993;88(suppl):I-371A.
176. Guzman RJ, Lemarchand P, Crystal RG, et al. Efficient and selective adenovirus-mediated gene transfer into vascular intima. *Circulation*. 1993;88:2838–2848.
177. Ono T, Gordon D, San V, et al. Gene therapy for vascular smooth muscle cell proliferation after arterial injury. *Science*. 1994;265:781–784.
178. Losordo DW, Pickering JG, Takeshita S, et al. Use of the rabbit ear artery to serially assess foreign protein secretion after site-specific arterial gene transfer in vivo. *Circulation*. 1994;89:785–792.
179. Riessen R, Isner JM. Prospects for site-specific delivery of pharmacologic and molecular therapies. *J Am Coll Cardiol*. 1994;23:1234–1244.
180. Moscatelli D, Rifkin DB. Membrane and matrix localization of proteinases: A common theme in tumor invasion and angiogenesis. *Biochem Biophys Acta*. 1989;948:67–85.
181. Hay E. *Cell Biology of Extracellular Matrix*. Second edition. New York, NY: Plenum Press; 1991.
182. Saksela O, Rifkin DB. Release of fibroblast growth factor-heparin sulfate complexes from endothelial cells by plasminogen activator mediated proteolytic activity. *J Cell Biol.* 1990;110:767–775.
183. Sato Y, Tsuboi R, Moses H, Rifkin DB. Characterization of the activation of latent TGF-B1 by co-cultures of endothelial and pericytes or smooth muscle cells: a self regulating system. *J Cell Biol.* 1990;111:757–763.
184. MacLeod DC, Strauss BH, de Jong M, et al. Proliferation and extracellular matrix synthesis of smooth muscle cells cultured from human coronary atherosclerotic and restenotic lesions. *J Am Coll Cardiol*. 1994;23:59–65.
185. Ferns GAA, Raines EW, Spruget KH, et al. Inhibition of neointimal smooth muscle accumulation after angioplasty by an antibody to PDGF. *Science*. 1991;253:1129–1132.

Chapter 19

Coronary Restenosis:
Insights from Animal Models

Robert S. Schwartz, MD,
Sanjay S. Srivatsa, MD,
Robert D. Simari, MD, and
David R. Holmes, Jr, MD

Coronary restenosis currently remains the major limitation to angioplasty and continues to defy definitive therapy. Important new data about the multifactorial causes of restenosis are emerging. These data include cellular proliferation, arterial remodeling, and matrix production. Although cellular proliferation has been a central target of previous antirestenosis strategies, it may not be as important as previously emphasized. Recent studies in arterial remodeling suggest that restenosis may relate to the ability of an injured artery to enlarge in a manner that compensates for neointimal growth. Extracellular matrix provides the bulk of neointimal volume, so that strategies to limit matrix formation could provide novel therapeutic opportunities. Animal restenosis models have only recently been used to improve understanding of restenosis pathophysiology; prior animal studies generally failed to predict effective therapies in human clinical trials. This may relate to clear differences across species in the neointimal response to injury, differences in hemostatic responses, the use of very high drug doses in prior animal trials, and the fact that animal studies frequently use histopathologic end points rather than angiographic surrogates. The problem of restenosis will be solved through an improved understanding of the cellular and physical mechanisms. We can no longer afford to perform large clinical trials of agents that have not been adequately evaluated in animal studies. Effective strategies to solve the restenosis problem can best be designed

From Vetrovec GW, Carabello BA, (eds.) *Invasive Cardiology: Current Diagnostic and Therapeutic Issues.* Armonk, NY: Futura Publishing Company, Inc.: © 1996.

through study of appropriate animal models, and by complete understanding of the inherent strengths and limitations of each.

Although coronary restenosis has been a problem since the inception of angioplasty, it has recently attained even more importance. The reports of clinical trials (EAST, GABI, RITA, and CABRI) comparing bypass surgery with angioplasty document comparability between percutaneous transluminal angioplasty (PTCA) and coronary bypass surgery in terms of patient survival and myocardial infarction. These studies differ regarding the need for repeat interventions, and thus highlight the importance of restenosis.

Pharmacologic approaches have clearly failed.[1–12] As reported by the STRESS and BENESTENT trials, coronary stents have been demontrated as lessening restenosis, but still do not solve the problem completely. Other new revascularization technologies show small differences.[13–20] Recently, the CAVEAT trials offer further evidence of these minor effects. It is increasingly evident that our incomplete understanding of restenosis pathophysiology has prevented formulation of a truly effective therapy.

Coronary Restenosis: Neointimal Hyperplasia and the Response to Injury

The injured coronary artery heals after injury by forming neointimal hyperplasia. In humans, hyperplastic coronary arterial tissue consists of an intense fibrocellular response of variable density. The primary constituents of the hyperplastic response are a combination of vascular smooth muscle cells, fibroblasts, and cells of macrophage/monocyte origin (Figure 1). Ultrastructural studies indicate many cytoplasmic myofibrils with few organelles. The severity of arterial injury may largely determine the neointimal volume at an arterial injury site. Late lumen loss is proportional to acute luminal gain, and the risk of restenosis is inversely proportional to the preprocedural minimum luminal diameter (MLD), where smaller MLD requires larger dilatation, and larger vascular injury.[21,22]

Restenosis is related to factors other than neointimal hyperplasia. These include arterial remodeling, elastic recoil, thrombus at the injury site, medial smooth muscle cell proliferation and migration, and excessive extracellular matrix production. Although the exact contribution of each has not been established, each is being actively investigated as potential causes and also as a means of developing therapeutic strategies.

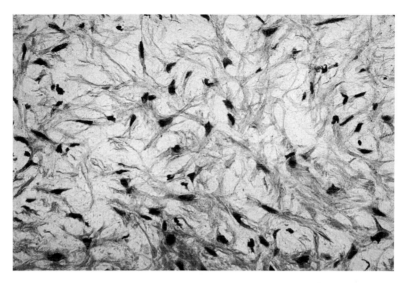

FIGURE 1. *Photomicrograph of restenotic human neointima. Cell density is rare, with much of the tissue volume being extracellular matrix. Hematoxylin/Eosin stain, magnification × 100.*

To better understand human restenosis, animal arterial injury models are playing an increasing, if controversial role in planning clinical strategies.[23] This chapter reviews the current state of animal restenosis models, and applies the implications of these models to the current treatment failures.

Specific Animal Restenosis Models

The Rat Carotid Artery Model

Historically, the rat carotid artery model was the first used to study the restenosis process. It was developed to understand atherosclerosis because a vigorous smooth muscle cell response to endothelial denudation occurs early after injury. Thus, the model became a standard for studying smooth muscle cell proliferation in response to arterial injury.[24] A major advantage of the rat carotid model lies in the comprehensive understanding of its molecular biology. Extensive immunohistochemistry and in situ hybridization studies make this the best characterized model, providing insights into molecular and genetic mechanisms of the arterial injury response.[24–30]

Either air desiccation[31-35] or balloon endothelial denudation[26,36,37] is used to injure the rate carotid artery. Endothelium is uniformly stripped from the vessel. While medial smooth muscle cell injury has been documented, laceration of the internal elastic lamina or media is rarely seen. Platelets deposit at the site of en-

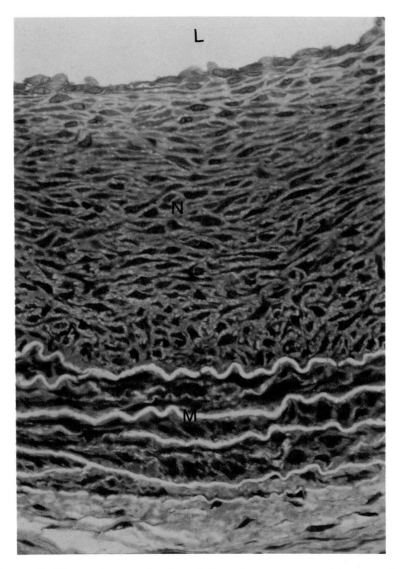

FIGURE 2. *Photomicrograph of neointima from a rat carotid artery after balloon denudation 14 days before the animal was killed. Note the thickness of this neointima is about twice that of the media. L, lumen; N, neointima; M, media. Hematoxylin/Eosin stain, magnification × 750. (Photo courtesy of Dr. Robert G. Johnson, West Point, PA.)*

dothelial denudation, although fibrin thrombi are not found. Within 2–3 weeks a smooth neointima covers the injury site (Figure 2). Neointimal thickness is typically comparable to media, about 50–100 μm, and results from migration and proliferation of medial smooth muscle cells.[38–41] Important studies in this model have used angiotensin converting enzyme (ACE) inhibitors to show potent inhibition of neointimal thickening, presumably through inhibition of smooth muscle cell proliferation.[42] Although two subsequent clinical studies failed to demonstrate a clinical effect of ACE inhibition,[11,43,44] interest in the role of angiotensin II continues.[37,42,43,45–51] The possible causes of these discrepancies are discussed later in this chapter.

Hypercholesterolemic Rabbit Iliac Artery Model

The response of the injured rabbit iliac artery has been extensively studied to test restenosis therapies and to understand the mechanisms of restenosis.[52,53] The rabbits are fed a hypercholesterolemic diet (1% to 2% cholesterol and 7% peanut oil), resulting in blood cholesterol levels of 1,000–2,000 mg%. Biochemical arterial injury is then supplemented by mechanical injury. Vascular injury is typically induced using a Fogarty balloon catheter inserted into both femoral arteries. This injury is generally superficial, and rarely damages deep arterial structures. Six weeks after initial arterial injury, both femoral arteries are examined arteriographically for stenoses. If a significant lesion is found, angioplasty is performed with standard balloon dilatation consisting of up to three inflations for 1 minute each (5–10 atm). Four weeks later, angiographic follow-up is performed, the animals are killed, and the arteries perfusion-fixed at physiologic pressures for histopathologic examination. Other successful injury methods include nitrogen desiccation.[32,34,35]

This model results in lipid laden foam cells in the media and outerportions of the neointima from macrophages that have ingested excessive lipid. Macroscopic and hemodynamically significant stenoses are reliably produced in this model.

Rabbit Ear Crush Injury Model

Another model using hypercholesterolemic New Zealand rabbits has been recently described.[54] Crushing pressure is applied at two sites of the central ear artery of rabbits maintained on a diet of 2.4% fat and 1% cholesterol. Neointimal thickening occurs along with smooth muscle cell proliferation (documented by bromodeoxyuridine) for 21 days. Area stenoses appear to be roughly 40%, with neointimal thickening beginning at day 5. The availability of the central artery makes it accessible for local treatments if desired.

Porcine Carotid Artery Injury Model

The response of injured porcine carotid arteries has been studied extensively and used to examine syndromes of accelerated atherosclerosis[55,56] and restenosis.[56-62]

A vigorous platelet thrombus forms after injury and is related to vessel injury depth, as well as to other factors such as local shear stress.[56,63] With deep vessel injury, exposure of collagen induces platelet aggregation and mural thrombosis, followed by migration and proliferation of smooth muscle cells. Neointimal formation occurs with deep injury.[59,64] However, neointimal volume is small, and rarely causes hemodynamically significant stenoses except in occasional cases of gross thrombus accumulation with subsequent organization.[57] Hypercholesterolemia is not necessary for this model. Proliferation in this model has been studied using bromodeoxyuridine. Growth fractions within the first 48 hours after injury may approach 30%.[64]

Porcine Coronary Artery Injury Models

Coronary arteries of normolipidemic domestic crossbred pigs respond to injury much like those of humans.[65] Hypercholesterolemia does not appear to influence these lesions in a substantive way.[66,67] In this model, the coronary arteries are injured either by a coronary angioplasty balloon alone[65,68] or by delivering an oversized metal coronary stent to the artery. Both methods create an injury that results in a thick neointima within 20–28 days (Figure 3). The histopathologic features of this neointima are identical to human restenotic neointima. Specimens from balloon-only injury typically show a single laceration of media, filled at 28 days by a variable thickness of neointima (Figure 4).

Vessels injured by oversized stents show multiple injuries in each section. Each injury site may be quantitated in the porcine oversized stent injury model as a mean injury score that is ordinally proportional to injury depth (Table 1).[21,69] The amount of neointimal thickening is directly proportional to this score (Figure 5). This

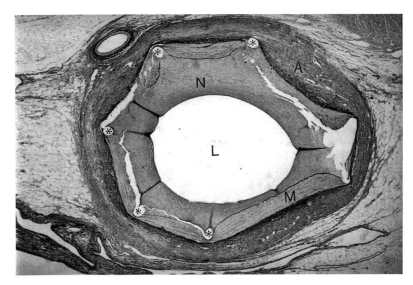

FIGURE 3. *Photomicrograph of a porcine coronary artery 28 days after oversized coil injury. Not all wires penetrated into the vessel media. Those wires that did elicited a significant neointimal response. Elastic van Gieson stain, magnification × 30. L, lumen; N, neointima; M, media; A, adventitia; *, holes from coil wires.*

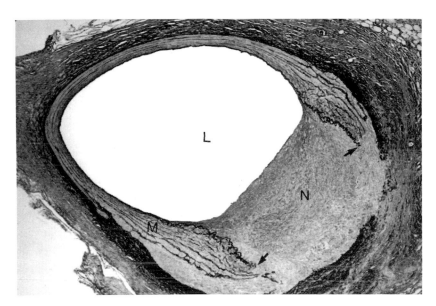

FIGURE 4. *Representative coronary artery section from a pig that underwent balloon inflation only, without coil implant. Note the neointima is only at the location of internal elastic laminalaceration. Elastic van Gieson stain, magnification × 3 0. L, lumen; NI, neointima; M, media; Arrows, location of IEL laceration.*

TABLE 1

Ordinal Histopathologic Injury Score
Ordinal Arterial Injury Score

Score	Description of Injury
0	Internal elastic lamina intact; endothelium typically denuded; media compressed, but not lacerated.
1	Internal elastic lamina lacerated; media typically compressed, but not lacerated.
2	Internal elastic lacerated; media visibly lacerated; external elastic lamina intact, but compressed.
3	External elastic lamina lacerated; typically large transluminal lacerations of media; coil wires sometimes residing in adventitia.

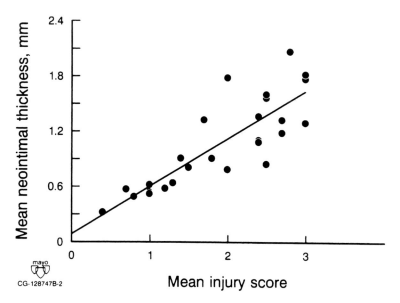

CG-128747B-2

FIGURE 5. *Scatterplot and regression line of mean neointimal thickness vs. mean injury score for porcine 26 coil-injured coronary artery segments. A statistically significant, proportional relationship clearly exists. The scatter increases for increasing mean depth of injury. (Adapted from Reference 21).*

permits creation of an injury-response regression line that can be used to quantitate the response to potential therapies.[70]

Smooth Muscle Cell Proliferation: Implications from Animal Models

Proliferation in the Injured Rat Carotid Artery

The current paradigm for coronary restenosis is based on migration and proliferation of medial smooth muscle cells. Many basic and clinical therapeutic strategies have concentrated on inhibiting smooth muscle cell proliferation to solve the problem. This concept evolved as a direct consequence of studies in the rat carotid artery,[40,71–76] where smooth muscle cell proliferation begins early after denudation (1 or 2 days), and proceeds for the following 14–30 days, at which time endothelial regrowth is complete. The studies by Clowes and colleagues[77] examined proliferation of smooth muscle cells in three groups of rats. These groups had hydrostatic arterial distension to 300 mm Hg, perfusion only without endothelial loss, and partial (50%) denudation of endothelium. Smooth muscle cell proliferation was evaluated using tritiated thymidine and showed labeling indices at 2 weeks of 24.5%±5.1% for the distended vessels (controls, 2.3%±4.4%), 1.2%±7.7% for the perfusion only group (controls 0.7%±1.0%) and with endothelial denudation, 33.8%±5.8%. Proliferation over time at 1, 2, 3, and 7 days was also examined in an earlier study. Thymidine labeling in the denudation group was 11.3%±13.8% (controls 2.7%±0.9%) at 3 days. The estimated DNA increase was 13% from medial proliferation alone, implying a single division for 15% of medial cells.

Proliferation in the Injured Porcine Coronary Artery

The proliferative behavior of neointimal formation in the porcine coronary artery is less well studied. Early studies show that a reliable vascular lesion results from directional atherectomy in normal porcine coronary arteries (Figures 6A and 6B). A full arc of media is removed by this procedure, leaving bare adventitia exposed to the flowing bloodstream as is seen in human directional atherectomy. A thick fibrin-rich thrombus appears to coat the injury site and also contains many platelets and loose platelet granules. This tissue was examined for proliferation using proliferating

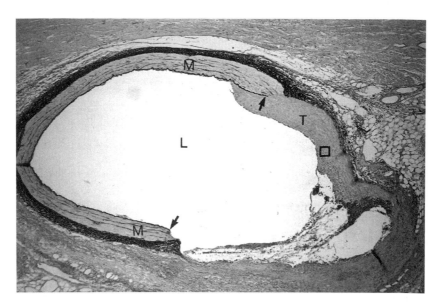

FIGURE 6A. *Photomicrograph of a previously normal porcine coronary artery subjected to a single cut from directional atherectomy. The lesion in this section is 2-days old. Note a thick layer of fibrin-thrombus attached to the injury site. There appears to be different densities to this fibrin, where the looser portions (arrows) may represent new thrombus, perhaps resulting from partial embolization of thrombus at this site. The thrombus is becoming organized with cells. Hematoxylin/Eosin stain, magnification × 30. Elastic van Gieson stain, magnification × 30. L, Lumen; NI, neointima; M, media; Arrows, location of atherectomy site; Box, location of transmission electron microscopy in Figure 6B.*

cell nuclear antigen (PCNA). PCNA is a highly conserved nuclear protein and cofactor of DNA polymerase-delta, and is expressed during the synthetic (S) phase of the cell cycle. It may also be present during G_1–S and G_2–M transition phases.

As shown by the specimen in Figure 6 (2 days after directional atherectomy) there was little or no medial proliferation near the injury site (Figure 7). Cells within the organizing thrombus also showed little PCNA expression. The adventitia of the vessel at the injury site as well as at sites opposite the injury show much PCNA expression (Figure 7). Whether subsequent time points will show substantial medial PCNA expression awaits further investigation.

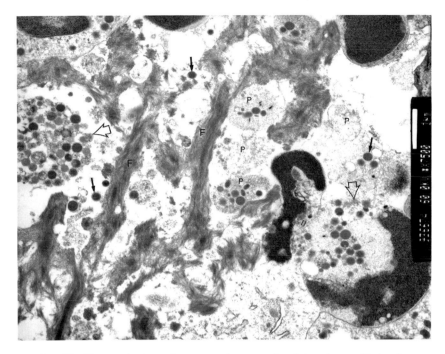

FIGURE 6B. *Transmission electron micrograph of the dense fibrin thrombus region noted in Figure 6A by square box. There are intact platelets present (marked P). Granulocytes (open arrows), and loose granules (closed arrows) are shown. Fibrin strands are also abundant (F). Magnification × 7500.*

These early results are interesting in the lack of early proliferation by medial cells.

Cellular Proliferation: General Considerations for Restenosis

The importance of smooth muscle cell proliferation in human restenosis has recently become controversial as well. Conflicting data about the fraction of proliferating cells in primary and restenotic lesions were examined by two studies.[78,79] Markedly different conclusions were reached concerning growth fractions in restenotic neointima by these studies.

Pickering[79] examined tissue samples obtained from directional

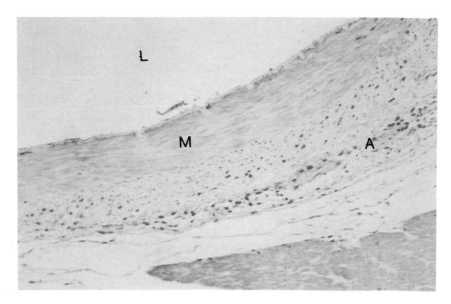

FIGURE 7. *Two-day old atherectomy section shown in Figure 6, except stained immunohistochemically with proliferating cell nuclear antigen (PCNA, PC-10). There is little staining of media smooth muscle cells in this section indicating little proliferation.*

atherectomy in 19 patients with coronary and peripheral restenosis. Tissue age ranged from 1.6 to 12.2 months after angioplasty. Proliferation was measured using immunohistochemistry and in situ hybridization to PCNA. In these restenotic lesions 20.6%±18.2% of cells were PCNA positive, with no statistical difference between peripheral and coronary lesions. No correlation with age of the restenotic lesion was found. The investigators concluded that antiproliferative therapy may be needed for a long time after angioplasty since even late lesions showed high levels of PCNA expression.

Conflicting data from the study by O'Brien[78] emerged from coronary restenotic lesions also obtained by directional atherectomy. One hundred lesions were studied with PCNA immunohistochemistry. Lesions ranged in age from 1 day to more than 1 year after angioplasty. In 74% of these restenotic lesions, *no* PCNA positive cells were detected. In the remaining 26% of lesions, <1% of cells stained for PCNA. There was no relation between PCNA positive cell count and time from angioplasty in this study, similar to the results of Pickering.[79] The authors suggest that the data do not refute the role of proliferation as a cause for restenosis. They indicated that while human cell kinetics may differ from rat carotid arteries, enhanced cell death, or low levels of proliferation for long periods could yield the hyperplastic lesion with enough volume to cause restenosis.

The low levels of proliferation evidenced by PCNA expression in humans and pigs leads to some interesting speculations. Cell proliferation has been studied extensively in relation to malignancies. The most malignant tumors (such as Burkitt's lymphoma) are known to have labeling indices of 20%–30%. Many mitoses are found when examining these tumors. Conversely, mitoses are extremely rare in restenotic lesions. Rapidly proliferating tumors (high labeling indices and growth fractions) are the most susceptible to antiproliferative chemotherapeutic interventions. Rapid and extensive cellular proliferation makes these tumors essentially curable. Similarly, the responsiveness to antiproliferatives of rat carotid artery must reflect the highly proliferative nature of this model. Conversely, antiproliferative agents such as methotrexate, lovastatin, colchicine, and external beam X-irradiation have shown little impact on neointimal thickening in pig and human coronary arteries.[7,10,70,80–83]

If the central pathophysiology of human restenosis is intense proliferation, it is then paradoxic that mitotic figures are rarely seen, and that antiproliferative strategies such as colchicine, angiotensin II inhibitors, and lovastatin have little or no effect. The low proliferative rates found by O'Brien[78] may thus explain the problem. Proliferation may not be the dominant pathophysiologic process of human restenosis, and alternative explanations for neointimal formation must be sought.

Restenosis: Arterial Remodeling in Patients and Animal Models

Recent evidence suggests that arterial remodeling may play an important part in the genesis of restenosis. Arterial remodeling was described earlier by Glagov and colleagues.[84,85] Atherosclerotic plaque mass causes an affected vessel to expand radially so that lumen area is preserved. Plaque volume causes stenosis only as a late event; at this time its volume is substantially larger than appreciated by angiography. The plaque causes outgrowth early, and ingrowth occurs late, causing stenosis.

After injury in the rat carotid artery, lumen size also tends to be maintained despite formation of neointimal hyperplasia. Neointima rarely causes stenoses in this model.

In the porcine coronary artery, remodeling also occurs. Stenoses regularly results from neointimal thickening. As thickening proceeds, the vessel's external diameter increases ("remodeling") at the same time lumen size decreases. To examine this phenomenon, 20 injured porcine coronary artery segments were studied 28 days after coronary injury by oversized metal wire stents. The internal elastic lamina and lumen size were planimetered, and neointimal thickness was measured. Remodeling was assessed by plotting lumen diameter and diameter of the IEL as a function of neointimal thickness (Figure 8). The results showed that pig coronary arteries remodel in response to neointimal thickening by simultaneously expanding and by narrowing the lumen. The vessel expands rapidly as the lumen narrows, evidenced by an inverse similarity in thickness-area slopes. Lumen size is thus preserved despite neointimal thickening, by outward growth of the vessel.

How does this homeostatic phenomenon happen? In vivo, the lumen is not an empty space, but is filled with pressurized blood. The vessel is driven outward by blood pressure as neointima forms. Blood pressure forces the gradual outward growth of neointima, until the circumferential wall tension is equal in magnitude. At this time, additional neointimal thickening grows inward, rapidly increasing the lumen stenosis.

Remodeling has also been reported in the rabbit iliac model.[86] In this important study, the lesions that caused luminal narrowing were those where compensatory enlargement failed in response to neointimal thickening. Thus, neointima obstructed the lumen earlier since the vessel could not dilate in response to its presence. The authors suggest that restenosis is due more to a failure of remodeling than to neointimal thickening.

Similar remodeling results occur following human angioplasty as well. Mintz and colleagues[87] reported 58 sequential patients undergoing revascularization using intravascular ultrasound, measuring neointimal thickness, plaque plus neointimal area, and external elastic lamina size. Results from this study indicated that 60% of late lumen loss may be due to a failure of the vessel to expand outward, or remodel.

The impact vessel's failure to appropriately remodel provides an interesting new explanation for the pathophysiology of restenosis. Further studies will be required, but strategies can be designed to enhance the vessel's remodeling capacity.

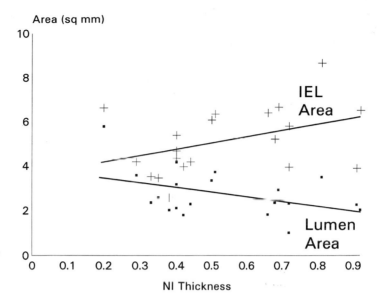

FIGURE 8A. *Graph showing the relationship between neointimal thickness, lumen diameter, and diameter of the internal elastic lamina (IEL) from normal pig coronary artery injured by oversized wire stent. The results show that the lumen tends to be preserved as neointima grows thicker, with the vessel growing larger to accomodate this thickening in a partially compensatory fashion.*

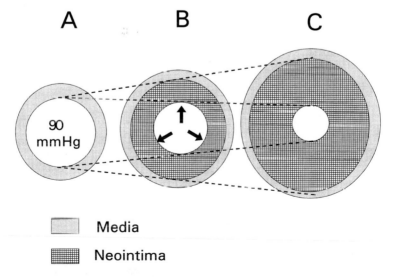

FIGURE 8B. *Schematic diagram of the remodeling paradigm in neointimal growth. Lumen size gradually decreases, but the vessel grows in proportion to maintain lumen size.*

Restenosis and Thrombus: Implications of Animal Models

Mural thrombus localizing to arterial injury sites differs substantially across species, and may explain observed differences in neointimal thickening. Thrombus has been studied extensively, and occurs regularly in humans not only after angioplasty, but also in acute clinical syndromes.[55]

After coronary injury in the pig a fibrin thrombus attaches to the site of injury and plays a substantial role in guiding the formation of neointima.[88-90] Within days, the thrombus is covered by endothelium, colonized by lymphocytes, monocytes/macrophages, and finally invaded by α-actin positive smooth muscle cells. These events have been categorized into three stages (Table 2) of which thrombus begins the cascade of events. Healing in the pig coronary artery occurs from the lumen outward toward adventitia. Smooth muscle cells at the injury site do not appear to participate actively in this model. The fibrin thrombus provides a biodegradable matrix serving as a scaffold into which the actin-positive cells migrate, possibly proliferate, and colonize.

TABLE 2

Three Histologic Stages of Arterial Response to Injury

Stage	Name	Description	Time
I	Thrombotic a. Platelet/fibrin b. Red cell/fibrin	· Local thrombus at injury site	6–24 hours
II	Cellular recruitment a. Endothelialization b. Mononuclear infiltration lysis begins	· Endothelium forms · Monocyte/lymphocyte infiltration · Fibrin/red cell debris	3–7 days
III	Proliferative a. Smooth muscle cells b. Fibroblasts	· Neointimal "Cap" forms on luminal surface · "Cap" thickens with time, matures · Resorption of fibrin/red cell debris · Volume increases over time—matrix synthesis · Vessel remodels over time	8–28 days

In rat carotid balloon endothelial denudation, little thrombus appears, and is typically limited to a thin layer of platelets at the injury site. Significant volume occupying fibrin-rich thrombus is virtually never found in this model. In the rabbit iliac model, macroscopic thrombus does occur, and has been characterized in a preliminary report.[91]

The question of mural thrombus volume and its relation to eventual neointimal volume is critical. Differences in mural thrombus volume in the days and weeks after angioplasty might contribute substantially to the development of restenosis. Differences of native thrombolytic potential across species could partially explain differences in mural thrombus. The distinction between "proliferation" and "thrombus" may blur as part of a spectrum since proliferation and colonization by cells may be guided by mural thrombus. The rat carotid artery may not generate substantial neointimal volume (and macroscopic stenoses) because it does not form macroscopic thrombus.

This suggests an alternative explanation for ineffective agents in human trials being effective in the rat carotid model. These agents might be very effective in reducing smooth muscle cell migration and proliferation, yet exhibit little effect on chronic mural thrombus deposition. The rat carotid injury model may be more "proliferative", while the rabbit and porcine models more "thrombotic".

Animal Restenosis Model Testing: Divergent Results from Clinical Trials

Many pharmacologic agents have been tested in the animal models described above, and representative results are summarized in Table 3. These data show agents effective in animal models are ineffective in human clinical restenosis trials. Why do many animal studies not reflect those seen in clinical trials of the same agents?

Elastic Arteries vs. Muscular Arteries

One significant difference relates to arterial microanatomy: medium-sized mammalian peripheral conductance vessels are elastic arteries. Elastin content of the aorta, carotid, and iliac arteries differs from the coronary arteries. The media of a conductance vessel is mostly elastin, folded into many fenestrated layers. There is

TABLE 3

Rat Carotid Model

Agent	Efficacy	References
Aspirin	++	(12, 62, 95–101)
Dipyridamole	++	(95, 98, 100–102)
Ticlopidine	++	(101)
Cilazapril	++	(42, 45)
Captopril	++	(42)
Anti-sense (c-myb)	++	(30)
Gamma interferon	++	(103)
Cyclosporin A	++	(104)
Heparin	++	(105)

Hypercholesterolemic Rabbit Iliac Model

Agent	Efficacy	References
Colchicine	++	(83)
Colchicine (local, intramural)	N	(82)
LMW heparin	++	(106)
Cilazapril	++	(45)
Doxorubicin	++	(107)
Heparin (systemic/local)	++	(108)
Heparin (local)	N	(109)
X-Irradiation	N	(110)
Gp IIb/IIIa Antibody	++, N	(111, 112)
Angiopeptin	++	(113)
r-TPA	++	(114, 115)
Cyclosporin A	N	(104)
Alpha Tocopherol	++	(116)
Losartin (AAI Antagonism)	N	(46)

Porcine Carotid Model

Agent	Efficacy	References
Methotrexate	N	(80)
Hirulog	N	(117)

Porcine Coronary Model

Agent	Efficacy	References
Angiopeptin	++	(68)
Lovastatin	N	(118)
Heparin		
Methotrexate	N	(81)
Probucol	++	(119)
Trandolapril	N	(93)
Captopril	N	(93)
Enalapril	N	(120, 121)
X-Irradiation	N	(70)
Microwave angioplasty	N	(122)

Key: ++ Effective in neointimal reduction; N not effective

essentially no autoregulatory control of vessel size by medial smooth muscle in the elastic artery.

Conversely, the coronary arteries are muscular vessels. They are primary distributing arteries, histologically similar to the brachial, radial, and femoral arteries. The media of the coronaries consists mostly of smooth muscle, permitting active vessel diameter change in response to end-organ need. It is tempting to hypothesize that vessels containing more smooth muscle might respond more vigorously to arterial injury.

Type and Severity of Arterial Injury

The type and severity of mechanical injury varies widely across animal models. In the rat carotid model, injury consists only of endothelial denudation. Major anatomic structures such as the internal elastic lamina, media, and external elastic lamina remain intact.

This mild injury is in contrast to balloon injury in the rabbit iliac and porcine coronary arteries. In the pig coronary model, significant neointimal hyperplasia results only if the internal elastic lamina is fractured (Figure 4).[69,92] Maintaining the structural integrity of the internal elastic lamina is essential to minimize neointimal hyperplasia in the pig. Injury to deeper structures causes proportionally more neointimal thickness, which rapidly increases as the media and external elastic lamina are lacerated.[21] Deep arterial injury in the rabbit and porcine coronary models is quite similar to that occurring in patients during balloon angioplasty.

Failure of Animal Models to Predict Clinical Results

Questions remain about studies of pharmacologic agents that show potent inhibition of neointimal hyperplasia in animals, yet fail to reduce restenosis in clinical trials. Several potential explanations exist for these discrepancies.

Drug Dosage and Timing Regimens

Uncertainty remains about how doses and timing of pharmacologic agents given to rodents and other small animals translate to comparable human doses. For example, in the studies of ACE inhibition described above, rats were treated with captopril 100 mg/kg or cilazapril 10 mg/kg body weight per day. This regimen caused an impressive reduction in percent neointimal coverage of the internal elastic lamina ($42\% \pm 11\%$ captopril treated vs. $111\% \pm 10\%$ control, and $35\% \pm 9\%$ cilazapril treated vs. $93 \pm 5\%$ control). The two cilazapril clinical trials (MERCATOR and MAR-CATOR) showed no impact on restenosis.[43,44] The highest cilazapril dose used in MARCATOR was 20 mg/day for 24 weeks. In a pateint weighing 70 kg, this corresponds to 0.29 mg/kg body weight, or only 2.5% of the dose reported effective in rats on a body weight basis. There was a marked discrepancy between the dose effective in rats compared to humans. Additionally, the most effective regimen in rats involved 6 days of drug pretreatment before injury. This pretreatment regimen was not used in either the MERCATOR or MARCATOR trials.

Methods of Efficacy Assessment

The outcome variable used in most clinical trials is quantitative coronary angiographic measurement of MLD change or percent luminal stenosis. Conversely, quantitative tissue measurements are generally the end points used in animal model studies, where much more information is available from microscopic histopathologic examination. The area of neointima, media, and residual lumen size can be measured precisely and compared across treatment groups in animal studies due to tissue availability. The above rat study of cilazapril would have reported a negative conclusion if MLD change had been applied to the histologic lumen diameter data, since the absolute difference between groups was <0.1 mm. Although the inhibition of neointimal thickness by cilazapril was 80%, the absolute inhibition was only 90 μm (0.09 mm). To better predict results in human trials when performing animal studies, angiographic equivalent measurements should be reported.

Interspecies Differences

A factor that could potentially be responsible for differences in animal model results and clinical trials is variability across species of arterial response to injury. ACE inhibition has been shown ineffective in pigs[93] and baboons at inhibiting neointimal formation.[94]

Are the mechanisms of neointimal formation in some animals the same as in patients? What is the role of interspecies variability in hemostasis and thrombosis, ie, the "thrombotic" vs. "proliferative" model characterizations? Few, if any, comparisons exist regarding these key questions. Preliminary data indicate that the amount of neointimal formation in dogs is markedly different than in pigs, despite similar degrees of arterial injury (Figure 9). Differences in arterial response can be expressed as the regression slope of injury and neointimal thickening. Treatments alter the y-intercept of this regression, but have less effect on the slope.[70] The slope is constant within a species,[90] so that differences across species demonstrate different injury-response regression slopes. The oversized stent response in baboon coronary arteries, for example, indicates that baboons have a lower, but nevertheless statistically significant relationship between injury and neointimal thickness (Figure 10). Dogs have an even lower injury-neointimal thickness response as discussed above.

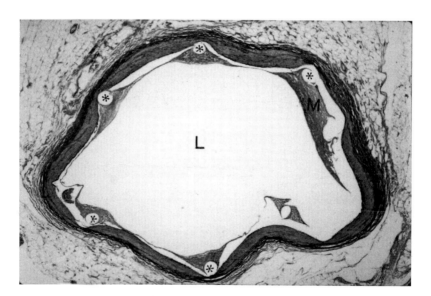

FIGURE 9. *Photomicrograph of a dog coronary artery after severe mechanical injury identical to that described for the porcine model. Despite the severe injury, the total volume of neointima is minimal and is clearly nonobstructive. L, lumen; M, media; N, neointima; *, wire hole sites; Elastic van Gieson stain, × 25. (Reproduced with permission from Reference 90.)*

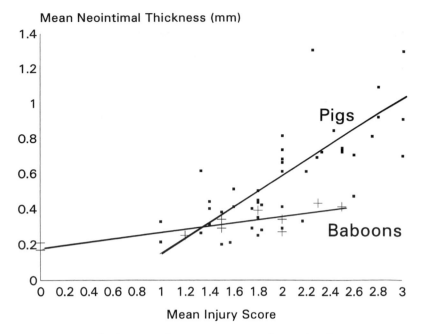

FIGURE 10. *Graph showing the quantitative relationship between ordinal injury and neointimal thickening, comparing pigs and baboons. As seen empirically, there is less overall response, and the differential response by baboons (manifested by the slope of these regression lines) is about 25% that of pigs. It is unclear where the human response would lie.*

Conclusions

Animal models have generated conflicting data regarding human restenosis. Many of these discrepancies can be explained on the basis of experimental methodology, or improper extensions of animal data to human trials. These problems can be summarized as follows:

1. An improved understanding of the role played by cell proliferation, vessel remodeling, thrombus, and matrix formation in human restenosis is critical. The role of cellular proliferation may have been overestimated previously in human restenosis.
2. The importance of using comparable drug doses and timing for animal models and clinical trials must be properly translated.
3. Different methods for data analysis may play a major role in

the variability of studies. The gold standard for clinical trials is coronary angiography, so that arterial lumen size (absolute, and relative or percent stenosis) must be evaluated when analyzing data from animal model studies.

4. The variability of injuries across models, and the volume of restenotic neointimal formation in different species is substantial.

Species at either end of the spectrum of neointimal volume should be carefully analyzed for clues explaining why some species generate very little neointima after coronary artery injury.

Finally, limitations of the animal models have been poorly understood because markedly divergent results with human studies have been common. A solution to restenosis must lie in a detailed understanding of the events causing neointimal thickening, cellular proliferation, arterial remodeling, and matrix formation. Once the contribution of these are understood, interventions can be strategically planned, demonstrated in animal models, and successfully translated to human therapy.

Acknowledgment

The authors wish to acknowledge the generous support of the J. Holden DeHaan Foundation, and Medtronic Inc. for their support of work in the causes and treatment of restenosis.

References

1. Austin GE. Lipids and vascular restenosis. *Circulation.* 1992;85:1613–1615.
2. Bell L, Madri JA. Original contributions: effect of platelet factors on migration of cultured bovine aortic endothelial and smooth muscle cells. *Circ Res.* 1989;65:1057–1065.
3. Bowles MH, Klonis D, Plavac TG, et al. EPA in the prevention of restenosis post PTCA. *Angiology.* 1991;42:187–194.
4. Califf R, Ohmann E, Frid D, et al. Restenosis: the clinical issues. In: Topol E, ed. *Textbook of Interventional Cardiology.* Philadelphia, PA: W.B. Saunders; 1990:363–394.
5. Faxon D, Spiro T, Minor S, et al. Enoxaparin, a low molecular weight heparin, in the prevention of restenosis after angioplasty: results of a double blind randomized trial. *J Am Coll Cardiol.* 1992;19:258A. Abstract.
6. Finci L, Hofling B, Ludwig B, et al. Sulotroban during and after coronary angioplasty. A double-blind, placebo controlled study. *Z Kardiol.* 1989;3:50–54.
7. Grines C, Rizik D, Levine A, et al. Colchicine angioplasty restenosis trial (CART). *Circulation.* 1991;84:II-365. Abstract.

8. Hoberg E, Schwarz F, Schomig A, et al. Prevention of restenosis by verapamil: the verapamil angioplasty study (VAS). *Circulation.* 1990;82: III-428. Abstract.

9. Israel DH, Gorlin R. Fish oils in the prevention of atherosclerosis. *J Am Coll Cardiol.* 1992;19:174–185.

10. O'Keefe J, McCallister B, Bateman T, Kuhnlein D, Ligon R, Hartzler G. Colchicine for the prevention of restenosis after coronary angioplasty. *J Am Coll Cardiol.* 1991;17:181A.

11. Serruys P, Hermans R. The new angiotensin converting enzyme inhibitor cilazapril does not prevent restenosis after coronary angioplasty: the results of the MERCATOR trial. *J Am Coll Cardiol.* 1992;19: 258A. Abstract.

12. Taylor R, Gibbons F, Cope G, et al. Effects of low dose aspirin on restenosis after coronary angioplasty. *Am J Cardiol.* 1991;68:874–878.

13. Garratt KN, Holmes DR Jr, Bell MR, et al. Restenosis after directional coronary atherectomy: differences between primary atheromatous and restenosis lesions and influence of subintimal tissue resection. *J Am Coll Cardiol.* 1990;16:1665–1671.

14. Hinohara T, Robertson GC, Selmon MR, et al. Restenosis after directional coronary atherectomy. *J Am Coll Cardiol.* 1992;20:623–632.

15. O'Neill WW. Mechanical rotational atherectomy. *Am J Cardiol.* 1992; 69.

16. Litvack F, Margolis J, Cummins F, et al. Excimer laser coronary (ELCA) registry: report of the first consecutive 2080 patients. *J Am Coll Cardiol.* 1992;19:276A. Abstract.

17. Anand RK, Sinclair IN, Jenkins RD, Hiehle JF Jr, James L, Spears JR. Laser balloon angioplasty: effect of constant temperature versus constant power on tissue weld strength. *Lasers Surg Med.* 1988;8:40–44.

18. Buchwald AB, Werner GS, Unterberg C, Voth E, Kreuzer H, Wiegand V. Restenosis after excimer laser angioplasty of coronary stenoses and chronic total occlusions. *Am Heart J.* 1992;123(4 Pt 1):878–885.

19. Ghazzal Z, Burton M, Klein L, et al. Predictors of restenosis following excimer laser: multicenter comprehensive angiographic analysis. *Circulation.* 1991;84:II-361. Abstract.

20. Margolis JR, Litvack F, Krauthamer D, Trautwein R, Goldenberg T, Grundfest W. Excimer laser coronary angioplasty: American multicenter experience. *Herz.* 1990;15:223–232.

21. Schwartz R, Huber K, Murphy J, et al. Restenosis and the proportional neointimal response to coronary artery injury: results in a porcine model. *J Am Coll Cardiol.* 1992;19:267–274.

22. Beatt KJ, Serruys PW, Luijten HE, et al. Restenosis after coronary angioplasty: the paradox of increased lumen diameter and restenosis. *J Am Coll Cardiol.* 1992;19:258–266.

23. Muller D, Ellis S, Topol E. Experimental models of coronary artery restenosis. *J Am Coll Cardiol.* 1992;19:418–432.

24. Guyton J, Rosenburg R, Clowes A, Karnovsky M. Inhibition of rat arterial smooth muscle cell proliferation by heparin. In vivo studies with anticoagulant and nonanticoagulant heparin. *Circ Res.* 1980;46:625–634.

25. Clowes AW, Clowes MM, Au YPT, Reidy MA, Belin D. Original contributions: smooth muscle cells express urokinase during mitogenesis

and tissue-type plasminogen activator during migration in injured rat carotid artery. *Circ Res.* 1990;67:61–67.

26. Fingerle J, Au YPT, Clowes AW, Reidy MA. Intimal lesion formation in rat carotid arteries after endothelial denudation in absence of medial injury. *Arteriosclerosis.* 1990;10:1082–1087.

27. Golden MA, Au YP, Kenagy RD, Clowes AW. Growth factor gene expression by intimal cells in healing polytetrafluoroethylene grafts. *J Vasc Surg.* 1990;11:580–585.

28. Reidy M, Clowes A, Schwartz S. Endothelial regeneration: V. Inhibition of endothelial regrowth in arteries of rat and rabbit. *Lab Invest.* 1983;49:569–575.

29. Simons M, Rosenberg R. Antisense approach to smooth muscle proliferation. *Circulation.* 1991;84:II-342.

30. Simons M, Edelman ER, DeKeyser J, Langer R, Rosenberg RD. Antisense c-*myb* oligonucleotides inhibit intimal arterial smooth muscle cell accumulation in vivo. *Nature.* 1992;356:62–65.

31. Ragosta M, Gimple L, Haber H, et al. Effectiveness of specific factor Xa inhibition on restenosis following balloon angioplasty in rabbits. *J Am Coll Cardiol.* 1992;19:164A. Abstract.

32. Sarembock I, Gertz D, Gimple L, Owen R, Powers E, Roberts W. Effectiveness of recombinant desulphatohirudin in reducing restenosis after balloon angioplasty of atherosclerotic femoral arteries in rabbits. *Circulation.* 1991;84:232–243.

33. Gellman J, Ezekowitz MD, Sarembock IJ, et al. Effect of lovastatin on intimal hyperplasia after balloon angioplasty: a study in an atherosclerotic hypercholesterolemic rabbit. *J Am Coll Cardiol.* 1991;17:251–259.

34. Haber H, Gimple L, Goldstein C, et al. The effect of oral terbinafine on restenosis following balloon angioplasty in rabbits. *Circulation.* 1991;84:II-332. Abstract.

35. LaVeau P, Sarembock I, Sigal S, Yang T, Ezekowitz M. Vascular reactivity after balloon angioplasty in an atherosclerotic rabbit. *Circulation.* 1990;82:1790–1801.

36. Au YP, Kenagy RD, Clowes AW. Heparin selectively inhibits the transcription of tissue-type plasminogen activator in primate arterial smooth muscle cells during mitogenesis. *J Biol Chem.* 1992;267:3438–3444.

37. Clowes AW, Clowes MM, Vergel SC, et al. The renin-angiotensin system and the vascular wall: from experimental models to man. Heparin and cilazapril together inhibit injury-induced intimal hyperplasia. *Hypertension.* 1991;18(Suppl):65–69.

38. Fingerle J, Johnson R, Clowes AW, Majesky MW, Reidy MA. Role of platelets in smooth muscle cell proliferation and migration after vascular injury in rat carotid artery. *Proc Natl Acad Sci USA.* 1989;86:8412–8416.

39. Gerdes J, Li L, Schlueter C, et al. Immunobiochemical and molecular biologic characteration of the cell proliferation-associated nuclear antigen that is defined by monoclonal antibody Ki-67. *Am J Pathol.* 1991;138:867–873.

40. Hanke H, Strohschneider T, Oberhoff M, Betz E, Karsch K. Time course of smooth muscle cell proliferation in the intima and media of arteries following experimental angioplasty. *Circ Res.* 1990;:651–659.

41. Hanke H, Strohschneider T, Oberhoff M, Betz E, Karsch KR. Time course of smooth muscle cell proliferation in the intima and media of arteries following experimental angioplasty. *Circ Res.* 1990;67:651–659.
42. Powell J, Clozel J, Muller R, et al. Inhibitors of angiotensin-converting enzyme prevent myointimal proliferation after vascular injury. *Science.* 1989;245:186–188.
43. Faxon DP. Angiotensin converting enzyme inhibition and restenosis: the final results of the MARCATOR Trial. *Circulation.* 1992;86:I-53. Abstract.
44. Does the new angiotensin converting enzyme inhibitor cilazapril prevent restenosis after percutaneous transluminal coronary angioplasty? Results of the MERCATOR study: a multicenter, randomized, double-blind placebo-controlled trial. *Circulation.* 1992;86:100–110.
45. Bilazarian S, Currier J, Haudenschild C, et al. Angiotensin converting enzyme inhibition reduces restenosis in experimental angioplasty. *J Am Coll Cardiol.* 1991;17:268A.
46. Bilazarian S, Currier J, Kakuta T, Huadenschild C, Faxon D. Angiotensin II antagonism does not prevent restenosis after rabbit iliac angioplasty. *Circulation.* 1992;86:I-187. Abstract.
47. Brozovich FV, Morganroth J, Gottlieb NB, Gottlieb RS. Effect of angiotensin converting enzyme inhibition on the incidence of restenosis after percutaneous transluminal coronary angioplasty. *Cathet Cardiovasc Diagn.* 1991;23:263–267.
48. Daemen MJ, Lombardi DM, Bosman FT, Schwartz SM. Angiotensin II induces smooth muscle cell proliferation in the normal and injured rat arterial wall. *Circ Res.* 1991;68:450–456.
49. Osterrieder W, Muller RKM, Powell JS, Clozel JP, Hefti F, Baumgartner HR. The Renin-angiotensin system and the vascular wall: from experimental models to man. Role of angiotensin II in injury-induced neointima formation in rats. *Hypertension.* 1991;18(Suppl):60–64.
50. Powell J, Muller R, Baumgartner H. Suppression of the vascular response to injury: the role of angiotensin-converting enzyme inhibitors. *J Am Coll Cardiol.* 1991;17:137B–142B.
51. Roux SP, Clozel JP, Kuhn H. The renin-angiotensin system and the vascular wall: from experimental models to man. Cilazapril inhibits wall thickening of vein bypass graft in the rat. *Hypertension.* 1991;18(Suppl):43–46.
52. Faxon DP, Weber VJ, Haudenschild C, Gottsman SB, McGovern WA, Ryan T. Acute effects of transluminal angioplasty in three experimental models of atherosclerosis. *Arteriosclerosis.* 1982;2:125–133.
53. Faxon DP, Sanborn TA, Weber VJ, et al. Restenosis following transluminal angioplasty in experimental atherosclerosis. *Arteriosclerosis.* 1984;4:189–195.
54. Banai S, Shou M, Correa R, et al. Original contributions: rabbit ear model of injury-induced arterial smooth muscle cell proliferation. Kinetics, reproductibility, and implications. *Circ Res.* 1991;69:748–756.
55. Ip JH, Fuster V, Badimon L, Badimon J, Taubman MB, Chesebro JH. Syndromes of accelerated atherosclerosis: role of vascular injury and smooth muscle cell proliferation. *J Am Coll Cardiol.* 1990;15:1667–1687.
56. Fuster V, Badimon L, Badimon JJ, Ip JH, Chesebro JH. The porcine

model for the understanding of thrombogenesis and atherogenesis. *Mayo Clin Proc.* 1991;66:818–831.

57. Steele P, Chesebro J, Stanson A, et al. Balloon angioplasty, natural history of the pathophysiological response to injury in a pig model. *Circ Res.* 1985;57:105–112.

58. Lam JY, Chesebro JH, Steele PM, et al. Antithrombotic therapy for deep arterial injury by angioplasty. Efficacy of common platelet inhibition compared with thrombin inhibition in pigs. *Circulation.* 1991; 84:814–820.

59. Chesebro JA, Lam JYT, Badimon L, Fuster V. Restenosis after arterial angioplasty: a hemorheologic response to injury. *Am J Cardiol.* 1987; 60:10B–16B.

60. Ip JH, Fuster V, Israel D, Badimon L, Badimon J, Chesebro JH. The role of platelets, thrombin and hyperplasia in restenosis after coronary angioplasty. *J Am Coll Cardiol.* 1991;17(suppl B):778–888.

61. Lam JYT, Chesebro JH, Steele PM, Dewanjee MK, Badimon L, Fuster V. Deep arterial injury during experimental angioplasty: relationship to a positive indium-111 labeled platelet scintigram, quantitative platelet deposition and mural thrombus. *J Am Coll Cardiol.* 1986;8: 1380–1386.

62. Webster MW, Chesebro JH, Fuster V. Platelet inhibitor therapy. Agents and clinical implications. *Hematol Oncol Clin North Am.* 1990;4:265–289.

63. Adams PC, Badimon JJ, Badimon L, Chesebro JH, Fuster V. Role of platelets in atherogenesis: relevance to coronary arterial restenosis after angioplasty. *Cardiovasc Clin.* 1987;18:49–71.

64. Webster M, Chesebro J, Grill D, Badimon J, Badimon L, Fuster V. The thrombotic and proliferative response to angioplasty in pigs after deep arterial injury: effect of intravenous thrombin inhibition with hirudin. *Circulation.* 1991;84:II-580. Abstract.

65. Schwartz RS, Murphy JG, Edwards WD, Camrud AR, Vlietstra RE, Holmes DR Jr. Restenosis after balloon angioplasty: a practical proliferative model in porcine coronary arteries. *Circulation.* 1990;82:2190–2200.

66. Rodgers GP, Minor ST, Robinson K, et al. Adjuvant therapy for intracoronary stents. Investigations in atherosclerotic swine. *Circulation.* 1990;82:560–569.

67. Rodgers GP, Minor ST, Robinson K, et al. The coronary artery response to implantation of a balloon-expandable flexible stent in the aspirin- and non-aspirin-treated swine model. *Am Heart J.* 1991,122: 640–647.

68. Santoian E, Foegh M, Gravanis M, et al. Treatment with angiopeptin inhibits the development of smooth muscle proliferation in a balloon overstretch swine model of restenosis. *J Am Coll Cardiol.* 1992;19:164A. Abstract.

69. Schwartz RS, Murphy JG, Edwards WD, Camrud AR, Vlietstra RE, Holmes DR Jr. Restenosis occurs with internal elastic lamina laceration and is proportional to severity of vessel injury in a porcine coronary artery model. *Circulation.* 1990;4:III-656.

70. Schwartz R, Koval T, Edwards W, et al. Effect of external beam irradiation on neointimal hyperplasia after experimental coronary artery injury. *J Am Coll Cardiol.* 1992;19:1106–1113.

71. Austin G, Ratliff N, Hollman J, Tabei S, Phillips D. Intimal proliferation of smooth muscle cells as an explanation for recurrent coronary artery stenosis after percutaneous transluminal coronary angioplasty. *J Am Coll Cardiol.* 1985;6:369–375.
72. Cariou R, Harousseau JL, Tobelem G. Inhibition of human endothelial cell proliferation by heparin and steroids. *Cell Biol Int Rep.* 1988;12: 1037–1047.
73. Clowes A, Reidy M, Clowes M. Kinetics of cellular proliferation after arterial injury: I. Smooth muscle growth in absence of endothelium. *Lab Invest.* 1983;49:327–332.
74. Conte JV, Foegh ML, Calcagno D, Wallace RB, Ramwell PW. Peptide inhibition of myointimal proliferation following angioplasty in rabbits. *Transplant Proc.* 1989;21:3686–3688.
75. Hirata S, Matsubara T, Saura R, Tateishi H, Hirohata K. Inhibition of in vitro vascular endothelial cell proliferation and in vivo neovascularization by low-dose methotrexate. *Arthritis Rheum.* 1989;32:1065–1073.
76. Karas SP, Gravanis MB, Santoian EC, Robinson KA, Anderberg KA, King SB3. Coronary intimal proliferation after balloon injury and stenting in swine: an animal model of restenosis. *J Am Coll Cardiol.* 1992;20:467–474.
77. Clowes A, Clowes M, Fingerle J, Reidy M. Kinetics of cellular proliferation after arterial injury. V. Role of acute distension in the induction of smooth muscle proliferation. *Lab Invest.* 1989;60:360–364.
78. O'Brien E, Alpers C, Stewart D, et al. Proliferation in primary and restenotic coronary atherectomy tissue. implications for antiproliferative therapy. *Circ Res.* 1993;73:223–231.
79. Pickering J, Weir L, Jekanowski J, Kearney M, Isner J. Proliferative activity in peripheral and coronary atherosclerotic plaque among patients undergoing percutaneous revascularization. *J Clin Invest.* 1993; 91:1469–1480.
80. Muller DWM Topol EJ, Abrams GD, Gallagher KP, Ellis SG. Intramural methotrexate therapy for the prevention of neointimal thickening after balloon angioplasty. *J Am Coll Cardiol.* 1992;20:460–466.
81. Murphy JG, Schwartz RS, Edwards WD, et al. Methotrexate and azathioprine fail to inhibit porcine coronary restenosis. *Circulation.* 1990; 82:III-429.
82. Wilensky RL, Gradus-Pizlo I, March KL, Sandusky GE, Hathaway DR. Efficacy of local intramural injection of colchicine in reducing restenosis following angioplasty in the atherosclerotic rabbit model. *Circulation.* 1992;86:I-52.
83. Currier J, Pow T, Minihan A, et al. Colchicine inhibits restenosis after iliac angioplasty in the atherosclerotic rabbit. *Circulation.* 1989;80:II-66. Abstract.
84. Glagov S, Weisenberg G, Zarins CK, Stankunavicius R, Kolettis GJ. Compensatory enlargement of human atherosclerotic coronary arteries. *N Engl J Med.* 1987;316:1371–1375.
85. Glagov S, Zarins CK, Masawa N, Xu CP, Bassiouny H, Giddens DP. Mechanical functional role of non-atherosclerotic intimal thickening. *Front Med Biol Eng.* 1993;5:37–43.
86. Kakuta T, Currier J, Horten K, Faxon D. Failure of intimal compensatory enlargement, not neointimal formation, accounts for lumen

narrowing after angioplasty in the atherosclerotic rabbit. *Circulation.* 1993;88:I-619. Abstract.

87. Mintz G, Kovach J, Javier S, Ditrano C, Leon M. Geometric remodeling is the predominant of late lumen loss after coronary angioplasty. *Circulation.* 1993;88:I-654. Abstract.

88. Schwartz R, Holmes D Jr, Topol E. The restenosis paradigm revisited: an alternative proposal for cellular mechanisms. *J Am Coll Cardiol.* 1992;20:1284–1293.

89. Schwartz R, Edwards W, Camrud A, Holmes DJ. Developmental stages of restenotic neointimal hyperplasia following porcinecoronary artery injury: a morphologic review. *J Vasc Med Biol.* In press.

90. Schwartz RS, Edwards WD, Huber KC, et al. Coronary restenosis: prospects for solution and new perspectives from a porcine model. *Mayo Clin Proc.* 1993;68:54–62.

91. Wilensky RL, Wong L, March KL, Sandusky GE, Hathaway DR. Immunohistochemical characterization of arterial injury and restenosis following angioplasty in the atherosclerotic rabbit. *J Am Coll Cardiol.* 1992;19:169A. Abstract.

92. Schwartz RS, Murphy JG, Edwards WD, et al. Coronary artery restenosis and the "virginal membrane": smooth muscle cell proliferation and the intact internal elastic lamina. *J Invasive Cardiol.* 1991;3:3–8.

93. Huber K, Schwartz R, Edwards W, et al. Effects of angiotensin converting enzyme inhibition on neointimal proliferation a porcine coronary injury model. *Am Heart J.* 1993;125:695–701.

94. Hanson S, Powell J, Dodson T, et al. Effects of angiotensin converting enzyme inhibition with cilazapril on intimal hyperplasia in injured arteries and vascular grafts in the baboon. *Hypertension.* 1991;18(Suppl 2):II-70–II-76.

95. Barnathan E, Schwartz J, Taylor L, et al. Aspirin and dipyridamole in the prevention of acute coronary thrombosis complicating coronary angioplasty. *Circulation.* 1987;76:125–134.

96. Ellis S, Roubin G, Wilentz J, Lin S, Douglas J Jr, King S III. Results of a randomized trl of heparin and aspirin vs. aspirin alone for prevention of acute closure (AC) and restenosis (R) after angioplasty (PTCA). *Circulation.* 1987;76:IV-213. Abstract.

97. Grigg LE, Kay TW, Valentine PA, et al. Determinants of restenosis and lack of effect of dietary supplementation with eicosapentaenoic acid on the incidence of coronary artery restenosis after angioplasty. *J Am Coll Cardiol.* 1989;13:665–672.

98. Koster JKJ, Tryka AF, HDoubler P, Collins JJJ. The effect of low-dose aspirin and dipyridamole upon atherosclerosis in the rabbit. *Artery.* 1981;9:405–413.

99. Mufson L, Black A, Roubin G, et al. A randomized trial of aspirin in PTCA: effect of high vs. low dose on major complications and restenosis. *J Am Coll Cardiol.* 1988;II-236A. Abstract.

100. Schwartz L, Bourassa MG, Lesperance J, et al. Aspirin and dipyridamole in the prevention of restenosis after percutaneous transluminal coronary angioplasty. *N Engl J Med.* 1988;318:1714–1719.

101. White C, Knudson M, Schmidt D. Neither ticlopidine nor aspirin-dipyridamole prevents restenosis post PTCA: results from a randomized placebo-controlled multicenter trial. *Circulation.* 1987;76:IV-213. Abstract.

102. Pirelli S, Danzi GB, Alberti A, et al. Comparison of usefulness of high-dose dipyridamole echocardiography and exercise electrocardiography for detection of asymptomatic restenosis after coronary angioplasty. *Am J Cardiol.* 1991;67:1335–1338.
103. Hansson GK, Holm J. Laboratory investigation: interferon gamma inhibits arterial stenosis after injury. *Circulation.* 1991;84:1266–1272.
104. McKenney P, Currier J, Haudenschild C, Heyman D, Faxon D. Cyclosporine A does not inhibit restenosis in experimental angioplasty. *Circulation.* 1991;84:II-70.
105. Clowes AW, Karnovsky MJ. Suppression by heparin of smooth muscle cell proliferation in injured arteries. *Nature.* 1977;265.
106. Timms I, Shlansky-Goldberg R, Healy H, Guo Y, Cope C. A novel form of non-anticoagulant heparin reduces restenosis following angioplasty in the atherosclerotic rabbit. *Circulation.* 1992;86:I-703.
107. Franklin SM, Kalan JM, Currier JW, et al. Effects of local delivery of doxorubicin or saline on restenosis following angioplasty in atherosclerotic rabbits. *Circulation.* 1992;86:I-52. Abstract.
108. Rogers C, Karnovsky MJ, Edelman ER. Intravenous and local perivascular heparin reduce endovascular stent thrombosis and intimal hyperplasia. *Circulation.* 1992;86:I-227. Abstract.
109. Gimple LW, Gertz SD, Haber HL, Powers ER, Roberts WC Sarembock IJ. Effect of "in situ" heparin delivery by a porous balloon catheter on restenosis following balloon angioplasty. *J Am Coll Cardiol.* 1992;19:169A. Abstract.
110. Gellman J, Healey G, Chen Q, et al. The effect of very low dose irradiation on restenosis following balloon angioplasty. A study in the atherosclerotic rabbit. *Circulation.* 1991;84:II-331. Abstract.
111. Azrin M, Todd M, Chen Q, Tselentakis M, Ezekowitz M. The effect of a monoclonal antibody to the platelet glycoprotein IIb/IIIa on restenosis after angioplasty in a rabbit model. *Circulation.* 1991;84:II-332.
112. Ling F, Chen Q, Migliaccio F, Tselentakis M, Azrin M, Ezekowitz M. The effect of prolonged platelet inhibition with multiple doses of an antiplatelet glycoprotein IIb/IIIa antibody on restenosis after angioplasty in the atherosclerotic rabbit. *Circulation.* 1992;86:I-226.
113. Hong M, Bhatti T, Matthews B, et al. Locally delivered angiopeptin reduces intimal hyperplasia following balloon injury in rabbits. *Circulation.* 1991;84:II-72. Abstract.
114. Kanamasa K, Ishida N, Hisaharu K, et al. tPA infusion for 7 days prevents restenosis following balloon angioplasty in atherosclerotic rabbit. *Circulation.* 1992;86:I-l85.
115. Gellman J, Sigal SL, Chen Q, Esquivel EL, Ezekowitz MD. The effect of tpa on restenosis following balloon angioplasty: a study in the atherosclerotic rabbit. *J Am Coll Cardiol.* 1991;17:25A.
116. Lafont A, Whitlow P, Cornhill J, Chisolm G. Alpha-tocopherol reduced restenosis after femoral artery angioplasty in a rabbit model of experimental atherosclerosis. *Circulation.* 1992;86:I-747.
117. Muller DWM, Golomb G, Gordon D, Maraganore JM, Levy RJ. Local adventitial hirulog delivery for the prevention of stent thrombosis and neotintimal thickening. *Circulation.* 1992;86:I-381.
118. Schneider J, Santoian E, Gravanis M, Gipolla G, Anderberg K, King

S III. Lovastatin fails to limit smooth muscle cell proliferation in nor-molipemic and hyperlipemic swine in an overstretch balloon injury model of restenosis. *J Am Coll Cardiol.* 1992;19:162A.

119. Schneider J, Berk B, Santoian E, et al. Oxidative stress is important in restenosis: reduction of neointimal formation by the antioxidant probucol in a swine model of restenosis. *Circulation.* 1992;86:I-186.

120. Santoian EC, Gravanis MB, Karas SP, et al. Enalapril does not inhibit smooth muscle cell proliferation in a balloon-injured coronary artery swine model of intimal hyperplasia. *Circulation.* 1991;84:II-70. Abstract.

121. Churchill DA, Siegel CO, Dougherty KG, Raizner AE, Minor ST. Failure of enalapril to reduce coronary restenosis in a swine model. *Circulation.* 1991;84:II-297.

122. Huber K, Schwartz R, Edwards W, Camrud A, Holmes D Jr. Severe medial cell injury does not prevent neointimal proliferation: histopathology following microwave angioplasty in a porcine coronary restenosis model. *J Am Coll Cardiol.* 1992;19:164A.

Chapter 20

The Clinical Biology of Restenosis

John W. Hirshfeld, Jr, MD

This chapter reviews the current restenosis knowledge base and discusses its application to the clinical management of patients with coronary artery disease in terms of choosing between coronary angioplasty and other alternative treatment strategies for the management of coronary disease. In particular, this chapter focuses on the impact of restenosis probability on:

1. The selection of patients and lesions for coronary angioplasty.
2. The conduct of a coronary angioplasty procedure.
3. The choice of a new device as opposed to conventional balloon angioplasty for a particular coronary lesion.

Events Causing Restenosis

The events that contribute to the restenosis process are well characterized. These include:

1. Elastic recoil, which is the early loss of lumen dimension within the first few minutes after the completion of an angioplasty procedure.[1,2]
2. Thrombus formation at the angioplasty site and its subsequent organization.[2]
3. Vascular wall remodeling.
4. Neointimal growth that is caused by the proliferation and phenotypic transformation of medial smooth muscle cells, their subsequent migration across the internal elastic lamina to the intima, and subsequent deposition of intracellular matrix within the intima causing loss of luminal dimension.

From Vetrovec GW, Carabello BA, (eds.) *Invasive Cardiology: Current Diagnostic and Therapeutic Issues.* Armonk, NY: Futura Publishing Company, Inc.: © 1996.

The current hypotheses concerning the mechanisms responsible for this process have been reviewed.[3-5]

Definition of Restenosis

One of the complexities of studying and characterizing restenosis is the lack of a single universally applicable definition. This is because it is impossible to distinguish completely between the restenosis process and its clinical consequences. Thus, there are both clinical and angiographic definitions of restenosis, and there are several different angiographic definitions of restenosis in common use.

Clinical Definitions of Restenosis

A clinical definition of restenosis is based on whether a clinical consequence of the restenosis process occurs. Such definitions are widely used to assess the overall clinical benefit of an angioplasty procedure. Because considerable asymptomatic restenosis occurs, clinical definitions of restenosis underestimate the frequency of angiographic restenosis.[6]

Angiographic Definitions of Restenosis

Angiographic definitions of restenosis characterize whether the restenosis processes has caused a particular decrease of lumen dimension in a lesion that has been treated with angioplasty. Given physicians' preference for variables that can be analyzed by non-parametric statistics, these definitions are categorical—defining boundaries that characterize whether restenosis is present or not. Such definitions are oversimplified characterizations of a multifactorial process that occurs in a graded fashion. In addition, given the complexity of characterizing the restenosis process in mathematical terms, a variety of definitions have been developed. Each definition measures a slightly different aspect of the restenosis process. The most commonly used definitions are:

1. Greater than 50% late loss of the acute gain in lumen dimension achieved by the angioplasty procedure.[7] This was Andreas Gruentzig's initial means of measuring the late loss of lumen dimension.
2. Greater than 0.72 mm lumen diameter decrease from the diameter achieved immediately after the angioplasty.[8] This definition is based on the variability of angiographic measurement of coronary dimensions and detects a measur-

able loss of lumen dimension. It does not, however, determine whether the loss of lumen dimension has clinical importance.
3. Greater than 50% diameter stenosis at follow-up angiography.[9] This definition is based on the physiologic principle that coronary artery obstruction achieves clinical importance when the artery is narrowed by more than 50% of its diameter. This definition has the weakness that a lesion that was 49% stenosed immediately after the angioplasty procedure and was 51% stenosed at follow-up would be considered restenosed, whereas a lesion that was 10% stenosed immediately after the procedure, but was 49% stenosed at follow-up would not.

The above cited definitions are useful for characterizing the state of an individual coronary lesion. These definitions may be used to compile aggregate descriptions of populations of lesions which may then be used for statistical analyses of group behavior to characterize the frequency and severity of restenosis. However, since this approach already involves a data reduction, another approach has recently been suggested. This approach characterizes a population of lesions as a cumulative frequency curve in which the cumulative frequency of a parametric variable related to stenosis severity such as stenosis diameter or percent stenosis is plotted as a function of the value of the variable.[10] This generates a sigmoid shaped-curve that characterizes the population of lesions (Figure 1). Different populations can be compared by comparing their

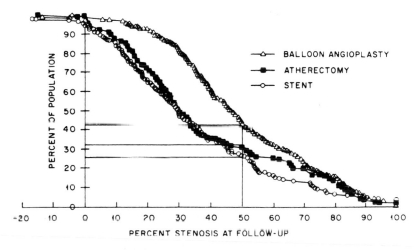

FIGURE 1. *Cumulative frequency distribution curve describing restenosis in a population of dilated coronary lesions. (Reproduced with permission from Kuntz RE, Gibson CM, Nobuyoshi M, Baim DS. Generalized model of restenosis after conventional balloon angioplasty, stenting, and directional atherectomy.* J Am Coll Cardiol. *1993;21:15–25.)*

curves. Although such curves contain more than tabulations of frequencies, their analysis is more complex intuitively and statistical comparison of such curves is more difficult. By comparing curves for two treatment populations the effect of a particular treatment on restenosis may be defined.

Frequency of Restenosis

The frequency with which restenosis occurs or the "restenosis rate" varies somewhat from series to series depending upon the definition used and the restudy rate. Overall, however, multiple series have confirmed that the frequency of angiographic restenosis ranges between 35% and 45%.[9,11,12]

Time Course of Restenosis

The time course of restenosis has been characterized by the meticulous studies of Nobuyoshi and Serruys.[12,13] These studies, which analyze serial angiographic examinations demonstrate two fundamental principles:

1. "Acute" restenosis is a misnomer. This term is often applied to early angioplasty failure occurring within the first few days after the procedure. These events do not represent actual restenosis, but are consequences of instability of a fresh angioplasty site.
2. The actual restenosis process takes place gradually over a period of 4–6 months. It causes a gradual loss of lumen dimension that generally becomes sufficiently narrow, causing return of ischemia in the distribution of the target vessel beginning about 3 months after the angioplasty. The loss of lumen dimension generally ceases after about 6 months and vascular dimension stabilizes at that point.

The time course of loss of lumen dimensions is charted in Figure 2.

Consequences of Restenosis

Restenosis produces sufficient lumen narrowing to cause ischemia sufficient to lead to the return of symptoms in 67% to 75% of patients who develop it. The remaining 25% to 33% of patients who do not develop symptoms either do not experience symptoms

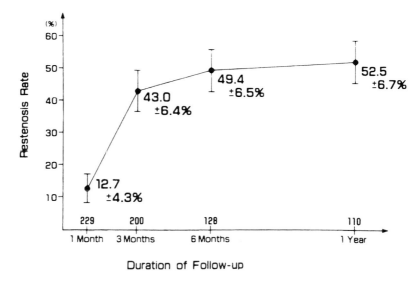

FIGURE 2. *Time course of the loss of lumen dimension after PTCA (single vessel disease) (Reproduced with permission from Reference 12.)*

when they have myocardial ischemia, or do not have ischemia that is severe enough to produce symptoms.[14]

These patients either have well-developed intercoronary collaterals, the recurrence of which, although severe enough to cross the definition threshold of restenosis, is not severe enough to produce symptoms. On average, the stenosis severity of lesions in patients with asymptomatic restenosis is less severe than in symptomatic patients.[6]

Restenosis has not been shown to have any impact on survival, probably because the majority of patients who are treated with coronary angioplasty have an excellent natural history for survival irrespective of the success or failure of their treatment. However, patients with asymptomatic restenosis are at risk of developing complications of coronary disease. In a series studied by Laarman et al[15], 41% of patients with single-vessel disease who had asymptomatic restenosis had a coronary event (defined as death, myocardial infarction, recurrent unstable angina, or requirement for revascularization) within 18 months.

Probability of Restenosis

The probability that a particular dilated coronary lesion will develop restenosis (according to a categorical definition) varies over a threefold range from one lesion to another. As will be discussed, this variable probability can form the underpinning of a strategy for selecting coronary lesions for angioplasty and determining the conduct strategy for managing them.

Patient Characteristics

Despite intensive study, very little relationship has been found between patient characteristics and restenosis probability. Margolis[16] found a weak relationship between the presence of diabetes and restenosis but did not successfully isolate it as a truly independent predictor. Other studies that used multivariate statistics have found little or no relationship between patient characteristics and restenosis.[17]

Lesion Characteristics (Table 1)

Gordon et al[18] measured the amount of late loss of lumen dimension (the difference between minimal lumen diameter immediately after a coronary angioplasty and at a 6-months post-coronary angioplasty angiogram) in a population of coronary lesions treated with stenting and found that the absolute amount of late loss varies considerably from lesion to lesion. The population of the magnitude of the late loss is normally distributed and is not related to patient characteristics. This explains why lesion characteristics are the best predictors of restenosis.

TABLE 1

Lesion Characteristics Associated with Increased Probability of Restenosis After Coronary Angioplasty

---

Preprocedural characteristics

  1) Lesion located in the left anterior descending artery or a saphenous vein graft.
  2) Increasing stenosis severity precoronary angioplasty (percent stenosis and/or minimal lumen diameter).
  3) Increasing lesion length.
  4) Decreasing arterial diameter.

Postprocedural characteristics

  1) Increasing stenosis severity postcoronary angioplasty (percent stenosis and/or minimal lumen diameter).

A number of angiographic characteristics of coronary lesions have been identified that correlate with the probability of restenosis. Of the many characteristics identified, the following have been found consistently in multiple series.[9,11,19,20] Lesion characteristics related to restenosis probability may be divided into two categories: preprocedural characteristics are known prior to the angioplasty procedure and their ability to predict restenosis may be used to select lesions under consideration for coronary angioplasty; postprocedural characteristics are, in part, related to the success of the angioplasty procedure. These characteristics are known only after the procedure has been completed.

Procedure Conduct

Little effect has been found for the influence of procedure conduct on the probability of restenosis. Roubin et al[21] studied the impact of deliberate balloon oversizing on the frequency of acute ischemic complications and restenosis. No effect on restenosis was found for balloon oversizing, but oversizing did cause an increased frequency of coronary dissection and acute ischemic events. However, it is not correct to conclude from these findings that procedure conduct has no influence on the probability of restenosis. Instead, it is likely that through experience, operators have identified the optimal technique for performing balloon angioplasty, and protocol defined modifications of technique do not offer further benefit.

Multivariate Prediction of Restenosis Probability

Because multiple lesion characteristics have independent ability to predict restenosis, the subject is ideally suitable for multivariate statistical modeling. Several authors have developed multivariate models from different data sets.[9,11,22] These models have a common theme in that they are dominated by measures of stenosis severity and length and also include stenosis location in the left anterior descending artery and in saphenous vein grafts. A representative model is summarized in Table 2.

A multivariate statistical model of restenosis can be used to calculate the probability of restenosis for a particular lesion. This is done by substituting the lesion's values for the significant variables into the equation defined by the model and solving for the probability of restenosis. Examples of such a calculation is shown

TABLE 2

A Multivariate Model to Predict Restenosis Probability After
Balloon Coronary Angioplasty

Variable	β	SE	Chi square
Intercept	−2.041		
Lesion length (mm)	0.077	0.024	10.23
Graft	1.602	0.494	10.54
LAD	0.596	0.191	9.71
% Stenosis post-PTCA	0.020	0.007	7.73
Vessel diameter	−0.385	0.153	6.38
% Stenosis pre-PTCA	0.211	0.009	5.48
"Optimal" balloon size	−0.398	0.189	4.43

Reproduced with permission from Reference 11.

in Table 3. This enables a physician to determine the likelihood that the benefit of a successful angioplasty will ultimately be frustrated by restenosis for a particular coronary lesion.

Unifying Concept to Explain Variability in Restenosis Probability

The overall observations that relate lesion characteristics to restenosis probability may be explained by the following unifying concept. Several of the lesion characteristics that correlate with restenosis probability describe reduced lumen dimension (percent stenosis precoronary angioplasty, minimal lumen diameter precoronary angioplasty, vessel diameter). Others are related to the extent of atheroma present within the lesion (lesion length, percent stenosis precoronary angioplasty and minimal lumen diameter precoronary angioplasty). Together these characteristics describe a circumstance in which increased atherosclerotic plaque burden and decreased vessel lumen diameter correlate with increased probability of restenosis. The correlation of postcoronary angioplasty percent stenosis and stenosis diameter has similar implications. Late loss of lumen dimension after coronary angioplasty is caused by a combination of elastic recoil and neointimal proliferation. This occurs to a variable degree from lesion to lesion, but a certain degree of late loss of lumen dimension following coronary angioplasty is inevitable. Thus, whether or not restenosis occurs depends on the amount of lumen dimension lost (the activity of the

TABLE 3

Examples of Restenosis Probability Calculations

Straightforward stenosis in a large RCA

Length:	2 mm
Location:	RCA
% Stenosis:	75
Eccentric:	No
Vessel Diam:	3.5 mm

$$y = -1.574, P = 17\%$$

Moderately Difficult Stenosis in Moderate-sized LAD

Length:	5 mm
Location:	LAD
% Stenosis:	80
Eccentric:	Yes
Vessel Diam:	2.7 mm

$$y = -.1258, P = 47\%$$

Very Difficult Stenosis in Heavily Diseased SVG

Length:	15 mm
Location:	SVG
% Stenosis:	90
Eccentric:	Yes
Vessel Diam:	3.2 mm

$$y = 1.572, P = 83\%$$

Reproduced with permission from Reference 11.

neointimal growth process which may be loosely determined by the amount of atheroma present) and the amount of space available in the vascular lumen to accommodate it (which is determined by the lesion dimensions). Consequently, restenosis is more likely in severe long stenoses in small vessels. The preponderance of restenosis in saphenous vein grafts may be explained by a greater degree of elastic recoil and a more aggressive neointimal proliferative process. The mechanism of the apparent preponderance of restenosis in the proximal left anterior descending artery has never been explained.

Prevention or Reduction of Restenosis

Pharmacologic Trials

To date, efforts to prevent or attenuate restenosis have been disappointingly ineffective. Considerable effort and expense have been applied to numerous trials assessing the efficacy of many different classes of pharmacologic agents. No convincing evidence of efficacy for any systemic drug therapy has surfaced to date. Although there have been a number of reports of success in individual studies, many of them have been limited by methodological problems and none have been substantiated by larger confirmatory trials. The underlying cause of failure of success of drug treatment is probably the perniciousness of the neointimal hyperplasia problem, and the inability to deliver sufficient concentrations of an active agent to the angioplasty site for a sufficient time period without incurring unacceptable toxicity.

New Interventional Devices

New interventional devices adopt one of two strategies to attempt to improve on the short-term result achievable by conventional balloon angioplasty: plaque removal and scaffolding the plaque away from the lumen. There are three basic strategies currently in use for plaque removal: plaque excision (directional atherectomy, extraction atherectomy); abrasive plaque destruction (Rotablator™, Heart Technologies, Bellevue, WA); and plaque vaporization (laser). Extraction atherectomy, rotational atherectomy, and laser angioplasty have each been demonstrated to be able to produce satisfactory short-term angioplasty results, however all have been plagued by restenosis rates that are indistinguishable from, if not greater than, restenosis rates for conventional balloon angioplasty.[23,24] Although it is possible that the lesions in these series had a greater restenosis probability than those in series of conventional balloon angioplasty, thus masking a beneficial effect of the device, no controlled trials have been performed and consequently, one must conclude from the currently available data that these devices have no beneficial effect on restenosis.

Directional atherectomy has been subjected to two controlled trials comparing it with conventional balloon angioplasty.[25,26] Directional atherectomy had a greater short-term complication rate than conventional coronary angioplasty, but had little positive impact on restenosis. Using a categorical definition of restenosis, the CAVEAT trial found a surprisingly high restenosis rate of 57% for conventional balloon angioplasty and a 50% restenosis for directional atherectomy. This occurred despite the fact that directional atherectomy yielded a larger lumen dimension immediately following the procedure (Table 4).

Several stent designs are in various stages of clinical evaluation. Only the Palmaz-Schatz stent (Johnson & Johnson Interventional

TABLE 4

Summary of Quantitative Coronary Angiographic Results
for Randomized Directional Atherectomy and
Stent vs. Balloon Angioplasty Trials

Directional Atherectomy (CAVEAT)		
Acute Result	DCA	PTCA
Min. lumen diam (mm):	1.89	1.66
% Stenosis:	33%	41%
Late Result		
Min lumen diam (mm):	1.35	1.23
% Stenosis:	52%	55%
Restenosis rate:	50%	57%
(>50% diameter stenosis)		
Stenting (Stress)		
Acute Result		
Min. lumen diam (mm):	2.47	1.92
% Stenosis:	19%	37%
Late Result		
Min lumen diam (mm):	1.77	1.53
% Stenosis:	41%	49%
Restenosis rate:	29%	43%
(>50% diameter stenosis)		

Data from Reference 25, CAVEAT Data Coordinating Center personal communication (RW
Califfe), and Reference 27.

Systems) has been compared with conventional balloon angioplasty
in a controlled trial. Two such trials have been conducted: the STent
REStenosis Study (STRESS), which was conducted predominantly
in the United States, and the Benestent Trial, which was conducted
predominantly in Europe.[27,28] The results of the two trials are con-
gruent and are summarized in Table 4 and Figure 3. Both data sets
demonstrate that stenting achieves a considerably larger minimal
lumen dimension acutely than does conventional balloon angio
plasty. However, stenting also suffers a greater late loss of lumen dimension over the succeeding 6 months. The increased late loss
partially offsets the greater gain achieved by stenting, but some of
the effect persists resulting in a significantly reduced categorical
restenosis rate (29% vs. 43%) and a 0. 2 mm difference in minimal
lumen diameter at follow-up. Stenting has also been evaluated as a
treatment for saphenous vein graft stenoses. In an uncontrolled
study, treatment with the Palmaz-Schatz stent yielded an angiographic restenosis rate of 26% considerably lower than any value reported for conventional balloon angioplasty.[29]

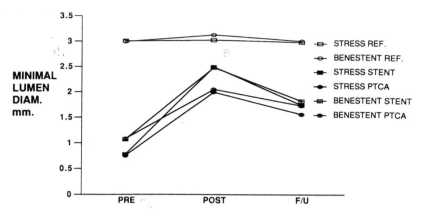

FIGURE 3. *Plot of the changes in minimal lumen diameter for two recently reported randomized trials comparing elective stenting with conventional balloon coronary angioplasty. The confidence interval bars have been deleted for clarity. (Reproduced with permission from Reference 27 [STRESS] and Reference 28 [BENESTENT].)*

Influence of Restenosis Probability on Selection of Patients for and the Conduct of Interventional Cardiac Procedures

In angioplasty's infancy, the principal determinant of whether angioplasty should be performed was the likelihood of executing the procedure effectively and safely. Current instrumentation has enhanced angioplasty's capability, greatly extending the range of lesions that can be successfully treated. However, there is little point to conducting angioplasty if the procedure's initial success is subsequently undermined by restenosis. Thus, the probability that restenosis will occur after a successful angioplasty should have an important influence on the decision to undertake the procedure and how it is to be conducted. This type of conceptual framework is applicable to several settings.

Single Vessel Disease with a High Restenosis Probability

Knowledge of the determinants of restenosis probability can be applied to the determination of the appropriateness of a particular coronary lesion for coronary angioplasty. The value to the patient of performing angioplasty in a circumstance in which the probability of a late failure of the procedure is greater than 50% must be carefully examined. Certain combinations of characteristics identify particular lesions as having restenosis probabilities in excess of 50%. Such characteristics include: 1) extreme lesion length (>15 mm); 2) small vessel diameter (>2.5 mm); 3) lesion location in saphenous vein grafts; 4) lesion geometry that precludes achieving a small postcoronary angioplasty percent stenosis.

The decision to undertake angioplasty in such circumstances must be made by balancing a number of competing issues that include the severity of the ischemia and the appropriateness of alternative treatment strategies. Small diameter vessels frequently have relatively small perfusion territories. Consequently, lesions in small vessels frequently do not cause severe ischemia. Thus, medical therapy is a viable alternative for many of these lesions. Conversely, although lesions in saphenous vein grafts have a high restenosis probability, the increased difficulty and hazard of repeat coronary surgery favors a catheter based approach if feasible. In long and geometrically complex lesions, careful consideration must be given to the appropriateness of other treatment strategies.

Multivessel Coronary Disease

Because the benefits of a revascularization procedure that does not require thoracotomy are seen as offsetting the detriment of a 30%–40% global restenosis rate, angioplasty is currently accepted as the treatment of choice for suitable single vessel coronary disease. However, the applicability of coronary angioplasty to multivessel coronary disease is less well defined because the lesion specific independent likelihood of restenosis means that the likelihood of at least one restenosis increases as the number of lesions dilated increases. Nobuyoshi[12] demonstrated that the probability of at least one restenosis in a patient who has three lesions dilated is >70% (Figure 4). The impact of the high frequency of restenosis after angioplasty for multivessel disease is illustrated by the findings of the Emory Angioplasty vs. Surgery Trial. This study found that 50% of patients with multivessel disease treated with angioplasty as an initial treatment strategy required at least one additional revascularization procedure within the first year after the initial procedure. This contrasted with 20% of the patients whose initial treatment strategy was bypass surgery. This requirement for revas-

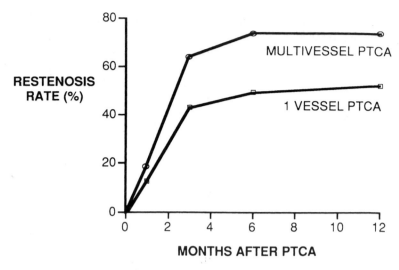

FIGURE 4. *Time course of the developement of at least one restenosis after PTCA as a function of the number of lesions dilated. (Reproduced with permission from Reference 12.)*

cularization in the angioplasty group is attributable to the high frequency of restenosis.[30]

Application of New Interventional Devices

Of the new interventional devices only stenting and directional atherectomy have been evaluated rigorously with respect to restenosis.

The Palmaz-Schatz stent has been shown to have a modest benefit to reduce restenosis when applied to vessels with diameters > 3. 0 mm and an apparent, but not yet conclusively proven benefit in saphenous vein grafts. Stents also achieve better short-term angiographic results than conventional balloon angioplasty. Its principal detriments are the requirement for a longer initial hospitalization and the risk of subacute thrombosis. It appears that stenting has the potential to reduce restenosis probability and should be considered for large native coronary vessels, saphenous vein grafts, and for lesions that respond poorly to conventional balloon angioplasty.

Directional atherectomy has been shown to date to have, at most, a very small impact on restenosis. However, directional atherectomy is highly effective at achieving superior acute angio-graphic results in certain anatomic situations such as highly ec-centric lesions, very proximal lesions, and aorto-ostial lesions. In these circumstances, a successful well executed directional atherec-tomy procedure may well reduce restenosis compared with con-ventional balloon angioplasty.

Summary

The elements of the current restenosis knowledge base are summarized in Table 5. They are organized into a conceptual framework that can be applied to clinical practice. A strategy for the application of this knowledge base to clinical practice is sum-marized in Table 6.

TABLE 5

Summary of the Current Restenosis Knowledge Base

---

1. Restenosis Probability:
   A. Some decrease of lumen diameter is inevitable following PTCA
   B. Restenosis is a lesion-specific entity
   C. The likelihood of restenosis is predictable and is influenced strongly by lesion characteristics
      · In multilesion PTCA, the likelihood of at least one restenosis increases with the number of lesions dilated
2. Clinical Impact of Restenosis:
   A. Whether the lumen loss following PTCA will cause symptoms is determined by the stenosis severity and the patient's characteristics
   B. Restenosis causes return of symptoms in two thirds of cases
      · The asymptomatic one third of patients with angiographic restenosis have a high likelihood of cardiac events within the next 2 years
   C. The increased likelihood of restenosis with multilesion PTCA is the major obstacle to extending PTCA to multivessel disease
      · Patients who undergo multilesion PTCA have a 50% likelihood of requiring additional revascularization procedures within 1 year
3. Means of Reducing Restenosis:
   A. Procedure conduct has little influence on the likelihood of restenosis
   B. To date: adjunctive drug therapy has no influence on the likelihood of restenosis
   C. Directional atherectomy and stenting improve the acute result of angioplasty, but are associated with a greater late loss of lumen diameter and more frequent complications
      · Directional atherectomy has little impact on restenosis
      · Stenting has a modest beneficial impact

TABLE 6

Strategy for Selecting Coronary Angioplasty and New Interventional Devices for Treating Particular Coronary Lesions

If Restenosis Probability <50%:

PTCA is appropriate for suitable lesions
- Consider DCA or stent if vessel diameter >3.5 mm and lesion access is straightforward
- Consider stent for SVBG if vessel diameter >3.0 mm.

If Restenosis Probability >50%

Appropriateness of PTCA diminishes unless patient requires revascularization and is a poor or inappropriate surgical candidate
- Consider DCA or stent if vessel diameter >3.0 mm
- Consider stent for SVBG if vessel diameter >3.0 mm.

References

1. Ardissio D, Di Somma S, Kubica J, et al. Influence of elastic recoil on restenosis after successful coronary angioplasty in unstable angina pectoris. *Am J Cardiol.* 1993;71:659–663.
2. Rensing BJ, Hermans WRM, Beatt KM, et al. Quantitative angiographic assessment of elastic recoil after percutaneous transluminal coronary angioplasty. *Am J Cardiol.* 1990;66:1039–1044.
3. Forrester JS, Fishbein M, Helfant R, Fagin J. A paradigm for restenosis based on cell biology: clues for the development of new preventive therapies. *J Am Coll Cardiol.* 1991;17:758.
4. Libby P, Schwartz D, Broi E, Tanaka H, Clinton SK. A cascade model for restenosis, a special case of atherosclerosis progression. *Circulation.* 1992;86(Suppl III):II-147-II-52.
5. Liu MW, Roubin GS, King SBI. Restenosis after coronary angioplasty: potential biological determinants and role of intimal hyperplasia. *Circulation.* 1989;79:1374–1387.
6. Vetrovec GW, DiSciascio F, Jugo R, et al. Comparative clinical and angiographic findings in patients with symptomatic and asymptomatic restenosis following angioplasty *J Am Coll Cardiol.* 1990;15(Suppl A):59A.
7. Thornton MA, Gruentzig AR, Hollman J, King SBI, Douglas JSJ. Coumadin and aspirin in the prevention of recurrence after coronary angioplasty: a randomized study. *Circulation.* 1984;69:721–727.
8. Reiber JH, Serruys PW, Kooijman CJ, et al. Assessment of short-, medium-, and long-term variations in arterial dimensions from computer-assisted quantitation of coronary cineangiograms. *Circulation.* 1985;71(2):280–288.
9. Leimruber PP, Roubin GS, Hollman J, et al. Restenosis after successful coronary angioplasty in patients with single vessel disease. *Circulation.* 1986;73:710–717.

10. Kuntz RE, Safian RD, Levine MJ, Reis GJ, Diver DJ, Baim DS. Novel approach to the analysis of restenosis after the use of three new coronary devices. *J Am Coll Cardiol.* 1992;19:1493–1499.
11. Hirshfeld JW, Schwartz JS, Jugo R, et al. Restenosis after coronary angioplasty: a multivariate statistical model to relate lesion and procedure variables to restenosis. *J Am Coll Cardiol.* 1991;18:647–656.
12. Nobuyoshi M, Kimura T, Nosaka H, et al. Restenosis after successful percutaneous transluminal coronary angioplasty: serial angiographic follow-up of 229 patients. *J Am Coll Cardiol.* 1988;12:616–622.
13. Serruys PG, Luuten R, Beatt KJ, et al. Incidence of restenosis after successful coronary angioplasty: a time-related phenomenon. *Circulation.* 1988;77:361–371.
14. Popma JJ, van den Berg EK, Dehmer GJ. Long-term outcome of patients with asymptomatic restenosis after percutaneous transluminal coronary angioplasty. *Am J Cardiol.* 1988;62:1298–1299.
15. Laarman G, Luitjen HE, van Zeyl LG, et al. Assessment of silent restenosis and long-term follow-up after successful angioplasty in single vessel coronary artery disease: the value of quantitative exercise electrocardiography and quantitative coronary angiography. *J Am Coll Cardiol.* 1990;16:578–585.
16. Margolis JR, Krieger R, Glemser E. Increased restenosis rate in insulin dependent diabetics. *Circulation.* 1984;70(Suppl II):II-75. Abstract.
17. Macdonald RG, Henderson MA, Hirshfeld JWJ, et al. Patient-related variables and restenosis after percutaneous transluminal coronary angioplasty—a report from the M-HEART Group. *Am J Cardiol.* 1990;66(12):926–931.
18. Gordon PW, Gibson CM, Cohen DJ, Carrozza IP, Kuntz RE, Baim DS. Mechanisms of restenosis and redilation within coronary stents—quantitative angiographic assessment. *J Am Coll Cardiol.* 1993;21(5):I-166-I-174.
19. Black AJR, Anderson HV, Roubin GS, Powelson SW, Douglas JSJ, King SBI. Repeat coronary angioplasty: correlates of a second restenosis. *J Am Coll Cardiol.* 1988;11:714–718.
20. Teirstein PS, Hoover CA, Lignon RW, et al. Repeat coronary angioplasty: efficacy of a third angioplasty for a second restenosis. *J Am Coll Cardiol.* 1989;13(2):291–296.
21. Roubin GS, Douglas JS Jr, King SB III, et al. Influence of balloon size on initial success, acute complications, and restenosis after percutaneous transluminal coronary angioplasty. *Circulation.* 1988;78:557–565.
22. Rensing BJ, Hermans WR, Vos J, et al. Luminal narrowing after percutaneous transluminal coronary angioplasty. A study of clinical, procedural, and lesional factors related to long-term angiographic outcome. Coronary Artery Restenosis Prevention on Repeated Thromboxane Antagonism (CARPORT) Study Group. *Circulation.* 1993;88(3):975–985.
23. Klein LW, Eigler N, Cummins F, Rothbaum D, investigators ftA. Long term clinical outcome and factors associated with adverse events after successful excimer laser coronary angioplasty (ELCA): A report from the multicenter ELCA registry. *Circulation.* 1993;88(Part 2):I-25. Abstract.
24. Buchbinder M, Warth D, Casale PN, Fenner J, Stenzer S. Cumulative 4 year experience from the Rotablator multicenter registry. *Circulation.* 1993;88(Part 2):I-150.

25. Topol EJ, Leya F, Pinkerton CA, et al. A comparison of directional atherectomy with coronary angioplasty in patients with coronary artery disease. *N Engl J Med.* 1993;329(4):221–227.
26. Adelman AG, Cohen EA, Kimball BP, et al. A comparison of directional atherectomy with balloon angioplasty for lesions of the left anterior descending coronary artery. *N Engl J Med.* 1993;329(4):228–233.
27. Fischman DL, Leon MB, Baim D, et al. A randomized comparison of coronary stent placement and balloon angioplasty in the treatment of coronary artery disease. *N Engl J Med.* In Press.
28. Serruys PW, deJaegere P, Kiemeneij F, et al. A comparison of balloon expandable stent implantation with balloon angioplasty in patients with coronary artery disease. *N Engl J Med.* In Press.
29. Leon MB, Ellis SG, Pichard AD, Baim DS, Heuser RR, Schatz RA. Stents may be the preferred treatment for focal aortocoronary vein graft disease. *Circulation.* 1991;84(Suppl II):II-249.
30. King SBI, Lembo NJ, Weintraub WS. Results from the Emory Angioplasty vs Surgery Trial (EAST) compared to the eligible non-randomized registry. *J Am Coll Cardiol.* 1994;22:469A.

Chapter 21

Approach to the High-Risk Interventional Patient

Alice K. Jacobs, MD

During the past decade, numerous technological advances have allowed percutaneous coronary revascularization procedures to be performed in higher risk patients with more complex coronary anatomy and comorbid disease. Patients and coronary lesions previously considered too high risk for an adverse outcome are now considered suitable for the procedure. This expansion in potential candidates for these higher risk procedures has created a role for both systemic and regional support modalities and the need for a particularly careful and thoughtful periprocedural management strategy.

The decision to perform percutaneous coronary revascularization in a high-risk setting is based on multiple factors and determined by the overall risk of the intervention. Certainly, prospective assessment of risk is difficult and there is no specific operational definition of "high risk". Patient factors and lesion factors have been evaluated. Patient factors that increase the risk of an adverse outcome include advanced age, left ventricular dysfunction, female gender, diabetes mellitus, and comorbid disease.[1] Lesion characteristics associated with abrupt closure have been previously described and are based on morphologic features such as lesion length, thrombus, eccentricity, tortuosity, and angulation.[2]

However, there is limited ability to predict the risk of hemodynamic compromise during coronary intervention, particularly if complicated by abrupt vessel closure. In a retrospective review of 28 clinical and angiographic variables in a group of consecutive patients undergoing coronary angioplasty, Bergelson and colleagues[3] reported that multivariate analysis identified multivessel disease, diffuse disease, myocardium at risk, and the severity of target le-

From Vetrovec GW, Carabello BA, (eds.) *Invasive Cardiology: Current Diagnostic and Therapeutic Issues.* Armonk, NY: Futura Publishing Company, Inc.: © 1996.

sion stenosis as independent predictors of hemodynamic compromise (defined as a decrease in systolic blood pressure ≥ 20 mm Hg to <90 mm Hg during balloon inflation). The regression coefficients of the variables on which this analysis was based were then used to create a 13-point weighted scoring system (Figure 1) that was prospectively applied to a separate group of consecutive patients undergoing coronary angioplasty. In using a risk score of ≥ 4 to define high risk for hemodynamic compromise, this scoring system had a sensitivity of 92% and a specificity of 92% (Figure 2).

Realizing that periprocedural pharmacologic therapy results in only a modest reduction in the ischemic response to percutaneous coronary intervention, systemic and regional support techniques have been gaining more widespread use. The goals of these modalities are to provide support to the systemic circulation, oxygenated blood to ischemic myocardium, and improved collateral blood flow into the ischemic region and to minimize oxygen consumption of ischemic tissue. When deployed properly and in an appropriate situation, these support modalities are quite effective. Which technique to use and whether to use it in a prophylactic or standby mode are current issues that face interventional cardiologists.

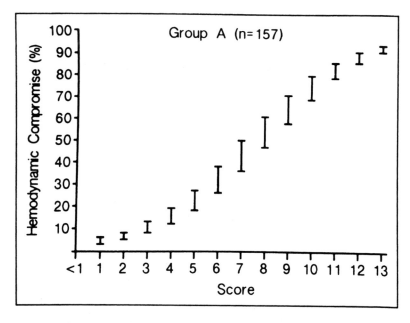

FIGURE 1. *The probability of hemodynamic compromise during percutaneous transluminal coronary angioplasty based on a weighted 13-point scoring system. (Reproduced with permission from Reference 3.)*

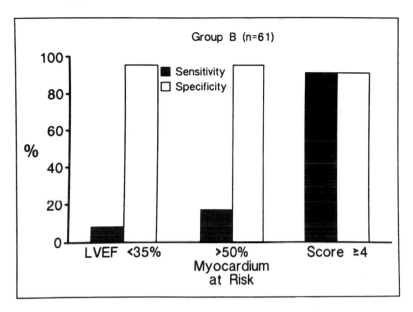

FIGURE 2. *The sensitivity and specificity of left ventricular ejection fraction (LVEF) < 35%, >50% viable myocardium at risk and a score ≥4 in the prediction of hemodynamic compromise during percutaneous transluminal coronary angioplasty. (Reproduced with permission from Reference 3.)*

Systemic Support Techniques

Intra-aortic Balloon Counterpulsation

Physiology

The intra-aortic balloon pump is the most widely used and simplest of the left ventricular assist devices that provide systemic (or global myocardial) support. Rapid expansion of a 40-cc elongated balloon in the descending thoracic aorta after the end of left ventricular ejection displaces 40 mL of blood, which increases perfusion pressure during diastole. Abrupt deflation just prior to the onset of ejection creates a relative decrease in intra-aortic blood volume of 40 mL that decreases afterload and the amount of work necessary to eject blood. This simple displacement of blood within the aorta produces a relatively passive augmentation of blood flow, rather than the active pumping from the left ventricle into the systemic circulation seen with the Hemopump. The overall hemodynamic effects of intra-aortic balloon counterpulsation are based, in

part, on the pathophysiologic state of the patient.[4] However, the reduction in systemic afterload results in a modest improvement in
stroke volume and cardiac output.

Special Considerations

Percutaneous placement of the intra-aortic balloon (at the bedside in patients without significant peripheral vascular disease) and
the use of smaller catheters and sheaths have improved the ease of
insertion and allowed the technique to be used in smaller patients
with moderate peripheral vascular disease. In fact, pediatric intra-
aortic balloons (30 cc, 8F, 30.5 inches long) have been effective in
providing the expected hemodynamic effects without compromis-
ing the peripheral arterial circulation in small/short patients with
peripheral vascular disease. Of note, aortic pressure should be
monitored proximal to the balloon because distal measurement of
aortic pressure will erroneously underestimate the degree of augmentation achieved. In addition, when the intra-aortic balloon is
deployed, the pump should be turned off when angioplasty or
atherectomy catheters are introduced or withdrawn (over a wire)
through the descending aorta.

Use of the intra-aortic balloon is limited to patients with a stable ventricular rhythm. Intra-aortic balloon counterpulsation does
not provide regional myocardial support during coronary balloon
inflation or after abrupt closure, although increased collateral
blood flow due to increased coronary perfusion pressure has been
reported.[5] Yet, extensive single center and anecdotal experience[6,7]
has suggested that the intra-aortic balloon is effective in providing
hemodynamic and clinical stability during percutaneous intervention (Figure 3), especially in the setting of decreased left ventricular function. In addition, use of the intra-aortic balloon to treat
recurrent acute closure of the target lesion has recently been reported.[8] Intra-aortic balloon counterpulsation may also provide a
valuable bridge to emergency coronary artery bypass surgery.

Cardiopulmonary Bypass

Physiology

By actively aspirating blood from the right atrium at the junc-
tion of the inferior vena cava and, after oxygenation, returning it to
the arterial system, the cardiopulmonary bypass system is capable

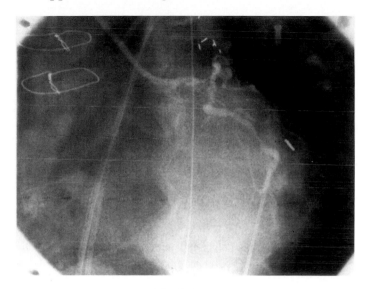

FIGURE 3A. *Cineangiograms of the left coronary artery (shallow left anterior oblique projection) illustrating a significant left main stenosis in an elderly patient with prior bypass surgery (patent graft to left anterior descending artery) no longer considered an operative candidate and in whom unstable angina was refractory to maximal medical management. Due to ongoing ischemia, the intra-aortic balloon (right) was inserted prior to angiography.*

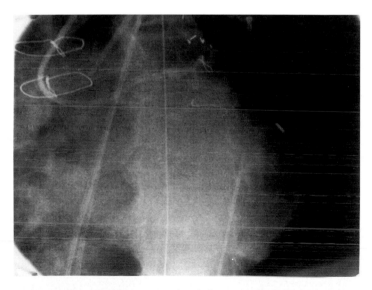

FIGURE 3B. *Balloon inflation in the left main coronary artery using a "kissing" balloon strategy and requiring the use of a left Amplatz guide for support.*

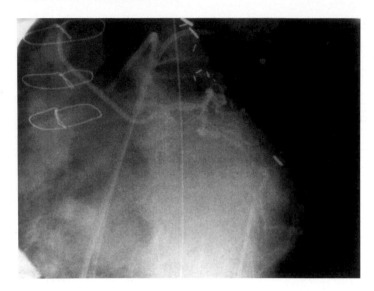

Figure 3C. *Follow-up cineangiogram illustrating an insignificant residual stenosis in the left main coronary artery.*

of total circulatory support, independent of cardiac rhythm, pulmonary vascular resistance, and function of the right side of the heart. Although it has been suggested that left ventricular venting may be critical for infarct salvage, in general, this has not been used. Left ventricular unloading appears to be adequate, particularly if sinus rhythm is maintained. Left ventricular pressure remains low and in the setting of decreased return to the left ventricle, it is likely that oxygen consumption is significantly reduced.

Special Considerations

Aorto-iliac angiography to exclude significant tortuosity or atherosclerosis should be performed prior to serial progressive local site dilation that allows insertion of large (18–20F) cannulas. The patient is fully anticoagulated (300 u/Kg of heparin) and the primed cardiopulmonary bypass system is attached to the cannulas. As bypass is initiated, intravenous fluid administration is frequently required to compensate for the fall in preload; subsequent fluid compensates for the fall in systemic pressure. After the interventional procedure, bypass is discontinued and the cannulas are removed percutaneously or under direct surgical repair. Hemostasis is achieved with an external groin clamp for several hours.

Up to 5 L/min of flow can be provided with a combination of 19F venous and 17F arterial cannulas and up to 3.5 L/min can be provided with 18F venous and 16F arterial cannulas. However, despite full support of the systemic circulation even during periods of cardiac arrest, there is no perfusion of the jeopardized myocardium during coronary balloon inflation or coronary occlusion.

The multicenter experience of 25 centers performing supported angioplasty has been collected in a national registry since March, 1988.[9,10] The morbidity and mortality associated with this technique, using a prophylactic or standby approach, as reported from the National Registry, are summarized in Table 1. Of note is that although overall mortality is similar in patients receiving prophylactic and standby support, mortality is significantly lower (7.0% vs. 13.0%, $P < 0.05$) in the group of patients with left ventricular ejection fraction $\leq 20\%$ in whom prophylactic support was undertaken. However, in the entire cohort of patients, the percent of patients receiving transfusions and experiencing vascular complications is significantly increased when prophylactic support is initiated.

Partial Left Heart Bypass

Physiology

Partial bypass to the left side of the heart provides oxygenated blood to the systemic circulation using a transseptal approach. Al-

---

TABLE 1

Cardiopulmonary Bypass: National Registry of Elective Supported Angioplasty: Morbidity and Mortality

	Prophylatic Support (n = 476)	Standby Support (n = 217)
Transfused (%)	31.0	14.0
Vascular complications	15.0	6.1
Acute Myocardial Infarction (%)	0.6	0.9
ECABG (%)	2.5	3.2
Death (%)	6.3	6.0
LVEF ≤20%	7.0	18.0
>20%	7.1	3.9

ECABG, emergency coronary artery bypass surgery; LVEF, left ventricular ejection fraction.

though the system is simple in comparison to cardiopulmonary by-pass in that a membrane oxygenator is not required, the physiology is similar. Oxygenated blood from the left atrium is pumped to a femoral artery cannula that provides support similar to the cardiopulmonary bypass system. Preload, cardiac work, and oxygen consumption are all reduced.

Special Considerations

Using a transseptal approach, a 14–20F catheter is placed in the left atrium. A 7F bidirectional arterial cannula has a separate port at the "heel" that allows blood to be directed down the leg, reducing the potential for lower limb ischemia.

To date, experience with this technique is limited. Preliminary reports suggest that hemodynamic support during coronary angioplasty can be provided.[11,12] However, the overall success of the technique and potential incidence of atrial septal defect is under active investigation.

Hemopump

Physiology

By using an axial flow pump to draw blood out of the left ventricle and expel it into the aorta, the Hemopump produces significant left ventricular unloading and reduces myocardial oxygen consumption. During left ventricular support, mean arterial pressure frequently exceeds left ventricular pressure throughout the duration of the cardiac cycle. Therefore, collateral blood flow into ischemic regions may be provided throughout the cardiac cycle, rather than during diastole alone.

Special Considerations

This innovative device consists of an Archimedes screw pump that rotates at 25,000 rpm to provide a flow rate of up to 3.5 L/min in a nonpulsatile fashion. The device requires a surgical cutdown and placement of a 12-mm Dacron™ graft for insertion into the femoral artery. Occasionally, peripheral angioplasty of the iliofemoral arteries may be necessary to allow passage of the 21F cannula. However, a 14F device is under development and can be percutaneously inserted through a modified 15F sheath. This 14F cannula is approximately 10 cm shorter than the 21F device and produces up to 2 L of flow per minute. The arterial cannula is passed retrogradely up the descending aorta, activated and advanced around the aortic arch and across the aortic valve using a prolapse technique similar to that used in a standard pigtail catheter insertion (Figure 4). Once inserted, the monitoring console is easily managed and does not require supervision by specialized perfusion teams.

The Hemopump output is independent of left ventricular func-

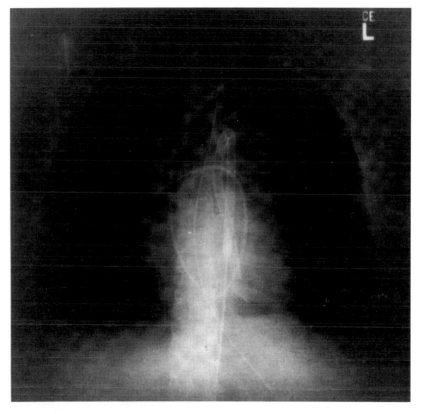

FIGURE 4. *Hemopump placement in a patient with acute myocardial infarction and subsequent pulmonary edema. The turbine rests in the descending aorta and the cannula tip rests across the aortic valve, just inferior to the mitral valve. (Reproduced with permission from Reference 31.)*

tion or cardiac rhythm and the device may be used for prolonged periods in compliant patients (without leg bending). It provides direct left ventricular decompression, but adequate filling of the left heart through the pulmonary circulation is required. Peripheral vascular disease, aortic valve disease, prosthetic aortic valves and left ventricular thrombus are contraindications to its use. Trials in small numbers of patients undergoing coronary angioplasty have reported favorable results.[13,14] A comparison of the systemic support devices is illustrated in Table 2.

Regional Support Techniques

Antegrade Perfusion

Recently, there has been an enormous interest in distal coronary artery perfusion during percutaneous intervention, based on the increased number of high-risk procedures being performed, as well as on the tendency to perform more prolonged balloon inflations in the setting of coronary artery dissection. Antegrade perfusion of the distal bed can be achieved by the active infusion of autologous blood using pumping systems or more easily by passive perfusion through catheter shaft side holes and the central lumen.

TABLE 2

Comparison of Systemic Modalities

	IAB	CPS	Hemopump
Size of Cannula/Sheath	8–12F	18–20F	21F (14–15F)
Type of Support	Passive	Active	Active
Level of Support	0.2–1.0 L/min	5.2 L/min	3.5 L/min (2.0 L/min)
Duration of Support	days–weeks	up to 8.5 hours	days–weeks
LV decompression	minimal	moderate	excellent
Stable rhythm acquired	yes	no	no
Limitation	AI, PVD	PVD	AS/AI RHF/PVD LV thrombus

AI, aortic insufficiency; AS, aortic stenosis; L/min, liters per minute; LV, left ventricular; PVD, peripheral vascular disease; RHF, right heart failure.

Perfusion Balloon Catheters

Physiology

During percutaneous intervention, transient coronary occlusion in patients without an adequate collateral circulation is very rapidly followed by regional myocardial dysfunction. In a majority of patients, coronary occlusion time is limited by angina, electrical instability or hemodynamic compromise. This ischemic response is dependent on the preprocedure target lesion stenosis, the size and viability of the myocardial territory distal to the target lesion, and the presence of collateral blood flow. If coronary occlusion time is brief, restoration of oxygenated blood rapidly reverses the ischemic response. Indeed, numerous experimental and clinical studies have demonstrated the efficacy of antegrade perfusion in reducing the manifestations of ischemia during coronary balloon inflation.[15-17]

In the passive perfusion systems, the aortic pressure serves as the driving force and the efficacy of the technique is based on the transcoronary "driving pressure" gradient. Flow rates are linearly proportional to proximal artery perfusion pressure and adequacy of hemoperfusion is dependent on catheter length, lumen diameter, and blood viscosity.

Special Considerations

The catheters are delivered as an over-the-wire or monorail system in routine fashion. Once the balloon is properly positioned, distal flow can be maximized by removing the guide wire, withdrawing the guiding catheter from the coronary ostium, and limiting inflation pressures so as not to encroach on the central lumen. Distal flow is limited by side branch occlusion, tandem lesions, small caliber vessels, and relative hypotension. However, by maintaining flow, these perfusion balloon catheters may be particularly useful during dilation of the more proximal lesion when performing a multilesion procedure in the same vessel. In addition, use of this technique should be considered when performing coronary angioplasty: 1) of a proximal lesion in a large vessel serving a large area of viable myocardium; 2) in the setting of hypertrophic cardiomyopathy, aortic stenosis and severe left ventricular hypertrophy; 3) in patients with reduced left ventricular function in whom the target lesion supplies viable myocardium (Figure 5); 4) in com-

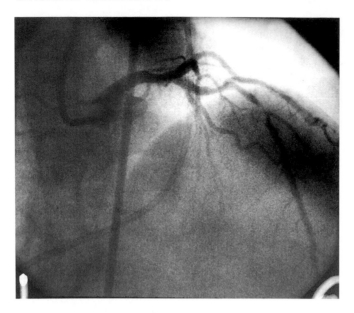

FIGURE 5A. *Cineangiogram in the right anterior oblique projection with cranial angulation illustrating a significant stenosis in the mid-left anterior descending artery that served viable myocardium in a patient with severely reduced left ventricular function.*

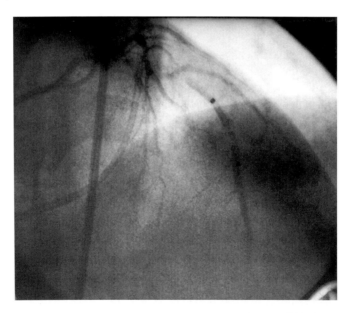

FIGURE 5B. *Cineangiogram in the same projection illustrating placement and inflation of a perfusion balloon catheter across the lesion. Contrast injection through the guiding catheter reveals flow in the distal artery as well as occlusion of a small diagonal artery adjacent to the balloon.*

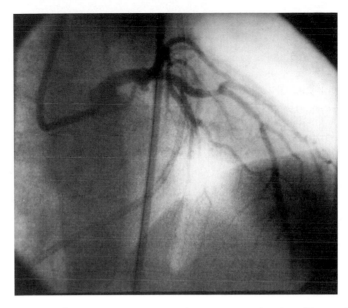

FIGURE 5C. *Final cineangiogram in the same projection illustrating an insignificant residual stenosis and restoration of flow in the diagonal artery.*

plex coronary lesion morphology, complicated by abrupt vessel closure/arterial dissection, and as a bridge to emergency surgery for a failed procedure.[18,19]

Retrograde Perfusion

In comparison to all of the support techniques, the retrograde perfusion modalities in general and specifically synchronized coronary sinus retroperfusion have undergone the most extensive experimental and preclinical evaluation.[20–23] The efficacy of these techniques is based on the unique microcirculation of the heart with its extensive arteriovenous and veno-venous anastomoses.[24] When used during coronary angioplasty, several studies have shown that synchronized coronary sinus retroperfusion is effective in reducing the ischemic response to coronary balloon occlusion as determined by the degree of angina, electrocardiographic changes, and left ventricular regional wall motion.[25–27]

Physiology

During synchronized retroperfusion, arterial blood is pumped via the coronary sinus during diastole and normal venous drainage occurs during systole. Therefore, myocardial edema, which occurs when venous drainage is impaired, is avoided. Inflation of a balloon catheter positioned in the coronary sinus avoids reflux into the right atrium and allows arterial blood to be pumped towards the ischemic myocardium. During synchronized retroperfusion, positron emission tomography has documented retrograde delivery of flow tracers and enhanced glucose metabolism in the risk region.[28] Although efficacy in reducing myocardial ischemia is based on direct delivery of arterial blood to the myocardium, enhanced myocardial washout may occur as well.[29]

Special Considerations

Coronary sinus catheterization requires fluoroscopic guidance and pressure monitoring and is most successful from the right internal jugular vein. Once the catheter enters the coronary sinus, contrast injection allows visualization of the anatomy (Figure 5) and placement of the catheter into the great cardiac vein is facilitated with a wire. After a short learning curve, successful cannulation of the cardiac vein is achieved in approximately 85%–90% of patients within 5 minutes.

The retroperfusion system consists of a coronary sinus catheter (8.5F triple lumen with a 10-mm diameter balloon at the tip), an arterial cannula (single lumen 7F or 8F catheter with distal end and side holes), a synchronized pneumatic pump triggered on the R wave of the electrocardiogram and an electropneumatic balloon inflation mechanism. The arterial cannula connects to the pumping console; arterial blood is delivered to the distal port of the coronary sinus catheter during balloon inflation that occurs during diastole. The pumping console maintains selected flow rates, provides balloon inflation with a fixed volume of gas in synchronization with each pump stroke, and allows monitoring of coronary sinus pressure from the distal port of the catheter. Maximum flow rates of 250 mL/min can be delivered, but flow rates are set so as not to exceed a coronary sinus systolic pressure of 60 mm Hg (in order to avoid microvascular damage).

Coronary sinus retroperfusion is usually reserved for patients undergoing high-risk procedures in the left anterior descending artery in whom severe peripheral vascular disease precludes systemic support modalities. In these patients, the pump and catheters are in a standby mode, but internal jugular venous cannulation with a 9F sheath prior to the procedure (and administration of heparin) should be performed. Synchronized retroperfusion is instituted for ongoing ischemia or an angiographic result necessitating prolonged coronary balloon inflation.

The advantages of retrograde perfusion during percutaneous revascularization are outlined in Table 3. This technique is effective in maintaining circulation to the arterial side branches that are otherwise compromised by angioplasty balloon catheters or coronary lesions. It is particularly useful when antegrade access to the artery is lost and can serve as a bridge to the operating room where the coronary sinus catheter can be used to rapidly institute coronary sinus retrograde cardioplegia.

The lack of efficacy in all patients (and the ability to predict which patients will benefit) limits the use of synchronized retroperfusion. This is probably due, in part, to the variable coronary venous anatomy, and in particular, to the extensive Thebesian circulation in some patients that shunts blood directly into the arterial and ventricular chambers (Figure 6). In addition, clinical experience with this technique has been obtained largely in the setting of disease in the left anterior descending artery, although positioning the balloon catheter in the proximal coronary sinus should theoretically provide similar efficacy in all myocardial regions. This hypothesis is supported by the fact that retrograde coronary sinus cardioplegia performed during cardiac surgery has not been shown to provide inadequate protection of the inferior and posterior wall of the left ventricle nor of the right ventricle.[30] A comparison of the regional support devices is illustrated in Table 4.

TABLE 3

Advantages of Retrograde Perfusion

1. Venous system is rarely diseased
2. Avoids manipulation of arterial system
3. Maintains access to ischemic microvasculature even when antegrade access to artery is lost
4. Provides access for retrograde infusion of pharmacologic agents.[32,33]
5. Coronary sinus pressure monitoring provides a continuous recording of left ventricular end-diastolic pressure.[34]
6. Serves as bridge to operating room

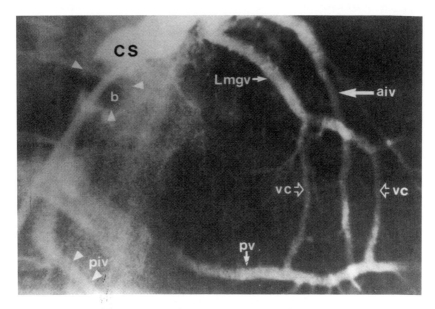

FIGURE 6. *Right anterior oblique projection of a coronary venogram. Manual contrast injection via the coronary sinus catheter during coronary sinus balloon inflation demonstrating large venous communications (vc) shunting contrast from the left marginal vein (Lmgv) to the posterior vein (pv) and potentially away from the anterior interventricular vein (aiv). b, retroperfusion catheter balloon; cs, coronary sinus; piv, posterior interventricular vein. (Reproduced with permission from Reference 27.)*

TABLE 4

Comparison of Regional Modalities

	Antegrade	Retrograde
Instrumentation	easy	moderate difficulty
	(less so with Fluosol)	
Success	>90%	85%
Limitations	side branchs	LAD distribution
	antegrade access	CS catheter
	hypotension	

CS, coronary sinus; LAD, left anterior descending artery.

Management Strategies

Periprocedural Approach to the Patient

The periprocedural approach to the patient is of critical importance and the overall strategy is outlined in Table 5.

Management Prior to the Procedure

In addition to considering patient factors, lesions factors, and the risk of hemodynamic compromise, the overall risk of the procedure is greatly influenced by the patient's candidacy for coronary bypass surgery and for systemic support techniques. The ability to support the systemic circulation (and regional myocardium if possible) and safely transport the patient to the operating room for emergency coronary bypass surgery is a major factor in the decision to perform the procedure. If the patient is not considered to be a surgical candidate under any circumstance and severe peripheral vascular disease precludes the use of the intra-aortic balloon, except in unusual circumstances, the patient should not be considered eligible for percutaneous revascularization in the setting of a high-risk lesion profile, particularly if the risk of hemodynamic compromise is also increased.

TABLE 5

Periprocedural Approach to the High-Risk Patient

Management Preprocedure

1. Risk assessment
2. Cardiac surgical consultation
3. Discussion with patient and family
4. Assessment of ability to use support modalities
5. Technical strategy

Management in the Intervention Laboratory

1. Peripheral angiography
2. Prophylactic vs. standby support
3. Hemodynamic monitoring

Management Postprocedure

1. Maintain anticoagulation
2. Observation in interventional unit

In the high-risk setting, prior to proceeding with percutaneous revascularization, formal cardiac surgical consultation should be obtained. Evaluation of the patient by the thoracic surgeon and the suitability of the patient for coronary bypass surgery either on an elective or emergency basis should be discussed. Occasionally, the patient is deemed to be a candidate for surgery on an elective basis, but not on an emergency basis, perhaps in the setting of multiple previous cardiac surgical procedures. If so, the optimal revascularization strategy should be reassessed.

In the patient deemed to be at high risk for an adverse outcome, the options for treatment and risks of the procedure should be discussed in detail with the patient and family and the likelihood of a major or minor complication explained in specific terms. In these high-risk circumstances, especially in the setting where surgical backup is refused, the support and understanding of both the patient and family is critically important.

When approaching a high-risk interventional procedure, preprocedural evaluation should include an assessment of the likelihood of successful placement of systemic and regional support devices. Peripheral vascular disease or other pathology such as aortic insufficiency which would preclude intra-aortic balloon placement should be noted. In addition, a detailed cineangiographic review will help determine the ability to maintain antegrade or retrograde perfusion, if necessary. As noted previously, in the patient in whom hemodynamic compromise during percutaneous revascularization is likely, candidacy for support technology should strongly influence the decision to perform the procedure.

It is also important that careful assessment of the dilatation and device strategy be undertaken. In the setting of multivessel disease, the order of the target lesions to be approached should be planned. Most often, the lesion deemed to be the "culprit" is approached first. However, in certain circumstances, revascularization of another lesion prior to the "culprit" lesion may provide collateral flow and thereby reduce the risk of the procedure. In this setting, a staged procedure should be considered, and, if possible, instrumentation of a second lesion when there is evidence of a dissection, thrombus, or suboptimal result in the first lesion should be avoided.

Management in the Interventional Laboratory

In all high-risk patients, and in particular in those patients at increased risk for hemodynamic compromise, it is prudent to prep femoral access sites. One femoral artery may be instrumented with a pigtail catheter and peripheral angiography of the aorto-iliac and common femoral arteries obtained. This aids in the decision to use one femoral site for the procedure and the other for the purpose of providing systemic support using large catheters. In these patients, it is important to consider routine instrumentation of the contralateral artery with a 5F sheath so as to ensure rapid deployment of support devices if necessary. Usually, the support modality is employed using a standby mode (with the exception of the above mentioned instrumentation of the contralateral femoral artery and perhaps of the right internal jugular vein). However, there are notable exceptions to this practice during which prophylactic support techniques may be instituted and include: 1) unprotected left main coronary angioplasty; 2) hemodynamic instability; 3) acute ischemia refractory to intravenous medical therapy; 4) stable but marginal hemodynamic profile with relative hypotension and elevated filling pressures; 5) severely reduced left ventricular function; 6) instrumentation of an artery supplying the only viable myocardium, particularly in the setting of poor left ventricular function; and 7) demonstrated hemodynamic compromise during previous revascularization of the same target lesion.

During all high-risk interventional procedures, hemodynamic monitoring with a pacing catheter positioned in the pulmonary artery should be considered. Importantly, prior to instrumenting the coronary artery, this allows arterial blood pressure, filling pressures and heart rate to be optimized with intravenous therapy including administration of fluids, nitroglycerin, pressor agents and lopressor.

Management Postprocedure

In most patients undergoing a high-risk procedure, heparin is continued until the following day when the sheaths are removed. If there is evidence of a dissection or residual thrombus, the sheaths may be removed on half-dose heparin and full-dose heparin resumed 2 hours after sheath removal and continued for a prolonged period (24–72 hours). Patients in whom abrupt closure would result in hemodynamic compromise or collapse should be observed in the interventional unit an additional 24–48 hours after sheath removal, preferably until heparin has been discontinued.

Systemic Support Techniques

During percutaneous coronary intervention, multiple factors determine which systemic support technique should be used in a given patient, but the following guidelines, based on published and anecdotal experience, should be considered. In patients with a left ventricular ejection fraction ≤20%, prophylactic cardiopulmonary bypass may be instituted. If the left ventricular ejection fraction is between 21%–30%, either standby cardiopulmonary bypass or intra-aortic balloon deployment should be instituted. In patients with a left ventricular ejection fraction between 30%–50%, the intra-aortic balloon should be used if the target lesion serves the only viable myocardium. In the setting of hemodynamic instability, either the intra-aortic balloon or cardiopulmonary bypass may be appropriate, considering the contraindications associated with each technique.

Regional Support

Similarly, consideration of specific patient factors as well as the advantages and disadvantages of antegrade and retrograde perfusion determines the optimal regional support technique. In the setting of proximal lesions serving a large territory, use of the perfusion balloon catheter as a primary strategy should be considered. Certainly, when the target lesion serves the only viable myocardium, perfusion balloon angioplasty (perhaps in combination with a systemic support modality) is an attractive strategy. However when vascular access is limited or antegrade access to the artery is lost, synchronized coronary sinus retroperfusion may be helpful.

Conclusion

Certainly, the efficacy of global and regional myocardial support techniques has allowed the expansion of percutaneous revascularization to high-risk patients with high-risk anatomy in whom the risk of death would have previously been considered prohibitive. However, in this situation, a thoughtful periprocedural management strategy is of utmost importance. After consideration of specific support modalities, detailed discussion with the patient, family, and thoracic surgeon, and detailed planning of the technical strategy, percutaneous revascularization can usually be performed safely and with a high rate of success. Therefore, the most difficult question currently is not whether the procedure is feasible, but whether is should be undertaken based on the procedural risk and the anticipated long-term outcome.

References

1. Holmes DR, Holubkov R, Vlietstra, RE, et al. Comparison of complications during percutaneous transluminal coronary angioplasty from 1977 to 1981 and from 1985 to 1986: The National Heart, Lung, and Blood Institute Percutaneous Transluminal Coronary Angioplasty Registry. *J Am Coll Cardiol.* 1988;12:1149–1155.
2. Ellis SG, Roubin GS, King SB III, et al. Angiographic and clinical predictors of acute closure after native vessel coronary angioplasty. *Circulation.* 1988;77:372–379.
3. Bergelson BA, Jacobs AK, Cupples LA, et a: Prediction of risk for hemodynamic compromise during coronary angioplasty. *Am J Cardiol.* 1992;70;1540–1545.
4. Weber KT, Janicki JS. Intra-aortic balloon counterpulsation: a review of physiological principles, clinical results, and device safety. *Ann Thorac Surg.* 1974;17:602–636.
5. Kern MJ. Intra-aortic balloon counterpulsation. *Coronary Artery Dis.* 1991;2:649–660.
6. Kahn JK, Rutherford BD, McConahay DR, et al. Supported "high risk" coronary angioplasty using intraaortic balloon pump counterpulsation. *J Am Coll Cardiol.* 1990;15:1151–1155.
7. Anwar A, Mooney MR, Stertzer SH, et al. Intra-aortic balloon counterpulsation support for elective coronary angioplasty in the setting of poor left ventricular function: a two center experience. *J Invasive Cardiol.* 1990;2:175–180.
8. Suneja R, Hodgson JM. Use of intraaortic balloon counterpulsation for treatment of recurrent acute closure after coronary angioplasty. *Am Heart J.* 1993;125:530–532.
9. Vogel RA. Initial report of the national registry of elective cardiopulmonary bypass supported coronary angioplasty. *J Am Coll Cardiol.* 1990;15:23–29.
10. Tommaso CL, Johnson RA, Stafford JL, et al. Supported coronary angioplasty and standby supported coronary angioplasty for high-risk coronary artery disease. *Am J Cardiol.* 1990;66:1255–1257.
11. Babic UU, Grujicic S, Djurisic Z, Vucinic M. Percutaneous left atrial aortic bypass with a roller pump. *Circulation.* 1989;80(suppl II):II-272 Abstract.
12. Glassman E, Chinitz L, Levite H, et al. Partial left heart bypass support during high-risk angioplasty. *Circulation.* 1989;80(suppl II):II-272 Abstract.
13. Loisance D, Duboise-Rande JL, Deleuze P, et al. Prophylactic intraventricular pumping in high risk coronary angioplasty. *Lancet.* 1990; 335:438–440.
14. Lincoff AM, Popma JJ, Bates ER, et al. Successful coronary angioplasty in two patients with cardiogenic shock using the Nimbus Hemopump support device. *Am Heart J.* 1990;120:970 972.
15. Cambell CA, Rezkalla S, Kloner RA, Turi ZG. The autoperfusion balloon angioplasty catheter limits myocardial ischemia and necrosis during prolonged balloon inflation. *J Am Coll Cardiol.* 1989;14:1045–1050.
16. Quigley PJ, Hinohara T, Phillips HR, et al. Myocardial protection during coronary angioplasty with an autoperfusion balloon catheter in humans. *Circulation.* 1988;78:1128–1134.

17. Leitschuh ML, Mills RM, LaRosa D, et al. Outcome after major dissection during coronary angioplasty using the perfusion balloon catheter. *Am J Cardiol.* 1991;67:1056–1060.
18. Sundram P, Harvey JR, Johnson RG, et al. Benefit of the perfusion catheter for emergency coronary artery grafting after failed percutaneous transluminal coronary angioplasty. *Am J Cardiol.* 1989;63: 282–285.
19. Tomaki H, Simpson JB, Philips HR, Stack RS. Transluminal intracoronary reperfusion catheter: a device to maintain coronary perfusion between failed coronary angioplasty and emergency coronary bypass surgery. *J Am Coll Cardiol.* 1988;11:977–982.
20. Mohl W, Glogar D, Mayr H, et al. Reduction of infarct size induced by intermittent coronary sinus occlusion. *Am J Cardiol.* 1984;53:923–928.
21. Jacobs AK, Faxon DP, Coats WD, et al. Coronary sinus occlusion: effect on ischemic left ventricular dysfunction and reactive hyperemia. *Am Heart J.* 1991;121:442–449.
22. Drury JK, Yamazaki S, Fishbein MC, et al. Synchronized diastolic coronary venous retroperfusion: results of a preclinical safety and efficacy study. *J Am Coll Cardiol.* 1985;2:328–335.
23. Yamazaki S, Drury JK, Meerbaum S, Corday E. Synchronized coronary venous retroperfusion: prompt improvement of left ventricular function in experimental myocardial ischemia. *J Am Coll Cardiol.* 1985; 5:655–663.
24. Wearn JT. The role of the thebesian vessels in the circulation of the heart. *J Exp Med.* 1928;47:293.
25. Kar S, Drury JK, Hajduczki I, et al. Synchronized coronary venous retroperfusion for support and salvage of ischemic myocardium during elective and failed angioplasty. *J Am Coll Cardiol.* 1991;18:271–282.
26. Nanto S, Nishida K, Hirayama A, et al. Supported angioplasty with synchronized retroperfusion in high-risk patients with left main trunk or near left main trunk obstruction. *Am Heart J.* 1993;125:301–309.
27. Incorvati RL, Tauberg SG, Pecora MJ, et al. Clinical applications of coronary sinus retroperfusion during high risk percutaneous transluminal coronary angioplasty. *J Am Coll Cardiol.* 1993;22:127–134.
28. O'Byrne GT, Nienaber CA, Miyazaki A, et al. Positron emission tomography demonstrates that coronary sinus retroperfusion can restore regional myocardial perfusion and preserve metabolism. *J Am Coll Cardiol.* 1991;18:257–270.
29. Chang BL, Drury KJ, Meerbaum S, et al. Enhanced myocardial washout and retrograde blood delivery with synchronized retroperfusion during acute myocardial ischemia. *J Am Coll Cardiol.* 1987;9: 1091–1098.
30. Menasche P, Piwnica A. Cardioplegia by way of the coronary sinus for valvular and coronary surgery. *J Am Coll Cardiol.* 1991;18:628–636.
31. Smalling RW. Percutaneous left ventricular assist. In: Topol EJ, ed. *Textbook of Interventional Cardiology.* Philadelphia, PA:W.B. Saunders; 1994:539–548.
32. Meerbaum S, Lang T, Provhitkov M, et al. Retrograde lysis of coronary artery thrombus by coronary venous streptokinase administration. *J Am Coll Cardiol.* 1983;51:1262–1267.
33. Karagueuzian HS, Ohta M, Drury KJ, et al. Coronary venous retroinfusion of procainamide: a new approach for the management of spon-

taneous and inducible sustained ventricular tachycardia during myocardial infusion. *J Am Coll Cardiol.* 1986;7:551–563.

34. Faxon DP, Jacobs AK, Kellett MA, et al. Coronary sinus occlusion pressure and its relation to intracardiac pressure. *Am J Cardiol.* 1985; 56:457–460.

Chapter 22

Management of Abrupt Closure

Mark Freed, MD and Robert D. Safian, MD

Abrupt Closure: Description of the Problem

Abrupt closure is the most important cause of procedural failure after percutaneous coronary intervention because of its association with patient morbidity and mortality. This chapter reviews the important considerations in the prevention and management of abrupt closure.

Classification of Abrupt Closure

Unfortunately, there are no standard definitions of abrupt closure. At William Beaumont Hospital (Royal Oak, MI), the following definitions are used for the Interventional Cardiology Quality Assurance Database: threatened abrupt closure (class 1): severe luminal narrowing (postintervention diameter stenosis <50%) and dissection, with TIMI flow=3 (Figure 1); Imminent abrupt closure (class 2): subtotal vessel occlusion postintervention, with TIMI flow=2 (Figure 1); and Definite abrupt closure (class 3): functional occlusion (99% stenosis) or total occlusion (100% stenosis) of the target lesion with TIMI flow ≤1 (Figures 2–4). The purpose of this classification is to distinguish frank abrupt closure from other "suboptimal" angioplasty results that are not associated with occlusion of the target lesion.

Given the importance of dissection as a risk factor for abrupt closure, dissections are also characterized angiographically by severity grade (0: no angiographic evidence for dissection; 1: minor intimal flap without luminal narrowing; 2: moderate dissection with luminal narrowing <50%; 3: significant dissection with luminal narrowing >50%; 4: severe dissection with total occlusion

From Vetrovec GW, Carabello BA, (eds.) *Invasive Cardiology: Current Diagnostic and Therapeutic Issues.* Armonk, NY: Futura Publishing Company, Inc.: © 1996.

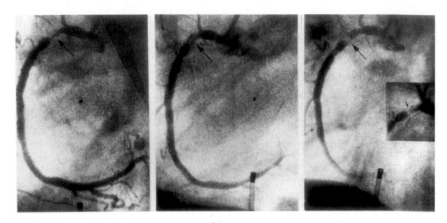

FIGURE 1. Right coronary angiogram demonstrates a focal proximal stenosis (**left panel,** black arrow). After balloon angioplasty (**middle panel**), there was a focal dissection with severe luminal narrowing (black arrow) with normal antegrade flow, consistent with threatened abrupt closure (class 1). Subsequent angiography (**right panel**) revealed progressive luminal narrowing (black arrow) with reduction in antegrade flow, consistent with imminent abrupt closure (class 2). This procedure was performed before the availability of new devices, and refractory abrupt closure was treated by emergency surgery. The morphology and extent of dissection would favor successful salvage by directional atherectomy or stenting. (Courtesy of Donald S. Baim, MD)

[99%–100% stenosis]) and morphology grade (0: no dissection; 1: focal dissection; 2: focal dissection with dye staining; 3: spiral dissection).

Etiology of Abrupt Closure

There are several potential mechanisms of abrupt closure including dissection, thrombus formation, elastic recoil, plaque separation, subintimal hemorrhage, and vasospasm. Unfortunately, contrast coronary angiography has a poor predictive value for distinguishing these mechanisms.[1] These data are supported by a recent angiographic study of abrupt closure, in which the cause of abrupt closure was indeterminate in 45% of cases.[2] Nevertheless, most interventional cardiologists believe that dissection is the major cause of abrupt closure; therefore, the treatment of abrupt closure continues to emphasize the treatment for dissection. These impressions are supported by the lack of utility of vasodilators or

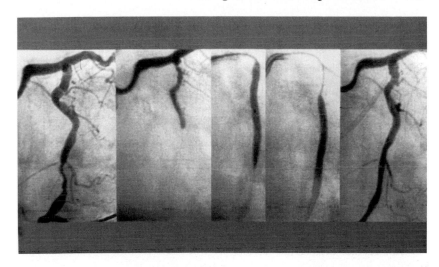

FIGURE 2. *Left coronary angiogram demonstrates a severe stenosis in the distal left circumflex, a large, dominant vessel (**first panel**). After angioplasty, there was class 3 abrupt closure (**second panel**), complicated by cardiogenic shock requiring a temporary pacemaker and an intra-aortic balloon pump. Because of proximal vessel tortuosity, a perfusion balloon catheter would not cross the lesion. A long (40 mm) balloon was inserted and multiple overlapping inflations were performed (**third** and **fourth** panel). Final angiography revealed no residual stenosis or dissection (**fifth panel**). The proximal vessel tortuosity and extent of dissection precluded directional atherectomy, and failure to pass a perfusion balloon catheter strongly suggested that stent delivery would have been unsuccessful.*

thrombolytic therapy alone, and the greater success of treatments that tack-up dissections or excise intimal flaps.

Incidence

The incidence of abrupt closure may vary depending on whether or not patients with threatened or imminent abrupt closure are included. Because abrupt closure is more common in patients with refractory unstable angina and acute myocardial infarction, the incidence of abrupt closure also depends on the characteristics of the study population. Despite these considerations, the incidence of abrupt closure has remained remarkably constant since 1979. In considering recently published series with

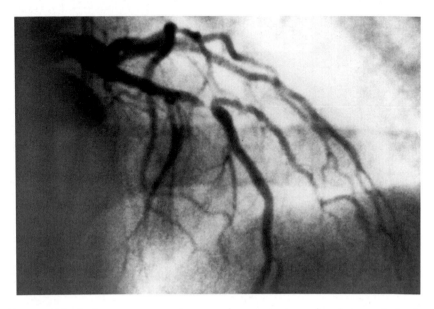

FIGURE 3A. *Left coronary angiogram demonstrates a focal stenosis in the proximal left anterior descending artery.*

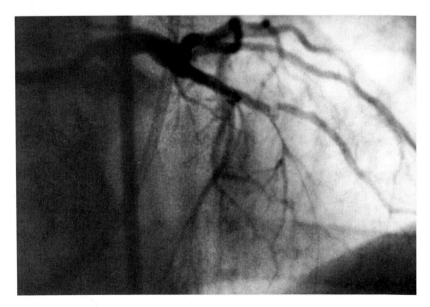

FIGURE 3B. *After angioplasty, there was frank abrupt closure (class 3).*

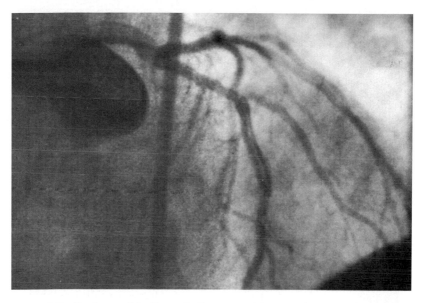

FIGURE 3C. *Prolonged balloon inflations with a perfusion balloon failed to reestablish vessel patency, but laser balloon angioplasty successfully saved the patient from emergency surgery. The residual dissection would lead us to prescribe empiric Coumadin for 6–8 weeks.*

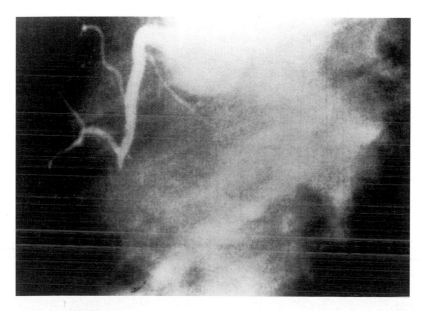

FIGURE 4A. *Right coronary angiogram demonstrates abrupt closure (class 3) after conventional angioplasty.*

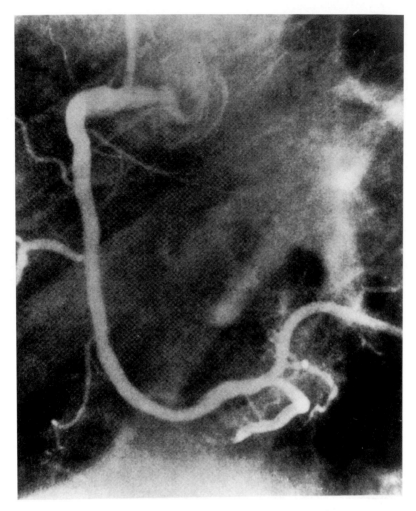

FIGURE 4B. *A single stent was placed, reestablishing normal flow with an excellent angiographic result. (Courtesy of Ulrich Sigwart, MD.)*

more than 500 patients, the overall incidence of abrupt closure was 4.6%, with a range of 2.0%–10.3%.[2-12]

Prevention of Abrupt Closure

Predictors of Abrupt Closure

With prevention as the goal, several studies have described clinical, angiographic, and procedural predictors of abrupt closure.[9,13,14] Using multivariate techniques, independent clinical correlates of abrupt closure include female gender (relative risk ~1.7) and unstable angina (relative risk ~1.6). Angiographic characteristics that seem to be associated with abrupt closure include the presence of multivessel disease (relative risk ~1.6–1.8), diffuse disease (relative risk ~1.8–2.6), intracoronary thrombus (relative risk ~1.7–2.9), bend >45° (relative risk ~2.0), and lesion at a vessel bifurcation (relative risk 1.9). However, the strongest correlates of abrupt closure are procedural variables,[14] including angiographic evidence of dissection (relative risk 2.7–5.2), a final translesional pressure gradient ≥20 mm Hg (relative risk ~4.2), and a final diameter stenosis ≥35% (relative risk ~1.9). Therefore, although certain preprocedural variables identify lesions at increased risk of abrupt closure, the strongest predictors can only be identified after the procedure has been completed. Despite the association of these variables with abrupt closure, PTCA has been performed safely and successfully even in "high-risk" lesions.[15] Furthermore, although differences in the incidence of abrupt closure may be statistically significant, the predictive accuracy is quite low for identifying the likelihood of severe complications in any given patient based on preprocedural characteristics.[16]

Medical Therapy

The development of abrupt closure is unpredictable, and reliable methods for preventing abrupt closure are not currently available. Recent studies indicate that when administered at least 24 hours prior to PTCA, aspirin alone, aspirin plus dipyridamole, and ticlopidine reduce the incidence of acute thrombosis and Q wave myocardial infarction.[17,18] Because of the importance of aspirin in preventing abrupt closure, we recommend deferral of elective interventional procedures in patients who have not received aspirin within 24 hours of the procedure. For urgent procedures in unstable patients, chewable aspirin with or without intravenous Dextran™ (Medisan Pharmaceuticals, Parsippany, NJ) should be considered in patients who have not received aspirin. Although ticlopidine may be a reasonable substitute for aspirin in patients with aspirin allergy, it should be administered for at least 4 days before intervention to achieve its full antiplatelet effect. Preliminary studies suggest a potential role for new thrombin inhibitors (eg, recombinant hirudin or hirulog) and experimental platelet inhibitors (eg, 7E3 antibodies) for decreasing the incidence of abrupt closure and improving the safety of percutaneous interventions.[19]

Technical Considerations

Modifications in the technique of angioplasty have been disappointing for preventing abrupt closure, including rapid versus slow balloon inflation, long versus short inflation time, and compliant versus noncompliant balloon material.[20] The benefits of oscillating versus steady balloon inflations are currently under investigation. The only technical consideration that has been demonstrated to impact on the incidence of abrupt closure is the selection of a properly sized balloon (balloon/artery ratio = 0.9–1.1); use of oversize balloons is associated with a fourfold higher incidence of abrupt closure.[21]

New Devices and Prevention of Abrupt Closure

The impact of new devices in preventing abrupt closure is an unresolved issue. Although one study[10] suggested a lower incidence of abrupt closure after stenting, directional atherectomy, and laser balloon angioplasty (1.8%) compared with PTCA (4.9%), Scott et al[12] reported no difference in the incidence of abrupt closure in the predevice era (4.8%) compared with the postdevice era (4.0%) in a nonrandomized study involving nearly 8,000 patients. Although there were significant decreases in the incidence of myocardial infarction and emergency bypass surgery during the new device era, these favorable results may have been due to increased operator experience, the use of perfusion balloon catheters, prolonged balloon inflations, better awareness of the importance of antiplatelet and anticoagulation therapy, as well as the use of stents and laser balloon angioplasty for salvaging some patients with abrupt closure. In a randomized study of PTCA versus directional atherectomy, there was no difference in the incidence of abrupt closure between the two groups.[22] Furthermore, the NACI Registry reported an abrupt closure rate of 4.3% in nearly 3,000 lesions, which is similar to the incidence of abrupt closure for conventional PTCA.[23] Other studies reported that the incidence of abrupt closure after transluminal extraction atherectomy and Rotablator™ (Heart Technologies, Bellwvue, WA) were 11.0% and 11.2%, respectively,[24,25] which may even be higher than the 2.0%–10.3% observed after PTCA.[2-12] Although stents may be useful for decreasing the incidence of abrupt closure due to dissection,[26] acute and subacute stent thrombosis may result in early vessel occlusion, thus negating some of the benefits of stents. Taken together, these data suggest that although new devices may be useful for reversing abrupt closure, they do not prevent abrupt closure.

Consequences of Abrupt Closure

Timing and Clinical Presentation

The clinical presentation of abrupt closure is usually not subtle. Most cases (75%) occur while the patient is still in the catheterization laboratory, while the remainder occur after the patient leaves the laboratory.[3,5,8,9,10,13] Although delayed abrupt closure has been reported even a week or more after intervention, over 90% of abrupt closures occur within 24 hours of the procedure. Once abrupt closure occurs, the clinical presentation includes chest pain (90%), ST segment elevation (75%), hypotension (16%–20%), ST segment depression (6%–13%), and ventricular fibrillation (0%–10%).[5,9] Circumstances in which abrupt closure may be clinically silent include previous intervention on a recent or chronic total occlusion, or closure of a target vessel that is well collateralized or supplies a small area of viable myocardium.

Early Outcome

Abrupt closure is the most important cause of procedure-related morbidity and mortality after percutaneous intervention. The incidence of hospital death (0%–8.3%), in-hospital bypass surgery (23%–40%), and myocardial infarction (13%–43%) are considerably higher than the incidence of death (1%), bypass surgery (3%), and myocardial infarction (2%) after interventions not resulting in abrupt closure.[2,3,5,8-10,13] Furthermore, data from the NHLBI Registry indicate that even when abrupt closure is successfully treated by repeat PTCA, substantial morbidity and mortality persist, including death (5%), bypass surgery (10%), and myocardial infarction (27%).[13] Although another study also suggested a high incidence of myocardial infarction after successful reversal of abrupt closure, the peak creatine kinase levels were significantly lower compared with patients with unsuccessful reversal of abrupt closure, suggesting smaller non-Q-wave myocardial infarctions in the former group.[8] Ellis et al[7] identified female gender, the presence of multivessel disease, and a target vessel supplying collaterals as independent correlates of mortality after abrupt closure.

Late Outcome

Late cardiovascular events appear to be more frequent in patients who suffer abrupt closure compared with those who do not.[13] In the NHLBI Registry, late events at 2 years included death (4%), myocardial infarction (9%), and late repeat PTCA or bypass surgery (30%).

For patients with abrupt closure successfully treated in the catheterization laboratory, late events at 2 years included death (8%), myocardial infarction (29%), and late revascularization (42%). For patients with abrupt closure who required emergency bypass surgery, late events at 2 years included death (9%), myocardial infarction (60%), and late PTCA (5%). Compared with patients without abrupt closure, those with abrupt closure (successfully treated or not) were found to have significantly higher in-hospital and 2-year mortality. In contrast, differences in the rate of myocardial infarction were no longer significant after hospital discharge.[13] Other studies have corroborated the adverse effects of abrupt closure on clinical outcome.[5,8,9]

In addition to the adverse impact of abrupt closure on clinical events, restenosis rates appear to be higher as well. One angiographic study reported a restenosis of 57% at 12 months after successful reversal of abrupt closure.[27] Clinical restenosis (the need for repeat revascularization by repeat PTCA, another percutaneous device, or bypass surgery) ranged from 24%–40% for successfully treated patients, whereas angina recurred in 15%–17% of patients after unsuccessful treatment for abrupt closure.[5,8,9]

Management of Abrupt Closure

Repeat PTCA

Emergency bypass surgery was originally recommended for all patients with abrupt closure after PTCA, but in 1984, Marquis et al[28] reported the feasibility of immediate repeat PTCA for "salvaging" patients from emergency surgery. Since that time, numerous studies have confirmed the efficacy of repeat balloon inflations (with or without a perfusion balloon catheter) with success rates of 40%–75%.[2,3,5,8–10,13] (Figure 2). In addition to repeat PTCA, several percutaneous devices have shown the ability to reverse abrupt closure (Figures 3 and 4).

Directional Atherectomy

Directional atherectomy was used as a salvage technique for abrupt closure or suboptimal PTCA in 102 lesions, with procedural success (final diameter stenosis ≤50% and no major complication) in 88%.[29] The final incidence of myocardial infarction (6%), bypass surgery (6%), and death (2%) compares favorably with the acute clinical outcome after successful salvage angioplasty (see above). However, directional atherectomy has several important limitations for treating abrupt closure, including its restricted use to relatively large vessels (≥2.5mm), its failure to negotiate proximal vessel tortuosity, and the inability to guide atherectomy cuts. This latter limitation is particularly important because of the potential for unintended deep tissue resection and the risk of coronary perforation. In fact, almost all of the severe coronary artery perforations after directional atherectomy have occurred after salvage atherectomy.

In practice, directional atherectomy may be considered for treatment of abrupt closure if all of the following characteristics are present: vessel diameter ≥2.5 mm, focal dissection (dissection length ≤10 mm), the presence of plaque separation or simple dissection without deep periadventitial dye staining, no obvious spiral dissection, and the presence of other proximal vessel characteristics that favor access to the target lesion (Figure 1). Directional atherectomy should not be used if the extent and length of dissection cannot be determined angiographically. Care should be taken to use properly sized (or slightly undersized) devices at low inflation pressures, and cuts should be directed away from the angiographically apparent normal wall, to minimize the risk of perforation. Further development of flexible housing devices, lower profile catheters, and ultrasound guidance may significantly enhance the use of directional atherectomy for treating abrupt closure. However, with currently available devices, it is unlikely that directional atherectomy will be suited for more than 5%–10% of abrupt closures.

Laser Balloon Angioplasty and Other Thermal Devices

In vitro studies have suggested that the combination of pressure and heat can successfully weld intima-media separations of human atherosclerotic tissue. In fact, this principle was applied to studies of laser balloon angioplasty for reversing abrupt closure after failed PTCA, in which Nd:YAG laser energy was used to heat the arterial wall to 110°C. In a multicenter international study of more than 100 patients with abrupt closure refractory to repeat PTCA, laser balloon angioplasty was able to reverse abrupt closure and avoid the need for emergency bypass surgery in 66% of patients (Figure 3).[30] Several anecdotal reports of removal and desiccation of thrombus suggest that thermal devices may have potential value for treating thrombus. Despite these dramatic acute results, the laser balloon was withdrawn from the market because of the development of restenosis in >70% of cases. The role of other thermal devices awaits further study; issues concerning the ideal tissue temperature for thermal sealing are still unresolved.

Stents

The recent FDA approval of the Cook Flexstent represents the most important therapeutic advance in the mechanical treatment of abrupt closure. Several studies have demonstrated the utility of stents for abrupt closure,[31-38] with rates of successful stent deployment exceeding 90%. Roubin et al[38] published the largest study of 115 patients with abrupt closure, with successful stent deployment in 100%, no instances of acute thrombosis, and subacute thrombosis in 6%. In this high-risk patient subset, the incidence of major complications was remarkably low, including non-Q-wave myocardial infarction (7%), Q wave myocardial infarction (4%), in-hospital bypass surgery (4.2%), and death (1.7%).

The indications for stenting have not been completely established. Although most operators agree with the use of stents for definite or imminent abrupt closure (class 2 and 3) (Figure 4), the use of stents for threatened abrupt closure (class 1) is more controversial. Lincoff et al[39] reported no differences in mortality or Q wave myocardial infarction between stented and unstented patients, but the incidence of emergency bypass surgery and non-Q-wave myocardial infarction was two- to fourfold higher in patients who did not receive a stent. However, no benefit was observed between stented and unstented patients for threatened abrupt closure.

There are several important limitations of stents for abrupt closure, including their limited role in small vessels (<2.5mm), the need for meticulous anticoagulation with the attendant risks of stent thrombosis and bleeding, and the requirement for a permanent metal implant. Future development of synthetic-polymer coated stents, biostable and biodegradable stents, and stents capable of drug delivery will very likely have a significant impact on expanding the use of stents for a variety of different indications, including abrupt closure.

Temporary Stents

Temporary stents are under investigation for treating dissections and abrupt closure. These devices may be useful for prolonged stenting of dissections without the need for a permanent implant. Temporary stents may be superior to perfusion balloon catheters for improving antegrade blood flow, ameliorating chest pain and ECG changes, and preserving flow to sidebranches. One such device (the Flow Support catheter) was recently withdrawn from the market, and another (HARTS, or heat-activated removable temporary stent), which applies heat and pressure to the arterial wall, has not yet entered large scale clinical evaluation.

Bailout Catheter

Placement of a bailout perfusion catheter is strongly recommended for refractory abrupt closure, improving blood flow to the distal vascular bed during preparation for emergency bypass surgery. Virtually any suitable infusion catheter with an endhole and multiple sideholes (including a perfusion balloon catheter) can be used for this purpose. Studies have confirmed a lower incidence of myocardial infarction and smaller peak creatine kinase elevations in patients who received a bailout catheter compared with those who received an intra-aortic balloon pump alone in preparation for emergency surgery.[10] If a bailout catheter cannot be inserted, the guide wire may be left in place (this alone may "stent" the vessel and allow some antegrade flow) and an intra-aortic balloon pump should be inserted.

Which Device for Abrupt Closure?

Unfortunately, there are no studies that directly compare all devices and treatment strategies for abrupt closure. In one study, the success rates for reversing abrupt closure were 48% for prolonged balloon inflations (balloon inflations ≥2 minutes), 78% for stenting, and 100% for directional atherectomy.[2] In contrast, the success rates for thrombolytic therapy alone was 0%, and for short-duration (<2 minutes) balloon inflations was only 5%. Independent correlates of successful reversal of abrupt closure were prolonged balloon inflations >2 minutes (odds ratio 5.11, *P*<0.001) and stenting (odds ratio 4.37, *P*<0.05). This study was limited by the small number of patients, and further studies are clearly needed to address this important question.

Adjunctive Treatments

Adjunctive measures for the treatment of abrupt closure include drug therapies, support devices, and technical adjuncts. Adjunctive drug therapy includes nitroglycerin, thrombolytic therapy, antiplatelet drugs, and calcium antagonists. Although pure coronary vasospasm is an unusual cause of abrupt closure after PTCA, it may be an important contributing factor after high-speed mechanical rotational atherectomy with the Rotablator. Routine use of intracoronary nitroglycerin (0.1–0.2 mg) is recommended in virtually all cases of abrupt closure to reverse any vasospasm that may be present.

Although thrombolytic agents are effective for acute myocardial infarction, their use in abrupt closure is less clearly established because of the difficulty in reliably identifying thrombus,[1] and since thrombolytic agents are usually used in conjunction with repeat PTCA.[40] However, since intracoronary thrombus may play an important role in patients with acute myocardial infarction, refractory unstable angina, or subtotal stenoses in saphenous vein bypass grafts, intracoronary Urokinase (250,000–500,000 U) or tPA (20 mg) may be a useful adjunct to repeat PTCA or other devices for abrupt closure associated with these clinical situations. However, it is unlikely that thrombolytic therapy alone will have a significant impact.

Apart from aspirin, which is routinely prescribed before PTCA, the antiplatelet agent most commonly used for abrupt closure is low molecular weight Dextran. Although anecdotal reports suggest some efficacy, there are no studies to confirm the utility of Dextran in this setting. Intracoronary calcium channel blockers may be useful in some patients with no-reflow, but their role in abrupt closure is unknown.

Support devices include the intra-aortic balloon pump and percutaneous cardiopulmonary bypass. Possible indications for balloon pumping in the setting of persistent abrupt closure include hemodynamic lability, need for redo bypass operation, failure to place a "bailout" perfusion catheter, final TIMI flow <3, and any final suboptimal angiographic result in a patient who is not a candidate for immediate bypass surgery. The routine use of intra-aortic balloon pumps after successful reversal of abrupt closure is controversial, although some preliminary studies suggest benefit. Percutaneous cardiopulmonary bypass should be considered in patients with cardiovascular collapse from any cause, but prompt surgical intervention is required to minimize myocardial injury. Technical modifications, such as overnight perfusion balloon inflations and/or infusions, have not been adequately tested, but some anecdotal reports suggest potential benefit.

Treatment Algorithm for Abrupt Closure

There is no widely accepted uniform method for treating abrupt closure. The approach currently used at William Beaumont Hospital is as follows (Figure 5):

For established or imminent abrupt closure (class 2 or 3), patients are immediately treated with intracoronary nitroglycerin, and additional heparin is administered to achieve an anticoagulation time (ACT) >300 seconds. The vessel is redilated for at least 5 minutes with a balloon matched to the diameter of the reference segment (balloon/artery ratio=0.9–1.1). For long, spiral dissections or dissections involving angulated segments of the vessel, a long (40-mm) balloon works well (Figure 2). For vessels supplying large territories, especially with hemodynamic compromise, a perfusion balloon catheter is preferred. Although slightly oversize balloons (balloon/artery ratio ~1.3) have reversed some abrupt closures, we have found this technique to be unpredictable because it may stabilize or extend the dissection. For this reason, oversize balloons are not routinely used, especially considering the availability of other more predictable methods for reversing abrupt closure.

If the vessel remains patent for at least 10 minutes and the lumen is stable, we generally prescribe an overnight infusion of heparin (maintain ACT ~200 seconds) with sheath removal the following morning. For persistent dissections with an adequate lumen (<50% stenosis), we empirically prescribe oral Coumadin™ (DuPont Pharma, Wilmington, DE) (international normalized ratio [INR] ~3.0–4.0) or subcutaneous heparin (10,000 U twice a day) for 6–8 weeks, in addition to aspirin (Figure 3).

If the angiogram suggests residual thrombus after prolonged balloon inflation, intracoronary urokinase is administered (250,000–500,000 U), with or without low molecular weight Dextran-40 (200-cc bolus and 30 cc/hour for 10 hours). If the vessel remains patent, the same guidelines are followed for overnight heparin and conversion to either oral Coumadin or subcutaneous heparin, as above.

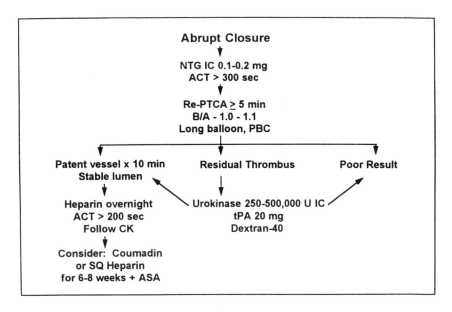

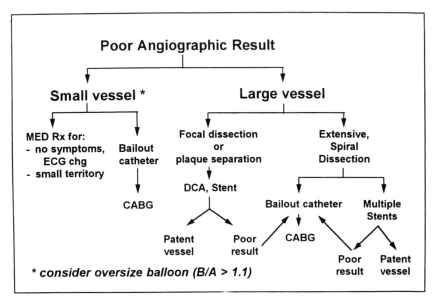

FIGURE 5. *A* and *B. Suggested algorithm for treatment of abrupt closure. NTG indicates nitroglycerin; IC: intracoronary; ACT: activated clotting time; PTCA: percutaneous transluminal coronary angioplasty; B/A: balloon/artery ratio; CK: creatine kinase; tPA: tissue plasminogen activator; U: units; SQ: subcutaneous; MED: medical; Rx: treatment; ECG: electrocardiogram; CABG: coronary artery bypass graft surgery; DCA: directional coronary atherectomy.*

If an unsatisfactory angiographic result is obtained after prolonged balloon inflations and the vessel is small (<2.3 mm), it will usually be redilated with an oversize balloon (balloon/artery ratio = 1.1–1.3 at low pressure for 10–20 minutes), and if a stable angiographic result is obtained, the treatment guidelines described above will be followed. If an unsatisfactory result persists, a bailout catheter will be inserted and the patient will be sent to emergency surgery. For patients with refractory abrupt closure in small vessels who experience no symptoms or ECG changes, or in whom there is only a small area of viable myocardium, medical therapy without bypass surgery will be strongly considered.

If an unsatisfactory result is obtained after prolonged balloon inflations in a large vessel, directional atherectomy or stenting will be considered (Figures 1, 3, and 4). The choice of atherectomy or stenting will depend on the experience of the operator, the depth of periadventitial dye staining, and the patient's ability to tolerate oral Coumadin. For experienced operators, directional atherectomy may be preferred for focal dissections without periadventitial contrast staining (Figure 1), since prolonged hospitalization and oral anticoagulation may be avoided. For less experienced operators, vessels with significant disruption of the vessel wall, or long spiral dissections, stenting (with one or more stents) should be performed immediately. For persistent abrupt closure, a bailout catheter should be inserted followed by immediate bypass surgery.

Conclusion

Abrupt closure is an important cause of procedure-related morbidity and mortality. Patient characteristics and lesion morphology have limited predictive value, and thus, abrupt closure remains largely unpredictable. The use of aspirin and selection of a properly sized balloon are effective in reducing the incidence of abrupt closure, but other technical aspects of the angioplasty procedure have limited utility for preventing abrupt closure. Although the availability of new interventional devices has not yet decreased the incidence of abrupt closure, directional atherectomy and stents are useful for treating many cases of abrupt closure refractory to prolonged balloon inflations, and may be useful for avoiding emergency surgery and decreasing patient morbidity. Future developments, such as new platelet and thrombin inhibitors, thermal devices, biodegradable stents, and vehicles for drug delivery, may have further impact on the prevention and management of abrupt closure.

References

1. White CJ, Ramee SR, Collins TJ, et al. Percutaneous coronary angioscopy: Application in interventional cardiology. *J Interven Cardiol.* 1993;6:61–67.
2. Lincoff AM, Popma JJ, Ellis SG, et al. Abrupt vessel closure complicating coronary angioplasty: clinical, angiographic, and therapeutic profile. *J Am Coll Cardiol.* 1992;19:926–935.
3. Hollman J, Gruentzig AR, Douglas JS Jr, et al. Acute occlusion after percutaneous transluminal coronary angioplasty—a new approach. *Circulation.* 1983;68:725–732.
4. Cowley MJ, Dorros G, Kelsey SF, et al. Acute coronary events associated with percutaneous transluminal coronary angioplasty. *Am J Cardiol.* 1984;53:12C–16C.
5. Simpfendorfer C, Belardi J, Bellamy G, et al. Frequency, management and follow-up of patients with acute coronary occlusions after percutaneous transluminal coronary angioplasty. *Am J Cardiol.* 1987;59:267–269.
6. Meyerovitz MF, Friedman RL, Ganz P, et al. Acute occlusion developing during or immediately after percutaneous transluminal coronary angioplasty: nonsurgical treatment. *Radiology.* 1988;169:491–494.
7. Ellis SG, Roubin GS, King SB III, et al. In-hospital cardiac mortality after acute closure after coronary angioplasty: analysis of risk factors from 8207 procedures. *J Am Coll Cardiol.* 1988;11:211–216.
8. Sinclair IN, McCabe CH, Sipperly ME, et al. Predictors, therapeutic options and long-term outcome of abrupt reclosure. *Am J Cardiol.* 1988;61:61G–66G.
9. de Feyter PF, van den Brand M, Jaarman GJ, et al. Acute coronary artery occlusion during and after percutaneous transluminal coronary angioplasty: frequency, prediction, clinical course, management, and follow-up. *Circulation.* 1991;83:927–936.
10. Kuntz RE, Piana R, Pomerantz RM, et al. Changing incidence and management of abrupt closure following coronary intervention in the new device era. *Cathet Cardiovasc Diagn.* 1992;27:183–190.
11. Tenaglia AN, Fortin DF, Frid DJ, et al. Long-term outcome following successful reopening of abrupt closure after coronary angioplasty. *Am J Cardiol.* 1993;72:21–25.
12. Scott NA, Weintraub WS, Carlin SF, et al. Recent changes in the management and outcome of acute closure after percutaneous transluminal coronary angioplasty. *Am J Cardiol.* 1993;71:1159–1163.
13. Detre KM, Holmes DR Jr, Holubkov R, et al. Incidence and consequences of periprocedural occlusion: The 1985–1986 National, Heart, Lung, and Blood Institute Percutaneous Transluminal Coronary Angioplasty Registry. *Circulation.* 1990;82:739–750.
14. Ellis SG, Roubin GS, King SB III, et al. Angiographic and clinical predictors of acute closure after native vessel coronary angioplasty. *Circulation.* 1988;77:373–379.
15. Myler RK, Shaw RE, Stertzer SH, et al. Lesion morphology and coronary angioplasty: Current experience and analysis. *J Am Coll Cardiol.* 1992;19:1641–1652.
16. Bergelson BA, Jacobs AK, Cupples LA, et al. Prediction of risk for he-

modynamic compromise during percutaneous transluminal coronary angioplasty. *Am J Cardiol.* 1992;70:1540–1545.

17. Barnathan ES, Schwartz JS, Taylor L, et al. Aspirin and dipyridamole in the prevention of acute thrombosis complicating coronary angioplasty. *Circulation.* 1987;76:125–134.

18. White CW, Chaitman B, Lassar TA, et al. Antiplatelet agents are effective in reducing the immediate complications of PTCA: report from the ticlopidine multicenter trial. *Circulation.* 1987;76(Suppl IV):IV-400. Abstract.

19. Topol EJ, Bonan R, Jewitt D, et al. Use of a direct antithrombin, hirulog, in place of heparin during coronary angioplasty. *Circulation.* 1993; 87:1622–1629.

20. Bach RG, Kern MJ, Aguirre FV, et al. Effects of percutaneous transluminal coronary angioplasty balloon compliance on angiographic and clinical outcomes. *Am J Cardiol.* 1993;72:904–907.

21. Roubin GS, Douglas JS Jr, King SB III, et al. Influence of balloon size on initial success, acute complications, and restenosis after percutaneous transluminal coronary angioplasty: a prospective randomized study. *Circulation.* 1988;78:557–565.

22. Topol EJ, Leya F, Pinkerton CA, et al. Comparison of directional atherectomy with coronary angioplasty in patients with coronary artery disease. *N Engl J Med.* 1993;329:221–227.

23. Safian RD, Lai SM, Buchbinder M, et al. Incidence and Management of Abrupt Closure After New Device Interventions: Report From the NACI Registry in 2988 Lesions. *Circulation.* 1993;88(Suppl I):I-585. Abstract.

24. Safian RD, May MA, Lichtenberg A, et al. Detailed clinical and angiographic analysis of transluminal extraction coronary atherectomy for complex lesions in native coronary arteries. *J Am Coll Cardiol.* 1995; 25:848–854.

25. Safian RD, Niazi KA, Strzelecki M, et al. Detailed angiographic analysis of high-speed mechanical rotational atherectomy in human coronary arteries. *Circulation.* 1993;88:961–968.

26. Schatz RA, Penn IM, Baim DS, et al. Stent restenosis study (STRESS): analysis of in-hospital results. *Circulation.* 1993;88(Suppl I):I-594. Abstract.

27. Ba'albaki HA, Weintraub WS, Tao X, et al. Restenosis after acute closure and successful reopening: implications for new devices. *Circulation.* 1990;82(Suppl III):III-314. Abstract.

28. Marquis JF, Schwartz L, Aldridge H, et al. Acute coronary artery occlusion during percutaneous transluminal coronary angioplasty treated by redilation of the occluded segment. *J Am Coll Cardiol.* 1984; 4:1268–1271.

29. McCluskey ER, Cowley M, Whitlow PL. Multicenter clinical experience with rescue atherectomy for failed angioplasty. *Am J Cardiol.* 1993;72:42E–50E.

30. Safian RD, Reis GJ, Jenkins RD, et al. Failed PTCA: salvage by laser balloon angioplasty. *Circulation.* 1990;82(Suppl III):III-673. Abstract.

31. Sigwart U, Urban P, Golf S, et al. Emergency stenting for acute occlusion after coronary balloon angioplasty. *Circulation.* 1988;78:1121–1127.

32. Goy JJ, Sigwart U, Vogt P, et al. Long-term clinical and angiographic

follow-up of patients treated with the self-expanding coronary stent for acute occlusion during balloon angioplasty of the right coronary artery. *J Am Coll Cardiol.* 1992;19:1593–1596.

33. de Feyter PJ, DeScheerder I, van den Brand M, et al. Emergency stenting for refractory acute coronary artery occlusion during coronary angioplasty. *Am J Cardiol.* 1990;66:1147–1150.

34. Burger W, Sievert H, Steinmann J, et al. Acute and mid-term experience with the Wiktor stent in acute complications and restenosis after coronary angioplasty. *J Interven Cardiol.* 1992;5:147–157.

35. Reifart N, Langer A, Storger H, et al. Strecker stent as a bailout device following percutaneous transluminal coronary angioplasty. *J Interven Cardiol.* 1992;5:79–83.

36. Haude M, Erbel R, Straub U, et al. Results of intracoronary stents for management of coronary dissection after balloon angioplasty. *Am J Cardiol.* 1991;67:691–696.

37. Kiemeneij F, Laarman GJ, van der Wieken R, et al. Emergency coronary stenting with the Palmaz-Schatz stent for failed transluminal coronary angioplasty: results of a learning phase. *Am Heart J.* 1993; 126:23–31.

38. Roubin GS, Cannon AD, Agrawal SK, et al. Intracoronary stenting for acute and threatened closure complicating percutaneous transluminal coronary angioplasty. *Circulation.* 1992;85:916–927.

39. Lincoff AM, Topol EJ, Chapekis AT, et al. Intracoronary stenting compared with conventional therapy for abrupt vessel closure complicating coronary angioplasty: a matched case-control study. *J Am Coll Cardiol.* 1993;21:866–875.

40. Schieman G, Cohen BM, Kozina J, et al. Intracoronary urokinase for intracoronary thrombus accumulation complicating percutaneous transluminal coronary angioplasty in acute ischemic syndromes. *Circulation.* 1990;82:2052–2060.

Chapter 23

Management of Cardiogenic Shock

Carl L. Tommaso, MD

Since the onset of the coronary care era, little progress has been made in the treatment of cardiogenic shock (CS). Previously, the diagnosis of CS was made based only on bedside parameters of low blood pressure, decreased urine output, and the presence of pulmonary congestion. In the early 1970s, with the advent of the pulmonary artery catheter, the diagnosis of CS could be made based on hemodynamic parameters, and several subsets of patients could be defined, namely, those with hypoperfusion with low filling pressures, patients with right ventricular infarctions, and those with other mechanical complications of myocardial infarction. The only treatment for CS was the use of vasopressor agents. The development of inotropic drugs with little vasoconstrictor actions, the use of vasodilators, and the use of the intra-aortic balloon pump became popular, but the mortality rate was essentially unchanged despite the intensive efforts to manage these patients with these therapies. Recently, the use of thrombolytic agents and coronary revascularization via interventional techniques has appeared and altered the frequency and mortality from CS.

Definition

CS is the development of state of hypoperfusion due to cardiac dysfunction (Table 1).[1] Most commonly, it develops because of dysfunction of the contractile function of the left ventricle as a result of significant damage to the left ventricle either by a single insult or as a result of multiple infarctions. It is recognized that when 40% or more of the left ventricle is irreversibly damaged, CS will occur.[2] Common clinical situations where shock occurs include the presence of multiple myocardial infarctions, multivessel coronary dis-

From Vetrovec GW, Carabello BA, (eds.) *Invasive Cardiology: Current Diagnostic and Therapeutic Issues.* Armonk, NY: Futura Publishing Company, Inc.: © 1996.

Table 1

Definition of Cardiogenic Shock by Clinical and Hemodynamic Criteria

Clinical	Hemodynmic
Poor perfusion	CO <2.2 L/m/m^2
Pulmonary congestion	PCW >18 mm Hg
Systolic BP <90 mm Hg	Systolic BP <80 mm Hg
Pulmonary edema	Urine <20 mL/hr
	PCW >12 mm Hg
	CVP >10 cm

ease, and occlusion of the proximal left anterior descending artery and the presence of a new left bundle branch block by ECG in conjunction with an infarction signaling the involvement of a large amount of myocardium. Although left ventricular pump dysfunction is the major cause of CS, mechanical complications of myocardial infarction such as ventricular septal defect, mitral valve dysfunction, ventricular rupture, or right ventricular infarction can cause CS.

Most commonly, CS is caused by myocardial infarction (Table 2), although rarely, other causes such as cardiac tamponade, aortic stenosis, primary mitral regurgitation, and overdose of negative inotropic drugs (barbiturates, calcium channel blockers, or β blockers) can cause CS.

Table 2

Causes of Cardiogenic Shock*

- Myocardial Infarction
- Complications of myocardial infarction
     Ventricular septal defect
     Papillary muscle dysfunction
     Right ventricular infarction
     Free wall rupture
- Aortic valve disease
- Mitral valve disease
- Overdose of negative ionotropic drugs
     β blockers
     Ca^{++} channel blockers
     Barbiturates
     Etc.

*Myocardial infarction is the most common cause.

The clinical recognition of CS is based on the usual parameters, evidence of poor perfusion noted by low blood pressure, cool extremities, reduced sensorium, reduced urine output, and the presence of evidence of pulmonary vascular congestion by examination or chest x-ray. Although many patients with myocardial infarction will manifest CS at or shortly after presenting at the hospital, most patients who develop it will do so 1 to 6 days after admission. In addition to the variable time on onset, there appears to be two subgroups of patients who develop CS (personal observation). One group includes those patients who develop a sudden change in clinical status, deteriorate rapidly, and often die within 60–90 minutes. Many of these patients probably represent sudden reocclusion of primary reperfused infarct related arteries. The other group includes those who develop increasing congestive heart failure and reduction in blood pressure over a period of hours.

Hemodynamically, the diagnosis of CS has been made by the use of the Swan-Ganz balloon flotation catheter. The combination of decreased perfusion as noted by a reduced cardiac output (<2.2 L/min/m^2) in the presence of high (or at least adequate) filling pressures (>18 mm Hg) is the commonly used hemodynamic definition.[3] O'Neill[4] suggests the use of the definition used in the 1973 multicenter intra-aortic balloon pump trial,[5] which is: 1) systolic arterial pressure <80 mm Hg intra-arterially; 2) urine output <20 mL/h; 3) left ventricular filling pressure >12 mm Hg and central venous pressure (CVP) >10 cm H$_2$O.

The use of the Swan-Ganz catheter has also allowed the recognition of the mechanical complications of myocardial infarction, right ventricular infarction, ventricular septal defect, papillary muscle dysfunction or rupture, and free wall rupture, to be differentiated from CS caused by left ventricular myocardial dysfunction.

Incidence and Outcome

The incidence of CS complicating myocardial infarction is usually reported as 5% to 15% (Table 3). The earliest reported series of patients with CS was in 1954, when Griffith et al[6] reported an 80% mortality rate for patients with CS after myocardial infarction. In 1978, Mirowski et al[7] reported on 1,246 patients admitted to a coronary care unit. They reported a 12% incidence of CS with a mortality rate of 87% in this patient group. In patients studied from 1965–1969, Scheidt et al[8] reported a 15% incidence of CS in pa-

Table 3

Incidence and Mortality of Cardiogenic Shock

Author (ref)	Incidence (%)	Mortality (%)
Conventional Therapy		
Griffith[7]	NA	80
Mirowski[8]	12	87
Killip[11]*	10	81
Gunnar[10]	NA	93
Goldberg[17]	7.5	78
IABP		
Scheidt[9]	15	86
Thrombolytics		
GISSI[18]*	NA	70
GUSTO[16]	8	NA
Kennedy[39]	NA	67
Angioplasty		
O'Neill[44]	NA	27
CABG		
Bolooki[45]	NA	34

Cardiogenic shock recorded on admission. NA, data not available. References 44 and 45 are pooled data. IABP: intra-aortic balloon pump; CABG: coronary artery bypasss graft surgery.

tients who presented with a myocardial infarction. The mortality rate in this group was 86%. Other studies reporting the mortality rate of patients with CS show that 80%–93% of patients with CS complicating myocardial infarction will die in-hospital.[9]

The cause of death in CS is reduced myocardial perfusion causing hemodynamic derangements, which cause cardiac and systemic metabolic derangements, leading to further reduction in myocardial perfusion and repeated hemodynamic derangements, leading to a downward spiral that results in poor tissue perfusion, acidosis, hypoxia, and death (Table 3).

Killip[10] was the first to document the mortality of a myocardial infarction related to the clinically determined hemodynamic status of patients. He noted four classes: class I patients had a normal physical examination and a mortality of 6%; class II patients had minimal rales and a mortality of 17%; class III patients had pulmonary edema with a normal blood pressure and a mortality of 38%; and class IV patients had CS, systolic blood pressure ≤90 mm Hg and a mortality of 81%.

In the study by Hands et al,[11] multivariate analysis indicated that independent predictors for in-hospital development of CS were age >65 years, left ventricular ejection fraction on hospital admission <35%, large infarct as estimated from serial enzyme determinations, history of diabetes mellitus, and previous myocardial infarction. It was noted in the same study that the increased frequency of these predictors was associated with a higher probability of developing CS. Patients with three, four, or five of these risk factors had a 17.9%, 33.7%, or 54.4% probability, respectively, of developing CS after hospital admission.

Bengtson et al[12] studied the Duke experience with CS. Variables with significant univariate association with in-hospital death, included patency of the infarct-related artery, patient age, lowest cardiac index, highest arteriovenous oxygen difference, and left main coronary artery disease. The most important independent predictors of in-hospital death were patency of the infarct-related artery, cardiac index, and peak creatine kinase-MB fraction. The mortality rate in patients with patent infarct-related arteries was 33% versus 75% in those with closed arteries and 84% in those in whom arterial patency was unknown. Patients who survived to hospital discharge were followed up for a median of 2 years, with a mortality rate of 18% after 1 year. These data suggest that the single parameter that can be altered and have an impact on the outcome is the patency of the infarct-related artery.

The 1980s ushered in the era of thrombolytic therapy and it is now important to note how the use of thrombolytics affects the likelihood of developing CS and the role of thrombolytics in patients with established CS. Mortality from myocardial infarction is due to a number of causes including CS, however, CS is the predominant cause of death. In our institution, over the last 5 years CS due to left ventricular dysfunction is responsible for 85% of the infarct mortality, with dysrhythmia causing 5%, RV infarction causing 5%, and other mechanical complications including wall rupture causing 5% (personal observation). Therefore, most of the mortality reduction found in the thrombolytic trials is due to the reduction of the incidence of CS.

The ISAM Study Group[13] found a reduction in infarct-related mortality from the use of streptokinase versus placebo in patients with myocardial infarction. The reduced mortality rate was due predominantly to the lower incidence of CS in the patients who had received streptokinase. They measured a 27% reduction of the incidence of CS.

The recently reported results of the GUSTO trial[14] documented the incidence of CS in patients receiving a lytic agent. In this trial, only 8% of patients (all of whom had received thrombolytic therapy) developed Killip class IV heart failure.

Goldberg et al,[15] however, described the trend of developing

CS from the prethrombolytic era into the thrombolytic era, 1975–1988. The incidence of CS complicating acute myocardial infarction remained relatively constant, averaging 7.5%. Although the patients who developed shock were much less likely to have received thrombolytic therapy than those who did not, the incidence of the use of thrombolytic therapy was small.

The GISSI Trial[16] demonstrated that patients admitted with Killip class III had a 30% mortality and patients admitted with class IV had a 70% mortality, and unlike patients in Killip class I or II where the benefit was great, there was no benefit from intravenous thrombolytic therapy.

Although there are anecdotal reports of the use of intravenous lytic agents reversing CS,[17] the above data from the large clinical thrombolytic trials suggest that the administration of thrombolytics to patients in severe heart failure or CS does not benefit these patients. Lower reperfusion rates, higher reocclusion rates, associated mechanical complications, or complete infarction are some possible explanations for the failure of thrombolytics in these patients.[18,19] Therefore, the significant lowering of overall mortality with the use of thrombolytics indicates that the risk of development of CS may be reduced by the use of these agents. However, in patients who either have CS at the time of presentation or develop CS during their hospitalization, thrombolytics do not alter the mortality.

Recent data have documented that primary angioplasty for the treatment of acute myocardial infarction has a better prognosis than the use of thrombolytics, however, none of the studies document a reduced incidence of CS.[20-22] However, since thrombolytics do not appear to alter the outcome in patients at high risk for the development of CS, immediate angioplasty should be considered in patients with advanced age, anterior infarction, or other indicators of high-risk infarction.[23]

Treatment

Pharmacologic Therapy

The earliest treatment for CS was the inotropic adrenergic agonist catecholamines, epinephrine and norepinephrine. Although these drugs were successful in elevating blood pressure, the marked vasoconstriction caused by them and the negative effect on myocardial oxygen demand may have caused more deleterious effects than beneficial ones.[24] They are rarely used as first-line agents now, and their use in the management of the patient with CS after myocardial infarction is limited to the severely refractory hypotensive patient.

Other inotropic drugs, particularly dopamine and dobutamine were developed, and had less effect on systemic vascular resistance. Holzer et al[25] documented an increase in urine output, a decrease in left ventricular filling pressures, a decrease in heart rate, and an increase in blood pressure in survivors of CS treated with dopamine. In a small number of patients, Ruiz et al[26] demonstrated that a response to dopamine infusion, increased blood pressure, cardiac index, and urine output separated survivors from nonsurvivors, suggesting that a response to dopamine is of prognostic value. Similarly, it has been demonstrated that the response to dobutamine also determined prognosis as reported by Tan and Littler.[27] Francis et al[28] compared the hemodynamic effects of dopamine and dobutamine and found both agents caused an increase in cardiac index, stroke work index, and a decrease in systemic vascular resistance in lower doses. At higher doses, dopamine caused a significantly higher systolic blood pressure and left ventricular filling pressure. The combination of dopamine and dobutamine was noted to have a synergistic effect. When combined, a significant increase in arterial pressure occurs; however, when dobutamine is combined with dopamine, the left ventricular filling pressure is reduced.[29]

Some investigators have demonstrated adverse effects of high-dose dobutamine. Moulopoulos et al[30] reported a protracted high-dose administration of dobutamine may adversely affect the survival of patients with postmyocardial infarction CS.

Other selective β_2-agonists such as salbutamol have also been investigated in CS. Salbutamol appears to have similar effects to dopamine,[31] although some investigators have demonstrated a significant increase in cardiac index without increasing arterial pressure.[32] Amrinone and milrinone have been used in the treatment of CS. In a study of patients with severe heart failure and CS after myocardial infaction, milrinone caused the cardiac index to increase by 106% after 30 minutes. Pulmonary capillary wedge pressure decreased after 30 minutes and the heart rate showed an overall tendency to decrease. The systolic blood pressure tended to increase.[33]

In order to counter the increase in systemic vascular resistance and increase in left ventricular filling pressures seen with the adrenergic agonists and to improve left ventricular emptying, many investigators have evaluated the use of vasodilators in combination with the inotropic agents. The most commonly used agents are nitroglycerin and nitroprusside.[34] When added to dopamine, nitroprusside causes an improvement in left ventricular filling pressure, an increase in cardiac index, and a decrease in systemic pressure.

McGhie and Golstein[35] reported on the use of pharmacologic agents in the treatment of CS. They classified patients into three groups: 1) patients with a high left ventricular filling pressure (>18 mm Hg) and a cardiac index <2.2 L/min/m², but systolic arterial pressure >100 mm Hg; 2) patients with a systolic arterial pressure <90 mm Hg, left ventricular filling pressure >18 mm Hg, and cardiac index <2.2 L/min/m²; and 3) patients with an elevated right ventricular filling pressure (>10 mm Hg) and cardiac index <2.2 L/min/m² and a systolic arterial pressure <100 mm Hg. Patients in the first subset usually require the use of vasodilator therapy and/or dobutamine. The choice of inotropic agent in patients in the second hemodynamic subset depends on the degree of systemic hypotension; dopamine is usually preferred initially because it increases arterial pressure in addition to improving cardiac output. Once the systemic blood pressure has been stabilized, dobutamine can be substituted for superior augmentation of cardiac output and its additional beneficial effects on the left ventricular filling pressure. Norepinephrine may be indicated in cases of severe systemic hypotension. Patients in hemodynamic subset 3, ie, right ventricular infarction, are treated with volume expansion and dobutamine.

Despite the improvement in hemodynamics, pharmacologic therapy does not appear to affect survival, therefore, survival rates remain low. However, the use of pharmacologic therapy in conjunction with the the early use of hemodynamic monitoring may determine outcome or predict the need for heroic therapies such as transplantation or suggest significant degrees of cardiac reserve so that revascularization can be predicted as successful.

Intra-aortic Balloon Pump and Other Mechanical Support Devices

The intra-aortic balloon pump (IABP) was developed in the 1960s and has been used extensively for patients with CS.[36,37] Because of the reduction in afterload and the presence of diastolic augmentation of coronary flow in nonseverely stenotic vessels, IABP is well suited to the treatment of patients in CS. Most patients can be hemodynamically stabilized by the use of IABP,[37] however, as demonstrated by Scheidt et al[6] the mortality of patients in CS treated with IABP remained in excess of 80%, which was unchanged from pre-IABP studies. Therefore, although IABP is excellent for stabilizing patients in CS, it does not affect mortality and should therefore, be considered only a temporizing measure until more definitive therapy can be instituted.

In addition to IABP (Table 4), there are several other devices that have been used in patients in CS to stabilize them and allow catheterization, angioplasty, or cardiac surgery to be performed. Gacioh et al[38] reported the University of Michigan experience with the use of IABP, Hemopump,[39] percutaneous cardiopulmonary bypass, and a ventricular assist device for adjunctive use in patients with CS undergoing invasive procedures. Although their numbers were not large enough to compare these technologies, it appears that patients who underwent a successful procedure had a significantly improved survival, and that each of these technologies contributed to enabling at least temporary stabilization that allowed a procedure to be performed. Shawl et al[40] reported on eight patients in profound CS, including two in full cardiac arrest, in whom percutaneous cardiopulmonary bypass and angioplasty were performed. Seven patients were alive at 1-year follow-up.

Unfortunately, none of the experience with these other devices is large enough to demonstrate superiority over IABP, and at this time IABP remains the treatment of choice for most patients. There are, however, some patients who are refractory to IABP, or who have rhythm disturbances that render IABP ineffective in whom percutaneous cardiopulmonary bypass or the Hemopump may be alternate forms of support.

It has also been demonstrated that IABP treatment after per-

TABLE 4

Devices of Hemodynamic Support Used as Adjunctive Therapy in Treatment of Cardiogenic Shock

Device	Advantages	Disadvantages
IABP	Familiar 8.5F insertion size Unloads Augments coronary flow Operated by nurse	Requires controlled regular rhythm
CPS	>5 L/min output Independent of rhythm Unloads	Unfamilar Large cannulae Require perfusionist Short time support
Hemopump	2–5 L/min output Independent of rhythm Unloads Used for several days	Unfamilar Large cannulae

cutaneous transluminal coronary angioplasty (PTCA) in hypotensive patients will have an improved short-term patency rate, therefore, IABP support after PTCA for CS is important adjunctive therapy.

Thrombolytic Agents

As noted, there is evidence that the thrombolytic drugs are not effective when given intravenously in patients who present or develop CS even when administered early. Data on the use of intracoronary lytic agents were reported by Kennedy et al[41] who reported treatment of 34 patients in CS with intracoronary streptokinase. Despite successful reperfusion, the in-hospital mortality remained 67%, probably because of similar reasons for the failure of intravenous lytic agents.

Angioplasty

The use of coronary angioplasty in the treatment of CS was first used in the early 1980s. Lee et al[42] reported that from 1982 to 1985, 69 patients were treated with emergency angioplasty in an attempt at reperfusion of the infarct-related artery. Balloon angioplasty was successful in 71%. Initial clinical and angiographic findings in the groups with unsuccessful and successful angioplasty were similar with respect to age, infarct location, and gender. Hemodynamic variables were similar. Patients with unsuccessful angioplasty had a short-term survival rate of 20%, compared with 69% in patients successfully dilated. Thirty-eight patients survived the hospital period and were followed up for 24 to 54 months. Twenty-four month survival was significantly better in successfully dilated patients (54%) versus the unsuccessful patients (11%).

In another study, Lee et al[43] reported a retrospective review of 87 patients with CS complicating acute myocardial infarction from 1975 to 1985. Patients treated with conventional therapy were compared with patients treated with conventional therapy and angioplasty. Extent of coronary artery disease, infarct location, and incidence of multivessel disease were similar between the groups. Hemodynamic variables including cardiac index, mean arterial pressure, and pulmonary capillary wedge pressure were also similar. The 30-day survival was significantly improved for patients who underwent angioplasty (50% versus 17%). Survival in patients with successful angioplasty was 77%. The findings suggest that angioplasty improves survival in CS compared with conventional therapy with survival contingent on successful reperfusion of the infarct-related artery.

Moosvi et al[44] studied the effects of coronary revascularization by percutaneous transluminal coronary angioplasty or coronary bypass grafting, or both on survival. Eighty-one patients with CS complicating acute myocardial infarction were evaluated. Thirty-two patients had successful revascularization and 49 patients had unsuccessful or no revascularization. Revascularization was achieved by coronary angioplasty in 22 patients, coronary bypass surgery in 2 and angioplasty followed by bypass surgery in 8. The in-hospital survival was significantly better in those patients with revascularization (18 of 32 or 56%) than in the patients without revascularization (4 of 49 or 8%). At 2-year follow-up, this survival difference remained consistent, ie, 16 of 32 patients (50%) with revascularization survived versus 1 of 49 patients (2%) without revascularization. The mean time from the onset of shock to revascularization differed significantly between survivors and nonsurvivors with the time to revascularization being 12 hours. In the revascularization group, the in-hospital survival rate was 77% (17 of 22) when revascularization was performed within 24 hours, but only 10% when it was performed after 24 hours. Therefore, not only was revascularization successful, but the shorter the time to revascularization the higher the likelihood of survival.

Hibbard et al[45] reviewed the records of all patients at the Mayo Clinic who underwent angioplasty for acute myocardial infarction complicated by CS, retrospectively, to determine whether coronary angioplasty improved survival. Of the 45 patients, 62% had successful dilation of the infarct-related artery and 38% had unsuccessful angioplasty. The groups were similar in the extent of coronary artery disease, infarct location, incidence of multivessel disease, and hemodynamic variables. The hospital survival rate was 71% in patients successfully treated and 29% in the unsuccessful group. At a mean follow-up interval of 2.3 years, the survival rate was 80% in patients surviving to hospital discharge.

The reported success of PTCA in these patients is less than that in other cohorts of patients. PTCA trials for acute myocardial infarction have reported in excess of 90% success, and although there have been reports as high as 88% success, the overall success in these patients is probably in the range of 65%.[46] These studies have almost always used balloon angioplasty exclusively; the use of other interventional devices has not been reported in patients with CS and could alter this success rate.

Although, these studies are not randomized, it does appear that angioplasty does alter the mortality of CS. It must be applied early and appears to have an excellent long-term outcome. Randomized trials are unlikely to be forthcoming due to the reluctance of investigators, and probable unethical nature of not perusing aggressive therapy at this time.[42]

Cardiac Surgery

Bolooki[47] reviewed the published experience spanning the last 20 years of the surgical experience of patients in CS. The data indicate that 66% of patients survive after emergency myocardial revascularization for acute myocardial infarction and CS. If cardiac damage is overwhelming and irreversible, selected patients may be "bridged" with mechanical biventricular circulatory assist devices and receive a transplant. Infarctectomy for acute myocardial infarction remains controversial and unproven; successful repair of free left ventricular wall rupture is uncommon. In patients with CS, operations for acute postinfarction ventricular septal defect or mitral insufficiency have operative survival rates of 45% and 54%, respectively. Long-term (>2 year) survival for patients after repair of acute postinfarction ventricular septal defect is 84%. However, 5-year survival after successful operation for acute postinfarction mitral insufficiency complicated by CS is only 40%. Pennington[48] notes that the surgical mortality is a function of age and that the mortality for patients 80 years and older is 67% to 75% and that as such octogenarians should not undergo bypass surgery for CS. This is similar to the recommendation offered by O'Neill[42] for aggressive nonsurgical therapy where, because there were no survivors over 75 years of age treated by PTCA, aggressive therapy was not warranted.

Recommendations for Therapy

Based on the available data (Figure 1), it appears that the optimal treatment for patients in CS would include early clinical identification, with confirmation made by a Swan-Ganz catheter to rule out other causes. Resuscitative efforts with correction of acidosis and hypoxia should be undertaken. Therapy with inotropic agents to restore blood pressure should be instituted and the use of a vasodilator agent begun if pulmonary congestion is significant and the blood pressure will tolerate. Other resuscitative efforts including restoring proper acid-base balance, correcting hypoxia, and ventilatory support should be instituted as necessary. The treatment of dysrhythmias pharmacologically or by cardioversion is

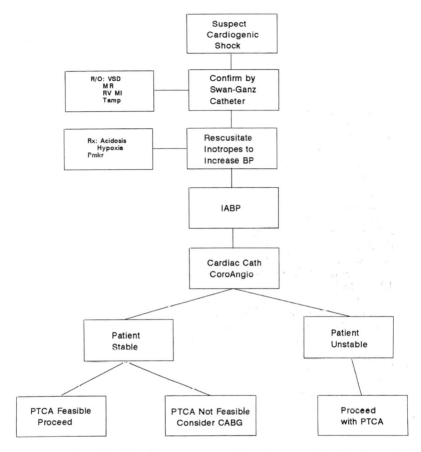

FIGURE 1. *Algorithm for the treatment of cardiogenic shock. If possible, all steps after the first could be performed in the cardiac catheterization laboratory. VSD, ventricular septal defect; MR, mitral regurgitation; RVMI, right ventricular infarction; Tamp, cardiac tamponade; PMKR, pacemaker; IABP, intra-aortic balloon pump; CoroAngio, coronary arteriography; PTCA, angioplasty or other interventional procedure; CABG, coronary artery bypass surgery.*

necessary, and if possible, the restoration of atrial-ventricular synchrony should be considered. These measures should be performed while readying the catheterization laboratory and all can be performed in the laboratory. An IABP should be inserted as soon as possible, and coronary arteriography performed. If the patient is hemodynamically stable and a feasible lesion is present, coronary angioplasty should be undertaken at that time. If, due to anatomy, the lesion is not feasible, emergent cardiac surgery should be undertaken. If the patient cannot be stabilized by use of pharmacologic therapy and IABP, use of other mechanical device may be warranted or attempt at a very high risk PTCA may be undertaken.

References

1. Weil MH, von Plotz M, Reckow EC. Acute circulatory failure (shock). In: Braunwald E, ed. *Heart Disease: A Textbook of Cardiovascular Medicine*. Philadelphia, PA: WB Saunders; 1988:561–590.
2. Harnarayan C, Bennett MA, Pentecost BL, Brewer DB. Quantitative study of infarcted myocardium in cardiogenic shock. *Br Heart J.* 1970; 32:728–732.
3. Forrester JS, Diamond G, Chatterjee K, Swan HJC. Medical therapy of acute myocardial infarction by application of hemodynamic subsets. *N Engl J Med.* 1976;295:1356–1362, 1404–1413.
4. O'Neill WW. Management of cardiogenic shock. In Topol E, ed. *Acute Coronary Intervention*. New York, NY: Alan R. Liss, Inc.; 1988:195–213.
5. Scheidt S, Wilner G, Mueller H, et al. Intra-aortic counterpulsation in cardiogenic shock. Report of a co-operative clinical trial. *N Engl J Med.* 1973;288:979–984.
6. Griffith GC, Wallace WB, Cochran B, et al. The treatment of shock associated with myocardial infarction. *Circulation.*1954;9:527–532.
7. Mirowski M, Israel W, Antonopoulos G, et al. Treatment of myocardial infarction in a community hospital coronary care unit. *Arch Intern Med.* 1978;138:210–215.
8. Scheidt S, Ascherian R, Killip T. Shock after acute myocardial infarction. A clinical and hemodynamic profile. *Am J Cardiol.*1970;26:556–564.
9. Gunnar RM. Cardiogenic shock complicating acute myocardial infarction. *Circulation.* 1988;78:1508–1510.
10. Killip T, Kimball JT. Treatment of myocardial infarction in a coronary care unit. A two year experience with 250 patients. *Am J Cardiol.* 1967; 20:457–464.
11. Hands ME, Rutherford JD, Muller JE. The in-hospital development of cardiogenic shock after myocardial infarction: incidence predictors of occurrence, outcome and prognostic factors. The MILIS Study Group. *J Am Coll Cardiol.* 1989;14:40–46.
12. Bengtson JR, Kaplan AJ, Pieper KS. Prognosis in cardiogenic shock after acute myocardial infarction in the interventional era. *J Am Coll Cardiol.* 1992;20:1482–1489.
13. The I.S.A.M. Study Group. A prospective trial of intravenous streptokinase is acute myocardial infarction (l.S.A.M.). *N Engl J Med.* 1986; 314:1465–1471.
14. Cardiogenic shock during myocardial infarction: The GUSTO experience with thrombolytic therapy. *Circulation.* 1993;88:I-253.
15. Goldberg RJ, Gore JM, Alpert JS: Cardiogenic shock after acute myocardial infarction. Incidence and mortality from a community-wide perspective, 1975 to 1988. *N Engl J Med.*1991;325:1117–1122.
16. Gruppo Italiano Per Lo Studio Della Streptokinasi Nell'lnfarcto Miocardio (GlSSl). Effectiveness of intravenous thrombolytic treatment in acute myocardial infarction. *Lancet.* 1986;i:397–401.
17. Andrews WR, Arnold JM, Sibbald WJ. Threatened reinfarction. Effective therapy using streptokinase with reversal of cardiogenic shock. *Chest.* 1990;98:495–497.

18. Bates ER, Topol EJ. Limitations of thrombolytic therapy for acute myocardial infarction complicated by congestive heart failure and cardiogenic shock. *J Am Coll Cardiol.* 1991;18:1077–1084.
19. Becker RC. Hemodynamic, mechanical, and metabolic determinants of thrombolytic efficacy: a theoretic framework for assessing the limitations of thrombolysis in patients with cardiogenic shock. *Am Heart J.* 1993;125:919–929.
20. Grines CL, Browne KF, Marco J, et al. A comparsion of immediate angioplasty with thrombolytic therapy for acute myocardial infarction. *N Engl J Med.* 1993;328:673–679.
21. Zijlstra F, DeBoer MJ, Hoorntje JCA, et al. A comparsion of immediate coronary angioplasty with intravenous streptokinase in acute myocardial infarction. *N Engl J Med.* 1993;328:680–684.
22. Gibbons RJ, Holmes DR, Reeder GS, et al. Immediate angioplasty compared with the administration of a thrombolytic agent followed by conservative treatment for myocardial infarction. *N Engl J Med.* 1993; 328:681–685.
23. Lange RA, Hillis LD. Immediate angioplasty for acute myocardial infarction. *N Engl J Med.* 1993;328:726–728.
24. Gunnar RM, Cruz A, Boswell J. Myocardial infarction in shock: hemodynamic studies and results of therapy. *Circulation.* 1966;33:753–762.
25. Holzer J, Karliner JS, O'Rourke RA. Effectiveness of dopamine in patients with cardiogenic shock. *Am J Cardiol.* 1973;32:79–84.
26. Ruiz CE, Weil MH, Carlson RW. Treatment of circulatory shock with dopamine. Studies on survival. *JAMA.* 1979;242:165–168.
27. Tan LB, Littler WA. Measurement of cardiac reserve in cardiogenic shock: implications for prognosis and management. *Br Heart J.* 1990; 64:121–128.
28. Francis GS, Sharma B, Hodges M. Comparative hemodynamic effects of dopamine and dobutamine in patients with acute cardiogenic circulatory collapse. *Am Heart J.* 1982;103:995–1000.
29. Richard C, Ricome JL, Rinailho A, et al. Combined hemodynamic effects of dopamine and dobutamine in cardiogenic shock. *Circulation.* 1983;67:620–626.
30. Moulopoulos SD, Stamateolopoulos SF, Nanas JN. Effect of protracted dobutamine infusion on survival of patients in cardiogenic shock treated with intraaortic balloon pumping. *Chest.* 1993;103:248–252.
31. Fowler MB, Timmis AD, Crick JP et al. Comparison of haemodynamic responses to dobutamine and salbutamol in cardiogenic shock after acute myocardial infarction. *Br Med J.* 1982;284:73–76.
32. Timmis AD, Fowler MB, Chamberlain DA. Comparison of hemodynamic response to dopamine and salbutamol in cardiogenic shock complicating myocardial infarction. *Br Med J.* 1981;282:7–9.
33. Klocke RK, Mager G, Kux A. Effects of a twenty-four-hour milrinone infusion in patients with severe heart failure and cardiogenic shock as a function of the hemodynamic initial condition. *Am Heart J.* 1991; 121:1965–1973.
34. Keung EC, Ribner HS, Schwartz W, et al. Effects of combined dopamine and nitroprusside therapy in patients with severe pump failure and hypotension complication in acute myocardial infarction. *J Cardiovasc Pharmacol.* 1980;2:113–119.
35. McGhie AI, Golstein RA. Pathogenesis and management of acute heart failure and cardiogenic shock: role of inotropic therapy. *Chest.* 1992; 102(Suppl 2):626S–632S.

438   *INVASIVE CARDIOLOGY*

36. Kantrowitz A, Krahover JS, Rosenbaum A, et al. Phase shift balloon pumping in medically refractory cardiogenic shock. *Arch Surg.* 1969; 739–743.
37. Dunkman WB, Leinbach RC, Bulkley MJ, et al. Clinical and hemodynamic results of intra-aortic balloon pumping and surgery for cardiogenic shock. *Circulation.* 1972;46:465–477.
38. Gacioch GM, Ellis SG, Lee L. Cardiogenic shock complicating acute myocardial infarction: the use of coronary angioplasty and the integration of the new support devices into patient management. *J Am Coll Cardiol.* 1992;19:647–653.
39. Lincoff AM, Popma JJ, Bates ER. Successful coronary angioplasty in two patients with cardiogenic shock using the Nimbus Hemopump support device. *Am Heart J.* 1990;120:970–972.
40. Shawl FA, Domanski MJ, Hernandez TJ, Punja S. Emergency percutaneous cardiopulmonary bypass support in cardiogenic shock from acute myocardial infarction. *Am J Cardiol.* 1989;64:967–970.
41. Kennedy JW, Gensini GG, Timmis GC, et al. Acute myocardial infarction treated with intracoronary streptokinase. A report of the Society for Cardiac Angiography. *Am J Cardiol.* 1985;55:871–875.
42. Lee L, Erbel R, Brown TM. Multicenter registry of angioplasty therapy of cardiogenic shock: initial and long-term survival. *J Am Coll Cardiol.* 1991;17:599–603.
43. Lee L, Bates ER, Pitt B. Percutaneous transluminal coronary angioplasty improves survival in acute myocardial infarction complicated by cardiogenic shock. *Circulation.* 1988;78:1345–1351.
44. Moosvi AR, Khaja F, Villanueva L. Early revascularization improves survival in cardiogenic shock complicating acute myocardial infarction. *J Am Coll Cardiol.* 1992;19:907–914.
45. Hibbard MD, Holmes DR Jr, Bailey KR. Percutaneous transluminal coronary angioplasty in patients with cardiogenic shock. *J Am Coll Cardiol.* 1992;19:639–646.
46. O'Neill WW. Angioplasty therapy of cardiogenic shock: are randomized trials necessary. *J Am Coll Cardiol.* 1992;19:915–917.
47. Bolooki H. Emergency cardiac procedures in patients in cardiogenic shock due to complications of coronary artery disease. *Circulation.* 1989;79(suppl):I-137-I-148.
48. Pennington DG. Emergency management of cardiogenic shock. *Circulation.* 1989;79(suppl I):l-149-I-151.

Chapter 24

State of the Art on Balloon Aortic Valvuloplasty: What Are the Indications for this Treatment in Aortic Stenosis?

Brice Letac, MD and Alain Cribier, MD

It is well known that severe aortic stenosis has a disastrous spontaneous evolution. This has been shown by at least two published series. In the series by O'Keefe,[1] the 1-year mortality rate was 44% and even higher—60%—in the series by Turina.[2] It is also well established that aortic valve replacement has an excellent as well as a long-lasting result. However, surgery cannot be performed in all cases, particularly in those at high risk and in some cases it cannot be performed at all. Because the only effective treatment for aortic stenosis is to open the aortic orifice to permit unobstructed blood flow from the left ventricle into the aorta, balloon aortic valvuloplasty had been proposed as another form of treatment for aortic stenosis.[3,4] This procedure generated a lot of enthusiasm in the initial 2 years of use, but in recent years it has been criticized and has been almost abandoned by many centers over the world. Our group at Rouen, France has performed balloon dilatation in over 600 cases of aortic stenosis and we continue to treat about 50 cases a year. The following summarizes our experience.

Case Example

As an illustrative example of what balloon valvuloplasty can sometimes do, we first describe the case of one of our recently dilated patients. This is a 67-year-old woman who had mitral valve replacement in 1987 and who became totally incapacitated over the

From Vetrovec GW, Carabello BA, (eds.) *Invasive Cardiology: Current Diagnostic and Therapeutic Issues.* Armonk, NY: Futura Publishing Company, Inc.: © 1996.

last 6 months because she developed aortic stenosis. The patient had been hospitalized repeatedly in another city during the last few months. Catheterization and echocardiography showed severe aortic stenosis with a valve area of 0.3 cm² and an ejection fraction of 22%. Additionally, there was marked tricuspid regurgitation. Cardiac surgeons refused to operate on this patient. We agreed to attempt an aortic dilatation in spite of her poor general condition. The patient was transferred by air to our hospital and was taken to the catheterization laboratory the morning after her arrival. Dilatation with a 20-mm diameter balloon, increased the valve area to 0.7 cm², which by itself is significant aortic stenosis, but represents a 130% increase in valve area for this patient. The recovery was quite spectacular. Seven days after the procedure, the patient was able to go shopping for some necessary items; 2 days later she flew to Nice, France, where her children were living, to have aortic valve replacement. Surgery took place 2 weeks later and the patient now leads a normal active life. Of course, not all cases are as spectacular as this one.

Clinical Results in Octogenarians

As the vast majority of our patients are elderly patients aged 80 or older, we present our results from a series of 86 consecutive patients in this group treated over a 3-year period from 1989 to 1991. We selected this particular subset of patients because they are commonly seen in clinical practice because of the increasing older population, and because these patients are the most fragile, therefore, higher complication rates should be expected. Also, we selected this time period because the technical aspects of the procedure had improved and become standardized and therefore reflect our current experience in aortic balloon valvuloplasty.

The mean age of these 86 consecutive patients was 84 ± 3 years, ranging from 80 to 92. All were highly symptomatic, 70% were in NYHA Class III to IV. One third of the patients had a markedly depressed left ventricular function with an ejection fraction <40%. One third of them had coronary artery disease, with 12% having three vessel coronary disease. Twelve percent had associated noncardiac disease. Only 7 patients (8%) were surgical candidates because they were otherwise healthy except for their aortic stenosis, but they refused surgery. Therefore, the patients in this group not only are elderly, but the vast majority of them also had associated adverse conditions that markedly increased the surgical risk or that made them unsuitable surgical candidates.

Balloon dilatation resulted in a decrease in the mean peak-to-peak gradient from 68 to 27 mm Hg and an increase of the aortic valve area from 0.52 to 0.97 cm^2, a 91% increase in area. All the results are not as uniform and a good result is not always obtained. A valve area of ≤ 1 cm^2 is considered a good result; this was obtained in 33% of cases. However, the valve area remained below 0.7 cm^2 in 13 cases (15%) and this could be considered a poor result. When the result is expressed as percent increase in valve area, a good result with an increase in valve area $\geq 75\%$ was obtained in more than half of the patients (55%). An increase in valve area between 50% and 75% was observed in 26% of the cases. Therefore, a poor result with an increase in valve area <50% was obtained in <20% of the cases and a complete failure, ie, an increase in <25% was found in only one case.

The following comments on the overall results can be made. An area of 0.9 or 1 cm^2 remains less than the >2 cm^2 area obtained with an artificial valve and thus, this area represents a residual degree of aortic stenosis. However, when the patient is 80 years or older, this may be sufficient improvement to lead a normal active life. Likewise, even in a younger patient, for instance aged 60, an aortic valve area of 1 cm^2 may represent a significant increase from a 0.5 cm^2 area, which is often sufficient enough to make the patient completely free of the usual symptoms of aortic stenosis such as pulmonary edema or anginal chest pain.

Similarly, when the increase in valve area is only 30% or 40%, it is usually an insufficient result as compared to what could have been expected, but this may be sufficient for an individual patient. For instance, if the patient had pulmonary edema with an aortic valve area of 0.5 cm^2, he or she may be completely relieved of his symptoms with a 0.7 cm^2 valve area, although the increase in valve is only 40%.

Although these data concern a series of elderly patients with most in frail condition, the complication rate was low (Figure 1). Two patients, one of whom was 84 years old and the other 86 years old, died during the procedure, representing a 3% mortality rate. The total rate of complications was 6.7% and it must be emphasized that there were no demonstrated calcium emboli or myocardial perforation. There were no serious local vascular complications at the puncture site, except for a benign local hematoma in a few patients. In-hospital stay was short; 40% of patients were discharged 2 to 3 days after valvuloplasty. The mean duration of hospital stay for the group was 6±5 days.

Follow-up, which is always difficult to obtain in elderly patients, was available in 87% of those who were discharged from the

PROCEDURE - RELATED COMPLICATIONS

- **In - hospital death (per-procedure)**   **2   (2.3%)**
- **Permanent AV block**   **1   (1.1%)**
- **Aortic insufficiency (Grade 3)**   **1   (1.1%)**
- **Myocardial infarction**   **1   (1.1%)**
- **Transient stroke**   **1   (1.1%)**

➡ TOTAL :   *6   (6.7%)*

☐ **Mean post-BAV hospital stay : 72 hrs (2 - 25 days)**

FIGURE 1.

hospital. Mean follow-up was 13 months. Eight patients of 84 patients (10%) had aortic valve replacement after improvement, after a mean of 8 months, with 2 patients dying in the immediate postoperative period. Four patients required repeat valvuloplasty 12 months later for recurrence of symptoms related to restenosis. Of these 4 patients, 3 improved with a mean increase in valve area from 0.57 to 1.4 cm^2 and 1 died within a few weeks because of severe heart failure.

During the follow-up period of 13 months, 27 patients died, a mortality rate of 33%. Death occurred at a mean of 9 months after the initial procedure. The mean age of the patients who died was 86 years. Actuarial survival rate, evaluated in 73 patients who did not have aortic valve replacement, was 73% at 1 year, a figure that compares favorably with the survival rates of 56% in the O'Keefe series and the 40% reported in the Turina series. Both of these were natural history studies, and included patients who were on average 20 years younger than the patients in our series (Figure 2).[1,2]

The main drawback of balloon valvuloplasty is the high restenosis rate. From our first 406 consecutive patients, 97 patients were able to have repeat catheterization within 7±5 months. The restenosis rate on an actuarial basis was 60% at 1 year.[5] Of note, the hemodynamic restenosis definition, ie, a loss of 50% of the gain obtained in the valve area after dilatation, does not correlate with the clinical definition, ie, the recurrence of symptoms in all the patients. Many patients remain clinically improved although they have hemody-

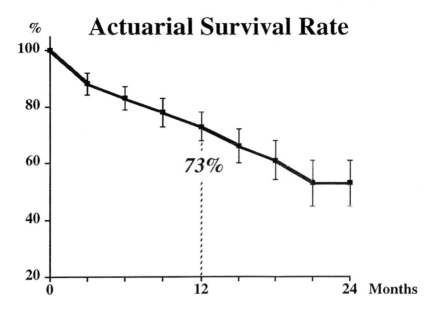

Actuarial Survival Rate

73%

One year spontaneous survival :   *O' Keeffe : 56%*
                                      Turina :   40%

FIGURE 2.

namic restenosis. This has also been observed in other studies.[6,7]. Obviously, a patient who had an aortic valve area of 0.5 cm² initially and has a 1-cm² area opening after valve dilatation still remains clinically improved, when by definition he has a restenosis with a valve area of 0.7 cm². Furthermore, repeat valvuloplasty can be performed in case of restenosis.[8-10] This was performed in 67 patients in our series of 406 consecutive patients, at a mean interval of 10 months. The mean aortic area increased from 0.60 to 0.86 cm², a result that is slightly less satisfactory than the one obtained during the initial dilatation. This is despite the fact that bigger balloon size had been used for the redilatation procedure in 60% of cases.

Technical Considerations

The important technical points of the procedure, which were standardized in 1988–1989 resulting in a low complication rate and maximal opening of the stenosed aortic valve, are as follows:

1) The balloon catheters to be used are double size balloons 15–20 mm or 18–23 mm in diameter with a double lumen to

allow recording the ventriculo-aortic gradient at each stage and with a soft pigtail tip, eliminating the risk of myocardial perforation.

2) The use of a 14F introducer with a valve reducing arterial injury and blood loss.

3) The use of an extra stiff guide wire that helps maintain stability of the balloon across the aortic valve during maximal balloon inflation.

4) Inflations must be performed rapidly so that the time between initiation of inflation and deflation and the removal of the balloon from the aortic orifice is not more than 30 to 40 seconds, particularly if there is a drop in blood pressure during inflation, in order to avoid brain and myocardial ischemia. It is particularly important to avoid lengthy inflations in cases of coronary artery disease and in cases of altered left ventricular function because a reduction in coronary blood flow and increased afterload strongly depress left ventricular function in a way that, even after complete deflation of the balloon, a return to a stable hemodynamic status may be slow, and low cardiac output may persist and brain damage may occur.

5) It is better to perform progressive dilatation. Begin with three inflations with the 15-mm segment of the balloon and proceed with three more inflations with the 20-mm segment. If at control, the increase in the aortic valve area obtained is <80 to 100%, the 20-mm balloon must be exchanged for a 23-mm balloon and inflations repeated with the bigger balloon. A 18–23-mm diameter balloon may be used for patients with large body surface area.

6) Most importantly, balloon inflations must be performed at the maximal pressure, ie, at or near the bursting point. This point cannot be stressed enough. Maximal inflation has a precise meaning: the point when the balloon would burst with an additional milliliter or half-milliliter of the liquid medium used for inflation. It is only at that point that the balloon becomes as stiff as a cylinder made of metal or of stone. At that moment, a 20-mm diameter balloon occupies an area of 3.14 cm^2 and a 23-mm diameter an area of 4.15 cm^2. If the balloon bursts, usually longitudinally, it does so without any deleterious consequence, and provides the best proof that it had reached and possibly even surpassed its maximal diameter. It is only when the balloon is really maximally inflated with no waist seen on the balloon at fluoroscopic screen, that it can push apart the leaflets of the valve and therefore enlarge the orifice. There is, however, a strong recoil phenomenon because the best aortic valve areas obtained in live patients or found in fresh post-mortem specimens from those patients in whom we performed dilatation are usually around 1.5 cm^2.

The mechanisms by which dilatation works are many.[11] Balloon dilatation breaks the calcified frame of the cusps or even breaks huge calcified nodules. It renders the cusps supple, often without producing an aortic regurgitation or increasing a previously existing regurgitation. It also tears the fused commissures, if present. It is important to note that balloon dilatation does not produce calcium embolism, probably because calcified deposits are enclosed in the frame of the cusps and remain covered by the endothelium.

Comparative Results of Aortic Valve Surgery

Before discussing the indications for balloon aortic valvuloplasty, which can be expected to stem mainly from contraindications to surgical aortic valve replacement, we have to examine the results of surgery for aortic valve replacement in situations where the surgical risk is higher than in usual patients, excluding those where surgery is absolutely contraindicated. As already noted, the largest subset of patients who are at increased surgical risk are elderly patients. This group is important to consider because excluding congenital and rheumatic forms, aortic stenosis is mainly a degenerative process most commonly involving the elderly population.

There are relatively few published series on the results of surgical aortic valve replacement for aortic stenosis in octogenarian patients. It is commonly said that age alone is not a contraindication to aortic valve surgery, and that patients older than 80 years can undergo surgery. It is, however, interesting to note that in concert with the introduction of aortic balloon valvuloplasty, surgical treatment of patients aged 80 years and over increased. Before 1986, there were only a few patients older than 80 who had surgery for aortic valve replacement, but the number of such operations increased up to tenfold after 1987. For instance, in the Deleuze series,[12] a mean of 3 patients a year aged 80 or more had aortic valve replacement before 1987, whereas this number increased to 14 patients a year in 1987, 1988, 1989. In the Olsson series,[13] there were only a few patients aged 80 or more operated on before 1987 and the number was 10 to 15 higher in 1989. At our institute, only about 1 patient more than 80 years old was operated on each year before 1987, whereas a mean of 10 patients underwent surgery each year in 1987, 1988, and 1989.

There is no doubt that patients older than 80 years with aortic stenosis undergo surgery with an acceptable risk when they are otherwise healthy. The surgical risk for aortic valve replacement in the otherwise normal patient <70 years old is 2% to 4%. However, based on nine surgical series found in the literature, the surgical risk in octogenarians is not only markedly higher, but is strikingly different from one series to another ranging from a minimal mortality of 6% in the Cullingford and Levinson series to 30% in the Edmunds series.[12–20] The approximate average surgical risk of the nine series is 14%. However, these surgical series concern octogenarian subjects who were carefully selected, and generally except for the aortic stenosis were otherwise healthy. Therefore, they do not represent the majority of elderly patients presenting with aortic stenosis, a fact that is recognized by several authors of these papers. The strict selection of patients aged 80 or over for surgical valve replacement is also strongly suggested by the small number of cases reported in most surgical papers. For instance, there were only 20 such patients in Turina's group (Zurich) in a 7-year period, ie, fewer than two patients a year.[20] The patients from these surgical series are not comparable with the patients who where treated with balloon aortic valvuloplasty in our series because we accepted all types of patients, many of whom were in poor condition. Half of our patients were not considered at all for surgery and balloon valvuloplasty was the only therapeutic possibility. In the other half, surgery was rejected because of a high surgical risk, which was estimated at 30% or higher. The presence of coronary artery disease also increases the surgical risk, particularly in elderly patients. Thus, in four surgical series, the surgical risk in octogenarians increased respectively from 6% to 30%; 8% to 17%; 6% to 19%; and from 11% to 21% when comparing patients who had aortic valve replacement alone with those who had coronary artery bypass surgery along with the valve replacement.[12,15,16,18,19] In our series of octogenarian patients, one third had coronary artery disease with no increased risk of the procedure, although no treatment of the coronary stenosis was undertaken. However, in our patients, angina pectoris was remarkably relieved by aortic dilatation alone. There are also indications that the surgical risk is markedly increased when surgery is performed in patients who have a marked decrease in left ventricular function.[12] In a recent report, Brogan et al[21] reported that the mortality rate was 33% in a series of 18 patients who had a low ventriculo-aortic gradient resulting from depressed left ventricular function, but whose mean age was 68 years, ie, almost 20 years younger than the patients in our series.[21] However, one must take into consideration that the cited surgical series are probably partially outdated because the surgical risk has decreased in recent years.

It is not a question of balloon aortic valvuloplasty versus surgery, and to quote Pasic,[20] percutaneous aortic valvuloplasty ". . . is a palliative procedure for a population of inoperable patients, but it is not an alternative to valve replacement".

Balloon aortic valvuloplasty should be considered in all patients in whom surgery cannot be performed because of absolute contraindications. This is because without any intervention to remove the mechanical obstacle to the left ventricular ejection, aortic stenosis has a disastrous outcome. This includes elderly patients with morbid cardiac or extracardiac conditions and younger patients with contraindications to surgery such as respiratory insufficiency, cancer, and severe or inoperable coronary disease.

In some situations, because of low cardiac output or profound shock the patient has such a poor clinical status that balloon dilatation is performed as a last resort. Despite the poor clinical status, the result may be quite good with prompt improvement.[22-25]

Things are probably more complex in those patients for whom surgery is not completely contraindicated, but who are at high risk. This group includes mostly older patients who are often in poor overall condition, who often have associated diseases, who have coronary disease, and who may have profound left ventricular dysfunction. It is often difficult to choose between surgery that is often high risk, but can have excellent long-term results if the patient survives compared with aortic balloon dilatation, which is low risk, but has a high restenosis rate. The prospective assessment of surgical risk is extremely difficult and uncertain. It is also difficult to define what an acceptable surgical risk is: is it 10%, or 20%, or 30%?

Another indication for considering balloon aortic valvuloplasty is as a bridge to surgery when there are temporary comorbid condition or when there is a pronounced left ventricular dysfunction that may improve after dilatation.[26,27] In our opinion, balloon aortic dilatation should be performed when one hesitates because of an evaluated high surgical risk that is secondary to a potentially reversible condition. This is particularly the case when there is a markedly depressed ejection fraction. In most cases, balloon valvuloplasty produces a sufficient enough improvement to allow the patient to have surgery later on in much better condition.[28,29]

Another indication for balloon aortic valvuloplasty is congenital aortic stenosis in young adults. The procedure is the treatment of choice in children, but it also produces excellent results in young adults, at an age where changing the native valve for a prosthesis is a problem.[30]

Balloon Aortic Valvuloplasty: Responses to the Criticism

Balloon aortic valvuloplasty has often been poorly represented. In Brogan et al,[21] although the mortality rate was 33% in patients with a mean age of 68, the authors concluded that they recommended surgery and did not even mention balloon valvuloplasty. In Bernard et al,[31] the result of balloon dilatation in a series of 46 patients was particularly poor possibly due to technical inadequacies. An increase in valve area of only 34% was obtained. Therefore, the authors decided to stop performing balloon valvuloplasty.[31] Furthermore, a recent editorial by cardiac surgeons referred to aortic valvuloplasty "off the wagon."[32]

To evaluate the merits of balloon aortic valvuloplasty objectively, it would be interesting to examine the results in series others than our own, ie, in series performed recently and that have benefited from improvements in the technique. Unfortunately, after an initial period of enthusiasm, it seems that balloon aortic valvuloplasty is not routinely performed in most catheterization centers and perhaps not at all in some. An average of 39 abstracts on balloon aortic valvuloplasty was presented each year at the American College of Cardiology and American Heart Association meetings in 1987, 1988, 1989, and a average of only 4 per year at the same meetings in 1990, 1991, 1992, and 1993. Some of the papers published in these last years have rated balloon aortic valvuloplasty unfavorably. This is true of often-cited series, the Mansfield Scientific Registry, which included 674 patients.[33,34] This series is a heterogeneous series, consisting of multiple operators many of whom with only limited experience with the procedure before the technical aspects had been standardized. This may also explain a high complication rate. Similarly, several other series raise questions of technical inadequacies in performing the procedure, as the increase in valve area was low, equal to, or less than 50% in which balloon inflation pressure was not documented, which explains the less than ideal results.[6,31,35–38]

Another clue that technical inadequacy results mainly from insufficient pressure exerted during balloon inflation is given by Robicsek et al.[39] This surgical group carefully examined with caliper measurements the effect of balloon inflation on aortic stenosis during open heart surgery, before excising the stenosed valve prior to replacement. The authors found that balloon inflation did not enlarge the orifice. To compare these results with our own clinical experience raises questions regarding technique. Our technique is to dilate using near rupture pressures. The authors utilized the recommended pressure inflation as indicated by the manufacturer, but this pressure is calculated in such a way that more than 99% of the balloons would have not burst at this pressure. For aortic dilatation, this pressure may be too low to affect the valve.

However, other centers continue to perform aortic valvuloplasty, including the group from the Massachusetts General Hospital in Boston.[40] This center recently reported a series of 310 patients, whose mean age was 79±1, who underwent balloon aortic valvuloplasty because they were either very high risk or nonsurgical candidates. The increase in valve area was from 0.5 to 0.8, a 74% increase, which confirms that the procedure can affect changes in valve area. The 8.6% mortality rate may reflect severely ill patients and/or patients who were treated during the "learning curve."

Abandonment of the technique in many centers before optimal technical experience had been attained may have limited the opportunity to compare valvuloplasty with surgery in high-risk patients.

How Many Patients Would Benefit from Aortic Valvuloplasty?

To determine whether aortic valvuloplasty deserves a place in all catheterization interventional centers or whether it should be limited to centers able to develop operator experience by performing a sufficient number of cases, we examined our own experience.

In the 3-year period from 1990 to 1992, we performed 177 valvuloplasties. Bearing in mind that while we consider aortic valve replacement the gold standard for the treatment of aortic stenosis, only 114 patients were operated on (64%) and 63 (36%) had balloon aortic valvuloplasty. As shown in Figure 3, only a few patients <70 years (11%) could not be operated on and had to be dilated. Conversely, in the group of patients aged 80 or older, only 30% were operated on while the rest (70%) were dilated. These figures confirm that elderly patients are the main subset of patients who have to be treated by balloon dilatation. Thus, we performed aortic balloon valvuloplasty in a average of 50 to 60 patients per year. Since our institute is the only referring hospital for approximately 1.6 million people in our region, and assuming that almost all patient with aortic stenosis were sent to us (which certainly may not be the case), we can deduce that about 40 to 50 patients per million of the population have to be treated each year by balloon aortic

**Age wise distribution of patients operated on or dilated
Mean number of patients (1990,1991,1992) = 177 per year**

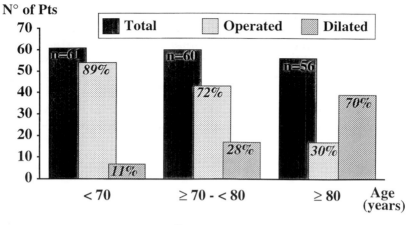

FIGURE 3.

valvuloplasty. Thus, in our center, the procedure is not performed in ". . . the most unusual of circumstances."[32] Nonoperable patients are seen by cardiologists and decisions of how to treat these patients must be addressed particularly for such patients who are significantly symptomatic. Balloon valvuloplasty may often provide significant symptomatic improvement, even if the result is not long lasting in many cases.

References

1. O'Keefe JH, Vlietstra RE, Bailey KR, Holmes DV. Natural history of candidates for balloon aortic valvuloplasty. *Mayo Clin Proc.* 1987; 62:976–991.
2. Turina J, Hess O, Sepulcri F, Krayenbuehl HP. Spontaneous course of aortic valve disease. *Eur Heart J.* 1987;8:471–483.
3. Letac B, Cribier A, Koning R, Bellefleur JP. Results of percutaneous transluminal valvuloplasty in 218 adults with valvular aortic stenosis. *Am J Cardiol.* 1988;62:598–605.
4. Cribier A, Savin Th, Saoudi N, et al. Percutaneous transluminal valvuloplasty of acquired aortic stenosis in elderly patients. An alternative of valve replacement? *Lancet.* 1986;1:63–67.
5. Letac B, Cribier A, Eltchaninoff H, Koning R, Derumeaux G. Evaluation of restenosis after balloon dilatation in adult aortic stenosis by repeat catheterization. *Am Heart J.* 1991;122:55–60.
6. Kuntz RE, Tosteson ANA, Berman AD, et al. Predictors of event-free survival after balloon aortic valvuloplasty. *N Engl J Med.* 1991;325:17–23.
7. Block PC, Palacios IF. Clinical and hemodynamic follow-up after per-

cutaneous aortic valvuloplasty in the elderly. *Am J Cardiol.* 1988;62: 760–763.

8. Ross TC, Banks AK, Collins TJ, Ramee SR, White CJ, Moore JW. Repeat balloon aortic valvuloplasty for aortic valve restenosis. *Cathet Cardiovasc Diagn.* 1988;18:96–98.

9. Feldman T, Glagov S, Chiu YC, Carroll JD. Second dilatation for restenosis following successful balloon aortic valvuloplasty: results, pathology and mechanism. *J Am Coll Cardiol.* 1989;13:2, 17A. Abstract.

10. Koning R, Cribier A, Asselin C, Mouton-Schleifer D, Derumeaux G, Letac B. Repeat balloon aortic valvuloplasty. *Cathet Cardiovasc Diagn.* 1992;26:249–254.

11. Letac B, Gerber L, Koning R. Insights on the mechanism of balloon valvuloplasty in aortic stenosis. *Am J Cardiol.* 1988;62:1241–1247.

12. Deleuze P, Loisance D, Besnainou F, et al. Severe aortic stenosis in octogenarians: is operation an acceptable alternative? *Ann Thorac Surg.* 1990;50:226–229.

13. Olsson M, Granstrom L, Lindblom D, Rosenqvist M, Ryden L. Aortic valve replacement in octogenarians with aortic stenosis: a case-control study. *J Am Coll Cardiol.* 1992;20:1512–1516.

14. Edmunds LH, Stephenson LW, Edie RN, Ratcliffe MB. Open-heart surgery in octogenarians. *N Engl J Med.* 1988;319:131–136.

15. Levinson JR, Akins CW, Buckley MJ, et al. Octogenarians with aortic stenosis. Outcome after aortic valve replacement. *Circulation.* 1989;80(Suppl I):I-49-I-56.

16. Bashour TT, Hanna ES, Myler RD, et al. Cardiac surgery in patients over the age of 80 years. *Clin Cardiol.* 1990;13:267–270.

17. Logeais Y, Leguerrier A, Rioux C, Delambre JF, Fasquel JL, Langanay T. Rétrécissement aortique calcifié chez les octogénaires. Résultat du traitement chirurgical. *Arch Mal Coeur.* 1990;83:1397–1399.

18. Cullinford A, Galloway A, Colvin S, et al. Aortic valve replacement for aortic stenosis in persons aged 80 years and older. *Am J Cardiol.* 1991; 67:1256–1260.

19. Freeman W, Schaff H, O'Brien P, Orszilak T, Naessens J, Tajik A. Cardiac surgery in the octogenarians: peri-operative outcome and clinical follow-up. *J Am Coll Cardiol.* 1991;18:29–35.

20. Pasic M, Carrel T, Laske A, et al. Valve replacement in octogenarians: increased early mortality but good long-term results. *Eur Heart J.* 1992;13:508–510.

21. Brogan WC, Grayburn PA, Lange RA, Hillis LD. Prognosis after valve replacement in patients with severe aortic stenosis and a low transvalvular pressure gradient. *J Am Coll Cardiol.* 1993;21:1657–1660.

22. Cribier A, Remadi F, Koning R, Rath P, Stix G, Letac B. Emergency balloon valvuloplasty as initial treatment of patients with aortic stenosis and cardiogenic shock. *N Engl J Med.* 1992;9:646.

23. Friedman HZ, Cragg DR, O'Neill WW. Cardiac resuscitation using emergency aortic balloon valvuloplasty. *Am J Cardiol.* 1989;63:387–388.

24. Cribier A, Lafont A, Eltchaninoff H, et al. La valvuloplastie aortique réalisée percutanée en dernier recours chez les patients atteints de rétrécissement aortique en état critique. *Arch Mal Coeur.* 1990;83: 1783–1790.

25. Desnoyers MR, Salem DN, Rosenfield K, et al. Treatment of cardiogenic shock by emergency aortic balloon valvuloplasty. *Ann Intern Med.* 1988;108:833–835.

26. Roth RB, Palacios IF, Block PC. Percutaneous aortic balloon valvulo-plasty: its role in the management of patients with aortic stenosis requiring major noncardiac surgery. *J Am Coll Cardiol.* 1989;13:1039–1041.
27. Levine MJ, Berman AD, Safian RD, Diver DJ, McKay RG. Palliation of valvular aortic stenosis by balloon valvuloplasty as preoperative preparation for non cardiac surgery. *Am J Cardiol.* 1988;62:1309–1310.
28. Berland J, Cribier A, Savin T, Lefebvre E, Koning R, Letac B. Percutaneous balloon valvuloplasty in patients with severe aortic stenosis and low ejection fraction. Immediate results and 1 year follow-up. *Circulation.* 1989;79:1189–1196.
29. Safian RD, Warren SE, Berman AD, et al. Improvement in symptoms and left ventricular performance after balloon aortic valvuloplasty in patients with aortic stenosis and depressed left ventricular ejection fraction. *Circulation.* 1988;78:1181–1191.
30. Sandhu SK, Lloyd TR, Crowley DC, Mendelsohn AM, Fedderly RT, Beekman RH. Balloon valvuloplasty in young adults with congenital aortic stenosis. *Circulation.* 1993;88(Part 2):I-341.
31. Bernard Y, Etievent J, Mourand LL, et al. Long-term results of percutaneous aortic valvuloplasty compared with aortic valve replacement in patients more than 75 years old. *J Am Coll Cardiol.* 1992;20:796–801.
32. Isom OW, Rosengart TK. Percutaneous aortic valvuloplasty: off the bandwagon, again. *J Am Coll Cardiol.* 1992;20:804–805.
33. Eeder GS, Nishimura RA, Holmes DR, et al. Patient age and results of balloon aortic valvuloplasty: the Mansfield Scientific Registry experience. *J Am Coll Cardiol.* 1991;17:909–913.
34. NHLBI Balloon Valvuloplasty Registry participants. Percutaneous balloon aortic valvuloplasty: acute and 30-day follow-up results in 674 patients from the NHLBI Balloon Valvuloplasty Registry. *Circulation.* 1991;84:2383–2397.
35. Grossetete R, Le Menager H, Paris D, Bar O, Leurent B, Crochet D. Valvuloplastie aortique percutanée: évolution à long terme à propos de 85 patients dilatés avec succés. *Arch Mal Coeur.* 1992;85:327–332.
36. Brady ST, Davis CA, Kussmaul WG, Laskey WK, Hirshfeld JW, Herrmann HC. Percutaneous aortic balloon valvuloplasty in octogenarians: morbidity and mortality. *Ann Intern Med.* 1989;110:761–766.
37. Legrand V, Beckers J, Fastrez M, Marcelle P, Marchal C, Kulbertus HE. Long-term follow-up of elderly patients with severe aortic stenosis treated by balloon aortic valvuloplasty. Importance of haemodynamic parameters before and after dilatation. *Eur Heart J.* 1991;12:451–457.
38. Rodriguez AR, Minor ST, West MS, et al. Balloon aortic valvuloplasty is not an effective long term therapy for calcific aortic stenosis with left ventricular dysfunction. *Eur Heart J.* 1990;11:387.
39. Robicsek F, Harbold NB. Limited value of balloon dilatation in calcified aortic stenosis in adults: direct observations during open heart surgery. *Am J Cardiol.* 1987;60:857–864.
40. Moreno PR, Jang IK, Block PC, Palacios IF. Long term follow-up of percutaneous aortic valvuloplasty in the elderly: The Massachusetts General Hospital Experience. *Circulation.* 1993;88(Part 2):I-340.

Chapter 25

Percutaneous Mitral Balloon Commissurotomy for Patients with Rheumatic Mitral Stenosis

Igor F. Palacios, MD

Since its introduction in 1984 by Inoue et al,[1] percutaneous mitral balloon commissurotomy (PMV) has been used successfully as an alternative to open or closed surgical mitral commissurotomy in the treatment of patients with symptomatic rheumatic mitral stenosis.[2-18] PMV produces good immediate hemodynamic outcome, a low complication rate, and clinical improvement in the majority of patients with mitral stenosis.[2-18] PMV is safe and effective, and provides sustained clinical and hemodynamic improvement in patients with rheumatic mitral stenosis. The immediate and long-term results appear to be similar to those of surgical mitral commissurotomy.[2-18] Currently, PMV is the preferred form of therapy for relief of mitral stenosis for a selected group of patients with symptomatic mitral stenosis.

Patient Selection

Selection of patients for PMV should be based on symptoms, physical examination, and two-dimensional and Doppler echocardiographic findings. The criteria required for patients to be considered for PMV includes:

1) symptomatic mitral stenosis (NYHA Class II or more),
2) no recent embolic event,
3) <2 grades of mitral regurgitation by contrast ventriculography (using the Seller's classification),
4) no evidence of left atrial thrombus on two-dimensional echocardiography.

From Vetrovec GW, Carabello BA, (eds.) *Invasive Cardiology: Current Diagnostic and Therapeutic Issues.* Armonk, NY: Futura Publishing Company, Inc.; © 1996.

Transthoracic and transesophageal echocardiography should be routinely performed before PMV. Patients in atrial fibrillation and patients with previous embolic episodes should be anticoagulated with warfarine with a therapeutic prothrombine time for at least 3 months before PMV. Patients with left atrium thrombus on two-dimensional echocardiography should be excluded. However, PMV could be performed in these patients if left atrium thrombus has resolved after warfarine therapy.

Technique of PMV

PMV should be performed in the fasting state under mild sedation. Antibiotics (dicloxacillin 500 mg given orally every 6 hours for 4 doses) are started before the procedure. Patients allergic to penicillin should receive 1 g vancomycin intravenously at the time of the procedure.

All patients carefully chosen as candidates for mitral balloon valvuloplasty should undergo diagnostic right and left and transseptal left heart catheterization. After transseptal left heart catheterization, systemic anticoagulation is achieved by the intravenous administration of 100 U/kg of heparin. In patients older than 40 years, coronary arteriography should also be performed.

Hemodynamic measurements, cardiac output, and cine left ventriculography are performed before and after PMV. Cardiac output is measured by thermodilution and Fick method techniques. Mitral valve calcification and angiographic severity of mitral regurgitation (Seller's classification) are grade qualitatively from 0 grade to 4 grades as previously described.[3] An oxygen diagnostic run is performed before and after PMV to determine the presence of left-to-right shunt after PMV.

There is not a unique technique of percutaneous mitral balloon valvuloplasty. Most of the techniques of PMV require transseptal left heart catheterization and use of the antegrade approach. Antegrade PMV can be acomplished using a single[2,3,6] or a double balloon techniques.[3,4,5,7] In this latter approach, the two balloons could be placed through a single femoral vein and single transseptal punctures[3,5,7] or through two femoral veins and two separate atrial septal punctures.[4] In the retrograde technique of PMV the balloons dilating catheters are advanced percutaneously through the right and left femoral arteries over guide wires that have been snared from the descending aorta.[19] These guide wires have been advanced transseptaly from the right femoral vein into the left atrium, the left ventricle, and the ascending aorta. A retrograde nontransseptal technique of PMV has also been described.[20–21]

The Antegrade Double Balloon Technique

In performing PMV using the antegrade double balloon technique (Figure 1) a 7F flow directed balloon catheter is advanced through the transseptal sheath across the mitral valve into the left ventricle.[22] The catheter is then advanced through the aortic valve into the ascending and then the descending aorta. A 0.038-inch, 260-cm long Teflon-coated exchange wire is then passed through the catheter. The sheath and the catheter are removed leaving the wire behind. A 5-mm balloon dilating catheter is used to dilate the atrial septum. A second exchange guide wire is passed parallel to the first guide wire through the same femoral vein and atrial septum punctures using a double lumen catheter. The double lumen catheter is then removed leaving the two guide wires across the mitral valve in the ascending and descending aorta. During these maneuvers care

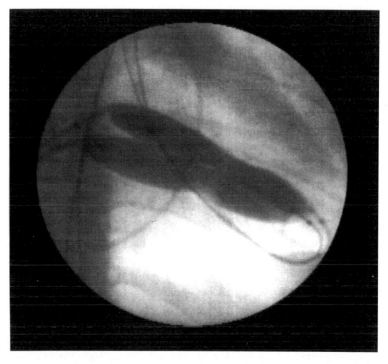

FIGURE 1. *Sequential steps of double balloon percutaneous mitral balloon commissurotomy (PMV). Two 0.038 guide wire are advanced into the ascending and descending aorta with the tip at the level of diaphragm. Two balloon catheters are placed straddling the stenotic mitral valve; markers identifying the proximal end of the balloons are inflated by hand until the waist produced by the stenotic valve disappears.*

should be taken to maintain large and smooth loops of the guide wires in the left ventricular cavity to allow appropriate placement of the dilating balloons. If a second guide wire cannot be placed into the ascending and descending aorta, a 0.038-inch Amplatz-type transfer guide wire with a preformed curlew at its tip can be placed at the left ventricular apex. In patients with aortic valve prosthesis both guide wires with preformed curlew tips should be placed at the left ventricular apex. When one or both guide wires are placed in the left ventricular apex, the balloons should be inflated sequentially. Care should be taken to avoid forward movement of the balloons and guide wires to prevent left ventricular perforation.

Two balloon dilating catheters, chosen according to the patient's body surface area, are then advanced over each one of the guide wires and positioned across the mitral valve parallel to the longitudinal axis of the left ventricle. The balloon valvotomy catheters are then inflated by hand until the indentation produced by the stenotic mitral valve is no longer seen. Generally one, but occasionally two or three inflations are performed. After complete deflation the balloons are removed sequentially.

The Inoue Technique of PMV

PMV can also be performed using the Inoue technique (Figure 2).[1,15-17] The Inoue balloon is a 12F, coaxial, double lumen catheter. The balloon is made of a double layer of rubber tubing with a layer of synthetic micromesh in between.

After transseptal catheterization, a stainless steel guide wire is advanced through the transspetal catheter and placed with its tip coiled into the left atrium and the transseptal catheter removed. A 14F dilator is advanced over the guide wire and used to dilate the femoral vein and the atrial septum. A balloon catheter chosen according to the patient's height is advanced over the guide wire into the left atrium. The distal part of the balloon is inflated and advanced into the left ventricle with the help of the spring wire stylet that has been inserted through the inner lumen of the catheter. Once the catheter is in the left ventricle, the partially inflated balloon is moved back and forth inside the left ventricle to assure that it is free of the chordae tendinae. The catheter is then gently pulled against the mitral plane until resistance is felt. The balloon is then rapidly inflated to its full capacity and then deflated quickly. During inflation of the balloon an indentation should be seen in its midportion. The catheter is withdrawn into the left atrium and the mitral gradient and cardiac output measured. If further dilatations are required, the stylet is introduced again and the sequence of steps described above

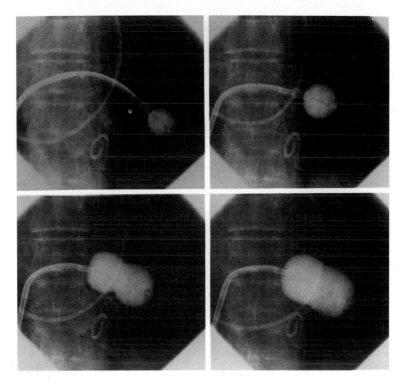

FIGURE 2. *Sequential steps of the Inoue technique of percutaneous mitral balloon commissurotomy (PMV). A partially inflated Inoue balloon catheter is placed into the left ventricle (**upper left,** it is then gently pulled against the mitral plane until resistance if felt (**upper right**). The balloon is then rapidly inflated by hand, an indentation is seen in the mid-portion of the balloon (**lower left**) straddling the stenotic mitral valve and inflated until the waist produced by the stenotic valve disappears (**lower right**).*

repeated at a larger balloon volume. After each dilatation its effect should be assessed by pressure measurement, auscultation and two-dimensional echocardiography. If mitral regurgitation occurs further dilation of the valve should not be performed.

Mechanism of PMV

The mechanism of successful PMV is splitting of the fused commissures toward the mitral annulus, resulting in commissural widening. This mechanism has been demonstrated by pathologic,[6,23] surgical,[23] and echocardiographic studies.[24] In addition, in patients with calcific mitral stenosis the balloons could increase mitral valve flexibility by the fracture of the calcified deposits in the mitral valve leaflets.[6] Although rare, undesirable complications such as leaflet tears, left ventricular perforation, tear of the atrial septum, and rupture of chordae, mitral annulus, and papillary muscle could also occur.

Immediate Outcome

Table 1 shows the changes in mitral valve area reported by several investigators using the double balloon and the Inoue techniques of PMV. In most series PMV is reported to increase mitral valve area from <1.0 cm^2 to ≥2.0 cm^2.[1-22,24-26]

Recently, the results from 564 patients with mitral stenosis who underwent PMV at the Massachusetts General Hospital between July, 1985 and September, 1992 were presented.[26] There were 460 females and 104 males with a mean age of 54±1 (range 13–87) years. Before PMV 71 patients (13%) were in New York Heart Association (NYHA) functional Class IV; 356 patients (63%) were Class III; 133 patients (24%) Class II; and 4 patients were Class I. One hundred and two patients had previously undergone surgical mitral commissurotomy and presented with mitral restenosis. Two hundred and ninety-one (52%) patients were in normal sinus rhythm and 273 (48%) had atrial fibrillation. Evidence of mitral valve calcification under fluoroscopy was present in 255 (45%) patients. A mild degree of mitral valve regurgitation (≤2 grades) was demonstrated by cine left ventriculography in 212 (39%) patients before PMV.

In this group of patients, PMV resulted in a significant decrease in mitral gradient from 15±1 to 5±1 mm Hg. The mean cardiac output increased from 3.9±0.1 to 4.5 L/min and the calculated mitral valve area from 0.9±0.1 to 2.0±0.1 cm^2. In addition, mean pulmonary artery pressure decreased from 37±1 to 28±1 mm Hg ($P<0.0001$). The mean left atrial pressure decreased from 25±1 to 16±1 mm Hg ($P<0.0001$) and the calculated pulmonary vascular resistances decreased significantly after PMV.

A successful hemodynamic outcome (defined as a post-PMV mitral valve area ≥1.5 cm^2, <2 grade increase in mitral regurgitation by angiography and a QP/QS < 1.5/1) was obtained in 79% of the patients. Although a suboptimal result occurred in 21% of the patients, a post-PMV mitral valve area ≤1.0 cm^2 (critical mitral valve area) was present in only 7% of these patients.

Univariate analysis demonstrated that the increase in mitral valve area with PMV is directly related to the balloon size used as they reflect in the effective balloon dilating area (EBDA) and inversely related to the echocardiographic score, the presence of

TABLE 1

Hemodynamic Results of PMV

Institution	Author	# of Patients	Age	Pre-PMV MVA	Post-PMV MVA
Mass General	Palacios et al	564	57±1	0.9±0.1	2.0±0.1
Tenon	Vahanian et al	1,058	44±1	1.0±0.2	1.9±0.3
Loma Linda	Ruiz et al	238	51±1	0.6±0.3	2.6±0.7
Beth Israel	Cohen et al	146	59±1	1.0±0.4	2.1±0.9
Takeda	Inoue et al	527	50±1	1.13±0.02	1.97±0.04
Chang Cung	Hung et al	204	44±1	1.0±0.3	2.0±0.7
George Washington	Chen et al	149	35±1	1.06±0.21	2.04±0.32
Kokura	Nobuyoshi	106	53±1	N/A	N/A
Guangdong	Chen CR et al	85		1.1±0.3	2.0±0.4
Athens University	Stefanadis et al	156	49±1	1.0±0.2	2.2±0.5
North American Multicenter Study	Herrmann et al	200	53±1	1.0±0.3	1.8±0.7
Inoue Balloon Registry	Feldman et al	290	54±1	1.0±0.3	1.7±0.6

atrial fibrillation, the presence of fluoroscopic calcium, the presence of previous surgical commissurotomy, older age, NYHA Class before PMV, and presence of mitral regurgitation before PMV. Multiple stepwise regression analysis demonstrated that the increase in mitral valve area with PMV is directly related to balloon size ($P<0.02$) and inversely related to the echocardiographic score ($P<0.0001$), presence of atrial fibrillation ($P<0.009$), and mitral regurgitation before PMV ($P<0.03$).

Predictors of the Increase in Mitral Valve Area with PMV

The Echocardiographic Score

The echocardiographic score is the more important predictor of the immediate outcome of PMV. In this morphologic score, leaflet rigidity, leaflet thickening, valvular calcification, and subvalvular disease are each scored from 0 to 4.[24,27] A higher score would represent a heavily calcified, thickened and immobile valve with extensive thickening and calcification of the subvalvular apparatus. Among the four components of the echocardiographic score, valve leaflet thickening and subvalvular disease correlate the best with the increase in mitral valve area produced by PMV. The increase in mitral valve area with PMV is inversely related to the echocardiographic score (Figure 3). The best outcome with PMV occurs in those patients with echocardiographic scores ≤8. The increase in mitral valve area is significantly greater in patients with echocardiographic scores ≤8 than in those with echocardiographic score >8. Suboptimal results with PMV are more likely to occur in patients with valves that are more rigid, more thickened, and those with more subvalvular fibrosis and calcification.

Balloon Size and EBDA

The increase in mitral valve area with PMV is directly related to balloon size. This effect was first demonstrated in a subgroup of patients who underwent repeat PMV.[9] They initially underwent PMV with a single balloon resulting in a mean mitral valve area of 1.2 ± 0.2 cm^2. They underwent repeat PMV using the double balloon technique, which increased the EBDA normalized by body surface area (EBDA/BSA) from 3.41 ± 0.2 to 4.51 ± 0.2 cm^2/m^2. The mean mitral valve area in this group after repeat PMV was 1.8 cm^2±0.2

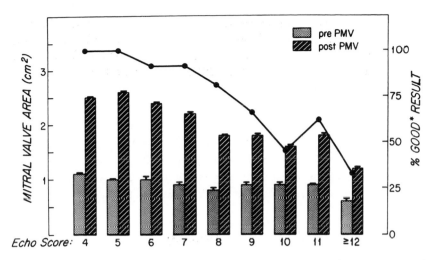

FIGURE 3. *Relationship between the echocardiographic score and change in mitral valve area after percutaneous mitral balloon commissurotomy (PMV) and relationship between the echocardiographic score and the percentage of patients who had a successful immediate hemodynamic outcome. (Modified with permission from Block PC, Palacios IF. Aorta and mitral valvuloplasty: the United States experience. In: Topol EJ, ed.* Textbook of Interventional Cardiology. *Philadelphia, PA: WB Saunders; 1993:1998.)*

cm^2. The increase in mitral valve area in 529 patients who underwent PMV at the Massachusetts General Hospital using the double balloon technique (EBDA of 6.4±0.03 cm^2) was significantly greater than the increase in mitral valve area achieved in 29 patients who underwent PMV using the single balloon technique (EBDA of 4.3±0.02 cm^2). The mean mitral valve areas were 2.0±0.1 and 1.4±0.1 cm^2 for patients who underwent PMV with the double balloon and the single balloon techniques respectively. However, care should be taken in the selection of dilating balloon catheters so as to obtain an adequate final mitral valve area and no change or a minimal increase in mitral regurgitation.

Mitral Valve Calcification

The immediate outcome of patients undergoing PMV is inversely related to the severity of valvular calcification seen by fluoroscopy. Patients without fluoroscopic calcium have a greater increase in mitral valve area after PMV than patients with calcified valves. Patients with either no or 1+ fluoroscopic calcium have a greater increase in mitral valve area after PMV (2.1 ± 0.1 and 1.9 ± 0.1 cm^2, respectively) than those patients with 2, 3, or 4$\pm$of calcium (1.7 ± 0.1, 1.5 ± 0.1 and 1.4 ± 0.1 cm^2, respectively).

Atrial Fibrillation

The increase in mitral valve area with PMV is inversely related to the presence of atrial fibrillation; the post-PMV mitral valve area of 291 patients in normal sinus rhythm was 2.1 ± 0.1 cm^2 compared with a valve area of 1.7 ± 0.1 cm^2 of 273 patients in atrial fibrillation.

Previous Surgical Commissurotomy

Although the increase in mitral valve area with PMV is inversely related to the presence of previous surgical mitral commissurotomy, PMV can produce a good outcome in this group of patients. The mean mitral valve area after PMV in 102 patients with previous surgical commissurotomy was 1.7 ± 0.1 cm^2 compared with a valve area of 2.0 ± 0.1 cm^2 in patients without previous surgical commissurotomy. In this group of patients an echocardiographic score ≤8 was again the most important predictor of a successful hemodynamic imnmediate outcome.

Age

The immediate outcome of PMV is directly related to the age of the patient. The percentage of patients obtaining a good result with this technique decreases as age increases. A successful hemodynamic outcome from PMV was obtained in only <50% of patients ≥65 years old.[14] This inverse relationship between age and the immediate outcome from PMV is due to the higher frequency of atrial fibrillation, calcified valves, and higher echocardiographic scores in elderly patients.

Mitral Regurgitation Before PMV

The presence and severity of mitral regurgitation before PMV is an independent predictor of unfavorable outcome of PMV. The increase in mitral valve after PMV is inversely related to the severity of mitral regurgitation determined by angiography before the procedure. This inverse relationship between presence of mitral regurgitation and immediate outcome of PMV is in part due to the higher frequency of atrial fibrillation, higher echocardiographic scores, calcified mitral valves under fluoroscopy, and older age in patients with mitral regurgitation before PMV.

Complications

Table 2 shows the complications reported by several investigators using the double balloon and the Inoue techniques of PMV.[1-20,24-27] Mortality and morbidity with PMV are low and similar to surgical commissurotomy. There is a <1% mortality. In the series from the Massachusetts General Hospital, there was a 0.5% mortality with no procedural death occurring in the last 400 patients undergoing this procedure. Thromboembolic episodes and stroke incidence of 0% to 3.1% has been reported. Severe mitral regurgitation (4 grades by angiography) has been reported in 1% to 5.2% of the patients. Some of these patients required in-hospital mitral valve replacement. Pericardial tamponade has been reported to occur in 0.2% to 4.1% of cases in these series. Pericardial tamponade can occur from transseptal catheterization and more rarely from ventricular perforation. PMV is associated with a 3% to 16% incidence of left-to-right shunt immediately after the procedure. However, the pulmonary to systemic flow ratio is ≥2:1 in only a minimum number of patients.

We have demonstrated that severe mitral regurgitation (grade 4 by angiography) occurs in about 2% of patients undergoing PMV.[27-29] An undesirable increase in mitral regurgitation (≥2 grades

TABLE 2

Complications of PMV

Institution	Mortality	Severe MR	Embolism/ Stroke	ASD	Tamponade
Mass General	0.5%	2.8%	1.0%	16%	0.8%
Tenon	0.5%	2.8%	3.1%	14%	0.7%
Loma Linda	1.0%	1.0%	1.0%	12%	1.2%
Beth Israel	0.6%	1.4%	2.1%		4.1%
Takeda	0.0%	1.9%	0.6%	12.8%	1.6%
Chang Gung	0.2%	5.2%	2.1%	10.2%	0.2%
George Washington	0.0%	1.4%	1.4%	2.7%	0.7%
Kokura	0.0%	4.8%	0.0%	4.8%	1.9%
Athens University	0.6%	4.5%	0.0%	0.0%	0.0%
North American Multicenter Registry	0.0%	2.4%	1.5%		1.0%
Inoue Balloon Registry	1.4%	3.8%	0.9%	3.1%	1.4%

by angiography) occurred in 12.5% of patients.[27–29] This undesirable increase in mitral regurgitation is well tolerated in most patients. Furthermore, more than half of the patients actually have less mitral regurgitation at follow-up cardiac catheterization. We have demonstrated that the ratio of the EBDA:BSA is the only predictor of increased mitral regurgitation after PMV. The EBDA is calculated using standard geometric formulas. The incidence of mitral regurgitation is lower if balloon sizes are chosen so that EBDA/BSA is ≤4.0 cm^2/m^2. The single balloon technique results in a lower incidence of mitral regurgitation, but provides less relief of mitral stenosis than the double balloon technique. Thus, there is an optimal balloon size between 3.1 and 4.0 cm^2/m^2 that achieves a maximal mitral valve area with a minimal increase in mitral regurgitation.[29]

Left-to-right shunt through the created atrial communication occurred in 3% to 16% of the patients undergoing PMV. The size of the defect is small as reflected in the pulmonary to systemic flow ratio of <2:1 in the majority of patients. Older age, fluoroscopic evidence of mitral valve calcification, higher echocardiographic score, pre-PMV lower cardiac output, and higher pre-PMV NYHA functional class are the factors that predispose patients to develop left-to-right shunt post-PMV.[30] Clinical, echocardiographic, surgical, and hemodynamic follow-up of patients with post-PMV left-to-right shunt demonstrated that the defect closed in 59%. Persistent left-to-right shunt at follow-up is small (QP/QS <2:1) and clinically well tolerated. In the series from the Massachusetts General Hospital there is one patient in whom the atrial shunt remained hemodynamically significant at follow-up. This patient underwent percutaneous transcatheter closure of her atrial defect with a clamshell device. Desideri et al[31] reported atrial shunting determined by color flow transthoracic echocardiography in 61% of 57 patients immediately after PMV. The shunt persisted in 30% of patients at 19±6 (range 9–33) months follow-up.[31] Independent predictors of the persistence of atrial shunt at long-term follow-up include the magnitude of the post-PMV atrial shunt(QP/QS >1.5:1), use of Bifoil balloon (two balloons on one shaft) and smaller post-PMV mitral valve area.

Follow-up

Clinical Follow-up

Follow-up studies after PMV are encouraging.[11,14–17,26,30–36] Following PMV, the majority of patients have marked clinical improvement and become NYHA Class I or II. The symptomatic, echocardiographic, and hemodynamic improvement produced by PMV persists in intermediate and long-term follow-up. The best long-term results are seen in patients with echocardiographic scores ≤8. When PMV produces a good immediate outcome in this group of patients, restenosis is unlikely to occur at follow-up.[11,14–17,26,30–36] Although PMV can result in a good outcome in patients with echocardiographic scores >8, hemodynamic and echocardiographic restenosis is frequently demonstrated at follow-up despite ongoing clinical improvement.[11,14–17,26,30–36]

Table 3 shows long-term follow-up results of patients undergoing PMV at different institutes. We recently reported an estimated 80-month survival rate of 75%±4% in a large cohort of patients undergoing PMV at the Massachusetts General Hospital.[26] Death at follow-up was directly related to age, post-PMV pulmonary artery pressure, pre-PMV NYHA functional class, and the echocardiographic score.

In the same group of patients, the estimated 80-month survival with freedom from mitral valve surgery (mitral valve replacement or mitral valve repair) was 46%±4%. The presence of mitral valve surgery at follow-up was directly related to post-PMV Seller's grade of mitral regurgitation, the history of previous surgical commissurotomy, pre-PMV NYHA class, and post-PMV mitral valve area.

The 80-month estimated event free survival of this patient's cohort (survival with freedom from mitral valve surgery and NYHA functional Class ≥ III) was 43%±4%. Events at follow-up were directly related to age, pre-PMV NYHA Class, post-PMV Seller's grade of mitral regurgitation, history of surgical mitral commissurotomy, post-PMV pulmonary artery pressure, and the echocardiographic score.

TABLE 3

Follow-up After PMV

Institution	Mean Follow-up	Survival	Event-free Survival
Mass General	32 ± 12 (6–84) months	81 ± 5% (7 years)	43 ± 4% (7 years)
Mass General	20 ± 12 (6–49) months	89 ± 5% (4 years)	66 ± 9% (4 years)
Tenon	18 ± 16 (1–72) months	92 ± 5% (4 years)	68 ± 7% (4 years)
Loma Linda	31 ± 22 (1–81) months		76% (6 years)
Beth Israel	36 ± 20 (2–69) months	76 ± 10% (5 years)	51 ± 10% (5 years)

Patients with echocardiographic scores ≤8 have a significantly greater survival, survival with freedom from mitral valve surgery, and event free survival (death, mitral valve surgery and NYHA Class ≥III) than those patients with echocardiographic scores >8. Patients with echocardiographic scores ≤8 have an 83%±6% 80-month survival. At 80 months follow-up, 58%±5% of patients were free of mitral valve surgery and 51%±6% of the patients were free of combined events. In contrast, patients with echocardiographic scores >8 have a 48%±8% 80-month survival. At 80 months follow-up, 25%±5% of patients were free of mitral valve surgery and only 22%±5% of them were free of combined events.[26]

Similar follow-up studies have been reported in other series with the double balloon technique and with the Inoue technique of PMV.[11,14–17,26,30–36] With the Inoue technique of PMV at intermediate long-term follow-up of 51 months, young patients with pliable valves, in sinus rhythm, and with no evidence of calcium under fluoroscopy were free of cardiovascular events. In contrast, 84% of patients with calcified valves and/or severe subvalvular disease were free of cardiovascular events at 48 months follow-up.[15–17] Cohen et al[18] reported the clinical follow-up of 146 patients undergoing PMV. The overall survival rate was 88% at 2 years and 76% at 5 years. Event free survival was 74% at 2 years and 51% at 5 years. Ninety-six percent of patients alive at follow-up were NYHA Class I or II. Independent predictors of longer event free survival were a lower echocardiographic score, lower left ventricular end diastolic pressure, and final mitral valve area post-PMV. Their lower 5-year event free survival can be explained by a larger number of patients with higher echocardiographic scores and mitral valve calcification. Furthermore, in that study 39% of the patients were considered to be high surgical risk candidates due to the presence of important coexisting conditions or advanced age.

Follow-up in the Elderly

Tuzcu et al[14] reported the outcome of PMV in 99 elderly patients (≥65 years of age). A successful outcome (valve area ≥1.5 cm² without ≥2+ increase in mitral regurgitation and without left-to-right shunt of ≥1.5:1) was achieved in 46 patients. The best multivariate predictor of success was the combination of echocardiographic score, NYHA functional class, and inverse of mitral valve area. Patients who had an unsuccessful outcome from PMV were in a higher NYHA functional class, had higher echocardiographic scores, and smaller mitral valve areas pre-PMV compared with those patients who had a successful outcome. Actuarial survival, and combined event free survival at 3 years were significantly better in the successful group. Mean follow-up was 16±1 months. Actuarial survival (79%±7% versus 62%±10%; $P=0.04$); survival without mitral valve replacement (71%±8% versus 41%±8%; $P=0.002$); and event free survival (54%±12% versus 38%±8%; $P=0.01$) at 3 years were significantly better in the successful group of 46 patients than the unsuccessful group of 53 patients. Low echocardiographic score was the independent predictor of survival and lack of mitral valve calcification was the strongest predictor of event free survival.

Follow-up of Patients with Calcified Mitral Valves

The presence of fluoroscopically visible calcification on the mitral valve influences the success of PMV. Patients with heavily (≥3 grades) calcified valves under fluoroscopy have a poorer immediate outcome as reflected in a smaller post-PMV mitral valve area and greater post-PMV mitral valve gradient. Immediate outcome is progressively worse as the calcification becomes more severe. The long-term results of percutaneous mitral balloon valvuloplasty are significantly different in calcified and uncalcified groups and in subgroups of the calcified group.[37] The estimated 2-year survival is significantly lower for patients with calcified mitral valves than for those with uncalcified valves (80% versus 99%). The survival curve becomes worse as the severity of valvular calcification becomes more severe. Freedom from mitral valve replacement at 2 years was significantly lower for patients with calcified valves than for those with uncalcified valves (67% versus 93%). Similarly, the estimated event free survival at 2 years in the calcified group became significantly poorer as the severity of calcification increased. The estimated event free survival at 2 years was significantly lower for the calcified than for the uncalcified group (63% versus 88%). The actuarial survival curves with freedom from combined events at 2 years in the calcified group became significantly poorer as the severity of calcification increased.[37] These findings are in agreement with several follow-up studies of surgical commissurotomy that demonstrate that patients with calcified mitral valves had a poorer survival compared to those patients with uncalcified valves.[38-40]

Follow-up of patients with Previous Surgical Commissurotomy

PMV also has been shown to be a safe procedure in patients with previous surgical mitral commissurotomy.[10,41,42] Although a good immediate outcome is frequently achieved in these patients, follow-up results are not as favorable as those obtained in patients without previous surgical commissurotomy.[41,42] Although there is no difference in mortality between patients with or without a history of previous surgical commissurotomy at 4-year follow-up, the number of patients who required mitral valve replacement (26% versus 8%) and/or were in NYHA Class III or IV (35% versus 13%) was significantly higher among those patients with previous commissurotomy. However, when the patients are carefully selected according to the echocardiographic score (≤ 8), the immediate outcome and the 4-year follow-up results are excellent and similar to those seen in patients without previous surgical commissurotomy.[10,41,42]

Echocardiographic and Hemodynamic Follow-up

Follow-up studies have shown that the incidence of hemodynamic and echocardiographic restenosis is low 2 years after PMV.[11,13,15–17,31] A study of a group of patients undergoing simultaneous clinical evaluation, two-dimensional Doppler echocardiography and transseptal catheterization 2 years after PMV reported 90% of patients in NYHA Classes I and II and 10% of patients in NYHA Class $\geq$ III.[13] In this study, hemodynamic determination of mitral valve area using the Gorlin equation showed a significant decrease in mitral valve area from 2.0 cm^2 immediately after PMV to 1.6 cm^2 at follow-up. However, there was no significant difference between the echocardiographic mitral valve areas immediately after PMV and at follow-up (1.8 cm^2 and 1.6 cm^2, respectively, P=NS). Although there was a significant difference in the mitral valve area immediately after PMV determined by the Gorlin equation and by two-dimensional echocardiography (2.0 cm^2 versus 1.8 cm^2), there was no significant difference between the mitral valve area determined by the Gorlin equation and the echocardiographic calculated mitral valve area (1.6 cm^2 for both) at follow-up. The discrepancy between the two-dimensional echocardiographic and Gorlin equation determined post-PMV mitral valve areas is due to the contribution of left-to-right shunting (undetected by oximery) across the created interatrial communication that results in both an erroneously high cardiac output and an overestimation of the mitral valve area by the Gorlin equation.[43] Desideri et al[31] showed no significant differences in mitral valve area (measured by Doppler echocardiography) at 19$\pm$6 (range 9–33) months follow-up between the post-PMV and follow-up mitral valve areas. Mitral valve areas were 2.2 ± 0.5 cm^2 and 1.9 ± 0.5 cm^2, respectively.[31] Echocardiographic restenosis (mitral valve area ≤ 1.5 cm^2 with $>50\%$ reduction of the gain) was seen in 21% of the patients.[34] Predictors of restenosis included age, smaller post-PMV mitral valve area, and higher echocardiographic score.[31]

With the Inoue technique, Chen et al[16] showed no significant differences in mitral valve area determined by two-dimensional Doppler echocardiography in 85 patients at a mean follow-up of 5 ± 1 years (range 43 to 79 months). Post-PMV and follow-up mitral valve areas were 2.0 ± 0.4 and 1.8 ± 0.5 cm^2, respectively (P=NS).

PMV versus Surgical Mitral Commissurotomy

Results of surgical closed mitral commissurotomy have demonstrated favorable long-term hemodynamic and symptomatic improvement from this technique. A restenosis rate of 4.2 to 11.4 per 1,000 patients per year was reported by John et al[44] in 3,724 patients who underwent surgical closed mitral commissurotomy. Survival after PMV is similar to that reported after surgical mitral commissurotomy. Although freedom from mitral valve replacement (87% versus 92%) and freedom from all events (67% versus 80%) after PMV are lower than reported after surgical commissurotomy,[26,31,39,40,44-52] freedom from both mitral valve replacement and all events in patients with echocardiographic scores ≤ 8 are similar to that reported after surgical mitral commissurotomy.[26,31,39,40,44-52]

Restenosis after both closed and open surgical mitral commissurotomy has been well documented.[44-51] Although surgical closed mitral commissurotomy is uncommonly performed in the United States, it is still used frequently in other countries. Long-term follow-up of 267 patients who underwent surgical transventricular mitral commissurotomy at the Mayo Clinic showed a 79%, 67%, and 55% survival at 10, 15, and 20 years, respectively. Survival with freedom from mitral valve replacement were 57%, 36%, and 24%, respectively.[53] In this study, age, atrial fibrillation, and male gender were independent predictors of death, while mitral valve calcification, cardiomegaly, and mitral regurgitation were independent predictors of repeat mitral valve surgery.[53] Because of similar patient selection and mechanism of mitral valve dilatation, similar long-term results should be expected after PMV. Indeed, prospective, randomized trials comparing PMV and surgical closed mitral commissurotomy have shown no differences in immediate and 3-year follow-up results between both groups of patients.[54-55] Furthermore, restenosis at 3-year follow-up occurred in 10% and 13% of the patients treated with mitral balloon valvuloplasty and surgical commissurotomy, respectively.[55] Results of randomized clinical trials comparing PMV and surgical open commissurotomy show similar results.

Conclusion

PMV produces a good immediate outcome and good clinical long-term follow-up results in a high percentage of patients with mitral stenosis. Patients with echocardiographic scores ≤8 have the best results, particularly if they are young, are in sinus rhythm, and have no evidence of calcification of the mitral valve under fluoroscopy. The immediate and long-term results of PMV in this group of patients are similar to those reported after surgical mitral commissurotomy. Patients with echocardiographic scores >8 have only a 50% chance of obtaining a successful hemodynamic result with PMV, and long-term follow-up results are less good than those from patients with echocardiographic scores ≤8. In patients with echocardiographic scores ≥12 it is unlikely that PMV could produce good immediate or long-term result. They preferably should undergo open heart surgery. However, PMV could be performed in these patients if they are not surgical candidates. Surgical therapy for mitral stenosis should be reserved for patients who have ≥2 grades of Seller's mitral regurgitation by angiography, which can be better treated by mitral valve repair and for those patients with severe mitral valve thickening and calcification or with significant subvalvular scarring to warrant valve replacement.

References

1. Inoue K, Owaki T, Nakamura T, Kitamura F, Miyamoto N. Clinical application of transvenous mitral commissurotomy by a new balloon catheter. *J Thorac Cardiovasc Surg.* 1984;87:394–402.
2. Lock JE, Kalilullah M, Shrivastava S, Bahl V, Keane JF. Percutaneous catheter commissurotomy in rheumatic mitral stenosis. *N Engl J Med.* 1985;313:1515–1518.
3. Palacios I, Block PC, Brandi S, et al. Percutaneous balloon valvotomy for patients with severe mitral stenosis. *Circulation.* 1987;75:778–784.
4. Al Zaibag M, Ribeiro PA, Al Kassab SA, Al Fagig MR. Percutaneous double balloon mitral valvotomy for rheumatic mitral stenosis. *Lancet.* 1986;1:757–761.
5. Vahanian A, Michel PL, Cormier B, et al. Results of percutaneous mitral commissurotomy in 200 patients. *Am J Cardiol.* 1989;63:847–852.

6. McKay RG, Lock JE, Safian RD, et al. Balloon dilatation of mitral stenosis in adults patients: postmortem and percutaneous mitral valvuloplasty studies. *J Am Coll Cardiol.* 1987;9:723–731.
7. McKay CR, Kawanishi DT, Rahimtoola SH. Catheter balloon valvuloplasty of the mitral valve in adults using a double balloon technique. Early hemodynamic results. *JAMA.* 1987;257:1753–1761.
8. Abascal VM, O'Shea JP, Wilkins GT, et al. Prediction of successful outcome in 130 patients undergoing percutaneous balloon mitral valvotomy. *Circulation.* 1990;82:448–456.
9. Herrman HC, Wilkins GT, Abascal VM, Weyman AE, Block PC, Palacios IF. Percutaneous balloon mitral valvotomy for patients with mitral stenosis: analysis of factors influencing early results. *J Thorac Cardiovasc Surg.* 1988;96:33–38.
10. Rediker DE, Block PC, Abascal VM, Palacios IF. Mitral balloon valvuloplasty for mitral restenosis after surgical commissurotomy. *J Am Coll Cardiol.* 1988;2:252–256.
11. Palacios IF, Block PC, Wilkins GT, Weyman AE. Follow-up of patients undergoing percutaneous mitral balloon valvotomy: analysis of factors determining restenosis. *Circulation.* 1989;79:573–579.
12. Abascal VM, Wilkins GT, Choong CY, Palacios IF, Block PC, Weyman AE. Echocardiographic evaluation of mitral valve structure and function in patients followed for at least 6 months after percutaneous balloon mitral valvuloplasty. *J Am Coll Cardiol.* 1988;12:606–615.
13. Block PC, Palacios IF, Block EH, Tuzcu EM, Griffin B. Late (two year) follow-up after percutaneous mitral balloon valvotomy. *Am J Cardiol.* 1992;69:537–541.
14. Tuzcu EM, Block PC, Griffin BP, Newell JB, Palacios IF. Immediate and long term outcome of percutaneous mitral valvotomy in patients 65 years and older. *Circulation.* 1992;85;963–971.
15. Nobuyoshi M, Hamasaki N, Kimura T, et al. Indications, complications, and short term clinical outcome of percutaneous transvenous mitral commissurotomy. *Circulation.* 1989;80:782–792.
16. Chen CR, Cheng TO, Chen JY, Zhou YL, Mei J, Ma TZ. Percutaneous mitral valvuloplasty with the Inoue balloon catheter. *Am J Cardiol.* 1992;70:1455–1458.
17. Hung JS, Chern MS, Wu JJ, et al. Short and long term results of catheter balloon percutaneous transvenous mitral commissurotomy. *Am J Cardiol.* 1991;67:854–862.
18. Cohen DJ, Kuntz RE, Gordon SPF, et al. Predictors of long-term outcome after percutaneous mitral valvuloplasty. *N Engl J Med.* 1991;327:1329–1335.
19. Babic UU, Pejcić P, Djurisic Z, et al. Percutaneous transarterial balloon valvuloplasty for mitral valve stenosis. *Am J Cardiol.* 1986;57:1101.
20. Stefanides C, Kouroklis C, Stratos C, Pitsavos C, Tentolouris C, Toutouzas P. Percutaneous balloon mitral valvuloplasty by retrograde left atrial catheterization. *Am J Cardiol.* 1990;65:650–654.
21. Stefanides C, Stratos C, Pitsavos C, et al. Retrograde nontransseptal balloon mitral valvuloplasty. Immediate results and long term follow-up. *Circulation.* 1992;85:1760–1767.
22. Palacios IF, Lock JE, Keane JF, Block PC. Percutaneous transvenous balloon valvotomy in a patient with severe calcific mitral stenosis. *J Am Coll Cardiol.* 1986;7:1416.

23. Block PC, Palacios IF, Jacobs M, et al. The mechanism of successful percutaneous mitral valvotomy in humans. *Am J Cardiol.* 1987;59:178.
24. Wilkins GT, Weyman AE, Abascal VM, Block PC, Palacios IF. Percutaneous mitral valvotomy: an analysis of echocardiographic variables related to outcome and the mechanism of dilatation. *Br Heart J.* 1988;60: 299–308.
25. Ruiz CE, Zhang HP, Macaya C, et al. Comparison of Inoue-single balloon versus double balloon techniques for percutaneous mitral valvotomy. *Am Heart J.* 1992;123:942–947.
26. Palacios IF, Block PC, Harrell L, Fisher G, Weyman AE. Long term follow up of patients undergoing percutaneous mitral balloon valvotomy: The Massachusetts General Hospital Experience. *Circulation.* 1993;88: I-340.
27. Abascal VM, Wilkins GT, Choong CY, Block PC, Palacios IF, Weyman AE. Mitral regurgitation after percutaneous mitral valvuloplasty in adults: evaluation by pulsed Doppler echocardiography. *J Am Coll Cardiol.* 1988;2:257–263.
28. The National Heart, Lung and Blood Institute Balloon Valvuloplasty Registry Complications and Mortality of Percutaneous Balloon Mitral Commissurotomy. *Circulation.* 1992;85:2014–2024.
29. Roth RB, Block PC, Palacios IF. Predictors of increased mitral regurgitation after percutaneous mitral balloon valvotomy. *Cathet Cardiovasc Diagn.* 1990;20:17–21.
30. Casale P, Block PC, O'Shea JP, Palacios IF. Atrial septal defect after percutaneous mitral balloon valvuloplasty: immediate results and follow-up. *J Am Coll Cardiol.* 1990;15:1300–1304.
31. Desideri A, Vanderperren O, Serra A, et al. Long term (9 to 33 months) echocardiographic follow-up after successful percutaneous mitral commissurotomy. *Am J Cardiol.* 1992;69:1602–1606.
32. Palacios IF, Tuzcu EM, Newell JB, Block PC. Four year clinical follow-up of patients undergoing percutaneous mitral balloon valvotomy. *Circulation.* 1990;(Suppl III):545.
33. Babic UU, Grujicic S, Popovic Z, et al. Percutaneous transarterial balloon dilatation of the mitral valve. Five year experience. *Br Heart J.* 1992;67:185–189.
34. The National Heart, Lung and Blood Institute Balloon Valvuloplasty Registry Participants. Multicenter experience with balloon mitral commissurotomy. NHLBI balloon valvuloplasty registry report on immediate and 30 day follow-up results. *Circulation.* 1992;85:448–461.
35. Pan M, Medina A, de Lezo JS, et al. Factors determinig late success after mitral balloon valvotomy. *Am J Cardiol.* 1993;71:1181–1185.
36. Herrmann HC, Kleaveland P, Hill JA, et al. The M-heart percutaneous balloon mitral valvuloplasty registry: initial results and early follow up. *J Am Coll Cardiol.* 1990;15:1221.
37. Tuzcu EM, Block PC, Griffin B, Dinsmore R, Newell JB, Palacios IF. Percutaneous mitral balloon valvuloplasty in patients with calcific mitral stenosis: immediate and long-term outcome. *J Am Coll Cardiol.* In press.
38. Harken DE, Ellis LB, Ware PF. The surgical treatment of mitral stenosis. I. Valvuloplasty. *N Engl J Med.* 1948;239:801.
39. Williams JA, Littmann D, Warren R. Experience with the surgical treatment of mitral stenosis. *N Engl J Med.* 1958;258:623–630.

40. Scannell JG, Burke JF, Saidi F, Turner JD. Five-year follow-up study of closed mitral valvotomy. *J Thorac Cardiovasc Surg.* 1960;40:723–730.
41. Medina A, Delezo JS, Hernandez E, et al. Balloon valvuloplasty for mitral restenosis after previous surgery. A comparative study. *Am Heart J.* 1990;120:568–571.
42. Davidson CJ, Bashore TM, Mickel M, et al. Balloon mitral commissurotomy after previous surgical commissurotomy. *Circulation.* 1992; 86:91–99.
43. Petrossian GA, Tuzcu EM, Ziskind AA, Block PC, Palacios IF. Atrial septal occlusion improves the accuracy of mitral valve area determination following percutaneous mitral balloon valvotomy. *Cathet Cardiovasc Diagn.* 1991;22:21–24.
44. John S, Bashi VV, Jairaj PS, et al. Closed mitral valvotomy: early results and long term follow up of 3724 patients. *Circulation.* 1983;68: 891 896.
45. Ellis LR, Harken DE, Black H. A clinical study of 1,000 consecutive cases of mitral stenosis two to nine years after mitral valvuloplasty. *Circulation.* 1959;19:803.
46. Elis FH, Kirklin JW, Parker RL, et al. Mitral commissurotomy; an overall appraisal of clinical and hemodynamic results. *Arch Intern Med.* 1954;94:774.
47. Hoeksema TD, Wallace RB, Kirklin JVV. Closed mitral commissurotomy. *Am J Cardiol.* 1966;17:825–828.
48. Kirklin JW. Percutaneous balloon versus surgical closed commissurotomy for mitral stenosis. *Circulation.* 1991;83:1450–1451.
49. Higgs LM, Glancy DL, O'Brien KP, Epstein SE, Morrow AG. Mitral restenosis: an uncommon cause of recurrent symptoms following mitral commissurotomy *Am J Cardiol.* 1970;26:34–37.
50. Glover RP, Davila JC, O'Neil TJE, Janton OH. Does mitral stenosis recur after commissurotomy? *Circulation.* 1955;11:14–28.
51. Hickey MSJ, Blackstone EH, Kirklin JW, Dean LS. Outcome probabilities and life history after surgical mitral commissurotomy: implications for balloon commissurotomy. *J Am Coll Cardiol.* 1991;17:29–42.
52. Scalia D, Rizzoli G, Campanile F, et al. Long-term results of mitral commissurotomy. *J Thorac Cardiovas Surg.* 1993;105:633–642.
53. Rihal CS, Schaff HV, Frye RL, et al. Long-term follow-up of patients undergoing closed transventricular mitral commissurotomy: a useful surrogate for percutaneous balloon mitral valvuloplasty. *J Am Coll Cardiol.* 1992;20:781–786.
54. Turi ZG, Reyes VP, Raju BS, et al. Percutaneous balloon versus surgical closed commissurotomy for mitral stenosis: a prospective, randomized trial. *Circulation.* 1991;83:1179–1185.
55. Turi ZG, Raju BS, Raju R, et al. Percutaneous balloon versus surgical mitral commissurotomy: three year follow-up of a randomized trial. *Circulation.* 1993;88:I 339.

Chapter 26

Cardiac Transplant Coronary Artery Disease:
Angiography and Interventions

George W. Vetrovec, MD

In the first year after cardiac transplantation, patient survival is determined by rejection, perisurgical complications, and infection. However, in subsequent years the risk of mortality is predominantly related to the relatively rapid development of transplant coronary artery disease and subsequent ischemic complications.[1-5] Transplant patients develop atherosclerosis of predominantly two types: proximal disease similar to typical atherosclerotic coronary disease plus a distal arteriopathy identified by irregular, often pruned or bluntly occluded vessels. The accelerated development of coronary artery disease is thought to be immunologically mediated vascular injury and to occur distinct from steroids, variations, and immunosuppression and/or lipids.[6] This chapter addresses the angiographic and intravascular ultrasound methods of diagnosis and the results of strategies to prevent or treat transplant atherosclerotic coronary artery disease.

Anatomical Definitions

Transplant coronary artery disease is common and is distinguished from typical atherosclerotic coronary artery disease by being more diffuse and involving distal, small vessels. Gao et al[6] have published the most extensive description of angiographically identified coronary artery disease in cardiac transplant patients. These authors define specific angiographic descriptions of transplant coronary artery disease (Figure 1) based on frequently recognized

From Vetrovec GW, Carabello BA, (eds.) *Invasive Cardiology: Current Diagnostic and Therapeutic Issues.* Armonk, NY: Futura Publishing Company, Inc.: © 1996.

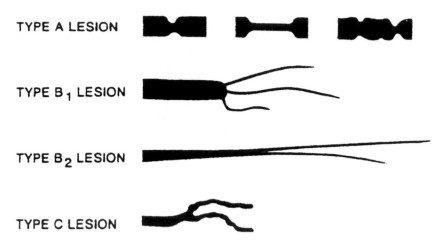

FIGURE 1. *Gao classification of cardiac transplant coronary disease. (Reproduced with permission from Reference 6.)*

anatomical abnormalities. These definitions define the more diffuse nature of transplant coronary artery disease, particularly involving distal vessels (types B_1, B_2, and C). Based on these definitions, the incidence of angiographically documented coronary artery disease ranged from 33% in patients on average 2.5 years posttransplant, to 42% in patients >5 years posttransplantation. Overall, more than 90% of patients have angiographic evidence of coronary artery disease by 5 years posttransplant (Figures 2 and 3).

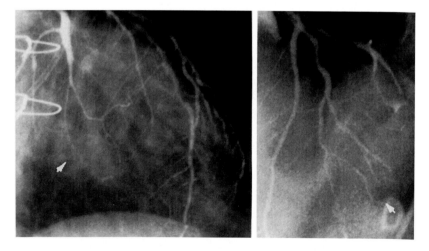

FIGURE 2. *Diffuse distal small vessel disease seen in the terminal posterior descending artery (**left**) and diagonal branches (**right**).*

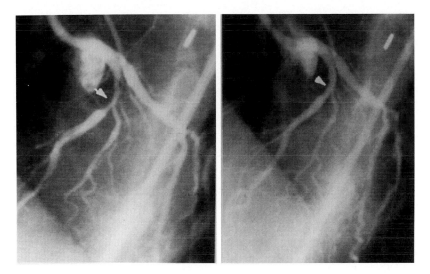

FIGURE 3. *Pre- and postballoon angioplast result for proximal left anterior descending and diagonal obstructions in a heart-lung transplant recipient. These lesions are chararcteristic of the more typical nontransplant, atherosclerotic coronary artery disease.*

Pathologic Correlations

The true incidence of transplant coronary disease is significantly greater when defined by light microscopy. This is based on pathologic evidence of the presence of vascular abnormalities in transplanted hearts whose recipients were autopsied a minimum of 14 months, but generally longer (mean 52 months) posttransplant.[4] Furthermore, Johnson et al[4] noted that type A lesions tended to be more lipid-rich, typical atherosclerotic lesions, while type B_1, B_2, and C represent more diffuse disease and appear much more fibrotic. Thus, the type A lesions appear to be more typical of nontransplant atherosclerotic coronary artery disease, presenting anatomically as predominantly proximal lesions, and presenting pathologically as lipid-rich. Furthermore, type A lesions were more commonly associated with thrombus and/or thrombotic occlusion, compared with distal lesions. Of transplant patients with angiographic coronary artery disease, 75% have one or more type A lesions. In contrast, type B_1, B_2 and C lesions are angiographically distinctive for transplant disease, are frequently seen earlier than type A lesions, and are universally identified in angiograms of transplant patients who develop coronary artery disease.

Coronary Collaterals

Despite diffuse, frequently occlusive transplant arteriopathy, collaterals are infrequent. Overall, 92% of occluded transplant vessels had absent or minimal angiographic collaterals compared with absence of collaterals in only 7% of nontransplant patients. Bajaj et al[7] have recently described a frequent "myocardial blush" pattern of collaterals associated with diffuse small vessel disease in transplant patients. Although less frequent than in nontransplanted coronary artery disease, type A lesions were more commonly associated with mature collaterals. These investigators suggested that microvascular ischemia may induce an angiogenic response to the diffuse distal arteriopathy, which is visualized angiographically as a contrast blush.

Nonangiographic Diagnosis of Transplant Coronary Artery Disease

Intravascular ultrasound provides an opportunity to assess early intimal changes in vivo. Investigators[8,9] have shown that intimal thickening occurs commonly by 1 year posttransplant and often before coronary angiographic abnormalities are present. Furthermore, other investigators[10] have demonstrated early intimal dysfunction measured by intracoronary acetylcholine testing performed 1 year after transplant in segments without evidence of intimal thickening on intravascular ultrasound.

Although intimal thickening progresses in severity and prevalence over time, even at 5 years posttransplantation, endothelial function is frequently normal even in thickened segments.[10] The latter suggests a reparative process of endothelial function despite intimal proliferation, which the authors[10] postulate may be normalized endothelial function resulting from episodic immune injury and subsequent healing. The impact of these findings in future preventive treatment is yet unknown, although the possibility exists that the response to immune injury may be modulated by more typical atherosclerotic risk factors.

Presentations of Transplant Ischemia

Although cardiac transplant coronary disease is frequent and often severe and diffuse, traditional angina symptoms are uncommon.[11] However, autonomic reinnervation occurs to varying degrees and, thus, some transplant patients develop angina.[12] More commonly, transplant coronary disease is diagnosed by routine screening, angiography, or by sequelae such as congestive heart failure secondary to ischemia or infarct-related myocardial damage. Noninvasive screening tests for ischemia are typically less reliable than in the nontransplant population.[13] However, recent studies using dobutamine echocardiography may provide more reliable information.[14]

Coronary spasm with typical transient ST segment elevations has been reported.[15] Although the pathophysiological mechanism of spasm in such patients is unknown, one expects that spasm occurs at sites with intimal abnormalities, even in the absence of coronary angiographic obstructive disease. Similar theories have been suggested as a mechanism for coronary artery spasm in patients without prior cardiac transplantation.

Prevention of Transplant Coronary Artery Disease

The prevention of transplant coronary artery disease, using the usual risk factor management for atherosclerosis, has been disappointing. Furthermore, even with advances in immunosuppression, coronary atherosclerosis remains a significant component of late clinical events in cardiac transplant patients. Recent reports[16,17] suggest that calcium channel blocking agents may retard the development of coronary vascular disease. Schroeder et al[16] reported minimal decreases in coronary artery luminal diameter in patients treated with diltiazem compared with transplant patients not receiving a calcium channel blocker. Over a 2-year follow-up period, patients who did not receive calcium channel blockers were more than twice as likely to develop new lesions, as well as lesions >50% diameter stenosis compared with treated patients. Finally, major events potentially attributable to coronary vascular disease (death, retransplantation) were also less frequent in diltiazem-treated patients.

Sheehan et al[17] reported a nearly 50% reduction in angiographic evidence of transplant coronary artery disease in patients treated with calcium channel blockers (predominantly nifidipine). The effect appeared to be principally in retarding diffuse disease development rather than preventing focal narrowings. Compounding atherosclerotic risk factors in both studies were relatively equal between groups, and thus, do not appear to account for these observations. These studies on transplant coronary artery disease are consistent with prior investigations that reveal a reduction in new coronary lesions in patients with nontransplant atherosclerosis.[18] More studies will be required to definitively document the benefit of calcium channel blocking agents in transplant coronary artery disease prevention, but current observations are encouraging.

Applications of Angioplasty

Attempts to treat transplant coronary atherosclerosis directly include bypass surgery, angioplasty, atherectomy, and retransplantation. The greatest experience in treating transplant coronary artery disease has been with percutaneous transluminal coronary angioplasty.[19-21] Halle et al[20] reported the largest experience in a multicenter, consecutive patient series from 11 transplant centers. In that report, 51 angioplasty procedures were performed in 35 patients, predominantly for angiographic evidence of coronary disease or documented ischemia. Dilated lesions were generally proximal and angiographically appeared similar to usual atherosclerotic coronary artery disease. Angiographic success ($\leq 50\%$ residual stenosis) was seen in 93% of lesions. One patient died immediately postprocedure. At follow-up, an average of 13 months postprocedure, 66% were alive without major vascular-related events. A major predictor of a favorable late outcome appears to be the absence of diffuse distal disease at the time of angioplasty.

Data on atherectomy is limited and does not suggest a major benefit over balloon angioplasty. Similarly, few patients have undergone elective bypass surgery posttransplantation, limiting any significant assessment of results. However, intuitively it would appear that the higher incidence of diffuse distal disease in transplant coronary artery disease might adversely affect a prolonged graft patency secondary to reduced distal flow.

Whether or not revascularization procedures affect long-term outcome is difficult to assess because the number of treated patients is small and multiple factors may affect outcome in patients with revascularization versus those not revascularized. Some interventional procedures have been performed to provide "vascular" stability while awaiting retransplantation. Overall, it would appear that angioplasty is best suited for those patients with proximal, relatively focal coronary disease with limited or absence of distal diffuse disease. In such patients an excellent short-term survival can be anticipated.

Summary

Coronary vascular disease remains a critical issue in the late outcome for cardiac transplant patients. This coronary vascular disease is diffuse, often occurring in the first year posttransplantation and is identified earliest in vivo by intravascular ultrasound. Angiographic disease recognition is less sensitive, but effectively identifies a frequent distal, diffuse small vessel disease component often associated with an angiographic blush phenomenon in the absence of usual collaterals, which are infrequently seen in transplant coronary disease. Endothelial activity may be abnormal early, but appears to potentially recover over time even in the setting of the development of diffuse intravascular thickening. The importance of endothelial dysfunction in the overall manifestation and management of transplant disease is undergoing further investigation.

From a preventive standpoint, routine treatment of atherosclerosis and changing immunosuppression seem to have had little impact on the development of transplant coronary disease. In contrast, recent reports suggest the possibility of a reduction in the development of new lesions with the use of calcium channel blocking agents. Finally, revascularization procedures, particularly coronary angioplasty, appear to be angiographically effective and associated with a good prognosis in those patients undergoing dilatation in the absence of diffuse distal disease. The issue of transplant coronary disease remains important as long-term outcome of transplant patients is clearly coupled with the high incidence of accelerated coronary vascular disease.

References

1. Jamieson SW, Oyer PE, Baldwin J, et al. Heart transplantation for end-stage ischemic heart disease: The Stanford experience. *Heart Transplantation*. 1984;3:224–227.
2. Bieber CP, Hunt SA, Schwinn DA. Complications in long-term survivors of cardiac transplantation. *Transplantation Proc*. 1981;8:207–211.
:3. Miller LW. Long-term complications of cardiac transplantation. *Prog Cardiovasc Dis*. 1991;33:229–282.
4. Johnson DE, Alderman EL, Schroeder JS, et al. Transplant coronary artery disease: histopathologic correlations with angiographic morphology. *J Am Coll Cardiol*. 1991;17(2):449–457.
5. O'Neill BF, Pflugfelder PM, Singh NR, et al. Frequency of angiographic detection and quantitative assessment of coronary arterial disease one and three years after cardiac transplantation. *Am J Cardiol*. 1989;63:1221–1226.
6. Gao S, Alderman EL, Schoeder JS, et al. Accelerated coronary vascular disease in the heart transplantation patient: coronary arteriographic findings. *J Am Coll Cardiol*. 1988;12(2):334–340.
7. Bajaj S, Shah A, Crandall C, et al. Coronary collateral circulation in the transplanted heart. *Circulation*. 1993;88(5)263–269.
8. Pinto FJ, St Goar FG, Fischell TA, et al. Nitroglycerin-induced coronary vasodilation in cardiac transplant recipients: evaluation with in vivo intracoronary ultrasound. *Circulation*. 1992;85:69–77.

9. St. Goar FG, Pinto FJ, Alderman EL, et al. Intracoronary ultrasound in cardiac transplant recipients: in vivo evidence of "angiographically silent" intimal thickening. *Circulation.* 1992;85:979–987.
10. Anderson TJ, Meredith IT, Uehata A, et al. Functional significance of intimal thickening as detected by intravascular ultrasound early and late after cardiac transplantation. *Circulation.* 1993;88(3):1093–1100.
11. Gao SZ, Schroeder JS, Hunt SA, et al. Acute myocardial infarction in cardiac transplant recipients. *Am J Cardiol.* 1989;64:1093–1097.
12. Stark RP, McGinn AL, Wilson RF. Chest pain in cardiac transplant recipients: evidence of sensory reinnervation after cardiac transplantation. *N Engl J Med.* 1991;324:1791–1794.
13. Smart FW, Ballantyne CM,. Cocanougher B, et al. Insensitivity of non-invasive tests to detect coronary artery vasculopathy after heart transplant. *Am J Cardiol.* 1991;67:243–247.
14. Akosah KO, Mohanty PK, Funai JT, et al. Non-invasive detection of transplant coronary artery disease by dobutamine stress echocardiography. *J Heart Lung Transplant.* In press.
15. Kushwaha JS, Mitchell AG, Yacoub MH. Coronary artery spasm after cardiac transplantation. *Am J Cardiol.* 1990;65:1515–1518.
16. Schroeder JS, Gao S, Alderman EL, et al. A preliminary study of diltiazem in the prevention of coronary artery disease in heart-transplant recipients. *N Engl J Med.* 1993;328(3):164–170.
17. Sheehan H, Vetrovec G, Graham S, et al. Calcium channel antagonists protect against the development of coronary artery disease following cardiac transplant. *J Am Coll Cardiol.* 1991;17(2):290A.
18. Lichtlen PR, Hugenholtz PG, Rafflenbeul W, et al. Retardation of angiographic progression of coronary artery disease by nifedipine: results of the International Nifedipine Trial on Antiatherosclerotic Therapy (INTACT). *Lancet.* 1990;335:1109–1113.
19. Vetrovec, GW, Cowley MJ, Newton CM, et al. Applications of percutaneous transluminal coronary angioplasty in cardiac transplantation. *Circulation.* 1988;98(suppl III):III-83–III-86.
20. Halle AA, Wilson RF, Massin EK, et al. Coronary angioplasty in cardiac transplant patients: results of a multicenter study. *Circulation.* 1992;86(2):458–462.
21. Halle AA, DiSciascio G, Wilson RF, et al. PTCA, directional atherectomy and coronary artery bypass surgery in cardiac transplant patients: multicenter findings. *J Am Coll Cardiol.* 1993;21(2):333A.

Chapter 27

Percutaneous Strategies for Management of Angina Pectoris After Coronary Bypass Surgery

John S. Douglas, Jr, MD

The treatment of recurrent symptoms of myocardial ischemia after coronary artery bypass surgery (CABG) remains one of the most difficult problems in contemporary cardiology. The frequency of this clinical malady relates to the huge pool of postsurgical patients, the progressive nature of the atherosclerotic process, and the abbreviated functional life span of veins interposed in the arterial circulation. This chapter focuses on the problem of recurrent angina pectoris after CABG, and the application of percutaneous revascularization strategies in its management.

Recurrent Angina Pectoris

Angina pectoris has been reported to recur in 4%–8% of patients annually after coronary bypass surgery.[1] This loss of the major palliative effect of the operative procedure was most often attributed to saphenous vein graft dysfunction that has been noted in over 5% of grafts before hospital discharge, about 20% within the first year, and 1%–2% per year for the next 6 years. In addition, significant new native coronary artery disease has been reported to occur in 5% of patients annually. Although arterial grafts are reported to have excellent long-term patency, perianastomotic stenoses and occlusions have been seen frequently in clinical practice (Figure 1). Whether the apparent higher than expected failure rate of arterial grafts is related to proliferation of cardiac surgical services (and reduced surgical expertise), or pressure felt by sur-

From Vetrovec GW, Carabello BA, (eds.) *Invasive Cardiology: Current Diagnostic and Therapeutic Issues.* Armonk, NY: Futura Publishing Company, Inc.; © 1996.

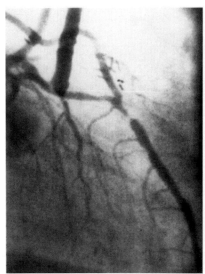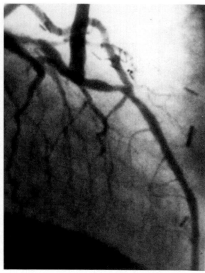

FIGURE 1. *Angina recurred within 2 months after coronary bypass surgery in a 38-year-old male. Coronary arteriography showed severe stenosis of the left anterior descending artery beyond left internal mammary artery insertion (**left,** right anterior oblique view). This lesion, which was clearly in the native left anterior descending coronary artery, was not present before surgery. Balloon angioplasty was successful (**right**). Restenosis occurred 4 months later and repeat angioplasty was successful. Follow-up catheterization 7 months later showed patent grafts and angioplasty site and the patient remained free of ischemic symptoms.*

geons to use marginally adequate arterial conduits, or perhaps placement of arterial grafts in vessels with noncritical stenoses cannot be determined.

Recurrent angina pectoris has resulted in increasing need for repeat revascularization procedures. At Emory University Hospital, reoperative CABG accounted for 5.4% of coronary surgery in 1982–1984, but 9.8% in 1985–1987, 13% in 1988–1990, and 15% in 1991–1992. Among 3,481 patients who underwent a first coronary bypass operation between 1978 and 1981 at Emory University Hospital, and were followed 12 years after CABG, 30% required reoperation.[2] Freedom from percutaneous transluminal coronary angioplasty (PTCA) at 5, 10, and 12 years was 0.98, 0.88, and 0.78, respectively. As the pool of postsurgical patients grows and ages, and as percutaneous methods evolve and mature, an increased use of percutaneous strategies is expected to relieve recurrent myocardial ischemia. Of special interest will be the impact of the increasing numbers of pediatric patients undergoing coronary artery surgical procedures for the treatment of Kawasaki's disease, coronary anomalies, and complex congenital heart disease. We recently intervened percutaneously to relieve postoperative ischemic symptoms in patients age 5 (correction of anomalous left coronary artery from pulmonary artery) and age 11 (coronary bypass for Kawasaki's disease).

Selection of revascularization strategies in postoperative patients has been encumbered by the well-known increased risk of reoperative coronary surgery. Even in the most experienced surgical centers, in-hospital death and nonfatal Q wave myocardial infarction rates were three times that of first operations[3] and reports of mortality rates of 7%–10% are not unusual. In addition, in the Cleveland Clinic experience, angina relief was less complete and graft patency at 5 years was 65% for saphenous vein grafts, and 88% for internal mammary artery grafts in patients who were recatheterized.[3] These observations and the unavoidable narrowing of therapeutic options accompanying each surgical procedure have caused most cardiologists to postpone reoperative surgery if safe, effective therapeutic options are available. In addition, there are many symptomatic patients with contraindications to surgery (pulmonary and renal failure, malignancy, advanced age) who are candidates for PTCA. Others with patent arterial grafts, limited myocardium in jeopardy, absence of venous or arterial conduits may also be approached percutaneously. In 1992, 467 patients who had had previous surgical revascularization underwent percutaneous intervention at Emory University Hospital, accounting for 27% of total percutaneous coronary interventions. In one-half of these patients, the site undergoing percutaneous intervention was in a saphenous vein graft.

Indications for Percutaneous Intervention

Patients who experience a recurrence of symptoms after coronary bypass surgery may have ischemia producing lesions in native coronary arteries, vein grafts, and/or arterial grafts. Selection for PTCA must be based on a careful analysis of multiple factors including the likelihood of a successful procedure, risk of complications, and probability of long-term symptomatic benefit compared to other options, specifically medical therapy and reoperation. The selection of percutaneous methods and the relative effectiveness of each are commonly influenced by the time that has elapsed since the coronary bypass operation. Consequently, indications for intervention will be discussed relative to postoperative interval.

Recurrent Angina Within One Year

The patient with recurrent symptoms within a few days or weeks of surgery commonly has venous graft thrombosis or stenosis at a graft-artery anastomotic site. Less commonly, an incomplete revascularization was achieved due to distal disease, inaccessible intramyocardial vessels, or bypass of the wrong vessel. Focal anastomotic lesions of arterial or venous grafts have been safely dilated in our experience even a few days postoperatively, but balloon sizing should be conservative. If a vein or arterial graft is thrombosed or if a functionally important vessel was not bypassed, the native vessel stenosis should be the target for intervention if possible. If the native vessel is not a reasonable target, angioplasty of the thrombosed graft is occasionally effective. Unfortunately, intragraft and systemic thrombolytic therapy within a few days of surgery has been complicated by significant mediastinal bleeding in about one-third of patients. Emergency percutaneous revascularization has been reported to be lifesaving in the presence of cardiogenic shock due to perioperative graft occlusion.

Percutaneous methods can be quite effective in the group of patients with recurrent angina between 1 month and 1 year after surgery. Lesions at the distal anastomosis of saphenous vein or internal mammary artery grafts are commonly the cause of ischemia in this time period, and these lesions can be dilated with very low procedural risk and excellent long-term patency. However, lesions occurring at the aortic anastomosis of vein grafts have more elastic recoil and a higher restenosis rate with balloon angioplasty in our experience. Directional atherectomy, excimer laser angioplasty, and placement of Palmaz-Schatz stents have been effective at this site.[4–16] Lesions appearing in the midportion of venous grafts within a year of surgery are due to intimal fibrous hyperplasia (or extrinsic compression due to mediastinal fibrosis) and balloon dilatation (Table 1) or directional atherectomy can be performed safely, but recurrences are relatively common. The risk of distal embolization at this time after surgery is quite low with either strategy. More favorable outcome has been obtained with the use of the Palmaz-Schatz stent. Although excellent initial and long-term results have been obtained with angioplasty of anastomotic lesions in arterial grafts, the outcome of angioplasty at other internal mammary artery graft sites is unknown. Short-segment total occlusions of internal mammary artery grafts are uncommon, but in a limited experience, successful dilatation has been possible.[17] These discrete segmental occlusions can be visualized only by meticulous attention to late filming in order to demonstrate passage of contrast down the graft to the site of occlusion.

TABLE 1

Balloon Angioplasty of Aortocoronary Saphenous Vein Grafts. Reports of ≥50 Patients.

Author (Date)	Reference	Successful PTCA (%)	Coronary Emboli	Emergency CABG	Death	AMI Q	AMI Non-Q
Douglas et al (1983)	7	58/62 (94)	0	1	0	1	0
Douglas et al (1986)	8	216/235 (92)	7 (3%)	3 (1.3%)	0	1	—
Cote et al (1987)	9	86/101 (85)	2 (2%)	1	0	1	—
Pinkerton et al (1988)	10	93/100 (93)	—	—	—	—	—
Dorros et al (1988)	11	44/53 (83)	3 (6%)	—	1	1	—
Reed et al (1989)	12	47/52 (90)	0	—	0	0	0
Platko et al (1989)	13	92/101 (92)	—	4 (4%)	1	—	—
Plokker et al (1991)	14	409/454 (90)	—	6 (1.3%)	3 (0.7%)	—	—
Douglas et al (1991)	15	539/599 (90)	—	21 (3.5%)	7 (1.2%)	15 (2.5%)	—
Miranda et al (1992)	16	410/440 (93)	—	+	5 (1.1%)	+	+

+A total of 19 patients (5%) had AMI, urgent CABG, or in-hospital death.

Recurrent Angina After One Year

When angina recurs more than a year following CABG, culprit lesions are frequently present in native coronary arteries or graft conduits that are suitable for PTCA. When it is feasible, PTCA of native coronary arteries is preferred due to lower restenosis rates. For saphenous vein graft lesions appearing within 3 years of surgery, the risk of vein graft embolism complicating PTCA is low, except in the presence of hypercholesterolemia and/or diabetes. Vein graft lesions appearing more than 3 years after surgery frequently have atheromatous elements and angioplasty related coronary embolism (documented by creatine kinase elevation) is seen in 10%–20% of patients overall. Atherosclerotic lesions in saphenous vein grafts contain foam cells, cholesterol clefts, blood elements, and necrotic debris with less fibrous tissue and calcification than is present in native coronary arteries. Atherosclerotic lesions in older saphenous vein grafts are frequently larger and more friable than native coronary artery lesions and thrombus formation is common. Predictors of vein graft embolization in our experience include the presence of lesion-associated thrombus, eccentricity, irregular surface or lesion ulceration and diffuse disease in the vein graft.[18] In vein grafts in place for over 5 years, selection for percutaneous intervention must be made with the awareness that the entire lesion may embolize. Consequently, vein grafts with large atheroma mass are poor candidates for intervention. Elastic recoil is frequently noted following balloon angioplasty of vein grafts and improved initial luminal results have been reported with stent placement and with directional atherectomy. Results with the Palmaz-Schatz stent are particularly promising (Figure 2) with restenosis rates in de novo midvein graft sites of approximately 20% at 6 months compared to 40% with extraction atherectomy, 53% with directional atherectomy, and over 60% with excimer laser angioplasty.[17] A relatively low rate of coronary atheroembolization has also been noted with the Palmaz-Schatz stent, perhaps due to trapping of atherosclerotic debris between the stent and graft wall. Vein graft lesions occurring at the proximal and distal anastomotic sites three or more years following surgery are frequently atherosclerotic and the results of percutaneous intervention are similar to midvein graft sites.[15]

The status of the left anterior descending coronary artery and its graft should influence the choice of revascularization options. Reoperation is often selected for severe disease of a vein graft to an important left anterior descending artery, whereas a patent arterial graft to this vessel favors percutaneous intervention. Angioplasty of chronic native artery stenoses in previously operated patients can

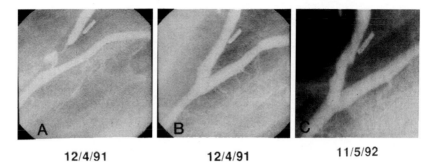

12/4/91   12/4/91   11/5/92

FIGURE 2. *A 74-year-old male presented in December 1991 with unrelenting chest pain. There was a history of bypass surgery (1981) and prior PTCA to the circumflex coronary artery and saphenous vein graft to the left anterior descending coronary artery. Coronary angiography revealed a complex stenosis of the saphenous vein graft to the left anterior descending coronary artery (A, left lateral view). Balloon angioplasty and deployment of a 3.5-mm Johnson & Johnson stent yielded an excellent angiographic result (B). Follow-up angiography 1 year later revealed only mild narrowing (C). The patient is asymptomatic 2 years after stenting. Younger patients with such complex saphenous vein graft lesions of left anterior descending coronary artery grafts are commonly referred for reoperation in our hospital.*

present challenging problems because of their fibrocalcific nature. Such lesions at the ostium of the right coronary artery and in the left main coronary artery frequently require nonballoon strategies such as Rotablator™ (Heart Technologies, Bellevue, WA), excimer laser, or directional atherectomy (Figure 3). Rotational atherectomy may be the only viable percutaneous option in lesions with heavy calcification. Recanalization of chronic total occlusions may be required when conduits are thrombosed or too diffusely diseased for rehabilitation. A need for more aggressive strategies with stiffer guide wires and high-pressure balloons may be expected in this patient subset.

Percutaneous intervention in vein grafts is generally not preferred when there is considerable thrombus formation. Prolonged intracoronary administration of thrombolytic agents has been used and initial results have been relatively favorable when thrombus was significantly reduced and treatment with extraction or directional atherectomy or balloon dilatation could be accomplished. We and others have used the Palmaz-Schatz stent if there was no residual thrombus apparent. Directional atherectomy has been commonly used for very eccentric lesions in this setting. Use of percutaneous intervention in the treatment of totally occluded saphe-

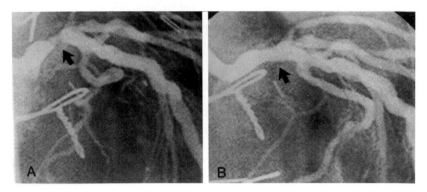

FIGURE 3. *A severe calcified stenosis of the left main coronary artery (**A**) was the culprit lesion in a 71-year-old female 8 years after CABG. The left anterior descending and right coronary arteries were occluded, but a left internal mammary artery to the left anterior descending coronary artery was patent. Rotational atherectomy (1.75 and 2.15 mm burrs) followed by a low-pressure balloon inflation yielded an excellent angiographic result (**B**) and relieved the patient's anginal symptoms.*

nous vein grafts is controversial. Balloon angioplasty alone has resulted in a high complication rate and low patency in our experience. Prolonged intragraft thrombolytic therapy has resulted in thromboembolic myocardial infarction, intracranial bleeding, intramyocardial hemorrhage, and the need for transfusion and femoral artery repair.[17] In the largest reported series, in-hospital complications occurred in one-third of patients and there were four late deaths. Of 13 grafts shown to be patent on follow-up angiography, less than one-half had been followed 6 months.[19,20] In a smaller series of 10 patients followed for a mean of 13 months, Levine and colleagues[21] showed that no patient was free of total occlusion and/or the clinical end points of myocardial infarction or death. These results should engender a relatively conservative approach to totally occluded vein grafts.

In our experience, saphenous vein graft lesions undergoing balloon angioplasty over 5 years following surgery have evidence of distal embolization in over 20% of patients, and the restenosis rate is relatively high, particularly for lesions that are >1 cm in length. In spite of these limitations, angioplasty is frequently helpful in the management of patients who have high-grade stenoses in grafts to arteries of moderate size and in patients in whom reoperation is not an excellent alternative. When a lesion in a graft conduit can be successfully dilated and the patient symptomatically benefited even for time periods as short as 1 year, this strategy may be reasonable as long as the risk to the patient is small. In some cases, the long-term patency of dilated grafts is surprisingly good. Even if restenosis occurs, the amount of time that has transpired may allow development of collateral flow sufficient to avoid infarction and/or disabling symptoms.

Initial Results

Although early series reported an increased risk of percutaneous strategies in the post-CABG patient, subsequent reports have not supported this finding. Procedural success rates of approximately 90% were reported for balloon angioplasty in the early 1980s with low morbidity and no mortality in carefully selected patients.[7] Many centers currently report procedural success of over 90% with Q wave infarction in 0%–2.5%, emergency coronary bypass surgery in approximately 2%–4%, and overall mortality rates of approximately 1%.[17]

The highest success and lowest complication rates occurred with angioplasty of lesions at the distal saphenous vein graft anastomotic site.[7,15,17] The most frequent complication of vein graft intervention in the Emory experience was non-Q wave myocardial infarction that occurred in over 10% of patients. The most common cause of in-hospital mortality in early series was embolic myocardial infarction after recanalization of totally occluded saphenous vein grafts.[17] Percutaneous intervention in older saphenous vein grafts has been associated with a higher complication rate, especially when there is associated thrombus. In recent studies from the Cleveland Clinic, directional and extraction atherectomy resulted in a 76% procedural success rate when graft thrombus was present, but in-hospital mortality exceeded 3% and myocardial infarction occurred in 24% of patients with diffuse saphenous vein graft disease, in spite of the fact that one-half of patients had been pretreated with urokinase.[22] Although the multicenter experience with extraction atherectomy in saphenous vein grafts is relatively favorable with angiographic success rates over 90% in 538 patients, in-hospital mortality rates were reported to exceed 3% and restenosis rates have been significant warranting thoughtful, conservative applications of this technique.[23] Although the use of atherectomy devices may have permitted broadening of indications in aging saphenous vein grafts, complications continue to be common and preliminary reports indicate that late cardiac events occur with higher frequency in this difficult subgroup of patients.

Favorable results have been reported from multicenter use of the Palmaz-Schatz coronary stent in saphenous vein grafts (Table 2). Stent deployment was successful in 98.7% of 626 patients.[24] Sin-

TABLE 2

In-hospital Results of Stent Implantation in Saphenous Vein Grafts, Selected Series, % of Patients.

Author (References)	N	Successful Implantation	Subacute Thrombosis	AMI	CABG	Death	Bleeding	Vascular Repair	Restenosis
Palmaz-Schatz Coronary Stent									
Leon[24]	626	98.7	1.3	1.9	3.9	2.3	7.7	8	27
Palmaz-Schatz Biliary Stent									
Piana[25]	54	97	0	0	0	2	—	14	—
Wong[26]	69	98	2.9	—	0	1.4	—	—	—
Knopf[27]	38	100	4	—	2	2	18	—	—
Hardigan[28]	31	100	19	—	—	2	—	14	—
Gianturco-Roubin Coil Stent									
Bilodeau[29]	37	100		14	0	0	22	—	35
Wiktor Stent									
Fortuna[30]	101	95	2	3	1	1	—	—	—
Wall Stent									
de Scheerder[31]	69	100	—	7	—	4	33	—	47

AMI, acute myocardial infarction; CABG, coronary bypass surgery.

gle stents were implanted in 82%, multiple single stents in 12%, and overlapping tandem stents in 6%. Myocardial infarction occurred in 1.9%, bypass surgery in 3.9%, and 2.3% died in-hospital. Acute or subacute stent thrombosis was noted in only 1.3% of patients. Bleeding requiring transfusion occurred in 7.7% and vascular surgery (arteriovenous fistula, psuedoaneurysm, or expanding hematoma) in 8%. Angiographic follow-up in 299 patients at 6.6 months revealed restenosis ($\geq$50%) in 27% overall. Restenosis was significantly lower in patients with de novo lesions, 18%, compared to those with previous PTCA at the stent site, 38% (P<0.001). The largest Palmaz-Schatz coronary stent distorts when expanded to a diameter greater than 4.5–5 mm and some investigators have explored the use of the FDA approved biliary stent in vein grafts 4.5–6 mm in diameter with favorable results (Table 2). The nonarticulated biliary stent has slightly thicker struts (improved fluoroscopic visibility, superior hoop strength) and provides more uniform coverage (no midstent gap), but is more difficult to deploy.

Excimer laser angioplasty use in vein grafts has been reported in multicenter registries with procedural success rates exceeding 90% (adjunctive balloon angioplasty in 80% of patients) with myocardial infarction and surgery rates comparable to that reported for balloon angioplasty (Q wave myocardial infarction 2.3%, CABG 0.7%, death 1%).[32] However, relatively high late cardiac event rates have been reported and restenosis rates appear similar to that achieved with balloon angioplasty.

Multicenter experience with directional atherectomy (DCA) in saphenous vein grafts reported an 87% initial success rate; non-Q wave infarction in 5.8%, Q wave infarction in 1.2%, bypass surgery in 1.2%, and in-hospital mortality in 0.8%.[33] Preliminary results of the CAVEAT II comparison of DCA with balloon angioplasty suggests somewhat better angiographic results with DCA, but more Q wave infarctions and similar restenosis. Although reported restenosis rates for de novo lesions appear comparable to balloon angioplasty (35%–65%), restenosis rates exceeding 80% have been reported following DCA of restenotic lesions.[33] Some operators favor DCA for ostial sites, eccentric lesions (Figure 4) and complex focal stenoses.[34,35]

The results of percutaneous intervention for internal mammary artery graft lesions, which usually occur at the anastomoses with native coronary arteries, are quite favorable and analogous to the distal anastomotic lesions of saphenous vein grafts. Of 177 patients reported, success was achieved in 164 (93%) and complications were minimal: one Q wave infarction and five dissections.[17] There were no reported in-hospital deaths. Although the vast ma-

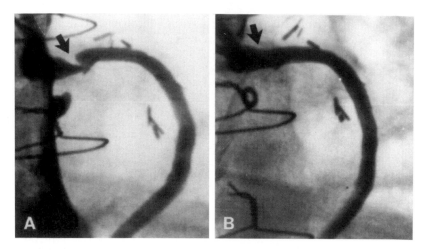

FIGURE 4. *Directional atherectomy was performed successfully for a very eccentric lesion (A) in a 4-year-old saphenous vein graft to the circumflex coronary artery in a 45-year-old male with unstable angina. In spite of the excellent result (B), restenosis occurred in 8 months and at that time, a Palmaz-Schatz stent was implanted. Recatheterization 6 months later showed excellent patency of the stent site, but a new lesion in the vein graft to the right coronary, which required balloon angioplasty. Fortunately, for the past 24 months the patient has been asymptomatic.*

jority of attempted lesions were at the graft to coronary artery anastomoses, 12 of 32 lesions in one report were midgraft lesions and at least 2 lesions were in the ostium or extremely proximal portion of internal mammary artery grafts. Use of balloon mounted stents has been reported for left and right internal mammary artery grafts. In patients with subclavian artery stenosis or occlusion, balloon angioplasty has been used successfully to improve internal mammary artery flow in patients before and after coronary bypass surgery.

Complications

Given the well-recognized increase in risk of coronary artery reoperation, emergency reoperation for failed angioplasty is clearly an undesirable outcome. At Emory University, 1,200 consecutive patients with prior coronary artery bypass surgery underwent percutaneous coronary intervention, and 3.6% required reoperation for failed PTCA[36] Three patients died in-hospital (mortality rate of 6.5%) and 24% had nonfatal Q wave myocardial infarction. Actuarial survival at 3 years was 91%. Colleagues at the Mid America Heart Institute reported three in-hospital deaths in 19 patients requiring emergency reoperation for failed PTCA (16% mortality), and 25% of survivors had Q wave myocardial infarction.[37] Although some have advocated the use of percutaneous cardiopulmonary bypass in patients with poor left ventricular function and/or a large ischemic potential, we have found intra-aortic balloon pumping to be adequate for intervention in a broad spectrum of patients with prior coronary bypass surgery.

Although abrupt closure occurs in approximately 4% of patients undergoing native vessel angioplasty, it is relatively uncommon following angioplasty of saphenous vein grafts. It was reported to occur in 1.5% of 448 procedures in five published reports.[17] Systematic analysis of predictors of this complication in native coronary arteries has been reported in detail, but predictors of this complication in vein graft intervention have not been reported. In our experience, thrombus, bulky lesions, and infarct-related lesions have an increased risk.

Coronary embolization is a rare complication of native vessel PTCA that is most often seen in patients with intracoronary thrombus (acute infarction, unstable angina, total occlusions). Iatrogenic air embolism is usually recognized by transient chest pain and ST segment elevation after injections of contrast media, whereas atheroembolism is suspected when ischemia unaccountably develops and persists immediately after dilatation of a lesion. In general, the clinical consequences of coronary embolization are proportional to the volume of embolic material. In native vessel interventions, minimal or no myocardial necrosis is the rule. The same is not necessarily true in vein grafts where atheroma are larger, more friable, and thrombus formation is common. We observed seven coronary emboli during 235 vein graft angioplasty procedures, a 3% occurrence rate. However, in vein grafts in place for over 5 years, over 25% developed creatine kinase elevations greater than three times normal.[17] This potential for coronary embolization is a major limiting factor in selecting old vein grafts for intervention. The frequency of this complication can be minimized by careful selection of patients, avoidance of large and eccentric vein graft lesions or thrombus laden lesions. Treatment once embolization has occurred is generally of a supportive nature (heparin, intravenous nitroglycerin, morphine, intra-aortic balloon pumping if needed), but intragraft thrombolytic therapy may be successful in selected patients.

Coronary artery perforation is a potential complication of all coronary interventions. Perforation during native vessel balloon angioplasty has been related to guide wire penetration, inflation of a balloon catheter in a subintimal location, and balloon oversizing. Saphenous vein graft perforation was noted in 0.5% of 235 balloon angioplasties and this complication limits balloon oversizing, a potential strategy to overcome elastic recoil in saphenous vein grafts. Prolonged balloon inflations at the site of perforation and reversal of anticoagulation is usually effective in stabilizing a limited perforation in our experience. A perfusion balloon catheter is best if technically feasible. In spite of the mediastinal scarring that is present in the postoperative patient, excessive hemorrhage and cardiac tamponade may occur requiring emergency catheter drainage of the mediastinum or surgery. Coronary artery perforation is more common with new devices and has been reported in 1%–2% of patients undergoing excimer laser angioplasty and extraction, directional and rotational atherectomy.[38] Perforation is less frequent (<1%) when these devices are used in saphenous vein grafts.

Long-term Results

The long-term outlook of patients who have undergone successful percutaneous coronary intervention after coronary bypass surgery is dependent on a number of factors including patient age, extent of coronary and graft atherosclerosis, left ventricular function, and the probability of restenosis of the sites treated. Investigators at the Mid-America Heart Institute reported their experience with native vessel PTCA in over 1,500 patients, noting actuarial survival at 6 years of 81% and event-free survival of 55%.[16] Multivariate predictors of survival were ejection fraction <40%, age greater than 70, unstable angina pectoris, and multivessel disease. At Emory, approximately 600 patients were followed after balloon angioplasty of saphenous vein grafts; 5-year survival was 81% and myocardial infarction-free survival 62%.[15] Myocardial infarction-free, repeat revascularization-free survival was 31% at 5 years. Restenosis was significantly related to the time elapsed between surgery and angioplasty. Restenosis occurred in 32% of vein grafts dilated within 6 months of surgery, but 43% from 6 months to 1 year, 61% from 1 to 5 years, and 64% when the interval was over 5 years (*P*<0.02). Restenosis occurred in 45% of lesions at the distal anastomosis, 61% of midvein graft lesions, and 68% of lesions at the proximal anastomosis (*P*<0.06). Survival at 5 years was 67% for proximal lesions, 72% for midvein graft lesions, and 92% for distal lesions (*P*<0.0001). Because of the higher restenosis rates encountered with balloon angioplasty of older saphenous vein grafts, nonballoon percutaneous approaches have been explored. However, restenosis was reported in 60% of patients following excimer laser angioplasty of saphenous vein grafts, and 50% of patients after directional and extraction atherectomy of de novo vein graft lesions and 80% after directional atherectomy of restenotic vein graft lesions. Whether encouraging low restenosis reported after Palmaz-Schatz stent placement in vein grafts will persist with longer follow-up remains to be determined.

Conclusion

The growing arsenal of coronary artery interventional strategies has perhaps its greatest challenge in the heterogeneous group of patients with previous coronary bypass surgery. In selecting therapy for these patients, the clinician must carefully weigh potential risks and benefits with the aim of achieving the most effective revascularization possible at the lowest risk to the patient. Patients best suited for percutaneous intervention are those with focal stenoses of native vessels, arterial grafts, or distal vein graft anastomotic site lesions. Those best suited for repeat surgery have multiple complex lesions and/or degenerated saphenous vein grafts.

References

1. Campeau L, Lesperance J, Hermann J, Corbara F, Grondin CM, Bourassa MG. Loss of the improvement of angina between 1 and 7 years after aortocoronary bypass surgery. *Circulation.* 1979;60(suppl I):I-1–I-5.
2. Weintraub WS, Jones EL, Craver JM, et al. Incidence of repeat revascularization after coronary bypass surgery. *J Am Coll Cardiol.* 1992;19:98A.
3. Loop FD, Lytle BW, Cosgrove DM, et al. Reoperation for coronary atherosclerosis. *Ann Surg.* 1990;212:378–386.
4. Kuntz RE, Piana R, Schnitt SJ, et al. Early ostial vein graft stenosis: management by atherectomy. *Cathet Cardiovasc Diagn.* 1991;24:41–44.
5. Eigler NL, Weinstock B, Douglas JS Jr, et al. Excimer laser coronary angioplasty of aorto-ostial stenoses: results of the Excimer Laser Coronary Angioplasty (ELCA) Registry in the first 200 patients. *Circulation.* 1993; 88:2049–2057.
6. Tierstein P, Stratienko AA, Schatz RA. Coronary stenting for ostial stenoses: initial results and six month follow-up. *Circulation.* 1991;84:II-250.
7. Douglas JS Jr, Gruentzig AR, King SB III, et al. Percutaneous transluminal coronary angioplasty in patients with prior coronary bypass surgery. *J Am Coll Cardiol.* 1983;2:745–754.
8. Douglas J, Robinson K, Schlumpf M. Percutaneous transluminal angioplasty in aortocoronary venous graft stenoses: immediate results and complications. *Circulation.* 1986;74(suppl II):II-281.

9. Cote G, Myler RK, Stertzer SH, et al. Percutaneous transluminal angioplasty of stenotic coronary artery bypass grafts: 5 years' experience. *J Am Coll Cardiol.* 1987;9:8–17.

10. Pinkerton CA, Slack JD, Orr CM, et al. Percutaneous transluminal angioplasty in patients with prior myocardial revascularization surgery. *Am J Cardiol.* 1988;61:15G–22G.

11. Dorros G, Lewin RF, Mathiak LM, et al. Percutaneous transluminal coronary angioplasty in patients with two or more previous coronary artery bypass grafting operations. *Am J Cardiol.* 1988;61:1243–1247.

12. Reed DC, Beller GA, Nygaard TW, et al. The clinical efficacy and scintigraphic evaluation of post-coronary bypass patients undergoing percutaneous transluminal coronary angioplasty for recurrent angina pectoris. *Am Heart J.* 1989;117:60.

13. Platko WP, Hollman J, Whitlow PL, et al. Percutaneous transluminal angioplasty of saphenous vein graft stenosis: long-term follow-up. *J Am Coll Cardiol.* 1989;7:1645–1650.

14. Plokker HW, Meester BH, Serruys PW. The Dutch experience in percutaneous transluminal angioplasty of narrowed saphenous veins used for aortocoronary arterial bypass. *Am J Cardiol.* 1991;67:361–366.

15. Douglas JS Jr, Weintraub WS, Liberman HA, et al. Update of saphenous graft (SVG) angioplasty: restenosis and long term outcome. *Circulation.* 1991;84(suppl II):II-249.

16. Miranda CP, Rutherford BD, McConahay DR, et al. Angioplasty of older saphenous vein grafts continues to be a sound therapeutic option. *J Am Coll Cardiol.* 1992;19(suppl A):350:A.

17. Douglas JS Jr. Percutaneous intervention in patients with prior coronary bypass surgery. In: Topol EJ, (ed.) *Textbook of Interventional Cardiology.* Second Edition, Philadelphia, PA: WB Saunders; 1993;339–354.

18. Liu MW, Douglas JS Jr, Lembo NJ, et al. Angiographic predictors of a rise in serum creatine kinase (distal embolization) after balloon angioplasty of saphenous vein coronary artery bypass grafts. *Am J Cardiol.* 1993;72:514–517.

19. Hartman J, McKeever L, Teran J, et al. Prolonged infusion of urokinase for recanalization of chronically occluded aortocoronary bypass grafts. *Am J Cardiol.* 1988;61:189–191.

20. Hartman JR, McKeever LS, Stamato NJ, et al. Recanalization of chronically occluded aortocoronary saphenous vein bypass grafts by extended infusion of urokinase: initial results and short-term clinical follow-up. *J Am Coll Cardiol.* 1991;18:1517–1573.

21. Levine DJ, Sharaf BL, Williams DO. Late follow-up of patients with totally occluded saphenous vein bypass grafts treated by prolonged selective urokinase infusion. *J Am Coll Cardiol.* 1992;19:292A.

22. Guzman LA, Villa AE, Whitlow P. New atherectomy devices in the treatment of old saphenous vein grafts: are the initial results encouraging? *Circulation.* 1992;86:I-780.

23. O'Neill WW, Kramer BL, Sketch MH Jr, et al. Mechanical extraction atherectomy: report of the U.S. transluminal extraction catheter investigation. *Circulation.* 1992;86(suppl I):I-779.

24. Leon MB, Wong SC, Pichard AD. Balloon-expandable stent implantation in saphenous vein grafts. In: Hermann HC, Hirshfeld JW, (eds.) *Clinical Use of the Palmaz-Schatz Intracoronary Stent.* Mount Kisco, NY: Futura Publishing Company Inc.; 1993;11.

25. Piana RN, Moscucci M, Kugelmass AD, et al. Treatment of large saphenous vein grafts and native coronary stenoses using the Palmaz-Schatz biliary stents: acute results. *Circulation.* 1993;88:I-307.
26. Wong SC, Chuang YC, Kent KM, et al. "Old" coronary or "new" biliary stent designs for treating saphenous vein graft lesions? *Circulation.* 1993;88:I-308.
27. Knopf WD, Lembo NJ, Cates CU, et al. Treatment of complex saphenous vein graft disease and suboptimal native coronary angioplasty result with biliary stenting: a promising new technique. *Circulation.* 1993;88:I-308.
28. Hardigan KR, Strumpf RK, Eagan JT, et al. Single-center Palmaz biliary stent experience in coronary arteries and saphenous vein grafts. *Circulation.* 1993;88:I-308.
29. Bilodeau L, Iyer S, Cannon AD, et al. Flexible coil stent (Cook Inc.) in saphenous vein grafts: clinical and angiographic follow-up. *J Am Coll Cardiol.* 1992;19:264A.
30. Fortuna R, Heuser RR, Garratt KN, et al. Wiktor intracoronary stent: experience in the first 101 vein graft patients. *Circulation.* 1993;88:I-139.
31. de Scheerder IK, Strauss BH, de Feyter PJ, et al. Stenting of venous bypass grafts: a new treatment modality for patients who are poor candidates for intervention. *Am Heart J.* 1992; 123:1046–1054.
32. Untereker WJ, Palacios IF, Hartzler G, et al. Excimer laser coronary angioplasty of saphenous vein grafts. *Circulation.* 1992;86(suppl I):I-780.
33. Ghazzal ZMB, Douglas JS, Holmes DR, et al. Directional coronary atherectomy of saphenous vein grafts: recent multicenter experience. *J Am Coll Cardiol.* 1991;17:219A.
34. Cowley MJ, DiSciascio G. Directional coronary atherectomy for saphenous vein graft disease. *Cathet Cardiovasc Diagn.* 1993;(suppl I)I:10–16.
35. Kerwin PM, McKeever LS, Marek JC, et al. Directional atherectomy of aorto-ostial stenoses. *Cathet Cardiovasc Diagn.* 1993;(suppl I)I:17–25.
36. Weintraub WS, Cohen CL, Curling PE, et al. Results of coronary surgery after failed elective coronary angioplasty in patients with prior coronary surgery. *J Am Coll Cardiol.* 1990;16:1341–1347.
37. Kahn JK, Rutherford BD, McConahay DR, et al. Outcome following emergency coronary artery bypass grafting for failed elective balloon coronary angioplasty in patients with poor coronary bypass. *Am J Cardiol.* 1990;66:285–288.
38. Ellis SG, Arnold AZ, Raymond RE, et al. Increased coronary perforation in the new device era: incidence, classification, management and outcome. *Circulation.* 1992; 86:I-787.

Chapter 28

Cardiac Catheterization in the Adult with Congenital Heart Disease

Larry A. Latson, MD

An increasing number of patients with congenital heart defects are either surviving into adulthood or are being recognized by new and more sensitive noninvasive tests. It has been estimated that there are 200,000 to 300,000 people in the United States between the ages of 21 and 40 with some type of congenital heart defect.[1] This number is projected to increase to over 500,000 within the next 10 years. In spite of this, the percentage of patients followed in a typical adult cardiology practice who have congenital heart disease as the major indication for continuing cardiac evaluation is small. This chapter reviews some of the major principles and techniques for optimal cardiac catheterization evaluation of congenital heart defects in adult patients. Emphasis is placed on considerations and caveats that may not be well known to personnel in laboratories that do not have the opportunity to routinely study large numbers of patients with congenital heart defects.

Primary Indications for Diagnostic Catheterization in Adult Patients with Congenital Heart Disease

The role of diagnostic catheterization in assessing congenital heart disease has decreased over the last 10 years because of the development of noninvasive methods for assessing many anatomical and physiologic details accurately enough for therapeutic planning.[2-4] Familiarity with the capabilities and limitations of nonin-

From Vetrovec GW, Carabello BA, (eds.) *Invasive Cardiology: Current Diagnostic and Therapeutic Issues.* Armonk, NY: Futura Publishing Company, Inc.: © 1996.

vasive techniques, especially echocardiography and magnetic resonance imaging (MRI) is vital when evaluating adult patients for possible diagnostic catheterization. Patients in whom diagnostic cardiac catheterization may still be needed after noninvasive evaluation fall into one of three major groups: 1) a group of older adult patients who are about to undergo a surgical procedure for a congenital heart defect may need catheterization because of the risk of concomitant significant coronary artery disease; 2) in another group, there are hemodynamic questions that can only be reasonably answered by cardiac catheterization measurements; 3) a final group includes those in whom noninvasive techniques may not adequately illustrate some anatomical details important to the surgeon.

Assessment of Coronary Artery Disease in Adult Patients with a Congenital Heart Defect

For most congenital heart defects, development of coronary artery disease appears to follow the same time course and patterns as in patients with structurally normal hearts.[5] Adult patients who require surgery for a congenital defect can therefore be evaluated with techniques and for indications that would routinely be used to evaluate adult patients preoperatively for more familiar problems, such as valvular disease. Because these techniques are well known in adult cardiology practices, we will not discuss them further. It is not yet known whether neonatal patients undergoing recently developed surgical procedures involving translocation of coronary arteries (such as the arterial switch procedure for transposition of the great vessels) will eventually develop more coronary artery problems as adults.

Hemodynamic Assessment in Adult Congenital Heart Disease

Primary hemodynamic parameters to be evaluated in typical cases of adult congenital heart disease are assessments of pressures and flows (and calculated resistances) in basal conditions and often after some type of pharmacologic or mechanical intervention. The sampling catheter(s) must be maneuvered into all appropriate chambers (or portions of chambers) and vessels in order to record pressures and obtain samples for oxygen saturation (and/or oxygen content) analysis. Therefore, one must have a good idea of the underlying anatomy in order to know where to place the catheter for a complete catheterization study. For instance, measurement of pressures in the right ventricular body and main pulmonary artery are not sufficient to characterize patients with a double chambered right ventricle, who may have very high pressures in the apex of the right ventricle, or patients with distal pulmonary artery branch stenosis, who may have high pressures in the central pulmonary arteries, but not arteriolar disease. These patients may still be candidates for surgery or balloon angioplasty.

Hemodynamic measurements are generally performed before angiograms. Small hand injections may be needed to identify unusual channels or unanticipated catheter positions, but as long as the amount of contrast is small, hemodynamics are not generally altered. Nonionic contrast agents alter hemodynamics less than traditional ionic agents, and thus may be preferred for complicated cases.[6]

In many catheterization laboratories, the standard method for measuring cardiac output is by the thermodilution technique. Unfortunately, this is not an accurate technique for measuring systemic cardiac output in the presence of intracardiac shunts, unless specialized curve analysis capability is available. The most practical way of measuring flows in the pulmonary and systemic circulations in patients with a shunt lesion is the Fick method (Appendix 1). At a minimum, oxygen saturations must be measured (or estimated) from sites best representing the blood on either side of both the pulmonary and systemic capillary beds. A congenital defect allowing a shunt results in a change in the oxygen saturation from the immediate postcapillary bed to the succeeding prearteriolar bed at the anatomical site of the shunt (ie, the saturation of blood in the right ventricle and pulmonary arteries will be higher than the saturation of right atrial blood in the presence of a ventricular septal defect [VSD]). As a routine, therefore, blood samples should be obtained for oxygen saturation determination in the innominate vein, superior vena cava (SVC), right atrium, inferior vena cava (IVC), right ventricle, main and both branch pulmonary arteries, and femoral artery. If indicated, samples may also be taken in the ascending aorta, left ventricle, left atrium, and pulmonary veins. Facilities must be available to analyze the oxygen saturation from samples immediately in each of these sites because unexpected changes in saturation from one site to another may indicate the site of a shunt and the need for additional catheter manipulations or angiograms.

In some patients being evaluated for a congenital heart defect, it may be adequate for surgical planning purposes to simply evaluate the ratios of pulmonary to systemic flow (Qp/Qs) and resistance (Rp/Rs). For instance, a minimally symptomatic patient with a VSD and a Qp/Qs of 2.5:1 with an Rp/Rs < 0.33 would meet generally accepted criteria for surgical intervention. If the patient is breathing room air, these ratios can be quickly calculated without measuring oxygen consumption (Appendix 1). In most cases, however, it is more appropriate to determine the actual flows and resistances. Calculations for these determinations require that oxygen consumption be measured or estimated. If at all possible, it is preferable to measure the oxygen consumption because errors of up to 50% in measurements of pulmonary blood flow have been found when comparing calculations using measured versus assumed oxygen consumption.[7] Similarly, for patients breathing room air, the contribution of dissolved oxygen to the calculated oxygen content of blood is small and can reasonably be ignored. However, when a patient is breathing high concentrations of oxygen, ignoring the dissolved oxygen in calculations of oxygen content in blood samples with a pO_2 over 100 can result in clinically significant errors.[8]

Numerous studies have shown higher early and late mortality in patients with left-to-right shunts and elevated pulmonary vascular resistance.[9,10] In the early days of open heart surgery, it was found that baseline pulmonary arteriolar resistances >7–8 units – M^2 were associated with long-term mortality of >50%.[11] Further studies have shown that some patients with elevated levels of basal pulmonary vascular resistance may not have irreversible pulmonary vascular disease if they continue to demonstrate the ability to react to pulmonary vasodilators. More recent studies have shown that patients in whom pulmonary resistance can be induced to fall to <7 units – M^2 by administration of a pulmonary vasodilator such as isoproterenol, still have an excellent prognosis for surviving surgical repair.[7] Vasodilator effects on pulmonary resistance have also been found to be predictive of early mortality after heart transplantation.[12] Accurate measurements of both pressure and cardiac output are therefore critical to correctly classify patients and testing of pulmonary vascular reactivity should be considered a routine part of the catheterization procedure for patients with borderline hemodynamics.

In some patients, it may be possible to directly test the probable effects of closure of a shunt by maneuvers in the diagnostic catheterization laboratory setting. Surgical shunts or systemic to pulmonary collaterals can often be temporarily occluded by the balloon of a standard flow directed catheter.[13] Changes in saturations, pressures, and cardiac output can be measured by additional catheters to better predict the outcome of permanent occlusion. We have used larger vascular occlusion balloons to temporarily close small atrial septal defects associated with right-to-left shunting after right ventricular myocardial infarction or pneumonectomy. Patients who tolerate these temporary occlusions without a significant fall in cardiac output will likely tolerate surgical or permanent transcatheter occlusion of their defects.

Anatomical Assessment of Congenital Heart Defects by Cardiac Catheterization

Prior to undertaking a diagnostic catheterization for anatomical assessment of congenital heart defects, the physician should consider his or her own knowledge and experience in this field. Thirty years ago, over 80% of adult patients undergoing cardiac catheterization had a simple left-to-right shunt or isolated valvular disease. In more recent years, over half of such patients in one center had complex or multiple defects or had previously undergone surgery for a congenital heart defect.[5] Reasonable assessment of these patients requires knowledge of the typical pathologic anatomy and additional defects that may commonly be associated with a known or suspected major defect. Indeed, the primary reason for diagnostic catheterization is often to rule out associated defects (such as anomalous pulmonary venous return) in patients with a readily appreciated primary defect (such as atrial septal defect). The physician may also be faced with patients following surgical procedures that have drastically altered the normal anatomy and connections (such as the Mustard procedure or Fontan procedure). Knowledge of the present and historical approaches to surgical corrections may be essential to guiding the catheter manipulations in such patients. The catheterization thus may specifically require manipulation of nonflow-directed catheters into vascular channels and through intracardiac communications not present in the vast majority of adult patients who are reasonably assumed to have structurally normal hearts. Knowledge of the orientation of possible abnormal structures is necessary in order to determine the optimal angulations for angiographic studies. This is especially important because large volumes of contrast media may be needed in complex cases.

For delineation of anatomical details, the primary factors to be considered are the delivery of sufficient contrast rapidly enough that excellent opacification is obtained while recording the images in the best projections. In order to reasonably opacify relatively normal size cardiac chambers in most adults, injection of approximately 40 mL of contrast is usually adequate. Larger volumes of contrast may be required to opacify enlarged cardiac chambers, especially in the presence of large intracardiac shunts. This amount of contrast should be delivered in the span of a single heart beat, if possible. Especially in the presence of a shunt, slow injections result in opacification of adjacent cardiac chambers and important details may be obscured. The use of large diameter catheters (8–11F) from the venous approach allows injection of contrast at rapid rates with lower pressures. The use of low injecting pressure lessens the risk of arrhythmias or myocardial staining. In many instances, the presence of transient injection produced arrhythmias may be tolerable if the primary purpose of the catheterization is to assess anatomical detail rather than the ventricular size or function.

In a significant percentage of diagnostic catheterizations the reason for the procedure may be to make precise angiographic measurements. Therefore, the method of magnification correction is critical. The angulations needed to demonstrate congenital defects angiographically tend to be complex. This may make traditional flat calibrated grids difficult to position accurately. Most often, the anatomical structures to be delineated are relatively large in comparison to catheter diameters. The use of catheter diameter as a reference for calibration is not appropriate if the structure to be measured is more than 3–4 times the diameter of the catheter. Angiographic marker catheters that have radiopaque bands along the length of the catheter may be used in many patients. Care must be taken to be certain that the marker catheter is in a position where it is not curved and the angulation of the patient or x-ray tubes does not result in foreshortening of the length between the markers. A calibration method that we have found advantageous is the use of a 2-cm diameter calibrated stainless steel sphere as a reference image. The sphere can be positioned on a small stand so that it is in the center of both planes of a biplane imaging system and provides accurate calibration at any angulation because of its shape.

The proper positioning of the image intensifiers is critical to good anatomical demonstration of congenital defects. The angulation must be chosen to maximize flow through the area or defect of interest with a minimum of foreshortening and overlap of other chambers or structures. Noninvasive evaluation may be helpful in estimating the best angulations in complex lesions. Table 1 lists typical angulations and injection sites used in our laboratory for assessing some common congenital defects. Further details are beyond the scope of this chapter, but may be found in other references.[14,15]

TABLE 1

Angiography of Typical Cases of Common Congenital Heart Defects

Defect	Preferred Injection Site	Typical Biplane View*	Comments
ASD	RUPV	LAO 15°–35°, cranial 30°–45°	Demonstrates location/type of defect but exact size better determined by transesophageal echo or "stretch diameter"
		Lateral	Some anterior defects seen well—relative RV and LV size illustrated
VSD	LV	LAO 35°–75°, cranial 20°–35°	Anterior defects better seen with more LAO angulation
		RAO 45°–90°, caudal 10°–25°	Demonstrates anterior muscular defects, profiles mitral valve
Right heart obstructions	RV, RVOT, or PA	LAO 0°–20°, cranial 30°–45°	Injection should be made as near obstruction as possible
		Lateral	Good for RV infundibulum and pulmonary valve
Left heart obstructions	LV	LAO 35°–75°, cranial 20°–35°	Demonstrates long axis of LV and LVOT
		RAO 45°–90°, caudal 10°–25°	Profile mitral valve and provides another view of LVOT
PDA	PDA or AO	Lateral	Injection in or near aortic end of PDA eliminates overlapping of ascending AO
		LAO 30°–45°, cranial 20°–35°	May profile some PDA's and shows aortic arch anatomy

*LAO and RAO angles referenced to image intensifier angle = 0° in straight anterior position. Cranial and caucal angles referenced to image intensifier angle = 0° when perpendicular to long axis of the body.

ASD, atrial septal defect; RUPV, right upper pulmonary vein; VSD, ventricular septal defect; LV, left ventricle; RV, right ventricle; RVOT, right ventricular outflow tract; PA, pulmonary artery; PDA, patent ductus arteriosus; AO, aorta.

Summary

The purpose of this chapter has been to review some of the important principles in the evaluation of adults with congenital heart disease. There is tremendous variability in the complexity of the lesions that may be found in this patient population. Some lesions are common enough that they are familiar to adult cardiologists who have an interest in congenital heart disease. However, patients with increasingly complex lesions are surviving into adulthood and the surgical and interventional catheterization procedures for treatment of congenital heart defects are becoming much more sophisticated in specialized centers. The number of adult patients with congenital heart disease is small enough that most adult cardiologists cannot be expected to be familiar with the nuances of modern diagnosis and treatment. Conversely, most pediatric cardiologists are very familiar with the anatomical and hemodynamic features of even complex congenital heart defects, but have very little familiarity with the general medical considerations, financial needs, or psycho-social aspects of taking care of adult patients. In most centers, the optimal assessment of adults with congenital heart disease is probably best done by a team that includes an internist or adult cardiologist in association with a pediatric cardiologist and a surgeon with special expertise in surgical management of congenital heart disease.[1,16] Use of this team approach can help to ensure that each patient is fully evaluated in a complete and cost-effective manner.

Appendix 1: Pulmonary and Systemic Flows by the Fick Principle

According to the Fick Principle, blood flow through the pulmonary (Qp) and systemic circulations (Qs) can be calculated if one knows the patient's oxygen consumption (VO_2) and the oxygen content (CON) of blood on both sides of the pulmonary and systemic capillary beds. VO_2 is either measured directly (the preferred method—see text) or estimated from a table of normal values.[17] The value of the VO_2 is usually indexed to body surface area, so that all subsequent computations are corrected for body size in order to facilitate comparison of values from patients of varying sizes.

In practice, the O_2 content of a blood sample is difficult to measure directly. In most centers, the O_2 content (measured in milliliters O_2 per liter of blood) is usually calculated from the hemoglobin concentration (in gm%), the O_2 saturation (O_2 SAT) measured by an oxymeter (with a value of 1 for blood in which the hemoglobin is 100% saturated), and the PO_2 by the formula:

$$O_2CON = hemoglobin \times 13.6 \times O_2SAT + (PO_2 \times 0.032)$$

In order to measure the appropriate O_2 contents, blood samples must be obtained from multiple locations. Pulmonary precapillary O_2 content is usually assumed to be the average of the O_2 content in samples from the distal pulmonary arteries (PAs). Pulmonary postcapillary O_2 content is best measured in the pulmonary veins (PV), left atrium, or a pulmonary capillary wedge sample. Systemic precapillary O_2 content is usually measured from a sample in a major systemic artery (SA). Systemic postcapillary O_2 content is the most uncertain value because different capillary beds and different parts of the body extract varying amounts of oxygen.[18] A commonly used method for estimating mixed venous O_2 content is:

$$MVO_2CON = (3 \times SVC\ O_2\ CON + IVC\ O_2\ CON)/4$$

Flows in the systemic and pulmonary circuits can be calculated as follows:

$$Qp = \frac{VO_2}{PV\ O_2\ CON - PA\ O_2\ CON}$$

$$Qs = \frac{VO_2}{SA\ O_2\ CON - MV\ O_2\ CON}$$

Effective pulmonary blood flow (Qep) is a measure of blood that flows appropriately to the pulmonary arteries and then is ejected into the systemic arteries:

$$Qep = \frac{VO_2}{PV\ O_2\ CON - MV\ O_2\ CON}$$

If there are no intracardiac shunts, then Qp, Qs, and Qep are all equal. If shunting is present, then the size of the left-to-right shunt is equal to:

$$Q_{L-R} = Qp - Qep$$

Size of the right-to-left shunt is:

$$Q_{R-L} = Qs - Qep$$

If a patient is breathing room air, then oxygen saturation alone is an excellent estimate of oxygen content. Even if oxygen consumption is not available, the ratio of pulmonary to systemic blood flow can be estimated as follows:

$$Qp/Qs = \frac{Ao\ SAT - MV\ SAT}{PV\ SAT - PA\ SAT}$$

References

1. Allen HD, Gersony WM, Taubert KA. Insurability of the adolescent and young adult with heart disease (Report From the Fifth Conference on

Insurability, October 3–4, 1991, Columbus, Ohio). *Circulation.* 1992; 86(2):703–710.

2. Sreeram N, Colli AM, Monro JL, et al. Changing role of noninvasive investigation in the preoperative assessment of congenital heart disease: a nine year experience. *Br Heart J.* 1990;63:345–349.

3. Kersting-Sommerhoff BA, Diethelm L, et al. Evaluation of complex congenital ventricular anomalies with magnetic resonance imaging. *Am Heart J.* 1990;120(1):133–142.

4. Kersting-Sommerhoff BA, Kiethelm L, Teitel DF, et al. Magnetic resonance imaging of congenital heart disease: sensitivity and specificity using receiver operating characteristic curve analysis. *Am Heart J.* 1989;118(1):155–161.

5. Flanagan MF, Leatherman GF, Carls A, Keane JF, Selwyn AP, Lock JE. Changing trends of congenital heart disease in adults: a catheterization laboratory perspective. *Cathet Cardiovasc Diagn.* 1986;12:215–218.

6. Girtz E, Wisneski J, Chiu D, Akin J, Hu C. Clinical superiority of a new nonionic contrast agent (iopamidol) for cardiac angiography. *J Am Coll Cardiol.* 1985;5:250–258.

7. Neutze JM, Ishikawa T, Clarkson PM, Calder AL, Barratt-Boyes BG, Kerr AR. Assessment and follow-up of patients with ventricular septal defect and elevated pulmonary vascular resistance. *Am J Cardiol.* 1989; 63:327.

8. Vargo T. Cardiac catheterization—hemodynamic measurements. In: Garson A Jr, Bricker T, McNamara, eds. *The Science and Practice of Pediatric Cardiology.* Volume 2. Malvern, PA: Lea & Febiger; 1990;913–945.

9. Allen HD, Anderson RC, Noren GR, Moller JH. Post-operative follow-up of patients with ventricular septal defect. *Circulation.* 1974;50:465–471.

10. Friedl B, Kidd BSL, Mustard WT, Keith JD. Ventricular septal defect with increased pulmonary vascular resistance. Late results of surgical closure. *Am J Cardiol.* 1974;33:403–409.

11. Moller JH, Patton C, Varco RL, Lillehei CW. Late results (30 to 35 years) after operative closure of isolated ventricular septal defect from 1954 to 1960. *Am J Cardiol.* 1991;68:1491–1497.

12. Murali, S, Kormos RL, Uretsky BF, et al. Preoperative pulmonary hemodynamics and early mortality after orthotopic cardiac transplantation: The Pittsburgh experience. *Am Heart J.* 1993;126(4):896–904.

13. Kopf GS, Kleinman CS, Hijazi ZM, Fahey TJ, Dewar ML, Hellenbrand WE. Fenestrated Fontan operation with delayed transcatheter closure of atrial septal defect. *J Thorac Cardiovasc Surg.* 1992;103(6):1039–1048.

14. *Angiocardiography of Congenital Heart Disease.* Freedom RM, Culham JAG, Moes CAF, eds. New York, NY: McMillan Publishing Company; 1984.

15. *The Science and Practice of Pediatric Cardiology.* Garson A Jr, Bricker JT, MacNamara DG. Malvern, PA: Lea & Febiger.

16. Perloff JK. The UCLA Adult Congenital Heart Disease Program. *Am J Cardiol.* 1986;57:1190–1192.

17. LaFarge CG, Mietternen OS. The estimation of oxygen consumption. *Cardiovasc Res.* 1970;4:23–30.

18. *From Cardiac Catheterization Data to Hemodynamic Parameters.* Yang SS, Bentivoglio LG, Maranhao V, Goldberg H, eds. Philadelphia, PA: F.A. Davis Company; 1978.

Chapter 29

Therapeutic Catheterization in the Adult with Congenital Heart Disease

Lee Benson, MD

Improvements in diagnostic accuracy and in surgical techniques have expanded the management options for patients with congenital cardiac malformations. These improvements have been paralleled by innovative techniques that have transformed the diagnostic cardiac catheterization laboratory into a therapeutic modality in neonatal, pediatric, and adult populations.[1] Interventional catheterization has become the preferred treatment or adjunct to surgical management for an increasing number of congenital malformations of the heart and circulation. At the Hospital for Sick Children, Toronto, fewer than 25 procedures were performed in 1985; currently over 270 (35%) of our total catheterization procedures are therapeutic. In contrast, the application of these techniques to the adult with congenital heart disease is a relatively new, but growing patient population. At the Toronto Hospital, Toronto General Division, The Centre for Congenital Heart Disease in the Adult supports 2,500 patients with congenital cardiac lesions. From this population, in 1993, 68 patients required cardiac catheterization with 19 interventional procedures (Dr. Peter McLaughlin, personal communication) from a total adult catheterization load of 6,600 cases per year. Yet, this is an expanding population with over 800 new referrals per year. This continually growing patient base will require that physicians develop expertise in the application of interventional techniques now frequently performed in the pediatric catheterization laboratories in the adult.

Interventional cardiac catheterization procedures may be classified as either corrective or palliative (Table 1).[2] Corrective proce-

From Vetrovec GW, Carabello BA, (eds.) *Invasive Cardiology: Current Diagnostic and Therapeutic Issues.* Armonk, NY: Futura Publishing Company, Inc.: © 1996.

Table 1

Lesions Amenable to Catheter-based Interventions

Amenable to repair

    Persistently patent ductus arteriosus (restrictive)
    Typical pulmonary valve stenosis
    Recurrent coarctation of the aorta

Potentially amenable to repair (unproven or in clinical trials)

    Patent foramen orvale (? stroke risk)
    Secundum atrial septal defect
    Muscular ventricular septal defect

Amenable to palliation—in lieu of surgery

    Aortic valve stenosis
    Postoperative systemic or venous obstructions
    Native coarctation of the aorta
    Obstructed prosthetic tissue valves/conduits
    Pulmonary arteriovenous malformations
    Pulmonary artery stenosis

Amenable to palliation—as an adjunet to surgery

    Systemic-to-pulmonary collaterals
    Systemic-to-pulmonary surgical shunts
    Venous obstructions (pulmonary, venous)
    Interatria communications (fenestrated Fontan)
    Pulmonary artery stenosis

(Modified with permission from Reference 2.)

---

dures such as balloon angioplasty in typical pulmonary valve stenosis, attain identical hemodynamic results as surgery and appear to be long lasting. Palliative interventions may be in lieu of surgery or a component of a broader management algorithm that includes surgical intervention. Such palliative interventions include balloon valvotomy of valvar aortic stenosis, nonsurgical coarctation of the aorta, or postoperative systemic or pulmonary venous obstructions. Similarly, procedures such as occlusion of systemic-to-pulmonary arterial collaterals, surgical shunts, or peripheral pulmonary arterial stenoses can simplify subsequent surgical procedures or expand surgical options in an individual patient.

    This chapter highlights the application of transcatheter closure of cardiac defects (eg, patent ductus arteriosus, atrial and ventricular defects, and vascular embolization) as well as balloon directed interventions (including endovascular stent implantation, aortic and pulmonary valvotomy aortic coarctation) and emphasises their application in the adult population.

Lesions Amenable to or Potentially Amenable to Repair

The Persistently Patent Ductus Arteriosus

The surgical ligation of a persistently patent ductus arteriosus by Gross and Hubbard in 1939 ushered in the era of surgical therapy for congenital heart disease, and represents one of the few curative operations.[3] Although generally an asymptomatic lesion, a persitently patent ductus arteriosus may produce symptoms caused by left ventricular volume overload and pulmonary hypertension. Surgical repair is safe and effective in infancy and childhood, but requires general anesthesia, thoracotomy, and a variable postoperative recovery. In the adult, surgical closure is less straightforward because of frequent ductal calcification, tissue friability, and aneurysmal dilatation.

Catheter closure of the ductus arteriosus was described by Porstmann and colleagues in 1971,[4] who used an 18F arterial sheath and a catheter positioned from the femoral artery retrograde across the ductus to the pulmonary artery. A guide wire was snared from the pulmonary artery and exteriorized from the femoral vein. A radiopaque polyvinyl alcohol plug (IVALON) was shaped to match the patient's ductal anatomy, introduced into the femoral artery, pushed along the guide wire, and positioned in the ampulla. Used primarily in adults due to the size of the delivery system, over 90% of ductus were occluded. Complications, however, were not uncommon (11%) and were primarily at the arterial cannulation site. Technical modifications have improved safety and applicability allowing successful occlusion in 95%–100% of adult patients (Figure 1).[5,6]

In 1976, Rashkind and Cuaso[7] described a method of umbrella closure of the ductus from the femoral artery applicable in the smaller child. Bash and Mullins[8] modified the technique for transvenous implantation, and it has become the most widely used ductal occluding device. The currently available device (USCI, Billerica, MA) is a spring-loaded double-disk umbrella of polyurethane foam, centrally welded to create opposing arm tension (Figure 2).

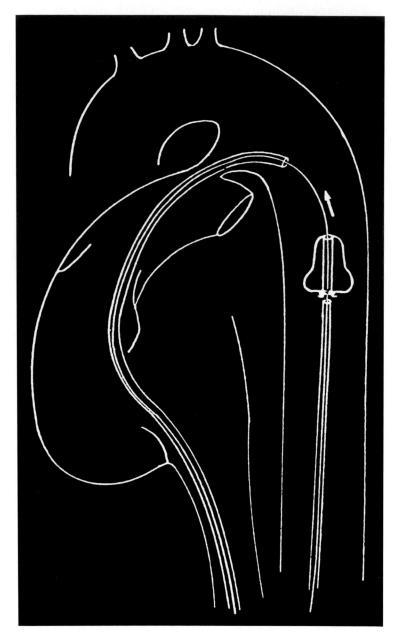

FIGURE 1. *Porstmann's transarterial plug method for closure of the patent ductus arteriosus. (Reproduced with permission from Reference 4.)*

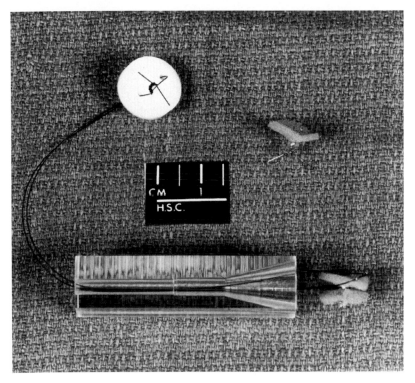

FIGURE 2. *The Rashkind^(TM) ductal occluder (USCI, Billerica, MA). Photograph shows opposing arms with and without foam covering. Below, plastic everting tube used to fold device into catheter pod is shown.*

Catheter Technique (Rashkind Occluder)

The device is locked to a wire release mechanism and collapsed into the distal pod of a specially designed 8F or 11F, 85-cm long delivery catheter. A long sheath is guided through the right side of the heart with an exchange length wire and placed across the ductal ampulla. The delivery system device is advanced through the sheath to the level of the tricuspid valve (Figure 3), and the collapsed device is then pushed from the delivery catheter pod into the sheath and guided to the ductus. The sheath is retracted over the device, opening the distal arms into the aorta. Holding the entire sheath-delivery catheter device firmly, it is pulled into the ductus to its pulmonary insertion (usually the narrowest portion of the ductus.[9] The long sheath is further retracted, opening the proximal arms in the pulmonary artery. Once satisfied that an adequate position has been attained, the device is released. Devices are avail-

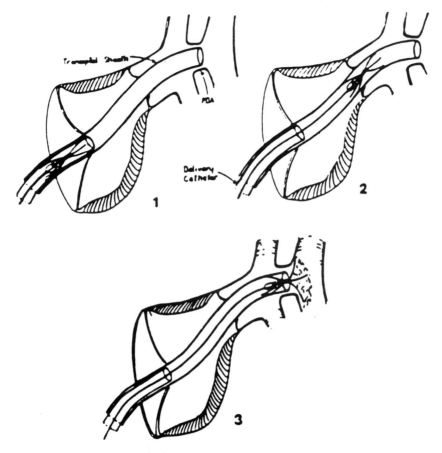

FIGURE 3. *Diagram of the transvenous technique for ductal umbrella placement. (Reproduced with permission from Reference 10.)*

able in 12-mm and 17-mm diameters adequate for occlusion of ductus up to 8 mm in diameter. Early experience with the device in a multicenter clinical trial (including single- and double-disk occluders) yielded successful closure in 66%. Persistent murmurs were present in 7%, postrelease embolization occurred in 13%, while decreasing to 3.6% during the final phase of the trial.[10] At The Hospital for Sick Children, Toronto there was a 99% implantation rate with 94% complete shunt obliteration in over 375 procedures as shown by color Doppler flow criteria[11] after 40 months of follow-up.

In an adult population at the Toronto Hospital, Toronto General Division, a similar experience with this technique has emerged.[12] Due to the difficulty in imaging the smaller 12-mm diameter device, the 17-mm diameter device has been exclusively used in suitably sized ductus. Twenty-five such implants have been accomplished, at a mean age of 40 years. At the time of discharge, there was no murmur in 24. There was normal Doppler flow in 15 of 21 at 30 months follow-up. Recently, Bridges et al[13] have reported the use of the "clamshell" atrial defect occluder in the adult with a large ductus arteriosus with excellent early success rates.

Presently, due to its ease of implantation, limited risks, and superb short- and long-term results, transcatheter closure is encouraged in all patients (>10 kg in weight) with an audible murmur. The procedures can be performed in the outpatient department, further reducing costs.

Valvar Pulmonary Stenosis

Catheter-directed therapy for valvar pulmonary stenosis was first performed by Rubio and Limon-Lason[14] in 1956 using a cutting-wire technique and later by Semb and colleagues[15] in 1979 using a balloon technique. The current technique of a static dilatation was first reported by Kan and associates[16] in 1982 and is the treatment of choice for typical doming pulmonary valve stenosis,[17] represented by fusion of the leaflet commissures. Dysplastic pulmonary valve stenosis with associated annular hypoplasia and small pulmonary trunk is less often associated with commissural fusion and not frequently amenable to correction by balloon dilation. Postprocedural dynamic right ventricular outflow obstruction is frequently observed, but generally regresses after successful dilation of the valve.

In neonates and infants with low cardiac output, congestion, or cyanosis, relief of valvar obstruction clearly improves outcome. However, in older patients, the natural history is less well defined. In patients with peak systolic ejection gradients of <40 mm Hg, progression of the obstruction is unlikely and therefore would not benefit from further gradient relief. Patients with critical obstruction and gradients ≥80 mm Hg are likely to have or develop cardiovascular compromise and should undergo prompt obstruction relief. The clinical course of patients with gradients between 40 and 80 mm Hg is more variable and in the asymptomatic individual, timing of intervention is unclear. If intervention is chosen, relief or prevention of symptoms, preservation of right ventricular function, and avoidance of gradient progression must be the goals. If such gradient relief can be achieved with minimal morbidity intervention would seem to be warranted.

Catheter Technique

The femoral vein or alternatively the internal jugular vein is entered percutaneously. Right heart hemodynamics and a biplane right ventriculogram are obtained to define the level of obstruction, anatomy of the outflow tract, and the pulmonary annulus diameter. A variety of techniques to safely and swiftly cross the pulmonary valve are available. In our institution, a right coronary catheter with an 0.035-inch guide wire to cross the valve is used. Once in the main pulmonary artery, the catheter is directed to the distal left pulmonary artery and removed over an exchange wire. A valvuloplasty balloon is chosen, 120% to 140% of the annulus diameter and generally 2 to 4 cm in length, and positioned across the valve. Longer balloons, although perhaps better positioned across the valve, may result in myocardial injury with inflation. Two side-by-side balloons may be used and inflated simultaneously to achieve an effective diameter of 140% of the pulmonary annulus. This technique is most common in older patients whose pulmonary annulus diameters are >20 mm.[18-20] Two balloons may also allow continued decompression of the right ventricle during inflation, avoiding excessive right ventricular hypertension (Figure 4). After dilation, postprocedure hemodynamics and angiography are obtained. Care must be taken to differentiate dynamic subpulmonary stenosis from residual valvar stenosis. The mechanism of gradient relief is by valve tearing along or parallel to the commissures or avulsion of the leaflets from the valve ring. Repeated dilations can be performed as necessary, a transvalvar gradient of <36 mm Hg considered a successful result.

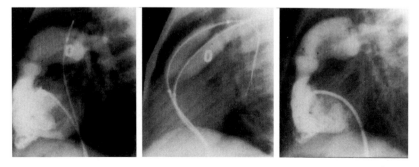

FIGURE 4. *Balloon angioplasty of valvar pulmonary stenosis using two balloons.* **Far left panel:** *prior to dilation;* **far right:** *postprocedure (note widened jet of contrast);* **Middle panel:** *the 2–15 mm ± 3 cm balloons during dilation.*

During balloon inflation, right ventricular pressure increases and tricuspid regurgitation is common. Right atrial pressure may rise transiently and a short lived right-to-left shunt may occur (through a patent foramen ovale or less commonly associated atrial septal defect). In the adult, such right-to-left shunting is infrequently of sufficient volume to support left ventricular filling, and transient hypotension frequently occurs; however, in the neonate and infant it may maintain systemic blood pressures during inflation, at the expense of the systemic saturation. Such shunting will provide a temporary egress for right atrial air or clots to the systemic circulation. Occasional premature contractions, prolongation of the QT interval and variable degrees of AV block have been noted.

The results of balloon dilation appear the same in children, adolescents, and young adults, although most experience is in the younger age groups. Most series have demonstrated excellent gradient relief with mean gradient reductions from 85 to 33 mm Hg. Short-term success was achieved in 98% of 784 procedures reported in the Valvuloplasty and Angioplasty of Congenital Anomalies Registry.[17] More recently, McCrindle and Kan[21] reported pooled results from multiple trials, and found an overall success rate of 80%. No change in mean gradient was observed over a 2-year follow-up period with a peak gradient remaining <36 mm Hg in 86% of their patient population.[21]

Non–life-threatening complications occurred in approximately 4% and included balloon rupture, vein perforation, and thrombosis. Procedural related mortality was <0.5%. Pulmonary insufficiency is generally mild and a hyperdynamic infundibular stenosis (without hemodynamic significance) noted in 20%.

The impact of balloon dilation in the older patient population is less well defined. Only 35 patients >20 years of age were present in the registry data,[17] although all had similar acute and short-term success rates. Balloon dilation has proved safe and effective for relief of obstruction in neonates and children and is the procedure of choice with severe obstructions of symptoms. Limited data are available in the adult population, although balloon dilation would appear a promising technique.

Recurrent Coarctation of the Aorta

A variety of methods exist for surgical repair that vary with morphologic form of coarctation of aorta, and include subclavian flap arterioplasty, overlay patch, or resection with end-to-end anastomosis. The incidence of residual obstruction or recoarctation also varies with type of coarctation and surgical repair, although is very low if performed beyond 3 years of age with end-to-end resection. Patients with residual or recoarctation require a second operation or balloon angioplasty.

Balloon angioplasty of recurrent or persistent aortic arch obstruction after surgical repair is now the procedure of choice with success rates >80% and low morbidity.[22] Although the use of balloon angioplasty in the setting of native coarctation remains controversial,[23] enough data have been accumulated to support its use as an alternative to surgery.

In the setting of recurrent coarctation, the best candidates are those with discrete lesions with a well-expanded isthmus and without transverse arch hypoplasia. The indications for intervention, in the absence of symptoms, are an arm-leg blood pressure gradient at rest of 20 mm Hg or more. For women of childbearing age, the merits of balloon angioplasty versus surgical repair of recurrent coarctation to reduce the risk of aortic rupture or dissection during pregnancy are not clear.

Catheter Technique

In the adult, after hemodynamic assessment, a biplane aortogram is obtained in the 20° left anterior oblique and lateral projections. An exchange wire is positioned across the narrowed segment and secured in the ascending aorta. A balloon dilating catheter is chosen to be three or four times the diameter of the obstruction (but <50% greater than the diameter of the native aorta), and positioned across the narrowing. The balloon is slowly inflated and the position monitored to avoid displacement. Generally, the balloon is left inflated for 30 to 45 seconds, deflated and removed over the stationary guide wire when hemodynamics and angiography are repeated. Patients frequently experience a painful sensation in the back or chest during dilation. A dilation is considered successful if the gradient is reduced 50% and angiographic diameter increased 30% or more.[24]

The application of this procedure is strongly supported in the setting of recurrent coarctation. Recent long-term surgical series have noted recurrent obstruction in 8% to 54% of patients, depending on repair technique, and reported mortality for reoperation has ranged from 7% to 20% with an associated risk of paraplegia. From the multicenter registry of balloon angioplasty,[22] 200 patient procedures were reviewed with 78.4% achieving <20 mm Hg gradients.

Procedure related deaths occurred in 2.5%, with one periprocedural stroke (0.5%). Intimal dissection was angiographically identified in 3 patients (1.5%) with operative repair required in one patient. Femoral arterial thrombosis requiring surgical intervention occurred in eight patients (4%).

From a single center experience, Hijazi and associates[25] reported 29 procedures in 26 patients (aged 4 months to 26 years). Acute gradient reduction to <20 mm Hg was achieved in 88%. There were no neurological sequelae or mortality. Hypoplasia of the transverse aortic arch in two children required ultimate surgical correction. Follow-up ranged from 1 to 7 years and no restenosis was found.

Balloon angioplasty for previously unoperated coarctation of the aorta is controversial. Surgical relief is associated with morbidity and mortality that varies with patient age and type of repair as well as comorbid lesions. Most surgical series report a 3% procedural mortality, although more recent techniques might reduce the mortality and paraplegia risk to 1%. Recurrent obstruction is a known risk, and as many as 33% may have true aneurysms of the repair site.[26] From the multicenter congenital anomalies angioplasty registry,[23] 141 native coarctations in 140 patients (age 3 days to 29 years) were dilated. Postprocedural gradients of <20 mm Hg were achieved in 76%. There was one procedure-related death, no strokes, and one patient required surgical relief of a persistent gradient. Femoral arterial complications were frequent (10%). Aneurysm formation at the dilation site occurred in 5%. Similar observations have been noted at the Hospital for Sick Children in 36 patients (1 year to 18 years), where aneurysm formations occurred in 6%. In 53 patients (0.1 to 19 years). Mendelsohn[27] reported a 68% success rate (gradient <20 mm Hg), with a 6% incident of aneurysm formation. Surgical repair was required in 3 of 4 unsuccessfully dilated lesions. Tyagi and colleagues[28] reported a series of 35 native coarctation dilation in an older population (14 to 37 years) with a success rate of 74% (gradient reduction <20 mm Hg). The majority of patients with unsuccessful procedures had associated transverse arch hypoplasia. Aneurysm formation occurred in 11.5% (3 patients) without clinical sequelae. Follow-up catheterizations in 26 patients (9 to 15 months postdilation) found recurrent lesions in 2 patients (8%).

These results indicate that balloon angioplasty of native coarctation is a potential alternative to surgical intervention. The critical issue is the degree of gradient relief that can be achieved by the technique. Late studies of such dilated patients will further define the role of this approach.

Lesions Potentially Amenable to Repair (Unproven or in Clinical Trials)

Secundum Atrial Septal Defect

Secundum atrial septal defects are common associated lesions occurring in 7% of all congenital lesions. Most adults with large shunt flows (<1.5:1) that were untreated until midlife will experience symptoms of dyspnea, congestive heart failure, or pulmonary hypertension, and may develop atrial arrhythmias or paradoxical emboli. Surgical therapy by suture or patch closure is one of the safest and effective forms of cardiac surgical therapy, particularly in childhood.[29] Despite safe surgical techniques, a significant perioperative morbidity occurs and includes atrial arrhythmias, emboli, hemorrhage pericardial inflammation, and a finite period of recovery.[30] Increasing age and pulmonary hypertension may also be independent risk factors for surgical mortality.

The concept of a catheter-based closure was proposed by King et al[31] and led Rashkind and colleagues[32] to develop an umbrella device that could engage the intra-atrial wall. Lock[33] expanded the concept of the double umbrella device for ductal occlusion and with modifications developed the double-umbrella or "clamshell" prosthesis (USCI, Billerica, MA). Four Dacron™ covered, spring-loaded hinged arms fold back on each other, grasping the septum (Figure 5).[33] Clinical trials in humans suggested that this approach is effective and safe if patients are properly selected.[34]

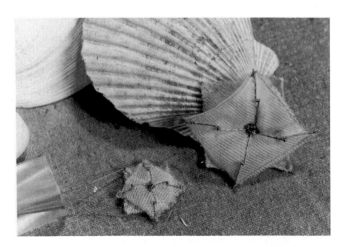

FIGURE 5. *Left,* The 17-mm diameter; ***right,*** 40-mm diameter *"clamshell" septal occluder (USCI, Billerica, MA). Note the Dacron covering supported by four spring-hinged arms used to grasp the septal wall on each disk. This design was later modified.*

Catheter Technique

The occlusion device is loaded onto the delivery catheter in a manner similar to that used for the ductal occluding device. A long sheath, placed in the left atrium is used to guide the delivery catheter to the right atrium, the occluder is pushed into the guide sheath, and brought to the end of the guide within the left atrium. The distal arms are opened within the left atrium (similar to the ductal device) and the entire device brought to the atrial septum. The position of the atrial wall is estimated by a preimplantation left arteriogram, although transesophageal echocardiography can more reliably assess atrial wall device relationships. Subsequently, the guide sheath is retracted, allowing the proximal (right atrial) arms of the device to open and fold into the atrial septum (Figure 6). The position of the device is confirmed and the device released. Low-dose aspirin and endocarditis prophylaxis is recommended for 6 months. The devices are available in five sizes: 17-, 23-, 28-, 33-, and 40-mm diameter and deployed with an 11F system. Sizing of the atrial defect is performed by a very flexible balloon, which stretches the defect while being pulled slowly from the left to the right atrium. Devices 1.8 to 2 times the measured diameter of the stretched defect are chosen for implantation.

During the initial clinical trial, 35 adult patients (aged 18 to 76 years) underwent attempted closure of their secundum atrial septal defect.[35] In two patients the defect was too large to close. One patient with a 27-mm diameter (stretched) defect had a 40-mm device implanted, but due to unstable positioning the device was with-

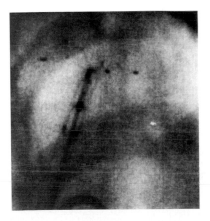 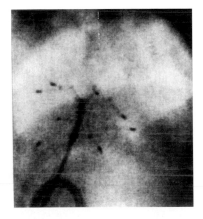

FIGURE 6. *Left panel,* the septal occluder positioned with the distal (left atrial) arms open and **right panel,** proximal arms open, grasping the intra-atrial septum.

drawn. The remaining 32 patients had successful implantations, with 5 significant residual leaks. In 3 of these patients, device arm herniation across the defect resulted in the residual shunt, while in 2 the device implanted was too small. A contrast reaction (1 patient) and pericarditis (1 patient) were the only procedural complications. No embolic events or bacterial endocarditis have occurred in 6 to 31 months of reported follow-up. Residual shunts (Doppler flow) have been documented in 32% at 1 year follow-up.

Due to fractures in the supporting arms of the clamshell prosthesis, clinical trials were suspended in June, 1991. These strut fractures seem to have occurred at the hinged arms of the device. Fracture incidence increases with device size (>50% incidence in devices 28 mm or greater). Such fractures have had no clinical sequelae and have not been correlated with residual leaks. In one patient, embolization of the broken device arm occurred to the right ventricle without adverse effect. Structural modifications of the device and animal testing are currently underway.

A double-disk "buttoned" device using a polyurethane foam disk with a counter-occluder arm is also undergoing early clinical trials.[36,37] This device, which is available in 25 to 40 mm diameters, may be implanted through 7F or 8F guide systems. In 46 patients (aged 1 to 63 years) with defect diameters (stretched) <23 mm, stable delivery was achieved in 74%. Surgical removal was required in 4, while device embolization occurred in 1. Device "unbuttoning" occurred in 1 patient during clinical follow-up. Clinical success (no more than a minor shunt at time of implantation) and a normal examination at follow-up occurred in 33 patients (1 to 12 months postprocedure). Echocardiographic residual shunting was noted in 39%.

Although surgical repair of the secundum atrial septal defect is effective, morbidity is not insignificant. The early results of these devices, although flawed, support further technical modifications and expanded clinical trials.

The Patent Foramen Ovale

The persistence of a flap valve communication between the left and right atria, the patent foramen ovale, may lead to right-to-left shunting during elevations in right atrial pressure. Cyanosis can develop in such patients with a patent foramen ovale whose right-sided filling pressures are chronically increased (right ventricular infarction, pulmonary emboli, etc.), or during transient elevations (Valsalva maneuvers, or thodioxia/platypnea syndrome). Since such patients are at risk for conventional surgery, device closure of the foramen ovale may be indicated.[38]

In idiopathic stroke, closure of the patent foramen ovale to prevent future paradoxical emboli remains controversial. Considerable circumstantial evidence is mounting incriminating such a pathophysiologic mechanism, at least in a few such patients. Lechat and colleagues[39] found the prevalence of patent foramen ovale in adult stroke patients <55 years (40%) significantly greater than controls (10%). The prevalence was particularly high in patients with no identifiable etiology. Since the prevalence of patent foramen ovale in the general population is high (20%–30%), a causal role in the etiology of idiopathic stroke is unclear. While anticoagulant therapy has been recommended as initial therapy, it carries a 1% to 4% risk of significant bleeding. Closure of the foramen ovale, either surgically or by transcatheter technique could, at least theoretically decrease the risk of such paradoxical emboli. In 36 patients with idiopathic stroke and associated patent foramen ovale, transcatheter closure was successfully undertaken. No subsequent strokes occurred in the 8.4-month follow-up,[40] although in the preprocedural period a significant incidence of secondary stroke occurred.

Postoperative Residual Defects and Fenestrated Fontan Procedure

Cardiac catheterization in the adult with congenital heart lesions is often precipitated by the need for assessment of residual defects after surgical "repair." For example, the patient who has a residual ventricular defect after surgery, has frequently undergone several attempts at closure. Poor ventricular function, arrhythmias, and comorbid lesions indicate that the patient is a poor surgical candidate. A number of such patients have successfully had their residual lesions closed or reduced significantly by intracardiac clamshell or ductal device implantations.

Other residual lesions successfully treated by catheter approach include central aorta to pulmonary shunts, systemic venous to pulmonary shunts, left superior or inferior cava to left atrium, intra-atrial baffle communications, systemic to pulmonary artery collaterals, valvular and paravalvular leaks, and coronary fistulae.[41–44]

In addition to their application in a variety of complex congenital lesions, in collaboration with new surgical techniques, transcatheter device closure allows more effective management of complex lesions. An example of one treatment algorithm for patients undergoing a Fontan procedure to palliate univentricular anatomy is the intentional creation of an intra-atrial shunt (baffle fenestration) to help modify the perioperative course by tempering the physiologic adjustment to an atrial dependent circulation.[45] At the time of the Fontan surgery, a 4- or 5-mm punch is made in the atrial wall. This creates an obligatory right-to-left shunt, temporarily increasing systemic output, although at the expense of a lower systemic oxygen saturation. In the postoperative period when hemodynamics stabilize, cardiac catheterization is performed, the defect test occluded, and permanently closed if right atrial pressure and cardiac output are acceptable. If the test occlusion is unsuccessful, either time or correction of secondary lesions (eg, pulmonary artery stenosis) will eventually lead to fenestration closure. Such fenestrations have been reported to reduce perioperative low cardiac output and death and reduce the risk of perioperative effusion.[46] Further study into the usefulness of the fenestrated Fontan concept is underway.

Ventricular Septal Defect

Transcatheter closure techniques have been applied to both congenital and acquired forms of ventricular septal defects in an attempt to eliminate the need for, or reduce the risk and complexity of surgical repair.[47,48] The majority of defects acquired because of myocardial infarction are distant from the aortic valve within the muscular septum or are at the apex. These have been closed using the clamshell device.

Lesions Amenable to Palliation In Lieu of Surgery

Valvar Aortic Stenosis

Balloon valvotomy for congenital aortic valve stenosis was first reported in children by Lababidi[49] in 1984, and subsequently applied to the adult population.[50] Because of the diverse nature of the morphologic substrate between congenital valve aortic stenosis and adult calcific aortic stenosis, the results obtained in children are considerably more successful. Since the risks of surgical valve replacement are low in the adult, while major complications of balloon aortic dilation are high, this application should be used cautiously.

In contrast, balloon aortic valvotomy has become the accepted therapy for children. Data from the Natural History of Congenital Heart Defects Study suggested[51] that if obstruction relief was achieved when the gradient was >50 mm Hg, surgical valvotomy was low risk and generally successful, with an 8% reoperation rate at 8 years (valve replacement) and 44% reoperation rate at 22 years.

Catheter Technique

After a right and left heart hemodynamic study is performed, biplane left ventriculography (right anterior oblique and long-axis oblique projections) and aortography are obtained to determine the aortic valve annulus diameter and degree of aortic regurgitation (if any). The balloon catheter may be advanced retrograde over a wire from the femoral or brachial vessels or across the atrial septum, left atrium and ventricle.[52,53] The diameter of the balloon should be 90% to 100% of the measured valve diameter and generally 5.5-cm long. If two balloons are required (diameter >20 mm), the combined balloon diameters should equal 1.3 times the measured valve diameter. Hemodynamics and aortography are repeated. If the gradient relief is inadequate and valve insufficiency not prohibitive a larger balloon diameter may be used (although the balloon/annulus ratio should be >1.1:1).

As suggested above, the response to balloon dilation differs appreciably according to valve morphology. Children and adolescents with mobile bicuspid stenotic valves achieve gradient reduction by splitting of the fused commissures.[49] This differs from the adult with fibrocalcific stenosis in the setting of a bicuspid, but nonfused valve. However, in the case of the adult with noncalcific bicuspid aortic stenosis recent data suggest that balloon dilation is a promising, effective palliation.[54] In the adult with calcific trileaflet aortic stenosis, selective application can improve orifice size, reduce gradient and improve (at least temporarily) symptoms, by producing fractures or fissures within the calcified leaflets, creating hinge points to improve valve mobility. The lack of improvement in calcific bicuspid aortic valve stenosis is thought to be caused by a lack of developing such hinge points.[55]

Success rates for patients of all ages approach 90% with mean gradient reduction from 69–77 mm Hg to 30–37 mm Hg.[56,57] Life-threatening complications occur in 5%, with fewer than 2%

periprocedural deaths. Aortic insufficiency develops in 10% to 30%, but generally not as severe.

Postoperative Venous Obstructions

Systemic and pulmonary venous obstructions may develop after atrial switch repair for transposition of the great arteries or the Fontan procedure. Balloon angioplasty may relieve caval, baffle, or pulmonary venous obstruction.[58] Recently, endovascular stents have been successfully used within these lesions with promising results.[59]

Prosthetic Tissue Valve Obstruction

Valved right ventricular-to-pulmonary artery conduits may become obstructed. Balloon dilation of the bioprosthetic valve has yielded modest success.[60] The procedure is palliative, but may postpone valve replacement for several years.

Intravascular Embolization-Pulmonary Arteriovenous Fistulae

Intravascular embolization techniques are commonly used in the catheter laboratory, given the frequently associated aorto-pulmonary collaterals, persistent surgical shunts, and pulmonary fistulae seen in congenital cardiac malformations. A variety of devices are used for vascular occlusion and include foam, glues, balloons, and coils.

Pulmonary arteriovenous fistulae are an example of such lesions, which lend themselves to catheter-directed therapies. They may occur as congenital or acquired, solitary or multiple, unilateral or bilateral, local or diffuse. The majority of such lesions involve the lower lobes or right middle lobe, eg, those associated after a classical Glenn (end-to-end superior vena cava to right pulmonary artery) anastomosis (Figure 7). Pulmonary angiography defines the lesion and allows planning for transcatheter occlusion. Occlusive devices include steel coils or detachable balloons. Because of the tendency for such fistulae to reoccur, the procedure is only palliative.[61] In the adult with such fistulae after a Glenn anastomosis, surgical creation of an axillary arteriovenous fistulae may allow regression, by supplying the pulmonary circulation a liver factor required for vessel integrity.[62]

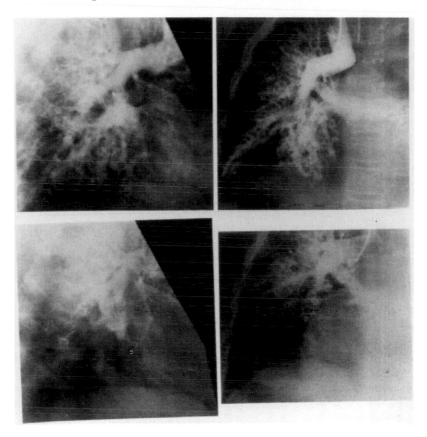

FIGURE 7. *A patient with arteriovenous malformations after a Glenn anastomosis.* **Upper panels** *(lateral/PA) (before) and* **lower panels** *(after) coil occlusion of the lower lobe fistulae.*

Interventional Catheterization as an Adjunct to Surgery

A number of lesions are amenable to occlusion procedures, performed as a planned adjunct to surgery (Table 1). Systemic-to-pulmonary collateral vessels, while preoperatively supporting pulmonary blood flow, will volume overload the left heart postprocedure and compromise perioperative care. Such collaterals should be ligated at the time of surgery, but when inaccessible, should be occluded early after repair.[63] In the preoperative patient, once each collateral vessel is identified, temporary occlusion is performed to determine if a hypoxic response is excessive (due to decreased pulmonary blood flow). If tolerated, the vessel may be occluded. Vessels that taper in diameter are easily occluded with coils or balloons placed directly through a guide catheter. Similarly, surgical shunts may be occluded with coil occluders, umbrellas, or balloons to avoid surgical intervention or a difficult dissection to ligate a shunt (particularly left-sided shunts) during surgical correction. The former is particularly useful if the patient has several sources of pulmonary blood flow, and can tolerate shunt obliteration for a short term, before repair.[63]

Pulmonary Artery Stenosis

The use of balloon angioplasty techniques for native or postoperative pulmonary arterial stenoses has improved survival and decreased morbidity in patients with either surgically untreatable (distal) or only fairly surgically relieved (proximal) stenoses. Such lesions consist of multiple patchy areas of intimal proliferation, and respond to enlargement through intimal and medial layer disruption. Peripheral pulmonary artery stenosis commonly coexists with lesions that restrict pulmonary blood flow in early life (such as Fallot's tetralogy) or occur near the site of previous surgical shunts or repairs (arterioplasties).

Patients considered candidates for intervention are symptomatic or cyanotic if related to restricted pulmonary blood flow, have stenoses that limit surgical or medical options, or lesions that produce right ventricular hypertension. Successful angioplasty results have been defined as vessel enlargements of >50%, or pressure gradient reductions of >30%, or increased flow to the affected lung.

Catheter Technique

After hemodynamic and angiographic definition, a balloon angioplasty catheter is positioned across the stenotic lesion, guided by a stiff exchange wire. Care must be taken, as in other angioplasty procedures, to avoid traversing a dilated (torn) lesion with an unguided catheter. Balloon diameters are chosen to be 3 to 4 times the narrow area and inflated initially at low pressures (4 atm) but gradually to high pressures (12 atm), if a persistent "waist" is present. Despite early encouraging results, recurrence has been frequent (17%) and either nondilatable or clinically nonsignificant caliber changes occur.[64] Nevertheless, this approach appears the initial form of therapy for such lesions.

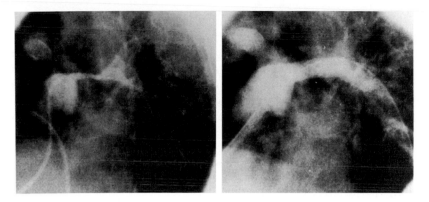

FIGURE 8. *A patient with severe left pulmonary artery stenosis after attempted surgical repair (**left panel**). Poststent implantation (**right panel**).*

Endovascular Stents

Due to nondilatable peripheral pulmonary artery stenosis, the concept of using an expandable endovascular stent to provide support that is resistant to recoil, for the vessel was tested in animal studies[65] and human clinical trials (Figure 8).[66,67] The Palmaz-Stent (Johnson & Johnson, New Brunswick, NJ) is the most widely applied stent for this application.

Catheter Technique

Prior to stent implantation, the lesion is dilated to ensure that it can be distended (if only transiently) and that recoil prevents simple balloon angioplasty. After a long 10F or 12F sheath is placed across the stenosis, a stent is "crimped" on the dilating catheter and the stent-catheter guided to the area of stenosis. The long sheath is withdrawn, the balloon dilated (very dilute contrast) and fixed into the vessel. Repeated dilations with larger balloons may be performed. Care is taken not to overdistend the vessel, creating a substrate for turbulent flow, a concept that determines ultimate balloon size. Low-dose heparin is administered for 24 hours and aspirin for 6 months (3–5 mg/kg per day).

Conduit Obstructions

Pulmonary or aortic homografts or composite conduits are commonly used to create continuity between the right ventricle and pulmonary arteries. Such vascular grafts may become obstructed within, or at the anastomotic sites. The use of balloon dilation and more recently stent implantation[66] (Figure 9) although palliative, has provided good short-term gradient relief to avoid surgical replacement. Long-term palliation in children is unlikely due to growth, although such approaches may afford the adult avoidance of surgery for longer periods. The inadvertent induction of pulmonary insufficiency may ultimately restrict long-term applications. The ultimate role for stent implantation in congenital heart disease is unclear, but early results are encouraging.

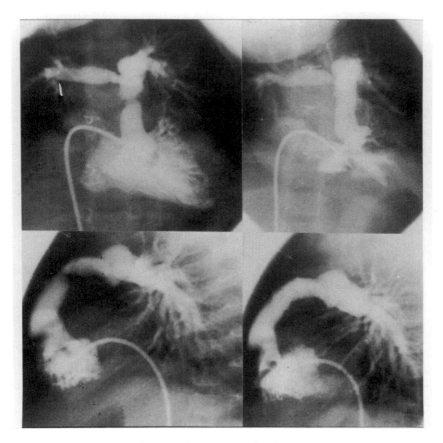

FIGURE 9. *A patient after conduit repair of pulmonary atresia, ventricular septal defect. Note severe conduit obstruction at the level of the conduit valve (aortic homograft)* (**left panels**) *(PA/lateral).* **Right panels,** *poststent implantation.*

Summary

Many of the catheter techniques discussed in this chapter are investigational or have had only early clinical applications. Nevertheless, a number of procedures are considered either: 1) **therapy or choice** (persistently patent ductus arteriosus occlusion, balloon angioplasty or stent implantation for peripheral pulmonary stenosis, balloon angioplasty for recurrent coarctation of the aorta, pulmonary balloon valvotomy, closure of right-to-left intra-atrial shunts, closure of muscular ventricular septal defects, fenestration closures, vascular (collateral) embolizations or 2) **alternatives to surgery** (atrial septal defect closure, balloon angioplasty of native coarctation of the aorta, conduit or baffle stent implantation, embolization of coronary fistulae). Unproven modalities (postmyocardial infarction ventricular defect closure, patent foramen ovale closure for stroke prevention, and stent implantation for pulmonary venous obstruction) require further study.

References

1. Allen, HD, Mullins CE. Results of the valvuloplasty and angioplasty of congenital anomalies registry. *Am J Cardiol.* 1990;65:772–774.
2. Jarmakani JM, Isabel-Jones J. Cardiac catheterization as a therapeutic intervention. In: Perloff JD, Child JD, eds. *Congenital Heart Disease in Adults.* Philadelphia, PA: WB Saunders; 1991;224–238.
3. Gross RE, Hubbard JP. Surgical ligation of a patent ductus arteriosus: report of first successful case. *JAMA.* 1939;112:729–731.
4. Porstmann W, Wierny L, Warnke H, et al. Catheter closure of patent ductus arteriosus—62 cases treated without thoracotomy. *Radiol Clin North Am.* 1971;9:203–218.
5. Wierny L, Plass R, Portsmann W. Transluminal closure of patent ductus arteriosus: long-term results of 208 cases treated without thoracotomy. *Cardiovasc Intervent Radiol.* 1986;9:279–285.
6. Bussman WD, Sievert H, Kohler KP, et al. Transfemoral plug closure of patent ductus arteriosus. *Z Kardiol.* 1987;76(Suppl VI):85.
7. Rashkind WJ, Cuaso CC. Transcatheter closure of patent ductus arteriosus: successful use in a 3.5 kilogram infant. *Pediatr Cardiol.* 1979;1: 3–7.
8. Bash SE, Mullins CE. Insertion of patent ductus arteriosus occluder by transvenous approach: a new technique. *Circulation.* 1984;70(Suppl II): II-285. Abstract.
9. Krichenko A, Benson LN, Burrows P, et al. Angiographic classification of the isolated, persistently patent ductus arteriosus and implications for percutaneous catheter occlusion. *Am J Cardiol.* 1989;63:877–900.
10. Rashkind WJ, Mullins CE, Hellenbrand WE, et al. Non-surgical closure of patent ductus arteriosus: clinical application of the Rashkind PDA occluder system. *Circulation.* 1987;75:583–592.

11. Hosking MCK, Benson LN, Musewe N, Dyck J, Freedom RM. Transcatheter occlusion of the persistently patent ductus arteriosus: 40 month follow up and prevalence of residual shunting. *Circulation.* 1991;84:2313–2317.
12. McLaughlin PR, Benson LN, Walters J. Umbrella closure of patent ductus arteriosus in the adult. *Can J Cardiol.* 1991;7:133A. Abstract.
13. Bridges ND, Perry SB, Parness I, et al. Transcatheter closure of a large patent ductus arteriosus with the clamshell septal occluder. *J Am Coll Cardiol.* 1991;18:1297–1302.
14. Rubio V, Limon-Lason R. Treatment of pulmonary valvular stenosis and of tricuspid stenosis using a modified catheter. Second World Congress on Cardiology, Washington, DC, Program Abstracts II, 1956.
15. Semb BKH, Tijonneland S, Stake G, et al. "Balloon valvulotomy" of congenital pulmonary valve stenosis with tricuspid insufficiency. *Cardiovasc Radiol.* 1979;2:239–241.
16. Kan JS, White RJ, Mitchell SE, et al. Percutaneous balloon valvuplasty: a new method for treating congenital pulmonary valve stenosis. *N Engl J Med.* 1982;307:540–542.
17. Stanger P, Cassidy SC, Girod DA, et al. Balloon pulmonary valvuloplasty: results of the valvuloplasty and angioplasty of congenital anomalies registry. *Am J Cardiol.* 1990;65:775–783.
18. Park JH, Yoon YS, Yeon KM, et al. Percutaneous pulmonary valvuloplasty with a double balloon technique. *Radiology.* 1987;164:715.
19. Al-Kasab S, Ribeiro P, Al-Zaibag M. Use of a double balloon technique for percutaneous balloon pulmonary valvatomy in adults. *Br Heart J.* 1987;58:136–141.
20. Rao PS. Balloon pulmonary valvuloplasty: a review. *Clin Cardiol.* 1989;12:55–74.
21. McCrindle BW, Kan JS. Long-term results after balloon pulmonary valvuloplasty. *Circulation.* 1991;83:1915–1922.
22. Hellenbrand WE, Allen HD, Golinko RJ, et al. Balloon angioplasty for aortic recoarctation: results of valvuloplasty and angioplasty of congenital anomalies registry. *Am J Cardiol.* 1990;65:793–797.
23. Tynan M, Finley JP, Fontes V, et al. Balloon angioplasty for the treatment of native coarctation: results of valvuloplasty and angioplasty of congenital anomalies registry. *Am J Cardiol.* 1990;65:790–792.
24. Lock JE, Bass JL, Amplatz K, et al. Balloon dilation angioplasty of aortic coarctation in infants and children. *Circulation.* 1983;68:109–116.
25. Hijazi ZM, Fahey JT, Kleinman CS, et al. Balloon angioplasty for recurrent coarctation of aorta. *Circulation.* 1991;84:1150–1156.
26. Pinzon JL, Burrows P, Benson L, et al. The morphology of the aortic arch after repair of coarctation of the aorta. *Radiology.* 1991;180:199–203.
27. Mendelsohn AM, Crowley DC, Koics KC, et al. Balloon angioplasty of native coarctation of aorta: eight year experience. *Circulation.* 1992;82:(Suppl I):I-633. Abstract.
28. Tyagi S, Arora R, Kaul VA, et al. Balloon angioplasty of native coarctation of the aorta in adolescents and young adults. *Am Heart J.* 1992;123:674–680.
29. Murphy JG, Gersh BJ, McGoon MD, et al. Long-term outcome after surgical repair of isolated atrial septal defect. *N Engl J Med.* 1990;323:1645–1650.
30. Horvath KA, Burke RP, Collins JJ, et al. Surgical treatment of adult

atrial septal defect: early and long-term results. *J Am Coll Cardiol.* 1992; 20:1156–1159.
31. King TD, Thompson SL, Steiner C, et al. Secundum atrial septal defect—non-operative closure during cardiac catheterization. *JAMA.* 1976;235:2506–2509.
32. Rashkind WJ. Transcatheter treatment of congenital heart disease. *Circulation.* 1983;67:711–716.
33. Lock JE, Rome JJ, Davis R, et al. Transcatheter closure of atrial septal defects—experimental studies. *Circulation.* 1989;79:1091–1099.
34. Latson LA. Transcatheter closure of atrial septal defects. In: Rao PS, ed. *Transcatheter Therapy in Pediatric Cardiology.* New York, NY: Wiley-Liss; pp 335–348.
35. Landzberg MJ, Bridges ND, van der Velde N, et al. Double umbrella closure of atrial septal defects in adults. *Circulation.* 1991;84:II-68. Abstract.
36. Sideris EB, Sideris SE, Fowlkes JP, et al. Transvenous atrial septal defect occlusion with a "button" double disk device. *Circulation.* 1990;81: 312–318.
37. Rao PS, Sideris EB. Transcatheter closure of heart defects: the role of "buttoned devices. In: Rao PS, ed. *Transcatheter Therapy in Pediatric Cardiology.* New York, NY: Wiley-Liss; 349–369.
38. Landzberg MJ, Bridges ND, Bittl JA, et al. Transcatheter closure of atrial septal defects in adults with orthodeoxia—platypnea syndrome. *J Am Coll Cardiol.* 1992;19:289A. Abstract.
39. Lechat PH, Max JL, Lascault G, et al. Prevalence of patent foramen ovale in patients with stroke. *N Engl J Med.* 1988;318:1148–1152.
40. Bridges ND, Hellenbrand W, Latson L, et al. Transcatheter closure of patent foramen ovale after presumed paradoxical embolism. *Circulation.* 1992;86:1902–1908.
41. Bailey LL, Freedom RM, Fowler RJ, et al. Non-operative management of late failure of a Glenn anastomosis. *J Thorac Cardiovasc Surg.* 1976; 71:371–375.
42. Beckman RH, Rocchini AP. Transcatheter treatment of congenital heart disease. *Prog Cardiovasc Dis.* 1989;32:1–30.
43. Hourihan M, Perry SB, Mandell VS, et al. Transcatheter closure of valvar and paravalvar leaks. *J Am Coll Cardiol.* 1992;20:1371–1377.
44. Lock JE, Cockerham JT, Keane JF, et al. Transcatheter umbrella closure of congenital defects. *Circulation.* 1987;75:593–599.
45. Bridges ND, Lock JE, Castaneda AR. Baffle fenestration with subsequent transcatheter closure—modification of the Fontan operation for patients at increased risk. *Circulation.* 1990;82:1681–1689.
46. Bridges ND, Castaneda AR. The fenestrated Fontan procedure. *Herz.* 1992;17:242–245.
47. Lock JE, Block PC, McKay RG, et al. Transcatheter closure of ventricular septal defects. *Circulation.* 1988;78:361–368.
48. Bridges ND, Perry SB, Keane JF, et al. Preoperative transcatheter closure of congenital muscular ventricular defects. *N Engl J Med.* 1991; 324:1312–1317.
49. Lababidi Z, Wm J, Walls JT. Percutaneous balloon aortic valvuloplasty results in 23 patients. *Am J Cardiol.* 1984;53:194–197.
50. Cribier A, Savin T, Berland J, et al. Percutaneous transluminal valvuloplasty of acquired aortic stenosis in elderly patients: an alternative to valve replacement? *Lancet.* 1986;1:63–67.

51. Wagner HR, Ellison RC, Keane JF, et al. Clinical course in aortic stenosis. *Circulation.* 1977;56(Suppl I):I-47-I-56.
52. Sholler GF, Keane JF, Perry SB, et al. Balloon dilation of congenital aortic valve stenosis. *Circulation.* 1988;78:351–360.
53. Safian RD, Berman AD, Diver DJ, et al. Balloon aortic valvuloplasty in 170 consecutive patients *N Engl J Med.* 1988;319:125–130.
54. Rosenfeld HM, Perry SB, Kean JF, et al. Balloon aortic valvotomy in young adults with congenital aortic stenosis. *Circulation.* 1990;82:III-29. Abstract.
55. Berdoff RL, Strain J, Crandall C, et al. Pathology of aortic valvuloplasty: findings after postmortem successful and failed dilations. *Am Heart J.* 1989;117:688–690.
56. O'Connor BK, Beekman RH, Rocchini AP, et al. Intermediate-term effectiveness of balloon valvuloplasty for congenital aortic stenosis. *Circulation.* 1991;84:732–738.
57. Rocchini AP, Beekman RH, Ben Shachar G, et al. Balloon aortic valvuloplasty. Results of the Valvuloplasty and Angiography of Congenital Anomalies Registry. *Am J Cardiol.* 1990;65:784–789.
58. Hosking MCK, Alshehri M, Murdison KA, et al: Transcatheter management of pulmonary venous pathway obstruction with atrial baffle leak following Mustard and Senning repair. *Cath Cardiovasc Diag.* 1993;30:76–82.
59. Chatelain P, Meier B, Friedli. Stenting of superior vena cava and inferior vena cava for symptomatic narrowing after repeated atrial surgery for D-transposition of the great arteries. *Br Heart J.* 1991;66:466–468.
60. Ensing GJ, Hagler DJ, Seward JB, et al. Caveats of balloon dilation of conduits and conduit valves. *J Am Coll Cardiol.* 1989;14:397–400.
61. Hoekenga DE, Stevens GF, Ball WS. Percutaneous angioplasty for peripheral pulmonary stenosis in the adult. *Am J Cardiol.* 1987;59:188–189.
62. Jonas RA. Invited letter concerning: the importance of pulsatile flow when systemic venous return is connected directly to the pulmonary arteries. *J Thorac Cardiovasc Surg.* 1993;105:173–174.
63. Perry SB, Radtke W, Fellows KE, et al. Coil embolization to occlude aortopulmonary collateral vessels and shunts in patients with congenital heart disease. *J Am Coll Cardiol.* 1989;13:100–108.
64. Hosking MCK, Thomaidis C, Hamilton R, et al. Clinical impact of balloon angioplasty for branch pulmonary artery stenosis. *Am J Cardiol.* 1992;69:1467–1470.
65. Benson LN, Hamilton F, Dasmahapatra H, et al. Percutaneous implantation of balloon expandable endoprosthesis for pulmonary artery stenosis: an experimental study. *J Am Coll Cardiol.* 1991;18:1303–1308.
66. Hosking MCK, Benson LN, Nakanishi T, et al. Intravascular stent prothesis for right ventricular outflow obstruction. *J Am Coll Cardiol.* 1992;20;373–380.
67. O'Laughlin MP, Perry SB, Lock JE, et al. Use of endovascular stents in congenital heart disease. *Circulation.* 1991;83:1923–1939.

Chapter 30

The Use of Direct Angioplasty in the Treatment of Acute Myocardial Infarction

Robert M. Califf, MD,
Robert A. Harrington, MD,
Richard S. Stack, MD, and
Harry R. Phillips, III, MD

The establishment of reperfusion as the cornerstone of the treatment of acute myocardial infarction (MI) has generally been accepted. The preferred method of establishing reperfusion is considerably less clear. Thrombolytic therapy saves 25–30 lives per 1,000 patients treated in the setting of ST segment elevation within 6 hours of symptom onset.[1] This benefit has been documented in clinical trials involving more than 100,000 patients in settings ranging from extremely sophisticated medical care facilities to rural hospitals with minimal ancillary support. After years of single center series purporting to demonstrate that direct angioplasty is an excellent therapy for MI, several small clinical trials in experienced hospitals generally serving as centers for direct angioplasty have shown dramatic advantages for this procedure over thrombolytic therapy.[2-4] This chapter systematically reviews the evidence in favor of each approach and attempts to present a balanced point of view. We begin with a discussion of conceptual issues, followed by an overview of available information from clinical trials, and a discussion of current research needs.

The fundamental issues that must be considered in the evaluation of therapy for acute MI are becoming increasingly evident. The central importance of TIMI grade 3 flow early in the course was so-

From Vetrovec GW, Carabello BA, (eds.) *Invasive Cardiology: Current Diagnostic and Therapeutic Issues.* Armonk, NY: Futura Publishing Company, Inc.: © 1996.

lidified by the results of the GUSTO trial.[5] In this study, the establishment of TIMI grade 3 flow at 90 minutes was associated with 4.3% mortality compared with 8% for TIMI grade 2 flow and almost 10% for TIMI grade 0 or 1 flow. Balanced against the preeminence of early achievement of TIMI grade 3 flow to preserve myocardium is the risk of reocclusion, which can negate the advantages of early reperfusion.[6] The issue of harm to organ systems other than the heart induced by this therapy must be addressed through careful observation of clinical outcomes in large numbers of patients. Even in the most skilled hands, the process of angioplasty itself is associated with a variety of complications, including thrombotic, mechanical and bleeding events. Thrombolytic therapy is also associated with a substantial risk of bleeding. In addition to the medical outcomes, the financial outcomes must also be considered. Increasingly, modest differences in the effects of treatment will be placed in the paradigm of cost effectiveness compared with other therapeutic choices. Finally, a minimum of 6 months of follow-up is required for comparison, to take into account the evolutionary processes of plaque and myocardial remodeling after the acute event, although a year of follow-up would be ideal.

Sources of Data

Until recently, the only available data for evaluating direct angioplasty consisted of single center observational case series. These series were criticized because they were most often reported by the individuals performing the procedures, raising questions about the objectivity of the reported outcomes. In the past several years, a series of small randomized trials has provided the most objective estimate of outcome. Table 1 outlines the design of each of these trials. The Primary Angioplasty in Myocardial Infarction Trial (PAMI)[2] compared "conventional" tissue plasminogen activator (tPA) administration with direct angioplasty in 395 patients, with the primary end point of combined incidence of death or reinfarction. The ongoing Dutch study[3] has compared standard streptokinase and direct angioplasty in 142 patients, with the primary end point of left ventricular ejection fraction on radionuclide angiography 6 weeks after the acute event. The Mayo study[4] enrolled only 97 patients because of the use of the sensitive end point of Tc-sestamibi infarct size. Finally, Ribiero et al[7] randomized 50 patients in a trial designed to evaluate a composite of clinical end points. All of these studies reported the critical clinical end points of death, reinfarction, recurrent ischemia, bleeding, and stroke.

Table 1

Strategies in Recent Randomized Trials of Direct PTCA vs. Thrombolysis

Trial	Patients	Thrombolytic	Primary End Point
PAMI[2]	395	tPA	Death ± reinfarction ± recurrent ischemia
Mayo[4]	97	tPA	Tc-sestamibi infarct size
Dutch[3]	142	SK	MUGA LV ejection fraction
Ribiero[7]	50	SK	Composite of clinical endpoints

PTCA, percutaneous transluminal coronary angioplasty; PAMI, Primary Angioplasty in Myocardial Infarction trial; tPA, tissue-plasminogen activator; SK, streptokinase; MUGA, multiple gated angiography; LV, left ventricular.

An additional multicenter registry, the Primary Angioplasty Registry (PAR),[8,9] which included 271 patients, had goals of developing objective parameters to describe clinical outcomes in a multicenter study and evaluating the effects of direct angioplasty on 6-month stenosis of the culprit artery and on left ventricular function. These results are supplemented by the findings of the Alabama Reperfusion in Myocardial Infarction Registry (ARMI),[10] which is an observational database at a number of medical centers in Alabama focusing on candidates for reperfusion therapy. In addition, the Myocardial Infarction Triage and Intervention (MITI) group[11] has established a database of all patients undergoing either thrombolytic therapy or direct angioplasty in Kings County, Washington.

Conceptual Issues

Feasibility

Proponents of direct angioplasty can now point to literature citing hundreds of cases with a high clinical success rate and a mortality rate similar to that of thrombolytic therapy. Claims that this procedure would not be feasible because of the illness of the patient or the complexity of the coronary lesion are no longer tenable. Two hundred and seventy-one patients in the PAR registry were identified in the emergency department as potential candidates for direct angioplasty; successful dilation of the infarct-related artery was achieved in 91%.[8] Most patients who were not considered candidates based on angiography experienced reperfu-

sion with TIMI grade 3 flow prior to consideration of direct angioplasty. Accordingly, over 90% of the patients had TIMI grade 3 flow
within several hours of the event. Furthermore, 88% had a reduction in residual stenosis to ≤50% luminal diameter as assessed by
an independent angiographic core laboratory.

Proponents of thrombolytic therapy can point to the huge
number of patients who have been entered into clinical trials in a
variety of clinical settings.[1,12,13] This therapy can be given with minimal medical supervision, although rapid and efficient administration requires a carefully organized community approach. In
comparison, direct angioplasty requires a carefully orchestrated effort by a highly qualified cardiologist and a technical staff capable
of manipulating complex equipment. Available literature points to
a substantial impact of the operator and hospital on the ultimate
outcome of the patient; inexperienced operators[14] and low volume
hospitals[15] have worse outcomes, including lower success rates,
higher mortality, and more emergency bypass surgery. The question of generalizing from the small, positive clinical trials remains
significant.

The simplicity of administration of thrombolytic therapy has
led many observers to conclude that time to reperfusion is shorter
with thrombolytic therapy than with direct angioplasty. This belief
would seem to be self-evident, given the fact that thrombolytic therapy can be administered in a variety of settings by the emergency
department staff, while direct angioplasty requires the assembly of
a sophisticated staff and movement of the patient to an appropriate facility. In fact, however, the 1-hour delay between emergency
department registration and treatment found in United States hospitals, coupled with the 45-minute time from treatment to reperfusion, can make the time to reperfusion using the two approaches
quite comparable (Figure 1).

Pathophysiologic Plausibility

The milieu of a culprit lesion in MI would seem to be inhos-
pitable to the use of mechanical therapy to establish reperfusion.
The disrupted plaque could make it difficult to negotiate the lesion.
Furthermore, studies of unstable angina have clearly established
that active atherosclerotic plaque is associated with an increased
risk of acute clinical events during and after angioplasty[16–18] and of
restenosis within 6 months after the procedure.[19] Pathological
studies have demonstrated that direct angioplasty or angioplasty

Time to Treatment

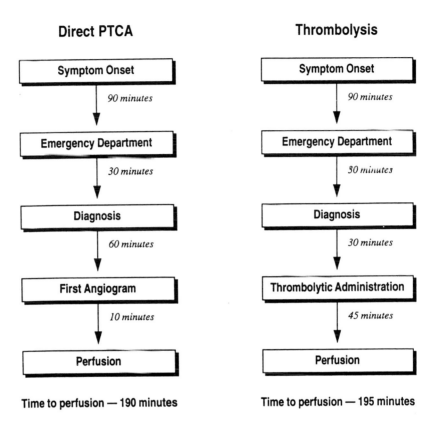

FIGURE 1. *Time to reperfusion for patients treated with PTCA and thrombolytics. PTCA, percutaneous transluminal coronary angioplasty.*

after thrombolytic therapy can be associated with extensive hemorrhage into the plaque.[20–22]

In contrast, the use of thrombolytic agents with associated antithrombin or antiplatelet therapy would seem to be a direct approach to counter the pathophysiologic mechanisms.

In a simpler fashion, however, mechanical agitation of the clot with relief of the underlying stenosis provides an attractive approach to the acute problem. Furthermore, a wider lumen should lower the risk of recurrent ischemia and rethrombosis of the culprit lesion, especially if accompanied by appropriate conjunctive antithrombotic therapy.

Physiologic Results

Thrombolytic therapy results in reperfusion of the infarct-related artery in 50%–85% of patients within the first 90 minutes of therapy, depending on the pharmacologic regimen chosen.[5,12,23] In 30%–55% of these cases, TIMI grade 3 flow is established in this time frame, with these patients having the lowest associated mortality. Over the next several hours, a steady-state perfusion rate of 80%–85% is observed with all of the available thrombolytic agents. Left ventricular function results have been disappointing with thrombolytic therapy, however, with an average difference of 2%–4% between patients who received thrombolytic agents and control patients in randomized trials.[12] A variety of reasons have been postulated for this modest effect, including frequent failure to establish early TIMI grade 3 reperfusion, common reperfusion-and-reocclusion cycles, and reperfusion injury.

Direct angioplasty achieves TIMI grade 3 flow in over 90% of patients in experienced centers. These results have now been duplicated in several multicenter studies, in addition to the many single center studies reported over the past decade. Uncontrolled studies with direct angioplasty have indicated that treatment is associated with a dramatic improvement in regional and global left ventricular function. Subsequent randomized trials have been less consistent. The Mayo study[4] found no difference in Tc-sestamibi estimated infarct size, proportion of area-at-risk salvaged or systolic left ventricular function. In contrast, the Dutch study[3] observed a substantial improvement in global left ventricular function in patients treated with direct angioplasty compared with patients treated with streptokinase.

Clinical Outcomes

Mortality

The use of direct angioplasty is associated with a substantial reduction in the risk of death in reported clinical trials (Table 2). This reduction (over 50% compared with thrombolytic therapy) would have a major impact on public health if these results were sustained with larger numbers of patients in multiple representative hospitals.

A variety of major concerns must be considered before these data are permitted to affect routine clinical practice. First, the centers participating in the trials had a long and dedicated interest in

Table 2

Direct PTCA vs. Thrombolysis: Mortality

	Thrombolysis		PTCA	
	n	Mortality # (%)	n	Mortality # (%)
PAMI[2]	200	13 (6.5)	195	5 (2.4)
Mayo[4]	50	2 (4)	47	2 (4.3)
Dutch[3]	70	4 (5.7)	72	0 (0)
Brazilian[7]	50	1 (2)	50	3 (6)
	370	20 (5.4)	364	10 (2.7)

PTCA, percutaneous transluminal coronary angioplasty; PAMI, Primary Angioplasty in Myocardial Infarction.

the use of direct angioplasty; thus the low mortality they realized may not be generalizable. Even within the Primary Angioplasty Registry, which included only dedicated sites, the mortality rate was almost double the observed mortality in the trials. Furthermore, Jollis and colleagues,[15] in an analysis of over 200,000 angioplasty procedures in the Medicare database, demonstrated a substantial incremental risk of death in centers performing fewer than 100 angioplasty procedures per year in Medicare patients. This relationship was even more pronounced in patients who underwent angioplasty in the setting of acute MI.

Secondly, the mortality of the thrombolytic treated patients in the PAMI trial, which to a large extent drives this overview, was inflated by the excessive rate of intracranial hemorrhage encountered in that trial. The rate of 1.3% is far outside the 95% confidence limits for the aggregate studies of tPA use.

The available trials used either standard-dose streptokinase or a 3-hour infusion of tPA as the comparative thrombolytic regimens. The Global Utilization of Streptokinase and Tissue Plasminogen Activator (GUSTO) trial,[24] however, demonstrated a relative 14% reduction in mortality with accelerated tPA compared with streptokinase, which had the same mortality as the 3-hour tPA infusion in several large trials. These data suggest that future studies should use accelerated tPA as the comparison group.

Finally, two observational studies have found a higher mortality rate in direct angioplasty patients than in thrombolytic-treated patients. In the state of Alabama, 107 patients treated with direct angioplasty had a mortality rate of 9.4% compared with 3.2% for 125 patients treated with thrombolysis.[10] After adjustment for baseline covariables, no significant difference was found in the mortality rate. Similarly, in a case control study in Seattle, Washington, in which patients were matched as to key baseline characteristics describing severity of the MI, the mortality rate was 11% with direct angioplasty and 8% with thrombolysis.[11]

In summary, the overview from small randomized trials demonstrates a provocative reduction in the risk of death. Whether these results will be stable in larger studies, which can provide more accurate statistical estimates and test therapies in a variety of clinical settings, remains to be seen. Currently, however, these data support the use of direct angioplasty in expert centers with efficient systems for performing the the procedure.

Reinfarction

The trials show a consistent and dramatic reduction in the rate of reinfarction with direct angioplasty compared with thrombolytic therapy (Table 3). Reocclusion leading to reinfarction is an expected outcome of thrombolytic therapy, since clot lysis is a dynamic process that induces a paradoxical prothrombotic state.[25] The unmasking of clot-bound thrombin by the gradual process of clot lysis precipitates recurrent thrombus formation, which, if inadequately opposed by endogenous mechanisms or pharmacotherapy, leads to recurrent occlusion. The achievement of a wide lumen with direct angioplasty leads to improved flow, thus eliminating one of the critical ingredients for intravascular thrombosis—impaired flow. The wide lumen could also be expected to increase the allowance for active thrombus formation on the surface of the plaque without occluding the lumen.

Improved conjunctive antithrombotic therapy with aspirin and

Table 3

Direct PTCA vs. Thrombolysis: Reinfarction

	Thrombolysis		PTCA	
	n	MI # (%)	n	MI # (%)
PAMI[2]	200	8 (4)	195	5 (3)
Mayo[4]	50	2 (4)	47	0 (0)
Dutch[3]	70	9 (13)	72	0 (0)
Brazilian[7]	50	0 (0)	50	0 (0)
	370	19 (5)	364	5 (1.4)

PTCA, percutaneous transluminal coronary angioplasty; MI, myocardial infarction; PAMI, Primary Angioplasty in Myocardial Infarction.

heparin or new antithrombotic agents[26-28] appears to have reduced reocclusion rates with thrombolytic therapy and angioplasty in recent trials. However, little information exists about the in-hospital angiographic follow-up in patients treated with direct angioplasty. Thus, the detection of reocclusion and reinfarction may not have been ideal in these trials. Although the new, more aggressive regimens may decrease the reinfarction rate with thrombolysis, direct angioplasty appears to have a significant advantage.

Stroke

The randomized trials demonstrate a remarkable absence of stroke in patients treated with direct angioplasty (Table 4). This finding is intuitively appealing—since no thrombolytic agent was administered, the risk of intracranial hemorrhage should have been essentially eliminated.

The total absence of stroke in these trials is clearly a statistical fluke, however. Nothing about direct angioplasty would be expected to eliminate the risk of thrombotic stroke, an outcome that occurs in 0.5% to 2% of patients with acute MI.[1,29,30]

In the PAR registry, three strokes occurred among 271 patients. One stroke was hemorrhagic, occurring in a patient who was treated with high-dose heparin during a complex procedure. Furthermore, as previously noted, the 3.2% risk of stroke observed in PAMI was far out of line with other experiences with thrombolytic therapy. Given the previously accumulated data, the likelihood of this result occurring is <0.1% (1 in 1,000).

TABLE 4

Direct PTCA vs. Thrombolysis: Stroke

	Thrombolysis		PTCA	
	n	Stroke # (%)	n	Stroke # (%)
PAMI[2]	200	4 (2)	195	0 (0)
Mayo[4]	50	0 (0)	47	0 (0)
Dutch[3]	70	2 (3)	72	0 (0)
Brazilian[7]	50	0 (0)	50	0 (0)
	370	6 (1.6)	364	0 (0)

PTCA, percutaneous transluminal coronary angioplasty; PAMI, Primary Angioplasty in Myocardial Infarction.

Recurrent Ischemia

The risk of recurrent ischemia closely tracks the risk of reinfarction; direct angioplasty produced a marked reduction compared with thrombolytic therapy in the clinical trials (Table 5). This result is consistent with the trials of routine angioplasty after thrombolytic therapy.[31-33]

Producing a wide lumen improves coronary flow and reduces the likelihood of reocclusion and stenosis to the point of recurrent ischemia. Symptomatic recurrent ischemia is a major problem with thrombolytic therapy, occurring in 25%–30% of patients. Asymptomatic ischemia or ischemia during later functional testing is also substantial. Recurrent ischemia is associated with a substantial incremental risk.[34,35]

Congestive Heart Failure

Almost no information exists comparing direct angioplasty with thrombolytic therapy with an end point of symptomatic congestive heart failure.

Longer Term Follow-up

Posthospital follow-up has been reported in direct comparisons[2,3] with maintenance or enhancement of the difference in outcomes observed over the first 6 weeks to 6 months after hospital discharge. In the PAR study,[9] the restenosis rate at 6 months of follow-up varied from 40% to 53% depending on the definition used.

Table 5

Direct PTCA vs. Thrombolysis: Recurrent Ischemia

	Thrombolysis		PTCA	
	n	# (%)	n	# (%)
PAMI2	200	56 (28)	195	20 (10)
Mayo4	—	—	—	—
Dutch3	70	27 (39)	72	6 (8)
Brazilian7	50	5 (10)	50	4 (8)
	320	88 (28)	317	30 (9)

PTCA, percutaneous transluminal coronary angioplasty; PAMI, Primary Angioplasty in Myocardial Infarction.

Clinical events after hospital discharge were rare, with a mortality rate of 2%, reinfarction rate of <5%, and a repeat revascularization rate of <25%. Reocclusion occurred in 13% of the cases after hospital discharge. No comparable data exist for thrombolysis, although the APRICOT study[36] reported a 25%–30% reocclusion rate within 3 months of successful thrombolysis.

Quality of Life

No direct comparisons exist with regard to quality of life during the first year after acute infarction in patients who undergo direct angioplasty. In TAMI 5[37] and PAR,[9] however, detailed information was gathered on multiple aspects of quality of life, including symptom status, employment, psychological status, and capacity to perform routine activities. As shown in Table 6, no substantial differences were observed between the two modes of therapy, nor would they be expected.

Cost

When the initial studies of angioplasty after thrombolytic therapy were reported, it seemed rational that the cost of routine angioplasty would exceed the cost of thrombolytic therapy (with revascularization reserved for patients meeting certain criteria). Direct comparisons performed thus far, however, have found no significant difference in cost, but a trend that favors the direct angioplasty strategy (Table 7). The underlying rationale for these findings is that performing an angiogram in the early phase of the infarction provides knowledge about the success of the initial reperfusion attempt while simultaneously allowing an accurate assessment of risk due to other underlying disease. This information allows the clinician to more expeditiously discharge the low-risk patient, while concentrating resources on the higher-risk patient. Furthermore, the beneficial reductions in recurrent ischemia and reinfarction offset the increased cost of the early procedure, because more subsequent procedures are needed to treat recurrent ischemia in patients treated with thrombolytic therapy.

Direct comparisons of cost are complex because of the variability of costs and charges from center to center. Charges traditionally have been fixed arbitrarily at each individual hospital[38] and have only an approximate relationship to the true cost of caring for the patient. Methods now exist for estimating true cost based on itemized billing or "microcosting systems," but these methods have

Table 6

Direct PTCA vs. Thrombolytics: Quality of Life

Rand MHI 5 (all/most of the time)	PAR (n = 251)	TAMI 5 (n = 443)
Happy	64%	57%
Calm, peaceful	52	48
Nervous	11	11
Downhearted, blue	6	8
In the dumps	3	4
Health interferes with social function	6	7
Health interferes with concentration	4	6
General Health Status		
Can do anything	22	20
Can do almost anything	55	55
Trouble with some activities	18	20
Trouble doing anything	6	6
Change from baseline		
Better	37	47
Same	50	41
Worse	37	47
Six-month Work Status		
Full/part-time	45	45
Sick leave	3	2
Laid off/unemployed	4	2
Retired/disabled	40	44
Homemaker	4	5
Change from baseline (working patients n = 136)		
Stopped work	9	—
Working more hours	3	—
Working fewer hours	9	—
Doing more strenuous work	1	—
Doing less strenuous work	3	—

PTCA, percutaneous transluminal coronary angioplasty; PAR, Primary Angioplasty Registry; TAMI 5, Thrombolysis and Angioplasty in Myocardial Infarction; MHI, mental health index.

not been applied to direct comparisons of angioplasty and thrombolytic therapy. Since charges related to invasive cardiology are generally disproportionately "marked up" to offset losses in other parts of the hospital, it is likely that a true cost comparison at the individual patient level would further favor direct angioplasty.

Another major issue in the discussion of costs for these ap-

Table 7

Direct PTCA vs. Thrombolytics: Costs

Study	Years of Enrollment	Study Type	n	Cost Measure	Time of Analysis	Hospital Days		Costs ($)	
						PTCA	Lytic Rx	PTCA	Lytic RX
De Wood[52]	N/A	RCT vs. tPA	54	Hospital charges	Initial hospitalization 1 year	N/A	N/A	14500 ± 5900	19000 ± 10800
O'Neil et al[53]	1988–1990	RCT vs. SK	122	Hospital charges	Initial hospitalization	7.7 ± 4	9 ± 5	18200 ± 7900 19643 ± 7250	25000 ± 12400 25191 ± 15368
Gibbons et al[4]	1989–1991	RCT vs. tPA	103	Hospital charges estimated costs	Initial hospitalization 6 months	7.7 ± 2.9	10.6 ± 8.1	16811 ± 8827 480 ± 3609	21400 ± 14806 2738 ± 7666
Grines et al[2]	1990–1992	RCT vs. tPA	358	Hospital charges MD fees	Initial hospitalization	N/A	N/A	24569	28235
Browne et al[54] Mark et al[55,56]	1990–1992	Prospective cohort	270	Hospital costs MD fees	Initial hospitalization 6 months Initial hospitalization 6 months	9.1	—	4239 ± 3260 12772 ± 8548 3563 ± 6543 5522 ± 2570 1144 ± 2426	3263 ± 10792 — — —

PTCA, percutaneous transluminal coronary angioplasty; RCT, randomized, controlled trial; tPA, accelerated tissue-plasminogen activator; N/A, not applicable; SK, streptokinase. (Adapted from Reference 38 with permission.)

proaches is the overall cost of building and maintaining facilities for percutaneous intervention and surgical backup. The fixed cost of providing every hospital with these facilities and the ongoing cost of equipment upgrade would be substantial and might not be reflected in the charges to the individual patient undergoing direct angioplasty, since these costs could be spread across other cardiovascular diagnoses. Regionalization of direct angioplasty would allow most patients in the United States to have access to direct angioplasty without increasing the total number of facilities, but such an approach is not feasible given the current structure of the health care system. Thus the charges to the individual patient may be lower on average with a strategy of direct angioplasty, but the proliferation of catheterization facilities would add substantially to the national budget for health care unless the facilities were carefully planned with regional access as a primary determinant of the need to open a facility.

Contraindications to Thrombolysis

A large number of patients with a diagnosis of acute MI and ST segment elevation have an absolute or strong relative contraindication to thrombolytic therapy. Perhaps the most frequent such contraindication is a recent history of stroke. In the GUSTO registry (Figure 2), 15% of patients with ST segment elevation had a clearcut exclusion criterion and 10% had other reasons to withhold thrombolytic therapy. Perhaps even more common is that patients will have multiple relative contraindications, making the practitioner uncertain about the risk/benefit ratio. The MITI group demonstrated that multiple factors were often involved in the decision not to give thrombolytic therapy to the elderly.[39]

Interestingly, Cragg and colleagues[40] demonstrated that these patients have an exceedingly high mortality, a finding that also was replicated in the GUSTO myocardial infarction registry.[24] Brodie and colleagues[41] have demonstrated satisfactory results in patients with contraindications to thrombolytic therapy, although no controlled or randomized studies in this population have been reported. Future studies should focus on controlled trials comparing a strategy of immediate angiography with conservative therapy in this population.

Cardiogenic Shock

Patients with cardiogenic shock on admission have an extremely high mortality that has not been significantly reduced by

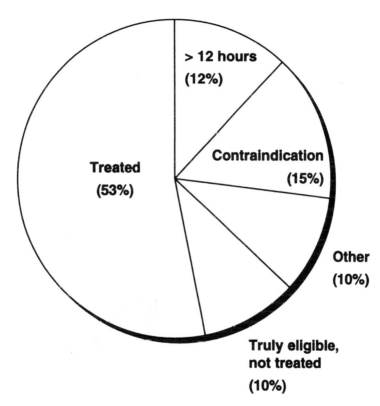

GUSTO MI Log
386 Patients with ST↑

- > 12 hours (12%)
- Contraindication (15%)
- Treated (53%)
- Other (10%)
- Truly eligible, not treated (10%)

FIGURE 2. *Contraindications to thrombolysis in patients with ST segment elevation.*

interventions such as hemodynamic monitoring, inotropic support, vasodilator therapy or intra-aortic balloon pumping.[42,43] Furthermore, clinical trials of thrombolytic therapy have been disappointing in patients with cardiogenic shock, with no definitive evidence of a mortality reduction in this group. However, because few patients with true cardiogenic shock were enrolled in thrombolytic trials, the confidence limits for the estimate of treatment effect on mortality in these patients overlap with the estimate for thrombolytics in general (25%–30% mortality reduction).[44] Some empirical data[45] and a reasonable theoretical rationale[46] have been advanced that associate this apparent limitation of thrombolytic therapy with a lower reperfusion rate. In the recently completed

GUSTO I trial, the overall mortality in the 315 patients presenting in cardiogenic shock was 58%: 61% of the patients with shock in the accelerated tPA group died compared with 57% of those in the streptokinase group.

In contrast, the outcomes with direct angioplasty appear to be substantially better than with thrombolysis. When reperfusion with direct angioplasty has been successful, the mortality has been <50% in-hospital[47] and long-term outcomes appear to be excellent.[43] When reperfusion is not achieved with direct angioplasty, the outcome is dismal. These observational studies must be interpreted with caution, however, because patients selected to undergo direct angioplasty may be quite different from the entire population of patients with cardiogenic shock. A recent observational study by Hochman and colleagues indicated that the most important prognostic factor in a cardiogenic shock population was the decision to go to the cardiac catheterization laboratory,[48] indicating that in observational studies the angioplasty procedure may simply be a marker for a lower risk, salvageable patient.

Other High-risk Groups

Analyses of the results of the published randomized trials of direct angioplasty versus thrombolytic therapy indicate that patients with the most to gain from direct angioplasty are those with the highest risk.[2] Thus, older patients with anterior infarction, large infarction or previous infarction may benefit the most; another important marker is hemodynamic compromise. This principal of benefit in proportion to underlying risk is common to many forms of revascularization, including bypass grafting and thrombolysis itself or the use of tPA instead of streptokinase.[49]

Non-ST elevation patients

Of patients with a final diagnosis of acute MI who die in-hospital, the majority never have ST segment elevation on the electrocardiogram.[41] Furthermore, in registries of acute MI, approximately half of the patients who eventually "rule in" do not have ST segment elevation. Currently available data indicate that thrombolytic therapy does not reduce mortality in these patients[1] and may even increase the risk of nonfatal reinfarction.[50]

The reasons for this paradox are unclear. Unfortunately, solid information about the strategy of immediate angiography with the intention of using direct angioplasty in these patients is not available.

Ongoing Trials

Two major ongoing trials should provide considerable insight into the generalizability of the currently available information developed at a select group of centers. The GUSTO II angioplasty substudy will randomize 1,200 patients to either direct angioplasty or accelerated tPA against a background of either heparin or hirudin antithrombin therapy (Figure 3). The SHOCK (Should We Revascularize Occluded Coronaries for Cardiogenic Shock?) trial will randomize patients presenting in cardiogenic shock to either immediate angioplasty or conservative care.

Clinical Protocol

Clinical protocols for direct angioplasty have a number of common elements. The patients in whom the indication is most firmly established are those with a large infarction with ST segment elevation. Time is considered equally important with the thrombolytic treatment, hence the workup needed to make a diagnosis and institute supportive treatment must be minimized.

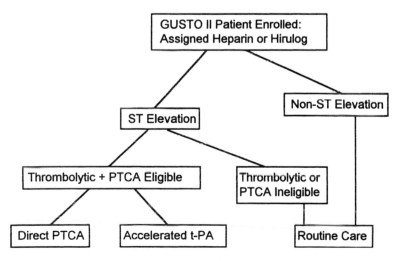

FIGURE 3. *GUSTO II angioplasty substudy design.*

Once a candidate for direct angioplasty is identified, the interventional cardiologist and the catheterization laboratory are immediately notified. Only when the diagnosis or strategy is in doubt should laboratory personnel wait for the interventional cardiologist's evaluation to prepare for the patient's arrival. The most important single issue is to ensure that a protocol is in place, so that the emergency department staff have no lost time due to confusion about whether to use thrombolysis or direct angioplasty or about whom to call to initiate the interventional process.

A different set of issues and problems arises when the patient reports to a hospital with no interventional cardiology facilities. Inordinate delays due to transport are unacceptable, yet in many situations an efficient transport team can move the patient while the staff is assembling at the interventional center. For the most part, routine transport of patients for direct angioplasty should be deferred until definitive studies comparing reperfusion approaches in a broader hospital base are completed.

The issue of "backup" surgery raises a similar series of concerns. The MITI group demonstrated that centers without surgical backup but with dedicated, experienced cardiologists and surgeons and an efficient, rapid system of interhospital transport can achieve excellent results.[51] This system involves a group of urban hospitals in close proximity to an efficient emergency medical system. Until more information is available, performing direct angioplasty without surgical backup is not recommended.

Conclusions

Direct angioplasty is an effective method of myocardial reperfusion when performed by experienced hands at experienced centers. The procedure is especially to be considered in patients with large infarctions or hemodynamic compromise. More research is needed for patients with thrombolytic contraindications and without ST segment elevation. Whether this technique should proliferate beyond dedicated interventional centers depends on the development of definitive treatment algorithms that, when applied at less experienced centers on a broad scale, do not result in decreased effectiveness of this treatment.

References

1. Fibrinolytic Therapy Trialists' (FTT) Collaborative Group. Indications for fibrinolytic therapy in suspected acute myocardial infarction: col-

laborative overview of early mortality and major morbidity results from all randomized trials of more than 1000 patients. *Lancet.* 1994; 343:311–322.

2. Grines CL, Browne KF, Marco J, et al. A comparison of immediate angioplasty with thrombolytic therapy for acute myocardial infarction. The Primary Angioplasty in Myocardial Infarction Study Group. *N Engl J Med.* 1993;328:673–679.

3. Zijlstra F, de Boer MJ, Hoorntje JC, et al. A comparison of immediate coronary angioplasty with intravenous streptokinase in acute myocardial infarction. *N Engl J Med.* 1993;328:680–684.

4. Gibbons RJ, Holmes DR, Reeder GS, et al. Immediate angioplasty compared with the administration of a thrombolytic agent followed by conservative treatment for myocardial infarction. The Mayo Coronary Care Unit and Catheterization Laboratory Groups. *N Engl J Med.* 1993;328:685–691.

5. The GUSTO Angiographic Investigators. The effects of tissue plasminogen activator, streptokinase, or both on coronary-artery patency, ventricular function, and survival after acute myocardial infarction. *N Engl J Med.* 1993;329:1615–1622.

6. Ohman EM, Califf RM, Topol EJ, et al. Consequences of reocclusion after successful reperfusion therapy in acute myocardial infarction. TAMI Study Group. *Circulation.* 1990;82:781–791.

7. Ribeiro EE, Silva LA, Carneiro R, et al. Randomized trial of direct coronary angioplasty versus intravenous streptokinase in acute myocardial infarction. *J Am Coll Cardiol.* 1993;22:376–380.

8. O'Neill WW, Brodie BR, Ivanhoe R, et al. Primary coronary angioplasty for acute myocardial infarction (The Primary Angioplasty Registry). *Am J Cardiol.* 1994;73:627–634.

9. Brodie BR, Grines CL, Ivanhoe R, et al. Six-month clinical and angiographic follow-up after direct angioplasty for acute myocardial infarction: final results from the primary angioplasty registry. *Circulation.* In Press.

10. Rogers WJ, Dean LS, Moore PB, et al, for the Alabama Registry of Myocardial Ischemia Investigators: outcome of patients managed with primary PTCA versus lytic therapy in a multicenter registry. *J Am Coll Cardiol.* 1993;21:330A. Abstract.

11. Martin JS, Litwin PE, Waxman DA, et al, for the MITI Project Investigators. Immediate and one year outcome following direct angioplasty versus thrombolytic therapy for acute myocardial infarction. *J Am Coll Cardiol.* 1993;21:331A. Abstract.

12. Granger CB, Califf RM, Topol EJ. Thrombolytic therapy for acute myocardial infarction. A review. *Drugs.* 1992;44:293–325.

13. Ohman EM, Califf RM. Thrombolytic therapy: overview of clinical trials. In: Gersh BJ, Rahimtoola SH, eds. *Acute Myocardial Infarction.* New York, NY: Elsevier; 1991:308–332.

14. Ritchie JL, Phillips KA, Luft HS. Coronary angioplasty; statewide experience in California. *Circulation.* 1993;88:2735–2743.

15. Jollis JG, DeLong ER, Collins SR, et al. The relationship between angioplasty volume and outcome in the elderly in the Medicare database. *Circulation.* 1993;88:I-480. Abstract.

16. Myler RK, Topol EJ, Shaw RE, et al. Multiple vessel coronary angioplasty: classification, results, and patterns of restenosis in 494 consecutive patients. *Catheterization Cardiovasc Diagn.* 1987;13:1–15.

17. Stammen F, De Scheerder I, Glazier JJ, et al. Immediate and follow-up

results of the conservative coronary angioplasty strategy of unstable angina pectoris. *Am J Cardiol.* 1992;69:1533.

18. Timmis AD, Griffin B, Crick JC, et al. Early percutaneous transluminal coronary angioplasty in the management of unstable angina. *Int J Cardiol.* 1987;14:25–31.

19. Hillegass WB, Ohman EM, Califf RM. Restenosis: the clinical issues. In: Topol EJ, ed. *Textbook of Interventional Cardiology.* Second editon. Philadelphia, PA: WB Saunders Company; 1993:415–435.

20. Duber C, Jungbluth A, Rumpelt H-J, et al. Morphology of the coronary arteries after combined thrombolysis and percutaneous transluminal coronary angioplasty for acute myocardial infarction. *Am J Cardiol.* 1986;58:698–703.

21. Colavita PG, Ideker RE, Reimer KA, et al. The spectrum of pathology associated with percutaneous transluminal coronary angioplasty during acute myocardial infarction. *J Am Coll Cardiol.* 1986;8:855–860.

22. Waller BF, Rothbaum DA, Pinkerton CA, et al. Status of the myocardium and infarct-related coronary artery in 19 necropsy patients with acute recanalization using pharmacologic (streptokinase, r-tissue plasminogen activator), mechanical (percutaneous transluminal coronary angioplasty) or combined types of reperfusion therapy. *J Am Coll Cardiol.* 1987;9:785–801.

23. Anderson JL, Karagounis LA, Becker LC, et al, for the TEAM-3 investigators: TIMI perfusion grade 3 but not grade 2 results in improved outcome after thrombolysis for myocardial infarction: ventriculographic, enzymatic, and electrocardiographic evidence from the TEAM-3 study. *Circulation.* 1994;87:1829–1839.

24. The GUSTO Investigators. An international randomized trial comparing four thrombolytic strategies for acute myocardial infarction. *N Engl J Med.* 1993;329:673–682.

25. Rapold HJ, Haeberli A, Kuemmerli H, et al. Fibrin formation and platelet activation in patients with myocardial infarction and normal coronary arteries. *Eur Heart J.* 1989;10:323–333.

26. The Epic Investigators. Use of a monoclonal antibody directed against the platelet glycoprotein IIb/IIIa receptor in high-risk coronary angioplasty. *N Engl J Med.* 1994. In press.

27. Topol EJ, Bonan R, Jewitt D, et al. Use of a direct antithrombin, hirulog, in place of heparin during coronary angioplasty. *Circulation.* 1993: 87;1622–1629.

28. van den Bos AA, Deckers JW, Heyndrickx GR, et al. Safety and efficacy of recombinant hirudin (CGP 39 393) versus heparin in patients with stable angina undergoing coronary angioplasty. *Circulation.* 1993; 88(1):2058–2066.

29. O'Connor CM, Califf RM, Massey EW, et al. Stroke and acute myocardial infarction in the thrombolytic era: clinical correlates and long-term prognosis. *J Am Coll Cardiol.* 1990;16:533–540.

30. Komrad MS, Coffey CE, Coffey KS, et al. Myocardial infarction and stroke. *Neurology.* 1984;34:1403–1409.

31. Topol EJ, Califf RM, George BS, et al, for the TAMI Study Group. A randomized trial of immediate versus delayed elective angioplasty after intravenous tissue plasminogen activator in acute myocardial infarction. *N Engl J Med.* 1987; 317:581–588.

32. Arnold AE, Simoons ML, Van de Werf F, et al. Recombinant tissue-type plasminogen activator and immediate angioplasty in acute myo-

cardial infarction. One-year follow-up. The European Cooperative Study Group. *Circulation.* 1992;86:111–120.

33. Rogers WJ, Baim DS, Gore JM, et al, for the TIMI II-A Investigators. Comparison of immediate invasive, delayed invasive, and conservative strategies after tissue-type plasminogen activator. Results of the Thrombolysis in Myocardial Infarction (TIMI) Phase II-A trial. *Circulation.* 1990;81:1457–1476.

34. Califf RM, Topol EJ, Ohman EM, et al, and the TAMI Study Group. Isolated recurrent ischemia after thrombolytic therapy is a frequent, important and expensive adverse clinical outcome. *J Am Coll Cardiol.* 1992;19(3):301A. Abstract.

35. Betriu A, Califf RM, Granger C, for the GUSTO Investigators. Importance of clinical findings during post-infarction angina in determining prognosis: results from the GUSTO trial. *J Am Coll Cardiol.* 1994:27A. Abstract.

36. Meijer A, Verheugt FWA, Werter CJPJ, et al. Aspirin versus coumadin in the prevention of reocclusion and recurrent ischemia after successful thrombolysis: a prospective placebo-controlled angiographic study. *Circulation.* 1993;87:1524–1530.

37. Califf RM, Topol EJ, Stack RS, et al. Evaluation of combination thrombolytic therapy and timing of cardiac catheterization in acute myocardial infarction. Results of thrombolysis and angioplasty in myocardial infarction—phase 5 randomized trial. TAMI Study Group. *Circulation.* 1991;83:1543–1556.

38. Mark D. Medical economics and health policy issues for interventional cardiology. In: Topol EJ, ed. *Textbook of Interventional Cardiology.* Second edition. Philadelphia, PA: W.B. Saunders; 1994:1323–1353.

39. Weaver WD, Litwin PE, Martin JS. Effect of age on use of thrombolytic therapy and mortality in acute myocardial infarction: the MITI Project Group. *J Am Coll Cardiol.* 1991;18:657–662.

40. Cragg DR, Friedman HZ, Bonema JD et al. Outcome of patients with acute myocardial infarction who are ineligible for thrombolytic therapy. *Ann Intern Med.* 1991;115:173–177.

41. Brodie BR, Weintraub RA, Stuckey TD, et al. Outcomes of direct coronary angioplasty for acute myocardial infarction in candidates and non-candidates for thrombolytic therapy. *Am J Cardiol.* 1991;67:7–12.

42. Goldberg RJ, Gore JM, Alpert JS, et al. Cardiogenic shock after acute myocardial infarction: incidence and mortality from a community-wide perspective, 1975 to 1988. *N Engl J Med.* 1993;325:1117–1122.

43. Bengtson JR, Kaplan AT, Pieper KS, et al. Prognosis in cardiogenic shock after acute myocardial infarction in the interventional era. *J Am Coll Cardiol.* 1992;20:1482–1489.

44. Califf RM, Bengtson JR. Cardiogenic Shock. *N Engl J Med.* 1994. In press.

45. Bates ER, Topol EJ. Limitations of thrombolytic therapy for acute myocardial infarction complicated by congestive heart failure and cardiogenic shock. *J Am Coll Cardiol.* 1991;18:1077–1084.

46. Becker RC. Hemodynamic, mechanical, and metabolic determinants of thrombolytic efficacy: a theoretic framework for assessing the limitations of thrombolysis in patients with cardiogenic shock. Editorial. *Am Heart J.* 1993;125:919–929.

47. O'Neill WW. Angioplasty therapy of cardiogenic shock: are randomized trials necessary?. *J Am Coll Cardiol.* 1992;19:915–917.

48. Hochman J, Boland J, Brinker J, et al, for the SHOCK investigators. Current spectrum of cardiogenic shock and effect of early revascularization on mortality: results of an international registry. *Circulation.* 1993;88:I-253. Abstract.
49. Califf RM, Simoons M, Lee KL, et al. Advantages of patient-specific predictions over subgroup analysis in defining differential treatment effects of tPA and streptokinase from the GUSTO trial. *J Am Coll Cardiol.* 1994:27A. Abstract.
50. TIMI Study Group. Early effects of tissue-type plasminogen activator added to conventional therapy on the culprit coronary lesion in patients presenting with ischemic cardiac pain at rest. The Thrombolysis in Myocardial Ischemia (TIMI IIIA) Trial. *Circulation.* 1993;87:38–52.
51. Weaver WD, Litwin PE, Maynard C, for the MITI Project. Primary Angioplasty for AMI Performed in hospitals with and without on-site surgical backup. *Circulation.* 1991;II:536. Abstract.
52. De Wood MA. Direct PTCA versus intravenous t-PA in acute myocardial infarction: results from a prospective randomized trial. 6th International Workshop on Thrombolysis and Interventional Therapy in Acute Myocardial Infarction, Dallas, TX, 1990.
53. O'Neill WW, Weintraub R, Grines CL, et al. A prospective, placebo-controlled randomized trial of intravenous streptokinase and angioplasty versus lone angioplasty therapy of acute myocardial infarction. *Circulation.* 1992;86:1710–1717.
54. Browne KF, Grines C, O'Neill W. Randomized trial of primary PTCA versus thrombolytic therapy in acute myocardial infarction (PAMI)—six month follow-up. *J Am Coll Cardiol.* 1993;21:176A. Abstract.
55. Mark DB, Brodie B, Ivanhoe R, et al. Effects of direct angioplasty on hospital costs in acute myocardial infarction: results from the multicenter PAR study. *Circulation.* 1991;II:257. Abstract.
56. Mark DB, Brodie B, Ivanhoe R, et al. Follow-up costs and other economic outcomes in patients treated with direct angioplasty for acute myocardial infarction. *J Am Coll Cardiol.* 1993;21:176A. Abstract.

Chapter 31

Indications for and Timing of Angiography After Thrombolysis

Robert A. O'Rourke, MD

In the past 25 years there has been a remarkable decrease in the early mortality after acute myocardial infarction.[1,2] This reduction in the age-adjusted mortality due to acute myocardial infarction is partially due to the widespread use of thrombolytic therapy to establish early reperfusion in patients presenting within the first 6 hours after the onset of symptoms.[1-3] Early myocardial reperfusion by means of primary coronary angioplasty has improved the mortality rate in many patients with myocardial infarction and its complications including those with cardiogenic shock.[3]

Adjunctive therapy with aspirin and anticoagulation has helped maximize the favorable effects of reperfusion therapy in patients whose infarct-related coronary artery is patent early after infarction.[4-7] Such patients have a lower mortality rate and better left ventricular function than do those in whom reperfusion therapy is unsuccessful.[4-7]

In the 70% of patients with acute myocardial infarction who do not receive thrombolytic therapy, risk stratification based on the patients preinfarction history, clinical characteristics observed during hospitalization, and noninvasive testing when indicated have resulted in a more aggressive diagnostic and therapeutic approach for those at high risk.[8] Secondary prevention by risk factor reduction and drug therapy is recommended for high- and low-risk postinfarction patients.[2,9]

Figures 1 and 2 outline a risk stratification approach to postinfarction patients who have undergone standard therapy. These figures emphasize the increased morbidity and mortality associated with recurrent myocardial ischemia, persistent left ventricular systolic dysfunction, late in-hospital ventricular tachyarrhythmias,

From Vetrovec GW, Carabello BA, (eds.) *Invasive Cardiology: Current Diagnostic and Therapeutic Issues.* Armonk, NY: Futura Publishing Company, Inc.: © 1996.

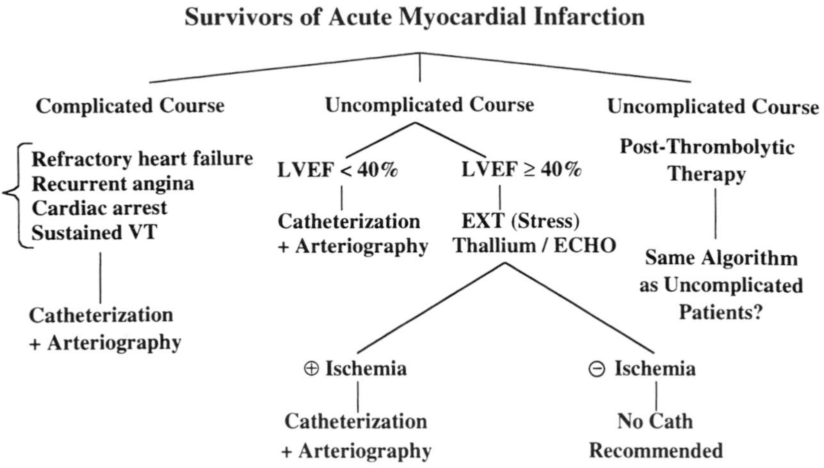

Survivors of Acute Myocardial Infarction

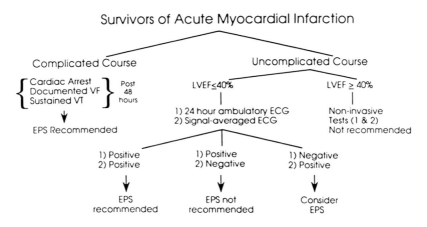

FIGURE 1. *A management strategy for survivors of acute myocardial infarction based on the patients clinical characteristics, the left ventricular ejection fraction (LVEF) and the presence or absence of inducible myocardial ischemia. VT, ventricular tachycardia. (Modified with permission from reference 10.)*

FIGURE 2. *Management strategy for survivors of acute myocardial infarction to determine the risk of ventricular tachyarrhythmias and sudden death during posthospital discharge follow-up. VF, ventricular fibrillation, VT, ventricular tachycardia, EPS, electrophysiological study, and LVEF, left ventricular ejection fraction. (Modified with permission from Reference 10.)*

and their combination.[10] The applicability of this approach to patients with acute myocardial infarction who have received thrombolytic therapy is currently being defined.

Considerable controversy exists concerning the indications for and the timing of coronary arteriography in patients with myocardial infarction who have been treated with thrombolytic therapy.[9] Several multicenter clinical trials have assessed routine coronary arteriography with coronary angioplasty of the infarct-related coronary artery when feasible in postthrombolytic patients as compared with a more conservative approach with coronary arteriography and PTCA reserved for patients with spontaneous or stress induced myocardial ischemia occurring after thrombolytic therapy.[11-18] In general, these studies have shown no advantage of routine cardiac catheterization with coronary angioplasty during the early hospital course after thrombolysis and a poorer prognosis and greater complication rate when immediate catheterization and angioplasty are performed within the first 2 hours after thrombolytic therapy.[11-18]

The accuracy of noninvasive testing for separating patients at high versus low risk after thrombolytic therapy for acute myocardial infarction remains to be determined. Several studies using one or more noninvasive tests to detect the presence of multivessel coronary artery disease and for determining the risk of subsequent major cardiac events have been disappointing.[9]

In this chapter, methods used to determine the need for and the timing of cardiac catheterization and coronary arteriography in patients with myocardial infarction undergoing standard therapy are delineated and the factors affecting patient management decisions after thrombolytic therapy emphasized.

Factors Affecting Management Decisions After Thrombolytic Therapy

Decisions concerning the management of patients who have received thrombolytic therapy for acute myocardial infarction are determined by several considerations. These include the presence or absence of high-risk patient characteristics before the index myocardial infarction or their appearance during in-hospital observation during or after thrombolytic therapy.[8,19] Also important are the results of studies in which early routine coronary arteriography/angioplasty and late routine coronary arteriography/angioplasty have been compared with a conservative strategy in which patients underwent catheterization with appropriate revascularization only when spontaneous or stress induced myocardial ischemia occur.[11-18] A third factor is the availability and reliability of noninvasive testing for further risk stratification of patients who appear clinically to be at low or moderate risk for recurrent cardiac events after thrombolytic therapy.[9] Also relevant is the likelihood of an open infarct related coronary artery and whether or not its patency status will affect the prognosis in specific patients with normal or depressed left ventricular function.[6,20]

Risk Factors Before and After Thrombolytic Therapy

In 3,339 patients enrolled in phase II of the Thrombolysis and Myocardial Infarction (TIMI) Trial, the presence of each of eight risk factors prior to the initiation of thrombolytic therapy was recorded.[19] These included: age ≥70 years, female gender, a history of diabetes mellitus or previous myocardial infarction, electrocardiographic evidence of evolving anterior infarction or atrial fibrillation, and evidence on physical examination of mild pulmonary congestion or hypotension and sinus tachycardia. The mortality rate at 6 weeks was only 1.5% in the 26% of patients who had none of these risk factors. In contrast, 5.3% of those with one or more risk factors died in 6 weeks ($P<0.001$). Among those with one or more risk factors, mortality at 6 weeks was related to the number of risk factors on admission; those with four or more had a 6-week mortality rate of 17.2%.[19]

In the TIMI Phase II Trial, the higher mortality in patients with prior myocardial infarction versus those without prior myocardial infarction using the conservative strategy suggests that early coronary arteriography and myocardial revascularization of these patients might be beneficial.[21] Conversely, the higher mortality in diabetics with the invasive strategy suggests that early aggressive management might not be suitable in this subgroup unless otherwise clinically indicated.[21]

The same clinical characterizations indicative of high risk in patients undergoing standard therapy likely apply to individuals receiving thrombolytic therapy for acute myocardial infarction. Evidence of recurrent myocardial ischemia, a depression in left ventricular ejection fraction below 40%, and late in-hospital ventricular arrhythmias also indicate a poor prognosis in postthrombolytic patients. In studies utilizing multivariant analysis to evaluate prognosis in patients after successful thrombolytic therapy, the mortality in the first year after discharge was low and appeared related to coronary anatomy, left ventricular function, and to a lesser extent age and history of previous infarction.[22-24] In one study, the mortality rate the first year after discharge was 8.2% in patients with an ejection fraction of <40% as compared with only 1.8% in those with an ejection fraction of ≥40%.[24]

McClements and Adgey[25] recently reported a consecutive series of 300 survivors of myocardial infarction (205 had received thrombolytic agents) who had signal-averaged electrocardiogram (ECG), Holter ECG monitoring, and radionuclide ventriculography prior to hospital discharge in an attempt to predict arrhythmic events (sudden death or sustained ventricular tachyarrhythmia) (Figure 3). During the mean follow-up of 1 year, 13 patients (4.3%) had an arrhythmic event, 11 with sudden death and 2 with sustained ventricular tachyarrhythmias. The signal-averaged ECG at discharge was 64% sensitive and 81% specific for predicting the arrhythmic events. High-grade ventricular ectopic activity on the Holter ECG was only 38% sensitive and 78% specific. A left ventricular ejection fraction <0.40 was the best test for prediction of arrhythmic events with a sensitivity of 75% and a specificity of 81%. These results suggest that the signal-averaged ECG and left ventricular ejection fraction each predict arrhythmic events after thrombolytic treatment for acute myocardial infarction and the Holter ECG results are less useful.

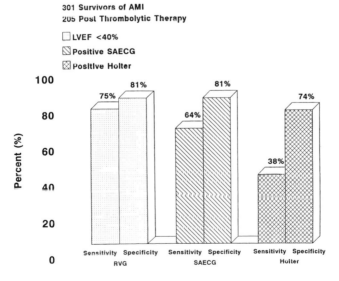

PREDICTION OF SUDDEN DEATH OR SUSTAINED VT BY NON-INVASIVE TESTING

FIGURE 3. *Sensitivity and specificity of three noninvasive techniques for detecting subsequent sudden death or sustained ventricular tachycardia (VT) in patients who survived acute myocardial infarction (AMI). LVEF, left ventricular ejection fraction; SAECG, signal-averaged electrocardiogram; Holter, ambulatory ECG recordings. (Modified with permisson from Reference 5.)*

Results of Conservative versus Aggressive Postthrombolytic Management

The effects on morbidity and mortality of early percutaneous transluminal coronary angioplasty (PTCA) performed in the immediate time period after thrombolysis therapy has been evaluated in three studies.[11-13] The TIMI-IIA study assessed whether immediate cardiac catheterization with PTCA, when appropriate, would confer an advantage over the same procedures performed 18 to 48 hours later.[11] All patients were treated with intravenous tPA within 4 hours of the onset of acute myocardial infarction. PTCA of the infarct-related artery was attempted in 72% of the 195 patients assigned to immediate PTCA; 84% of the attempts were considered to show improvement. Coronary angioplasty was attempted in 55% of the 194 patients assigned to 18 to 48 hours PTCA; 93% of the attempts were judged as showing improvement. No difference between the two PTCA groups were observed for left ventricular ejection fraction measured by contrast ventriculography prior to discharge. Immediate catheterization/angioplasty was associated with more frequent bleeding and more often with the need for coronary bypass surgery. Of patients undergoing PTCA within 2 hours after thrombolysis, 20% require blood transfusions as compared with 7.2% when PTCA was delayed ($P<0.001$). Coronary artery bypass graft surgery was necessary for 16.4% of the 2-hour PTCA group as compared with 7.7% of those undergoing later PTCA ($P < 0.01$).

In the Thrombolysis and Angioplasty in Myocardial Infarction (TAMI)-1 Trial, patients randomized to an immediate angioplasty approach had a higher mortality rate (4% vs. 1%) as compared with patients assigned to a deferred catheterization and angioplasty strategy.[12] There was also a greater need for emergency coronary bypass surgery (7% vs. 2%) and an increased transfusion requirement (21% vs. 14%) in those undergoing immediate angioplasty after intravenous thrombolysis.

In the European Cooperative Study,[13] patients randomized to immediate coronary arteriography and angioplasty of the infarct-related vessel had a high rate of immediate reocclusion and early recurrent ischemia. As compared with a control group, there was a higher mortality at 1 year (9.3% vs. 5.4%) in the group undergoing immediate angioplasty. All three of these studies indicate that routine immediate coronary angioplasty early after thrombolysis confers no additional benefit and may in fact be harmful.

Several clinical studies have evaluated the potential benefit of deferred coronary arteriography and angioplasty prior to hospital discharge as compared with a conservative approach with coronary arteriography and myocardial revascularization reserved for patients with spontaneous or provokable myocardial ischemia.[14–18]

In the TIMI Phase II Trial, patients receiving tPA were randomly assigned to treatment according to an invasive strategy consisting of coronary arteriography 18 to 48 hours after the administration of tPA followed by prophylactic coronary angioplasty when feasible, or to treatment according to a conservative strategy with arteriography and PTCA performed only in patients with spontaneous or exercise-induced myocardial ischemia.[14]

In the group assigned to the invasive strategy PTCA was attempted in 56.7% of cases; the procedure was arteriographically successful in 93.3%. In the group assigned to the conservative strategy, 13.3% of the patients underwent clinically indicated PTCA within 14 days of the onset of symptoms. Reinfarction or death within 42 days occurred in 10.9% of the group assigned to the invasive strategy and in 9.7% of those assigned to the conservative strategy (P=NS) (Figure 4). There was no significant difference between the two groups in the left ventricular ejection fraction at rest or during exercise either at hospital discharge or 6 weeks after ran-

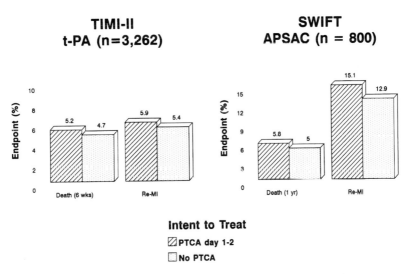

FIGURE 4. *Incidence of death and recurrent myocardial infarction at 6 weeks or 1 year after thrombolytic therapy in patients undergoing coronary angioplasty (PTCA) at 18–48 hours versus those undergoing no catheterization/angioplasty unless spontaneous or provokable myocardial ischemia occurred. (Modified with permission from References 14 and 15.)*

domization. Thus, an invasive strategy of coronary arteriography 18 to 48 hours after the onset of symptoms followed by prophylactic PTCA conferred no advantages in terms of reduction in mortality or reinfarction over a more conservative strategy according to which those procedures were provided only to patients with recurrent ischemia. The conservative strategy was also a less complex and less costly approach.

In the Should We Intervene Following Thrombolysis (SWIFT) trial, 397 patients were randomized to receive early arteriography plus appropriate intervention and 403 to receive conservative care.[15] Coronary arteriography and angioplasty were performed between 18 to 48 hours of randomization in the group being treated with interventional therapy (Figure 4). The mortality rate at 12 months was no different (5.8% vs. 5.0%) in the intervention group as compared with those undergoing conservative management. The reinfarction rate at 12 months (15.1% vs. 12.9%) were also similar in the two groups.

Two additional studies have compared patients undergoing cardiac catheterization with prophylactic coronary angioplasty at 3 or more days following intravenous thrombolysis with a group undergoing conservative management after thrombolytic therapy.

In a study from Israel,[16] 97 patients were randomized to an invasive group who underwent routine coronary arteriography and angioplasty 5±2 days after thrombolytic therapy, whereas 104 patients were randomized to a conservative group who underwent angiography only for recurrent postinfarction angina or exercise-induced ischemia (Figure 5). In the invasive group the total mortality after a mean follow-up of 10 months was 8 of 97 as compared with only 4 of 104 in the conservative group. A higher rate of rehospitalization was observed among patients assigned to the conservative group. The results of this study suggest that conservative treatment is preferable to invasive treatment, even when cardiac catheterization is delayed.

In the Treatment of Post-Thrombolytic Stenoses (TOPS) study,[17] 87 patients treated within 6 hours of onset of chest pain with thrombolytic therapy and with negative functional tests for inducible ischemia were randomized between PTCA to be performed 4 to 14 days after myocardial infarction versus no PTCA. PTCA was successful in 38 of 42 patients (88%), but resulted in non-Q wave myocardial infarction due to acute closure of the treated site in 3 of 42 (9.5%) (Figure 5). There was no difference in 6-week resting ejection fraction or increase in ejection fraction with exercise between the two groups. There were no deaths in either group. The actuarial 12-month infarct-free survival was 97.8% of the no PTCA

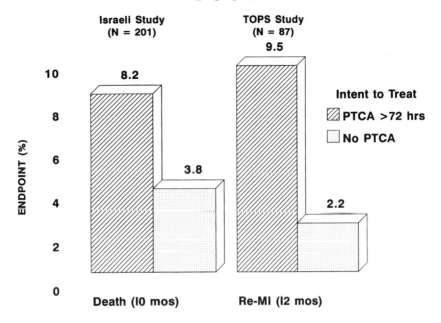

FIGURE 5. *Results of late deferred cardiac catheterization/angioplasty at >72 hours postthrombolytic therapy as compared with no catheterization or PTCA in a randomized group of patients. (Modified with permission from References 16 and 17.)*

group and 90.5% of the PTCA group (*P*=0.07). Thus, there was no functional or clinical benefit from routine late PTCA after myocardial infarction treated with thrombolytic therapy in this relatively low-risk cohort of patients.

To determine whether predischarge arteriography is beneficial in patients with acute myocardial infarction treated with tPA, heparin, and aspirin the outcomes were compared in 197 patients in the TIMI IIA study assigned to conservative management with routine predischarge coronary arteriography and in 1,461 patients in the TIMI IIB study assigned to conservative management without routine coronary arteriography unless ischemia reoccurred spontaneously or on predischarge exercise testing (Figure 6).[18] During the initial hospital study, coronary arteriography was performed in 93.9% of the routine catheterization group and 34.7% of the selective catheterization group (*P*<0.001), but the frequency of coronary revascularization was similar in the two groups (24.4% vs. 20.7%, *P*=NS). Coronary arteriograms showed a predominance of 0 or 1-vessel disease (stenosis>60%) in both groups.

PREDISCHARGE CORONARY ARTERIOGRAPHY (CA)
(TIMI - II)

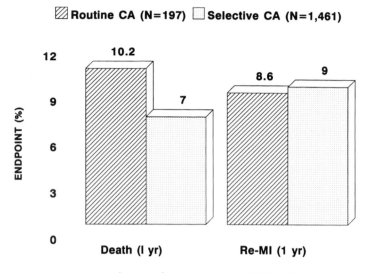

FIGURE 6. *A nonrandomized comparison of TIMI II patients treated with routine coronary arteriography versus those treated with selective coronary arteriography with death and recurrent myocardial infarction used as end points. (Modified with permission from Reference 18.)*

At the end of 1 year coronary arteriography had been performed one or more times in 98.9% of the routine catheterization group and 59.4% of the selective catheterization group ($P<0.001$) whereas death and nonfatal reinfarction had occurred in 10.2% vs. 7% ($P=0.10$) and 8.6% vs. 9.0% ($P=0.87$), respectively (Figure 6). The selective coronary arteriography strategy reduced by about 40%, the number of patients exposed to the small but definite risks and the cost of the procedure without changing the one year survival or reinfarction rates. Thus, it would seem to be the appropriate management strategy.

Accuracy of Risk Stratification by Noninvasive Testing

Many studies suggest that the positive and negative predictive accuracy of noninvasive tests designed to detect myocardial ischemia, depressed left ventricular performance, and recurrent ventricular tachyarrhythmias are less useful in patients undergoing successful thrombolytic therapy than in patients receiving standard therapy.[26-34] Nevertheless, as indicated, a conservative strategy excluding cardiac catheterization from patients without spontaneous or provokable ischemia on noninvasive testing has been associated with a favorable outcome in patients after thrombolytic therapy.

There are several possible reasons why noninvasive testing has been deemed less accurate in postinfarction patients having received thrombolytic therapy. First, patients undergoing coronary arteriography after thrombolytic therapy have had less extensive coronary artery disease and better left ventricular function than patients having undergone coronary arteriography prior to the advent of thrombolytic therapy.[2,9,35,36] Therefore, in general, such patients are at a relatively lower risk and noninvasive testing is likely to be less discriminating. Second, the relative mortality after successful thrombolytic therapy in hospital and over the long term is relatively low with a <4% postdischarge mortality during the first year of follow-up in many series.[37] Thus, if the major cardiac event rate is low the specificity of a noninvasive test for detecting high risk will also be relatively low, many patients having a false-positive test for high risk. Third, the end points used in many studies concerning the usefulness of noninvasive testing for risk stratification after thrombolytic therapy often include the development of unstable angina, the need for coronary angioplasty, and the use of coronary artery bypass surgery in addition to the stronger primary endpoints of cardiac death and nonfatal reinfarction. In many of the studies a positive test is followed by a subsequent therapeutic intervention that alters the natural history.

Finally, the stress utilized to demonstrate inducible myocardial ischemia or left ventricular dysfunction has frequently been low level.[33,34,38] In most studies, those at greatest risk were patients who were unable to undergo predischarge ECG exercise testing.[38] Noninvasive testing using near maximum exercise testing or pharmacologic stress plus isometric exercise might demonstrate ECG or myocardial imaging evidence of ischemia or regional left ventricular dysfunction that is not present with lesser degrees of stress. In many studies of patients evaluated after an acute myocardial infarction, near maximum exercise testing performed early after the event (4–7 days) defined many more patients as being at high risk than a lower degree of exercise performed at a later time period after the myocardial infarction.[39]

Detection of Myocardial Ischemia and Multivessel Disease

Electrocardiography, myocardial perfusion imaging, and regional wall motion assessment (echocardiography and radionuclide ventriculography) are the noninvasive methods commonly used to indicate the presence of myocardial ischemia during stress in the form of exercise, coronary vasodilator drugs (dipyridamole, adenosine), or positive inotropic agents (dobutamine).[39,40] Myocardial perfusion imaging with either thallium-201 or [99]m technetium sestamibi has been shown to be accurate in detecting stress-provokable myocardial ischemia with an improvement in the ischemic defect noted during subsequent rest.

In a study by Haber and associates,[33] the ability of exercise thallium-201 scintigraphy to detect inducible ischemia and thus identify multivessel coronary artery disease was evaluated in 88 consecutive postinfarction patients who received thrombolytic therapy and subsequently underwent predischarge noninvasive testing and coronary arteriography (Figure 7). Exercise-induced thallium-201 redistribution on quantitative scintigraphy was significantly more prevalent than exercise ST segment depression (48% vs. 14%, $P<0.001$). The sensitivity and specificity of exercise ST depression alone for identification of multivessel disease were 29% and 96%, respectively. The sensitivity and specificity of a remote thallium-201 defect for detecting multivessel coronary artery disease were 35% and 87%, respectively, not significantly different from values for ST depression alone. When considered as a single variable the presence of either ST segment depression or a remote thallium-201 defect was associated with a 58% sensitivity ($P<0.05$ compared with either ST segment depression or thallium-201 redistribution alone), but with a somewhat diminished specificity of 78%. There was no difference in the extent or severity of arteriographic coronary disease in patients with multivessel disease when related to the presence or absence of inducible ischemia.

In a study to determine whether low-level exercise thallium testing is useful for identifying high-risk patients after thrombolytic treatment for acute myocardial infarction, 64 patients who underwent early thrombolytic therapy for acute myocardial infarction and 107 patients without an acute intervention were evaluated by Tilkemeier and associates.[34] The ability of exercise ECG and thallium redistribution imaging to predict future events were compared in both groups of patients (Figure 8). After a mean follow-up of 374 days, cardiac events occurred in 25% of those with versus

IDENTIFICATION OF MULTIVESSEL CAD POST THROMBOLYSIS BY ECG & THALLIUM ETT (N=88)

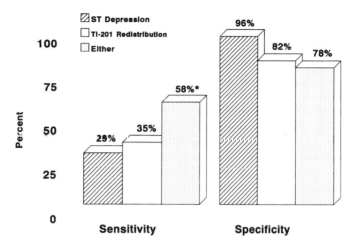

FIGURE 7. *The sensitivity and specificity of ST depression, thallium-201 redistribution or either test abnormal for detecting multivessel coronary artery disease (CAD) after thrombolytic therapy. The asterix indicates statistical significance as compared with ST depression or thallium redistribution. ETT, exercise treadmill thallium. (Modified with permission from Reference 33.)*

32% of those without acute intervention. These included: death, recurrent myocardial infarction, coronary artery bypass grafting, or angioplasty; 75% of the events occurred in the 3 months after the first infarction. The only significant predictors of outcome were left ventricular cavity dilatation in the thrombolytic therapy group and ST segment depression and increased lung uptake of thallium in the standard therapy group. The sensitivity of exercise thallium was 55% in the intervention group and 77% in the nonintervention group (P<0.05). Therefore, in the patients undergoing thrombolytic therapy for acute myocardial infarction, nearly half the events after discharge were not predicted by predischarge low-level exercise thallium testing.

In a preliminary report by Jaarsmar and associates[41] risk stratification after thrombolysis was relatively accurate utilizing dobutamine stress echocardiography. Forty-seven consecutive patients who had been treated with thrombolytic therapy for acute infarction underwent dobutamine stress echocardiography and cardiac

PROGNOSTIC VALUE OF ETT - THALLIUM IMAGING AFTER THROMBOLYTIC TREATMENT OF AMI

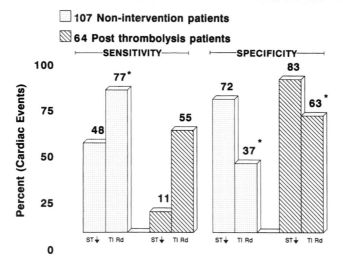

FIGURE 8. *The sensitivity and specificity of exercise treadmill ECG testing with thallium myocardial perfusion imaging in 107 nonintervention patients and 64 patients after thrombolytic therapy for determining the percentage of cardiac events during an average follow-up of 1 year. Differences between groups occurred for the sensitivity of ST segment depression and the specificity of both ST segment depression and thallium redistribution. Tl Rd: redistribution thallium. (Modified with permission from Reference 34.)*

catheterization 7 ± 2 days after myocardial infarction. During low-dose dobutamine (5–10 μg/kg per minute) infusion contractile reserve (viability) defined as improved wall motion in the infarct zone was assessed. High-dose dobutamine (30–40 μg/kg per minute) infusion then was performed until patients developed worsening or new wall motion abnormalities, angina, ST segment depression or to a predicted heart rate of 85%. New ischemic events during a mean follow-up of 9 months occurred in 19 of 25 patients with wall motion worsening at high-dose dobutamine for a positive predictive value of 76% and in only 4 of 22 patients without wall motion worsening for a negative predictive value of 84%.

Assessment of Ventricular Function

In postinfarction patients undergoing standard therapy there has been an inverse relationship between the left ventricular ejection fraction and 1-year survival. Recurrent cardiac events and an increased mortality rate are significantly more common in patients with a left ventricular ejection fraction below 40%.[3,8,25,42,43] The left ventricular ejection fraction is usually measured noninvasively by two-dimensional echocardiography or radionuclide ventriculography in postinfarction patients prior to discharge. In some patients, there will be significant improvement in left ventricular ejection fraction occurring during the first 2 weeks after myocardial infarction with the initial reduction in ejection fraction partially due to stunned myocardium.[44] Nevertheless, a predischarge ejection fraction of below 40% is associated with an increased morbidity and mortality. From an analysis of patients followed for 5 years after treatment of an acute myocardial infarction with thrombolytic therapy, the same relation between low ejection fraction and high risk for cardiac death and recurrent cardiac events seems applicable to patients treated with thrombolytic therapy.[22,24,37]

Detection of Ventricular Arrhythmias

In patients undergoing standard treatment for infarction, recurrent sustained ventricular tachycardia and sudden death are more likely in patients with certain characteristics.[8,41] These include a left ventricular ejection fraction of <40%, the presence of more than 10 premature ventricular depolarization, triplets, or nonsustained ventricular-tachycardiac on ambulatory ECG recordings, a positive signal-averaged ECG, a lack of normal heart rate variability, and exercise-induced ventricular tachycardia.[45] As indicated earlier,[24] the available data suggest that such markers of increased risk also pertain to patients after thrombolytic therapy. However, the patient undergoing thrombolytic therapy is less likely to have depressed left ventricular function, less likely to have severe multivessel residual coronary artery disease and the incidence of signal-averaged ECGs that are positive is significantly reduced when thrombolytic therapy has been successful.[46] This relative electrical stability is one of the factors relevant to the "open artery hypothesis" (see below).

The Open Artery Hypothesis

For patients with acute myocardial infarction, the clinical importance of a patent as opposed to an occluded infarct-related coronary artery (open infarct-related artery hypothesis) has become well accepted.[6,20] It is based on the principle that early reperfusion of the infarct-related coronary artery results in myocardial salvage that preserves ventricular function, the latter being responsible for improved survival. In the GUSTO trial the improved 30-day survival in tPA treated patients as compared with streptokinase treated patients appears to be related primarily to successful early reperfusion.[5] Earlier reperfusion also resulted in better left ventricular function.

Considering the higher mortality in patients with occluded or incomplete perfusion at 90 minutes, it is imperative to develop better noninvasive methods for determining the early success or failure of thrombolytic therapy so that patients who may benefit from immediate retreatment with the thrombolytic agent or urgent revascularization can be recognized at the earliest possible time.[6,14] Routine immediate coronary arteriography is not suitable for this purpose for reasons previously stated. Currently, several promising noninvasive techniques are being further evaluated for this purpose.[6] Continuous ST segment monitoring may provide an accurate marker of successful reperfusion and patent infarct-related arteries after thrombolytic therapy.[47] In the TAMI 7 Study,[47] continuous 12-lead ST segment recovery analysis was used as a noninvasive method for the real-time detection of failed myocardial reperfusion. All patients had 12-lead continuous ST segment monitoring and acute coronary arteriography. ST segment recovery and reelevation were analyzed up to the moment of arteriography at which time patency was predicted (Figure 9). Infarct-artery occlusion was seen on first injection in 27% of patients. The positive predictive value of incomplete ST recovery or ST reelevation by this method was 71% and negative predictive value 87% with 90% specificity and 64% sensitivity for coronary occlusion. ST recovery analysis predicted patency in 94% of patients with TIMI III flow versus 81% of patients with TIMI II flow and predicted occlusion in 57% of patients with collateralized occlusion versus 72% of patients with noncollateralized occlusion. In a regression model including other noninvasive clinical descriptors, ST recovery alone contained a vast majority of the predictive information about coronary artery patency.

A second noninvasive method concerns the use of the creatine kinase MM and MB isoforms that have been identified and separated electrophorethically into the two types found in cardiac muscle, MB_2 and MM_3.[48] After release into the serum, these isoforms are converted by the enzyme carboxypeptidase N to the serum isoforms MB_1 and MM_1. $CK-MB_2$ and $CK-MM_3$ are released more rapidly if reperfusion has occurred than if the artery remains occluded. An elevated ratio of MB_2/MB_1 and the rapid rate of rise in

DETECTION OF FAILED REPERFUSION BY ST-SEGMENT RECOVERY ANALYSIS
TAMI 7 STUDY

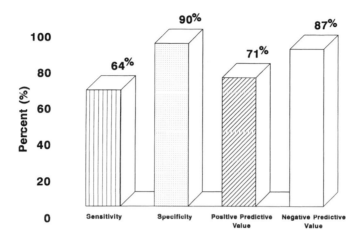

FIGURE 9. *Sensitivity, specificity, positive and negative predictive value of continuous ST segment monitoring for detecting failed reperfusion with thrombolytic therapy. (Modified with permission from Reference 47.)*

the concentration of MM_3 appear to correlate with an open infarct-related artery.[48]

Imaging with ^{99}M Tc-labeled sestamibi may also be useful for assessing postthrombolytic infarct-related coronary artery patency noninvasively.[49] Sestamibi, like thallium-201, rapidly accumulates in viable myocardial cells proportional to myocardial perfusion; however, unlike thallium, it does not redistribute significantly as a function of time. Therefore, sestamibi has been used to define myocardium at risk during the pretreatment phase of acute myocardial infarction and subsequently to determine myocardial perfusion and salvage after thrombolytic therapy.[6,49] Hopefully the use of such noninvasive indicators of coronary artery patency as well as others now being developed (eg, magnetic resonance imaging), will identify patients with acute myocardial infarction who do not respond to thrombolytic therapy initially or in whom reocclusion has subsequently occurred.

Recent basic and clinical experimental studies suggest that late reperfusion of an occluded coronary artery after the time period considered necessary for attaining myocardial salvage still favorably affects clinical outcome.[20] These effects may be considered to be the "time independent" effects of an open infarct-related artery.[20]

Routine Coronary Arteriography

Coronary arteriography provides important information concerning the pathologic anatomy of the coronary circulation. In general, the more severe the coronary artery stenosis (eg, >90%) and the more extensive the coronary artery disease the greater risk for future cardiac events. However, coronary arteriography performed early after myocardial infarction often fails to distinguish between the severity of the underlying coronary artery stenosis and the presence of partial thrombosis.[9] Coronary artery remodeling takes place during the several days after the acute cardiac event. Furthermore, patients undergoing thrombolytic therapy often have no significant residual stenosis or single vessel coronary artery disease.[9,11–18] Serial coronary arteriographic studies have shown that the angiographic status of the coronary artery circulation does not necessarily predict subsequent acute coronary events and which artery is likely to become the infarct-related coronary vessel.[50] Additionally, pathologic studies and studies utilizing intravascular ultrasound and coronary angioscopy indicate that coronary arteriography does not always accurately delineate the severity of coronary atherosclerosis.[9]

More importantly clinical studies utilizing catheterization routinely in patients after thrombolytic therapy show no advantage to this approach over a conservative strategy where patients undergo cardiac catheterization only if spontaneous or provokable myocardial ischemia is documented. The major benefit of routine coronary arteriography is to detect the 20% to 25% of patients whose infarct-related coronary artery is occluded despite thrombolytic therapy. As indicated previously, the currently available non invasive techniques are not always able to separate patients with a patent from those with a closed infarct-related artery.[9,20] A patent infarct-related coronary artery is associated with a better long-term prognosis, particularly in those with a left ventricular ejection fraction of <40%.[51]

It is not yet clear as to which patients with an occluded infarct-related artery will benefit from predischarge opening of the vessel at the time of coronary arteriography. It is likely to vary, depending on the site of infarction, the affected coronary artery, the collateral circulation, the status of left ventricular function and the amount of poststenosis viable myocardium. In TAMI-6 patients, PTCA of occluded infarct-related arteries 48 hours after onset of symptoms improved left ventricular ejection fraction over that in patients who did not receive this procedure; however, this improvement in systolic function was not maintained at 6-month follow-up.[52]

If routine cardiac catheterization and coronary arteriography are recommended as routine procedure in patients after thrombolytic therapy, coronary angioplasty or coronary artery bypass graft surgery should be reserved only for those with clinical indications such as provokable myocardial ischemia as demonstrated by noninvasive testing. Mortality rates range between 30% and 40% in patients after failed attempts at either direct or salvage PTCA, and thus, the importance of caution in the use of angioplasty in acute infarction patients.[53]

The role of coronary arteriography before hospital discharge after myocardial infarction was assessed in 1,043 hospital survivors of the Alteplase/placebo and the Alteplase/PTCA trials of the European Cooperative Study Group.[22,24] Forty-two of the 1,043 patients (4.0%) died between 1–489 days after predischarge coronary arteriography. In survivors, follow-up ranged from 34 to 1,106 days. In a stepwise multivariate regression model, the use of diuretics and/or digitalis, a history of previous infarction and age exceeding 60 years were retained in the model using clinical data only. In addition, inability to perform exercise testing and a <30 mm Hg exercise-induced systolic blood pressure increase were selected as significant risk factors by multivariate analysis. Large enzymatic infarct size, radionuclide left ventricular ejection fraction below 40%, and multivessel disease were also important determinants of mortality after hospital discharge.

The risk function that included coronary arteriography performed no better for late mortality prediction than the risk function based on clinical data and noninvasive testing. Patients without a history of previous infarction, not treated with diuretics and/or digitalis, and with a systolic blood pressure increase of 30 mm Hg or more during exercise had an excellent survival (98.6%) in the first year after hospital discharge, irrespective of whether symptoms of recurrent ischemia occurred. This low-risk group formed 47% of the total patient population and did not benefit from coronary arteriography.

A diagnostic strategy based on the European Cooperative Study Group update[22] is illustrated in Figure 10. With echocardiography or radionuclide ventriculography, patients with severe left ventricular dysfunction can be identified. Thallium scintigraphy

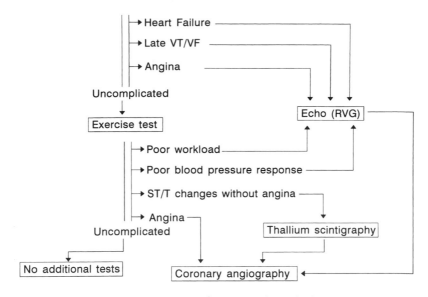

FIGURE 10. *Management approach to postthrombolytic myocardial infarction patients based on a multivariant analysis in 1,043 patients. See text. VT, ventricular tachycardia; VF, ventricular fibrillation; RVG, radionuclide ventriculography. (Modified with permission from Reference 22.)*

can be used to verify whether exercise-induced ST changes without angina represent a significant area of ischemia.

Selective Coronary Arteriography

Considering the data from multicenter trials discussed above, there are many reasons for recommending cardiac catheterization and coronary arteriography only for selected postthrombolytic patients. The data indicate that a conservative approach with catheterization reserved for selected patients at increased risk is as effective in reducing subsequent acute cardiac events as is a routine cardiac catheterization approach. The cost savings by avoiding 40% or more of the cardiac catheterizations and related unnecessary myocardial revascularization procedures are considerable.[54] Noninvasive testing utilizing a measurement of left ventricular systolic function and stress testing to evoke myocardial ischemia (Figure 1) is considerably less expensive than coronary arteriography, which provides only anatomical data and often results in unnecessary revascularization procedures for any documented residual stenosis in the infarct-related coronary artery even though the long-term outcome is likely to be favorable without the procedure.

As indicated previously, using the TIMI-II data, Rogers and colleagues[18] compared the strategy of predischarge catheterization with no angioplasty was compared with a conservative strategy of selective catheterization in TIMI-II patients. Although there was no difference in 1-year mortality, the high in-hospital mortality of 8% for patients receiving catheterization with no angioplasty compared with 4% for patients receiving selective catheterization (P = 0.01) is noteworthy.

The restricted use of postthrombolytic catheterization would facilitate continuity of care in local community centers and avoid the need for interhospital transfer for the purpose of doing predischarge arteriography.[9] Indeed, in the TIMI-II trial, the conservative strategy after thrombolytic therapy was equally effective in community hospitals despite the greater use of coronary arteriography/angioplasty at tertiary hospitals.[55] Thus, a strategy of selective arteriography is highly practical because it results in a decrease in the frequency of unnecessary procedures, transfers and PTCA as well as a decrease in cost and risk.[9]

Specifically, early coronary arteriography often is recommended for patients in whom continuous ST segment monitoring or a delayed serum CK enzyme peak and continuing pain suggest that thrombolysis has been unsuccessful.

After the initial 6–18 hours, but prior to predischarge evaluation, coronary arteriography is indicated in patients with recurrent episodes of ischemic chest pain, in patients with congestive heart failure that persists during intensive medical therapy and in patients with recurrent ventricular tachycardia, or ventricular fibrillation during intensive antiarrhythmic therapy.[3]

In patients with an uncomplicated myocardial infarction who have undergone thrombolytic therapy, predischarge cardiac catheterization and coronary arteriography are indicated in patients who have had episodes of postinfarction angina pectoris, in those that have provokable ischemia by noninvasive testing and in those who have a left ventricular ejection fraction of <40%.[3] It is likely in the latter group that a patent infarct-related coronary artery is most important for favorably influencing long-term prognosis and many of these patients will have severe multivessel disease with indications for coronary artery bypass surgery.

Summary

Based on the available data concerning the indications for the timing of angiography after thrombolysis, the inevitable conclusion is reached that conservative versus aggressive management is indicated for the 40% to 50% of patients at low risk who do not have spontaneous or provokable myocardial ischemia.

Factors to be considered in management decisions after thrombolytic therapy include risk factors before and after thrombolytic therapy, the result of studies assessing conservative versus aggressive postthrombolytic management, the accuracy of risk stratification by noninvasive testing and the relevance of the open artery hypothesis in decision making for low-risk patients with normal left ventricular function. While there are benefits of routine coronary arteriography relative to determining the severity of coronary artery disease and whether or not the infarct-related artery is patent, selective coronary arteriography is a more feasible and less expensive approach for appropriate patients. The low annual mortality rate with this approach is equal to that obtained when patients undergo routine coronary arteriography with myocardial revascularization based on the result of the routine procedure.

References

1. O'Rourke RA. Overview of trends in heart disease: changing prognoses after acute myocardial infarction. *Am J Epidemiology.* 1993;3:541–546.
2. Reeder GS, Gersh BJ. Modern management of acute myocardial infarction. *Curr Probl Cardiol.* 1993;2:81–156.
3. Gunnar RM, Bourdillon PDV, Dixon DW, et al. ACC/AHA Task Force Report. Guidelines for the early management of patients with acute myocardial infarction. *J Am Coll Cardiol.* 1990;16:249–292.
4. The GUSTO Investigators. An international randomized trial comparing four thrombolytic strategies for acute myocardial infarction. *N Engl J Med.* 1993;329:673–682.
5. The GUSTO Angiographic Investigators. The effects of tissue plasminogen activator, streptokinase or both on coronary-artery patency, ventricular function and survival after acute myocardial infarction. *N Engl J Med.* 1993;329:1615–1622.
6. Braunwald E. The open-artery theory is alive and well again. *N Engl J Med.* 1993;329:1650–1652.
7. Fuster V. Coronary thrombolysis. A perspective for the practicing physician. *N Engl J Med.* 1993;329:723–724.
8. O'Rourke RA. Non-invasive and invasive testing after myocardial infarction. *Curr Probl Cardiol.* 1991;11:727–763.
9. Topol EJ, Holmes DR, Rogers WJ. Coronary angiography after thrombolytic therapy for acute myocardial infarction. *Ann Intern Med.* 1991; 114;877–885.
10. Roberts R, Morris D, Pratt GM, et al. Pathophysiology, recognition and treatment of acute myocardial infarction and its complications. In: Schlant RC, Alexander RW, eds. *The Heart.* Eighth edition. New York, NY: McGraw-Hill Inc; 1994:1107–1184.
11. The TIMI Research Group. Immediate vs delayed catheterization and

angioplasty following thrombolytic therapy for acute myocardial infarction. TIMI II A results. *JAMA*. 1988;260:2849–2858.

12. Topol EJ, Califf RM, George BS, et al. A randomized trial of immediate versus delayed elective angioplasty after intravenous tissue plasminogen activator in acute myocardial infarction. *N Engl J Med*. 1987; 317:581–588.

13. Simoons ML, Arnold A, Betriu A, et al. Thrombolysis with rt- PA in acute myocardial infarction: no beneficial effects of immediate PTCA. *Lancet*. 1988;1:197–203.

14. The TIMI Study Group. Comparison of invasive and conservative strategies after treatment with intravenous tissue plasminogen activator in acute myocardial infarction. Results of the thrombolysis in myocardial infarction (TIMI) phase II trial. *N Engl J Med*. 1989;320:618–627.

15. SWIFT Trial Study Group. SWIFT trial of delayed elective intervention versus conservative treatment after thrombolysis with anistreplase in acute myocardial infarction. *Br Med J*. 1991;302:555–560.

16. Barbash GI, Roth A, Hod H, et al. Randomized controlled trial of late in-hospital angiography and angioplasty versus conservative management after treatment with recombinant tissue-type plasminogen activator in acute myocardial infarction. *Am J Cardiol*. 1990;66:538–545.

17. Ellis SG, Mooney MR, George BS, et al. Randomized trial of late elective angioplasty versus conservative management for patients with residual stenoses after thrombolytic treatment of myocardial infarction. *Circulation*. 1992;86:1400–1406.

18. Rogers WJ, Babb JD, Baim DS, et al. Selective versus routine predischarge coronary arteriography after therapy with recombinant tissue-type plasminogen activator, heparin and aspirin for acute myocardial infarction. *J Am Coll Cardiol*. 1991;17:1007–1016.

19. Hillis LD, Forman S, Braunwald E, et al. Risk stratification before thrombolytic therapy in patients with acute myocardial infarction. *J Am Coll Cardiol*. 1990;16:313–315.

20. Kim CB, Braunwald E. Potential benefits of late reperfusion of infarcted myocardium. The open artery hypothesis. *Circulation*. 1993;88:2426–2436.

21. Mueller HS, Cohen LS, Braunwald E, et al. Predictors of early morbidity and mortality after thrombolytic therapy of acute myocardial infarction. Analyses of patient subgroups in the thrombolysis in myocardial infarction (TIMI) trial, Phase II. *Circulation*. 1992;85:1254–1264.

22. Arnold AER, Simoons ML, Detry JMR, et al. Prediction of mortality following hospital discharge after thrombolysis for acute myocardial infarction: is there a need for coronary arteriography? *Eur Heart J*. 1993;14:306–315.

23. Schlant RC, O'Rourke RA, Collen D, et al. Reperfusion in acute myocardial infarction: International Society and Federation of Cardiology (ISFC) task force on myocardial reperfusion. In press.

24. Arnold AER, Simoons ML, Van de Werf F, et al. Recombinant tissue-type plasminogen activator and immediate angioplasty in acute myocardial infarction. One-year follow-up. *Circulation*. 1992;86:111–120.

25. McClements BM, Adgey AAJ. Value of signal-averaged electrocardiography, radionuclide ventriculography, Holter monitoring and clinical variables for the prediction of arrhythmic events in survivors of acute myocardial infarction in the thrombolytic era. *J Am Coll Cardiol*. 1993; 21:1419–1423.

26. Cleempoel H, Vainsel H, Dramaix M, et al. Limitations on the prognostic value of predischarge data after myocardial infarction. *Br Heart J.* 1988;60:98–103.
27. Touchstone DA, Beller GA, Nygaard TW, et al. Functional significance of predischarge exercise thallium-201 findings following intravenous streptokinase therapy during acute myocardial infarction. *Am Heart J.* 1988;116:1500–1507.
28. Marx B, Bertel O, Amann F. Late recurrent ischaemia in infarct patients with a normal predischarge exercise test after thrombolysis. *Eur Heart J.* 1990;11:897–902.
29. Sutton JM, Topol EJ. Significance of negative exercise thallium test in the presence of a critical residual stenosis after thrombolysis for acute myocardial infarction. *Circulation.* 1991;83:1278–1286.
30. Lette J, Laverdie[gr]re M, Cerino M, et al. Is dipyridamole-thallium imaging preferable to submaximal exercise thallium testing for risk stratification after thrombolysis? *Am Heart J.* 1990;119:671–672.
31. Beller GA. Noninvasive assessment of myocardial salvage after coronary reperfusion: a perpetual quest of nuclear cardiology. *J Am Coll Cardiol.* 1989;14:874–876.
32. Lavie CJ, Gibbons RJ, Zinsmeister AR, et al. Interpreting results of exercise studies after acute myocardial infarction altered by thrombolytic therapy, coronary angioplasty or bypass. *Am J Cardiol.* 1991;67:116–120.
33. Haber HL, Beller GA, Watson DD, et al. Exercise thallium-201 scintigraphy after thrombolytic therapy with or without angioplasty for acute myocardial infarction. *Am J Cardiol.* 1993;71:1257–1261.
34. Tilkemeier PL, Guiney TE, LaRaia PJ, et al. Prognostic value of predischarge low-level exercise thallium testing after thrombolytic treatment of acute myocardial infarction. *Am J Cardiol.* 1990;66:1203–1207.
35. Marshall JC, Waxman HL, Sauerwein A, et al. Frequency of low- grade residual coronary stenosis after thrombolysis during acute myocardial infarction. *Am J Cardiol.* 1990;66:773–778.
36. Muller DWM, Topol EJ, Ellis SG, et al. Multivessel coronary artery disease: A key predictor of short-term prognosis after reperfusion therapy for acute myocardial infarction. *Am Heart J.* 1991;121:1042–1049.
37. Simoons ML, Vos J, Tijssen JG, et al. Long-term benefit of early thrombolytic therapy in patients with acute myocardial infarction: 5 year follow-up of a trial conducted by the interuniversity cardiology institute of the Netherlands. *J Am Coll Cardiol.* 1989;14:1609–1615.
38. Chaitman BR, McMahon RP, Terrin M, et al. Impact of treatment strategy on predischarge exercise test in the thrombolysis in myocardial infarction (TIMI) II trial. *Am J Cardiol.* 1993;71:131–138.
39. Jain A, Myers GH, Sapin PM, et al. Comparison of symptom limited exercise stress test with heart rate limited exercise stress test early after myocardial infarction. *J Am Coll Cardiol.* 1993;22:1816–1820.
40. Verani M. Pharmacologic stress myocardial perfusion imaging. *Curr Probl Cardiol.* 1993;8:481–528.
41. Jaarsma W, Cramer JMJ, Suttorp MJ, et al. Risk stratification following thrombolysis in acute myocardial infarction with dobutamine stress echocardiography. *Circulation.* 1993;88:I-120. Abstract.
42. The Multicenter Post-infarction Research Group. Risk stratification and survival after myocardial infarction. *N Engl J Med.* 1983;309:331–336.

43. Gomes JA, Winters SL, Stewart D, et al. A new noninvasive index to predict sustained ventricular tachycardia and sudden death in the first year after myocardial infarction: based on signal-averaged electrocardiogram, radionuclide ejection fraction and Holter monitoring. *J Am Coll Cardiol.* 1987;10:349–357.

44. Zaret BL, Wackers FJ, Terrin ML, et al. Assessment of global and regional left ventricular performance at rest and during exercise after thrombolytic therapy for acute myocardial infarction: results of the thrombolysis in myocardial infarction (TIMI) II Study. *Am J Cardiol.* 1992;69:1–9.

45. Kjellgren O, Gomes JA. Current usefulness of the signal-averaged electrocardiogram. *Curr Probl Cardiol.* 1993;6:361–420.

46. Gang ES, Lew AS, Hong M, et al. Decreased incidence of ventricular late potentials after successful thrombolytic therapy for acute myocardial infarction. *N Engl J Med.* 1989;321:712–716.

47. Krucoff MW, Croll MA, Pope JF, et al. Continuous 12-lead ST-segment recovery analysis in the TAMI 7 study. Performance of a non-invasive method for real-time detection of failed reperfusion. *Circulation.* 1993; 88:436–446.

48. Roberts R, Kleinman V. Earlier diagnosis and treatment of acute myocardial infarction necessitates the need for "a new diagnostic mind set". *Circulation.* In press.

49. Wackers FJ, Gibbons RJ, Verani MS, et al. Serial quantitative planar technetium-99m isonitrile imaging in acute myocardial infarction: efficacy for noninvasive assessment of thrombolytic therapy. *J Am Coll Cardiol.* 1989;14:186–173.

50. Little WC, Downes TR, Applegate RJ. The underlying coronary lesion in myocardial infarction: implications for coronary angiography. *Clin Cardiol.* 1991;14:868–874.

51. Lamas GA, Flaker GC, Mitchell G, et al. Effect of captopril therapy on post MI outcome in patients with and without a patent infarct-related artery. *J Am Coll Cardiol.* 1993;21:44A. Abstract.

52. Topol EJ, Califf RM, Vandormael M, et al. , and the TAMI-6 study group. A randomized trial of late reperfusion for acute myocarial infarction. *Circulation.* 1992;85:2090–2099.

53. Ryan TJ, Bauman WB, Kennedy JW, et al. ACC/AHA Task Force Report. Guidelines for percutaneous transluminal coronary angioplasty. *J Am Coll Cardiol.* 1993;22:2033–2054.

54. Charles ED, Rogers WJ, Reeder GS, et al. Economic advantages of a conservative strategy for AMI management: rt-PA without obligatory PTCA. *J Am Coll Cardiol.* 1989;13:152A. Abstract.

55. Felt F, Mueller HS, Braunwald E, et al. Thrombolysis In Myocardial Infarction (TIMI) phase II trial. Outcome comparison of a "conservative strategy" in community versus tertiary hospitals. *J Am Coll Cardiol.* 1990;16:1529–1534.

Chapter 32

Should Everyone Have An Open Artery After Myocardial Infarction?

Eric R. Powers, MD

The benefits of reperfusion after acute coronary occlusion and the mechanisms responsible for observed benefits have been subjects of great interest for over a decade. In studies of patients with acute myocardial infarction, successful reperfusion has been reported to improve clinical outcome. However, incompletely answered questions include: "When after infarction is reperfusion of value?" and "What are the mechanisms of observed beneficial effects?"

The strategy of early reperfusion evolved from the pioneering work of Reimer and Jennings.[1,2] Their animal studies demonstrated that after coronary occlusion, myocardial infarction develops progressively in a "wavefront" fashion over a relatively short period of time (0–6 hours). Reperfusion at an early stage of the infarction process salvaged myocardium and the amount of salvage was determined by the interval between coronary occlusion and reperfusion. Myocardial salvage was thus a time-dependent phenomenon. These studies led to the hypothesis that early reperfusion after myocardial infarction in humans would also result in myocardial salvage and that this salvage would result in a preservation of ventricular function that in turn would be associated with an improvement in clinical outcome. This hypothesis has been extensively tested in humans and as is discussed, the value of early successful reperfusion has been clearly demonstrated.

Recently, however, it has become clear that myocardial salvage may not be the only mechanism of benefit of reperfusion. Available evidence strongly suggests that there are benefits of reperfusion and coronary patency that are independent of the time to reperfusion. These observations suggest that late reperfusion may be clinically valuable in some patients. This concept leads to the practical

From Vetrovec GW, Carabello BA, (eds.) *Invasive Cardiology: Current Diagnostic and Therapeutic Issues.* Armonk, NY: Futura Publishing Company, Inc.: © 1996.

question of whether a strategy of late reperfusion is rational for some patients, and if so, how can these patients be identified?

This chapter discusses the evidence supporting the hypothesis that early reperfusion and associated myocardial salvage is beneficial in humans, and also reviews the evidence that late coronary reperfusion and coronary patency, irrespective of the time to reperfusion, also improves clinical outcome in some patients. Possible mechanisms for the salutory effects of late reperfusion and coronary patency and the hypothesis that late reperfusion is particularly beneficial if myocardial viability has been maintained by collateral blood flow will be discussed.

Is Myocardial Salvage After Early Successful Reperfusion an Important Mechanism of Benefit of Reperfusion After Myocardial Infarction?

As described earlier, animal studies have clearly shown that reperfusion of the myocardium within a certain period of time after coronary occlusion results in myocardial salvage and preservation of ventricular function.[1,2] Furthermore, the extent of salvage is time dependent; the earlier the reperfusion after coronary occlusion, the greater the salvage. Clinical studies have demonstrated that mortality after myocardial infarction is closely related to left ventricular function. Thus, it has been hypothesized that the observed improvement in survival with reperfusion therapy after acute myocardial infarction is due to myocardial salvage and resultant preserved left ventricular function, and that the greatest improvement in survival would be seen with the earliest reperfusion.

Evidence that time to treatment can be an important determinant of the favorable effect of reperfusion therapy is compelling. The first major randomized controlled study of intravenous thrombolytic therapy using strepokinase, GISSI 1,[3] demonstrated a substantial decrease in mortality for patients treated early (within 1 hour of the onset of chest pain) cornpared to patients treated later after the onset of symptoms. Furthermore, no decrease in mortality was observed in patients treated 6 hours or more after the onset of symptoms. These data are consistent with the hypothesis that a major mechanism of benefit of reperfusion therapy is myocardial salvage. Recently, the GUSTO study[4] has provided important confirmatory evidence that time to reperfusion can be an important determinant of the favorable effects of reperfusion. Front-loaded tissue plasminogen activator (tPA) resulted in earlier reperfusion, but no greater coronary patency other than the tested thrombolytic regimens was found to be significantly superior improving survival. Furthermore, when survival benefit in GUSTO was related to time from onset of symptoms to treatment, improved left ventricular function and mortality with early treatment was demonstrated. The recently published EMIP study came to a similar conclusion.[5] This study and a meta-analysis of published studies, suggested that the administration of thrombolytic therapy prior to hospital arrival was associated with a significant improvement in survival when compared to in-hospital administration. Thus, shortening time to treatment contributes to the value of reperfusion in some patients. The mechanism responsible for this effect has not been positively identified, but may be myocardial salvage.

Some studies examining the relationship between time to treatment and preservation of left ventricular function have demonstrated better ventricular function with early reperfusion compared with later reperfusion.[4-6] This is particularly evident when "early" treatment is administered within the first hour after the onset of symptoms. However, other studies have not found a correlation between time to reperfusion and preservation of ventricular function.[8,9] Several trials, including the TIMI I[8] and TAMI[9] (Figure 1) studies, have demonstrated a poor or absent correlation

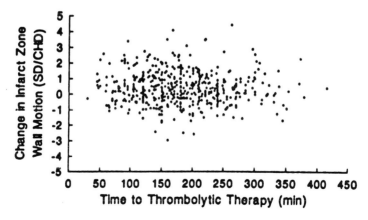

FIGURE 1. *The relationship between improvement in infarct zone regional wall motion and time to administration of thrombolytic therapy.[9] Scatterplot of change in infarct zone regional wall motion from early to the 7-day catheterization is shown as a function of time from symptom onset to the administration of intravenous thrombolytic therapy. No relation was observed between improvement in infarct zone regional wall motion and time to thrombolytic therapy. SD/CHD, standard deviations from the mean per chord.*

between time from symptom onset to initiation of thrombolytic therapy and preservation of left ventricular function. Similarly, the expected relationship between left ventricular function and survival[10] has not been consistently observed in patients receiving thrombolytic therapy.[11] In addition, studies have reported improved survival with reperfusion therapy, but have failed to demonstrate an associated benefit on preservation of left ventricular function.[12] These results have led to the hypothesis that the benefit of reperfusion may at least in part be explained by factors other than time to reperfusion and myocardial salvage.

Is There Evidence For Benefits of Late Reperfusion?

As described above, there are data that suggest that very early reperfusion may impact significantly on myocardial salvage and left ventricular function. However, in most patients time to reperfusion and changes in regional and global left ventricular function have little, if any correlation.[9] As shown in Figure 1, preservation of regional left ventricular function occurred in many patients with successful reperfusion, but was as likely to occur with late as with early reperfusion. Additional studies have demonstrated substantially better left ventricular function in patients with presumed late spontaneous reperfusion than those in whom late patency was not achieved. Thus, there appears to be a time-independent effect of successful reperfusion on left ventricular function in some patients.

A relationship between infarct artery patency and favorable long-term clinical outcome has been clearly demonstrated. The Western Washington Trial of intracoronary streptokinase demonstrated a striking improvement in survival in streptokinase treated patients compared to untreated controls despite similar estimates of infarct size and ejection fraction in the two groups.[13,14] Cigaroa and colleagues[15] reported a study of 179 patients with single vessel coronary artery disease. With a mean follow-up of almost 4 years, no patient with a patent infarct artery died compared with an 18% mortality in patients with an occluded infarct artery. In addition, other adverse clinical outcomes including unstable angina and congestive heart failure were less common in the group with a patent infarct related artery.

The TIMI I study compared the thrombolytic agents tPA and streptokinase with the primary end point being patency of the infarct-related artery 90 minutes after the onset of therapy. tPA was found to be twice as effective as streptokinase in producing 90-

minute reperfusion.[16] However, contrary to expectation, this difference in 90-minute patency did not translate into better left ventricular function or improved clinical outcome. However, when late survival was assessed based on patency of the infarct related rather than the specific thrombolytic agent administered, artery patency was a powerful predictor of survival despite the fact that reperfusion was achieved relatively late after the onset of infarction in this study (Figure 2).[17] Furthermore, left symptoms ventricular function was not different in the patent and occluded infarct artery groups. Thus, improved survival correlated with infarct artery patency rather than improvement in left ventricular function.

The previously reported relationship between survival and left ventricular function demonstrated in the prethrombolytic era[10] appears to be altered by the presence of a patent infarct related artery. In the TIMI II trial, survival was unexpectedly high in the group of patients with significant depression of ventricular function.[11] Furthermore, a recent study reported excellent survival in patients with large infarcts of the left ventricle (40% of left ventricular mass) in the presence of a patent infarct artery.[18] In previous studies, infarctions of this magnitude have been associated with cardiogenic shock and death in patients not receiving reperfusion therapy.

Thrombolytic therapy administered late after the onset of myocardial infarction, after the potential for myocardial salvage has been eliminated, has been shown to improve survival in some stud-

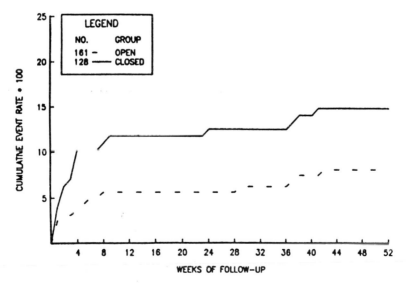

FIGURE 2. *TIMI Phase I. Life table cumulative mortality rates by perfusion status at 90 minutes.17*

ies. The ISIS II,[19] and LATE,[20] studies have demonstrated improved survival compared to untreated patients when thrombolytic therapy was administered more than 6 hours after the onset of symptoms.

Thus, these data suggest a time-independent effect of reperfusion on ventricular function and a close relationship between infarct artery patency and improved clinical outcome and support the hypothesis that late reperfusion after myocardial infarction may be beneficial.

Possible Mechanisms of Benefit of Late Reperfusion

Several possible mechanisms for the salutory effects of a patent infarct artery that are independent of myocardial salvage have been proposed. In animals and humans, infarct expansion and aneurysm formation may occur after myocardial infarction. A number of animal studies, including rat, pig, and dog models, have suggested that late reperfusion reduces ventricular dilation and aneurysm formation. In contrast, persistent occlusion of the infarct artery has been associated with ventricular dilation and aneurysm formation. In the TIMI I study, ventricular dilation occurred more frequently in patients with occluded than patent infarct-related arteries.[21] The TAMI-6 study[22] addressed the value of late reperfusion and enrolled patients between 6 and 24 hours after the onset of symptoms. Patients were randomized to tPA or placebo. At 6-month follow-up, placebo treatment was associated with an increase in left ventricular diastolic volume. In contrast, patients treated with thrombolytic therapy had no evidence of left ventricular dilatation. The absence of ventricular dilation and aneurysm formation has been associated with improved long-term clinical outcome in patients after myocardial infarction.

Another proposed mechanism for the benefit of a patent infarct artery and late reperfusion is an improvement in electrical stability and a decrease in serious ventricular arrhythmias. Several studies have demonstrated a lower incidence of abnormal signal-averaged electrocardiograms in patients treated with thrombolytic drugs compared to patients not treated.[23] Furthermore, in some but not all studies, thrombolytic therapy has been associated with a decrease in the incidence of inducible ventricular arrhythmias,[24] and a greater likelihood of suppressibility of inducible arrhythmias with drugs[25] Thus, available data suggest that early reperfusion results in an improvement in the signal-averaged electrocardiogram, and a decrease in the incidence and drug resistance of ventricular arrhythmias.

The effects of late reperfusion on the signal-averaged electrocardiogram and the incidence of ventricular arrhythmias remains uncertain. Several studies have looked at the influence of late reperfusion on the signal averaged electrocardiogram.[26,27] Different studies have shown different effects. In a study of 50 patients undergoing balloon coronary angioplasty of an occluded infarct related artery 2 days to 5 weeks after infarction, we found no effect of successful late reperfusion on the prevalence of late potentials.[26] Of interest, the absence of late potentials was associated with an improvement in ventricular function late after successful reperfusion. This finding suggests that the absence of abnormalities on the signal averaged electrocardiogram may be associated with the presence of myocardial viability within the infarct zone. To date, there are no convincing data demonstrating an effect of late reperfusion on clinically important ventricular arrhythmias or the inducibility of arrhythmias by electrophysiologic stimulation.

The benefits of reperfusion may, at least in part, be due to the restoration of antegrade blood flow to viable myocardium. We have examined the hypotheses that (1) viable myocardium in the infarct zone is common in patients late after acute infarction; (2) that this viable myocardium is associated with collateral blood flow; and (3) that restoration of antegrade blood flow late after infarction is associated with improvement in regional left ventricular function in the infarct zone.[28] We used the techniques of contrast echocardiography to assess collateral blood flow and two-dimensional echocardiographic changes in regional wall motion to assess viability and benefit of late reperfusion. Contrast echocardiography is illustrated in Figure 3. The top half of this figure demonstrates an image obtained after contrast microbubbles were injected into the left main coronary artery of a patient with recent inferior wall infarction and right coronary occlusion. As can be seen, there is a homogeneous pattern of contrast uptake throughout the left ventricular myocardium. The bottom half of the figure shows a frame from the contrast echocardiographic study performed after successful balloon angioplasty of the right coronary artery and the injection of contrast microbubbles into the patent right coronary artery. This defines the right coronary artery perfusion bed. A comparison between this image and the image in the upper half of the figure demonstrates that the entire right coronary artery perfusion bed was perfused by collaterals. We studied patients between 2 days and 5 weeks after myocardial infarction. All patients had total occlusion of the infarct-related artery. We first examined the extent of collateral flow. On average, greater than 70% of the perfusion bed of the infarct related artery was supplied by collaterals. Successful angioplasty was associated with an improvement in regional function in 25 of 34 patients, but in only 1 of 9 patients with

Before Angioplasty

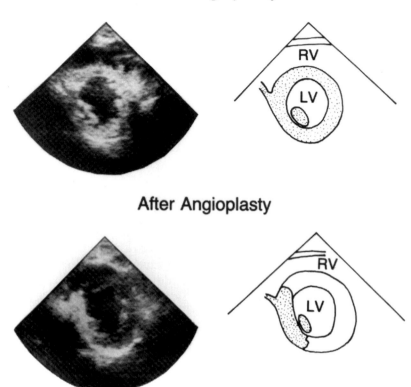

After Angioplasty

FIGURE 3. *Short-axis view of the left ventricle (LV) obtained by two-dimensional echocardiography in a patient with an occluded right coronary artery.[28] In the upper panel, sonicated diatrizoate sodium-diatrizoate meglumine was injected into the left main coronary artery before balloon angioplasty of the right coronary artery. Homogeneous opacification of the entire myocardium, including the occluded right coronary artery bed, is evident. In the lower panel, sonicate sodium-diatrizoate meglumine was injected selectively into the right coronary artery after successful angioplasty of that vessel. This injection defined the perfusion bed supplied by the right coronary artery. RV, right ventricle; LV, left ventricle.*

unsuccessful reperfusion. Similarly, regional wall motion score only improved significantly in patients with successful reperfusion. Improvement in regional wall motion at follow-up was strongly correlated with the extent of collateral blood flow to the infarct zone prior to reperfusion (Figure 4). We concluded that myocardial viability was common in infarct zones, that collateral blood flow

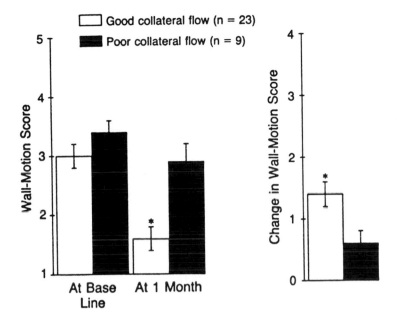

FIGURE 4. *Mean (± SEM) wall motion score in patients with good and poor collateral blood flow by myocardial contrast echocardiography.[28] Patients with >50% of the infarct bed supplied by collateral vessels were defined as having good collateral flow, and those patients with <50% of the bed supplied by collateral vessels were defined as having poor collateral flow. Patients with good collateral flow had significantly better function 1 month after successful balloon angioplasty than those with poor collateral flow (**left panel**). The improvement in wall motion score 1 month after angioplasty was also greater in patients with good collateral blood flow (**right panel**). Wall motion was scored as follows: 1, normal function; 2, mild hypokinesia; 3, severe hypokinesia; 4, akinesia; and 5, dyskinesia. The asterisk indicates a significant difference from baseline (P < 0.01).*

was associated with viability (and almost certainly maintained viability), and that successful late reperfusion resulted in improved function if collateral blood flow and viability were present.

The Importance of Collaterals for Maintaining Myocardial Viability After Myocardial Infarction

Although the functional and clinical significance of coronary collaterals in patients with coronary artery disease has been clearly established, some studies have expressed doubt about the importance of collaterals in the setting of acute myocardial infarction. This uncertainty may be due to the fact that the presence of collaterals has traditionally been evaluated by angiography. Angiography has a lower limit of resolution of 100 μm and many collaterals are smaller in size. In addition angiography only identifies epicardial collateral conduits that may not reflect collateral flow at the level of the myocardium. Other techniques such as contrast echocardiography and thallium-201 scintigraphy have clearly demonstrated the importance of collaterals for maintaining myocardial viability after coronary occlusion.

The prevalence of collaterals at the onset of acute myocardial infarction in man remains unclear. Angiographic studies early after infarction have demonstrated that 30% to 45% of patients have angiographic evidence of collateral flow. Our studies using contrast echocardiography,[28] show that collaterals were much more common at an average of 12 days after infarction.

Animal studies have clearly demonstrated the importance of collaterals in modifying infarct size after coronary occlusion. Several clinical studies have provided evidence that collaterals limit infarct size and are associated with preservation of left ventricular function and a reduction in aneurysm formation. Finally, as discussed earlier, our studies suggest that collaterals maintain myocardial viability and allow "hibernation" of the myocardium for prolonged periods following acute myocardial infarction.

Studies of Late Reperfusion

The potential clinical value of late reperfusion is suggested by a recent study demonstrating improved 3-year survival in patients with late reperfusion using balloon angioplasty.[29] Several studies have assessed the strategy of late administration of thrombolytic agents. In ISIS-2,[19] using streptokinase, cardiovascular mortality was reduced by 20% at 5 weeks in patients treated between 13 and 24 hours after the onset of symptoms. In the LATE study[20] tPA was administered 6 to 24 hours after the onset of symptoms. At 35-day follow-up, there was a significant (26%) reduction in mortality for patients treated 6 to 12 hours after the onset of symptoms. However, there was no mortality reduction for patients treated between 13 and 24 hours. In contrast, the EMERAS trial of streptokinase administration 6 to 24 hours after acute myocardial infarction[30] showed no significant benefit of therapy. The TAMI-6 study,[22] studied late thrombolysis using tPA and late balloon angioplasty in patients with persistent total occlusion of the infarct related artery. There was no improvement in systolic function at six months in those treated with or without thrombolytics or those treated with or without angioplasty.

Why did these studies fail to show consistent clinical benefits of late reperfusion? A possible explanation is that any potential long-term salutary effect of late reperfusion was nullified by reocclusion of the infarct artery. Reocclusion of the infarct artery late after treatment with thrombolytic therapy is common. This has been clearly demonstrated in a number of studies including the APRICOT study.[31] In TAMI-6,[22] late patency of the infarct-related artery was not significantly different in the thrombolytic, non-thrombolytic, angioplasty and nonangioplasty groups. Thus, it appears that our current strategies for maintaining coronary patency are inadequate. Late reperfusion may only be beneficial if coronary patency can be maintained.

There has been recent interest in new strategies to improve and maintain coronary patency. In particular, there has been great interest in new direct antithrombins including hirudin[32] and hirulog and antiplatelet agents including platelet receptor blockers. Preliminary data suggest that these therapies may be effective in promoting and maintaining coronary patency in patients undergoing reperfusion after acute myocardial infarction. Of interest, direct antithrombins are also being studied as adjunctive therapy at the time of coronary angioplasty to prevent restenosis.[33]

Summary

Early reperfusion remains an important goal for the treatment of patients with acute myocardial infarction. However, early reperfusion, early enough to result in significant myocardial salvage, may only be achieved in a minority of patients with acute myocardial infarction because of delays in initiation of therapy. Recent data suggests that late reperfusion may also be clinically valuable, the value being maximal in those patients with collaterals and maintained myocardial viability in the infarct zone. These concepts are illustrated in Figure 5. Reperfusion within 1–2 hours of the onset of symptoms results in myocardial salvage and is associated with maximal mortality reduction.

Reperfusion after 3 hours (the majority of treated patients) does not result in myocardial salvage, but is associated with reduced mortality. However, the benefits of both early and late reperfusion may be lost by coronary reocclusion. Thus, approaches to

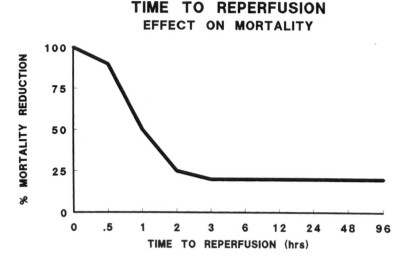

FIGURE 5. *Hypothetical relation between time to reperfusion and mortality. Maximal reduction in mortality occurs with successful reperfusion within 2 hours of the onset of symptoms and is due to myocardial salvage. The benefit of late reperfusion (the majority of patients) is due to factors other than myocardial salvage and is independent of time to reperfusion. (Adapted from Reference 34.)*

maintain coronary patency are crucial for the achievement of maximum benefit from any reperfusion strategy.

References

1. Reimer KA, Lowe JE, Rasmussen MM, Jennings RB. The wavefront phenomenon of ischemic cell death. I: myocardial infarct size vs duration of coronary occlusion in dogs. *Circulation.* 1977;56:786–794.
2. Reimer KA, Jennings RB. The "wavefront phenomenon" of myocardial ischemic cell death. II: Transmural progression of necrosis within the framework of ischemic bed size (myocardium at risk) and collateral flow. *Lab Invest.* 1979;40:633–644.
3. GRUPPO Italiano Per Lo Studio Della Streptochinasi Nell'Infarcto Miocardico (GISSI). Effectiveness of intravenous thrombolytic treatment in acute myocardial infarction. *Lancet.* 1986;1:397–401.
4. The GUSTO Angiographic Investigators. The effects of tissue plasminogen activator, streptokinase, or both on coronary artery patency, ventricular function, and survival after acute myocardial infarction. *N Engl J Med.* 1993;329:1615–1622.
5. The European Myocardial Infarction Project (EMIP Group). Prehospital thrombolytic therapy in patients with suspected acute myocardial infarction. *N Engl J Med.* 1993;329:383–389.

6. Mathey DG, Sheehan FH, Schofer J, Dodge HT. Time from onset of symptoms to thrombolytic therapy: a major determinant of myocardial salvage in patients with acute transmural infarction. *J Am Coll Cardiol.* 1985:6:518–525.
7. Sheehan FH, Doerr R, Schmidt WG, et al. Early recovery of left ventricular function after thrombolytic therapy for acute myocardial infarction: an important determinant of survival. *J Am Coll Cardiol.* 1988; 12:289–300.
8. Sheehan FH, Braunwald E, Canner P, et al. The effect of intravenous thrombolytic therapy on left ventricular function: a report on tissue-type plasminogen activator and streptokinase from the Thrombolysis in Myocardial Infarction (TIMI) Phase I Trial. *Circulation.* 1987;75: 817–829.
9. Harrison JK, Califf RM, Woodlief LH, et al. Systolic left ventricular function after reperfusion therapy for acute myocardial infarction: an analysis of determinants of improvement. *Circulation.* 1993;87:1531–1541.
10. The Multicenter Postinfarction Research Group. Risk stratification and survival after myocardial infarction. *N Engl J Med.* 1983;6:331–336.
11. Zaret BL, Walkers FJ, Terrin M, et al. Does left ventricular ejection fraction following thrombolytic therapy have the same prognostic impact described in the prethrombolytic era? Results of the TIMI II Trial. *J Am Coll Cardiol.* 1991;17:214A.
12. Van de Werf F. Discrepancies between the effects of coronary reperfusion on survival and left ventricular function. *Lancet.* 1989;1:1367–1369.
13. Kennedy JW, Ritchie JL, Davis KB, Fritz JK. Western Washington randomized trial of intracoronary streptokinase in acute myocardial infarction. *N Engl J Med.* 1983;309:1477–1482.
14. Kennedy JW, Ritchie JL, Davis KB, Stadius ML, Maynard C, Fritz JK. The Western Washington randomized trial of intracoronary streptokinase in acute myocardial infarction: a 12-month follow up report. *N Engl J Med.* 1985;312:1073–1078.
15. Cigarroa RG, Lange RA, Hillis LD. Prognosis after acute myocardial infarction in patients with and without residual anterogade coronary blood flow. *Am J Cardiol.* 1989;64:155–160.
16. Chesebro JH, Knatterud G, Roberts R, et al. Thrombolysis In Myocardial Infarction (TIMI) Trial, Phase I. A comparison between intravenous tissue plasminogen activatior and intravenous streptokinase; clinical findings through hospital discharge. *Circulation.* 1987;76:142–154.
17. Dalen JR, Gore JM, Graunwald E, et al. Six- and twelve-month follow-up of the phase I Thrombolysis in Myocardial Infarction (TIMI) Trial. *Am J Cardiol.* 1988;62:179–185.
18. McCallister BD, Christian TF, Gersh BJ, Gibbons RJ. Prognosis of myocardial infarctions involving more than 40% of the left ventricle after acute reperfusion therapy. *Circulation.* 1993;88:1470–1475.
19. ISIS-2 (Second International Study of Infarct Survival) Collaborative Group. Randomised trial of intravenous streptokinase, oral aspirin, both or neither among 17,187 cases of suspected acute myocardial infarction: ISIS-2. *Lancet.* 1988;2:349–360.
20. LATE Study Group. Late Assessment of Thrombolytic Efficacy (LATE) study with alteplase 6–24 hours after onset of acute myocardial infarction. *Lancet.* 1993;343:759–766.

21. Lavie CJ, O'Keefe JH, Chesebro JH, Clements IP, Gibbons RJ. Prevention of late ventricular dilatation after acute myocardial infarction by successful thrombolytic reperfusion. *Am J Cardiol.* 1990;66:31–46.
22. Topol EJ, Califf RM, Vandormael M, et al. A randomized trial of late reperfusion therapy for acute myocardial infarction. *Circulation.* 1992;85:2090–2099.
23. Gang ES, Lew AS, Hong M, Wang FZ, Siebert CA, Peter T. Decreased incidence of ventricular late potentials after successful thrombolytic therapy for acute myocardial infarction. *N Engl J Med.* 1989;321: 712–716.
24. Sager PT, Perlmutter RA, Rosenfeld LE, McPherson CA, Walkers FJ, Batsford WP. Electrophysiologic effects of thrombolytic therapy in patients with a transmural anterior myocardial infarction complicated by left ventricular aneurysm formation. *J Am Coll Cardiol.* 1988;12: 19–24.
25. Hii JTY, Traboulsi M, Mitchell LB, Wyse DG, Duff HJ, Gillis AM. Infarct artery patency predicts outcome of serial electropharmacological studies in patients with malignant ventricular tachyarrhythmias. *Circulation.* 1993;87:764–772.
26. Ragosta M, Sabia PJ, Kaul S, DiMarco JP, Sarembock IJ, Powers ER. Effects of late (1 to 30 days) reperfusion after acute myocardial infarction on signal-averaged electrocardiogram. *Am J Cardiol.* 1993;71: 19–23.
27. Lange RA, Cigarroa RG, Wells PJ, Mremers MS, Hillis LD. Influence of anterograde flow in the infarct artery on the incidence of late potentials after acute myocardial infarction. *Am J Cardiol.* 1990;65:554–558.
28. Sabia PJ, Powers ER, Ragosta M, Sarembock IJ, Burwell LR, Kaul S. An association between collateral blood flow and myocardial viability in patients with recent myocardial infarction. *N Engl J Med.* 1992;327: 1825–1831.
29. Bernardi MM, Whitlow PL. Reperfuson later than five days after acute myocardial infarction improves three-year survival. *Circulation.* 1991;84(Suppl II):II-232. Abstract.
30. EMERAS Collaborative Group. Randomised trial of late thrombolysis in patients with suspected acute myocardial infarction. *Lancet.* 1993; 342:767–772.
31. Meijer A, Verheught FWA, Werter CJPJ, Lie KI, van der Pol JMJ, van Eenige MJ. Aspirin versus coumadin in the prevention of reocclusion and recurrent ischemia after successful thrombolysis: a prospective placebo-controlled angiographic study. Results of the APRICOT study. *Circulation.* 1993;87:1524–1530.
32. Cannon CP, McCabe CH, Henry TD, et al. Hirudin reduces reocclusion compared to heparin following thrombolysis in acute myocardial infarciton: results of the TIMI-5 trial. *J Am Coll Cardiol.* 1993;21:136a. Abstract.
33. Sarembock IJ, Gertz SD, Gimple LW, Owen RM, Powers ER, Powers WC. Effectiveness of recombinant desulphatohirudin on restenosis following balloon angioplasty in rabbits. *Circulation.* 1991;84(1):232–243.
34. Gersh BJ, Anderson JL. Thrombolysis and myocardial salvage. Results of clinical trials and the animal paradigm-Parodoxic or predictable. *Circulation.* 1993;88:296–306.

Chapter 33

Coronary Angiography:
An Intervention Run Amok

Thomas B. Graboys, MD

We have witnessed a nearly 50% reduction in mortality from coronary artery disease over the three-decade period between 1950 and 1980.[1] This decline predated the widespread use of cardiovascular interventions such as coronary angioplasty (PTCA) and coronary bypass graft surgery (CABG). Despite these data, CABG procedures have increased from 180,000 in 1983 to 300,000 in 1986 and nearly 400,000 in 1993.[1]

Paralleling the exponential growth of bypass surgery has been the ever increasing popularity of coronary angioplasty. There has been a tenfold increase in the number of PTCAs performed from the 30,000 procedures done in 1983 to approximately 350,000 or more performed in 1993. PTCA has become a "cottage industry" despite the fact that there is not one study to date that has demonstrated superiority of PTCA over medical therapy in terms of survival or freedom from infarction among patients with chronic stable coronary disease. Thus, it appears that nearly three quarters of a million people in this country undergo either angioplasty or bypass surgery. How do we explain these figures given advances in pharmacotherapy and decreases in both the incidence and mortality of coronary disease? One answer can be found in the large number of coronary arteriographies undertaken. Indeed, once arteriography is carried out, revascularization with either PTCA or bypass surgery inevitably occurs. Catheterization then is the funnel to both procedures. Not withstanding that for patients with acute or unstable ischemic syndromes in whom revascularization may well be lifesaving, the majority of persons subjected to coronary arteriography in the United States have chronic stable angina. They undergo the procedure to "define the anatomy" or more likely to

From Vetrovec GW, Carabello BA, (eds.) *Invasive Cardiology: Current Diagnostic and Therapeutic Issues.* Armonk, NY: Futura Publishing Company, Inc.: © 1996.

find suitable coronary lesions to dilate. The threshold to catheterize in some geographic areas is so low that 20% to 45% of coronary angiograms do not disclose underlying coronary disease.[2] Either the procedure is being undertaken as a "routine" or physicians are simply not taking any type of detailed history.

What are the usual rationalizations for coronary arteriography?

Rationale 1: To Diagnose Coronary Disease

An angiogram is not required to diagnose underlying coronary disease. In fact, most patients present with either an acute myocardial infarction or angina pectoris. Indeed, in the vast majority of patients, the diagnosis of this disease is made primarily by a detailed history or a cardiac event. Only rarely are patients encountered in whom symptoms are sufficiently atypical or noninvasive studies so inconclusive that a coronary angiogram is necessary to define the presence or absence of atherosclerosis.

Rationale 2: To Begin Medical Therapy

Some argue that coronary arteriography is necessary in order to define a medical program, but one does not need the "anatomy" before initiating anti-ischemic medication. In fact, patients are frequently rendered symptom-free only to have a recurrence when medication is stopped prior to exercise testing.

Rationale 3: To Determine an Individual Patient's Prognosis

Sufficient data exist that shows that noninvasive assessment with echocardiography and exercise stress testing is sufficient to stratify patients in differing risk categories. It is the state of ventricular function, not the number of diseased vessels that predicts outcome.[3–5] Indeed earlier studies emphasized that a meticulous history used with an exercise test rendered sufficient information so that there was little added benefit from coronary arteriography.[6,7]

Rationale 4: A Coronary Angiogram Will Disclose a Seriously Stenosed Vessel That is Likely to Induce an Acute Cardiac Event or Myocardial Infarction

Studies by a number of investigators[8] including Little et al[9] emphasized the fact that coronary angiography did not predict the site of future coronary occlusions. In one study[9] investigators reviewed coronary angiograms in 42 consecutive patients and noted that in two thirds of patients, the "culprit vessel" had less than a 50% stenosis on the initial angiogram. In only one third of patients did the myocardial infarction occur in that vessel deemed most severely stenosed. Their conclusion was that ". . . assessment of the angiographic severity of coronary stenosis may be inadequate to accurately predict the time or location of a subsequent coronary occlusion that will produce a myocardial infarction."[9]

Rationale 5: Coronary Ateriography is Only Done on Patients Who Have Undergone Assessment of Functional Ischemia

It does not appear to be the case that coronary ateriography is only done on patients who have undergone assessment of functional ischemia. In a review of over 2,000 coronary angioplasties carried out in the state of Michigan by Topol and colleagues,[10] two thirds of those undergoing PTCA had not had an exercise treadmill study to assess "functional ischemia." One might then argue that these patients were too unstable to undergo exercise testing. However, that seemingly was not the situation inasmuch as nearly three quarters of these patients had as an admitting diagnosis chronic stable coronary disease. Indeed, in studies carried out by the Rand group assessing "appropriateness" of various cardiovascular interventions, chronic stable coronary disease is the most common coded diagnosis.[11,12]

Thus, if we do not need a coronary angiogram to diagnose angina, to initiate pharmacotherapy, to predict future infarction, or to prognosticate, under which circumstances should an angiogram be carried out? From the numbers presented elsewhere it is increasingly clear that this is a procedure that is a prelude to either angioplasty or bypass surgery. There would be no argument if the patient's clinical profile warrants either of those interventions. Given the fact that the majority of patients undergoing catheterization have "chronic stable" coronary disease as their admitting diagnosis,[11,12] and given the fact that a number of centers have a high fraction of normal coronary angiograms,[2] one can only conclude quite reasonably that this procedure is vastly overutilized.

What other factors substantiate this assertion? First, we have overtrained cardiologists and cardiovascular surgeons. Cardiovascular trainees conclude that without specialized training in angioplasty or electrophysiology, they are not "marketable." In a recent commentary, Topol and Calif[13] note that too many cardiologists are doing coronary interventions and too many cardiac surgeons are operating. They underscore this conclusion by citing that nearly half of members or fellows in the American College of Cardiology indicate that they are carrying out coronary angioplasty, but that the average interventional cardiologist in the United States does fewer than 25 PTCA cases per year. This is approximately half of the American College of Cardiology's "lenient guideline" that states that each physician must perform at least 50 interventions annually.[13–15] [*Editors' note:* The most recent guidelines recommend 75 per year.]

Second, we have spawned too many catheterization laboratories. Increases in the volume of coronary angiography is based in part upon the explosive growth of cardiac catheterization laboratories as documented by Nicod and coworkers[16] in the greater San Diego area as well as investigators in Seattle[17] who demonstrated that there was an approximately threefold higher rate of coronary angiography for patients after an acute myocardial infarction who were hospitalized at facilities with on-site catheterization laboratories. In fact, there was no difference in mortality among patients hospitalized at facilities with or without catheterization laboratories. The likelihood of further interventions, however, with either angioplasty or bypass surgery was significantly higher at hospitals which had the availability to carry out either procedure. The Lewis F. Bishop Lecture given by Gorlin[18] raised questions about the "inherent conflict of interest for both practitioners and hospitals in the performance of interventional procedures." Economic factors are compelling. Effectively, interventional cardiologists carry out angioplasty in a "closed loop" system, ie, initial evaluation of the patient, exercise treadmill test, thallium study, coronary angiogram, and finally, coronary angioplasty. One can only wonder that if a single fee were paid for the "inclusive management" of angina, how many catheterizations would be undertaken?

Third, the public, press, and frequently the physician perceive this disease as one of a "plumbing problem." Seduced by the technology and weaned on a quick fix, either a bypass or a balloon seem for many patients to be the logical and most compelling option.

Studies from our group[19,20] have raised questions as to the feasibility of second opinions for bypass surgery[19] and more recently, coronary angiograms.[20] Among 168 patients referred for a second opinion as to the need for coronary angiography, 134 (80%) were judged not to require that procedure. Indications for angiography were similar to those that emerged from the initial publication of CASS,[3] emphasizing stability of symptoms, intact ventricular function, and additionally a satisfactory exercise treadmill test. Thus, recommendations for coronary angiography included any of the following criteria:

1. A substantial drop in exertional blood pressure near peak exercise associated with signs of definitive angina or ST segment depression.
2. Angina at rest or requiring increasing amounts of medications in spite of a previously effective anti-ischemic drug program.
3. Presentation of angina as pulmonary edema.
4. Intolerance of medication.
5. Angina in the setting of malignant ventricular arrhythmia, ie, sustained ventricular tachycardia or primary (noninfarction-related) ventricular fibrillation.

After a nearly 4-year follow-up there were 11 deaths, 7 of which were cardiac, for an annualized cardiac mortality of 1.1%. Nineteen patients experienced new myocardial infarction (2.7% annualized rate). Twenty-seven of the 168 patients (4.3%) developed unstable angina and 26 patients were referred for coronary angiography or CABG. Among the 21 patients undergoing CABG at a mean of 29 months from initial presentation there was one fatality.

Conclusion

Current noninvasive procedures allow us to assess risk among patients presenting with coronary artery disease. In the stable patient coronary angiography adds little to a noninvasively determined "prognostic index." Evidence that coronary angiography is overutilized is underscored by 1) the high fraction of normal coronary arteriograms in many centers; 2) the overtraining of interventional cardiologists; 3) the enhanced likelihood of ordering arteriography if there is an on-site catheterization laboratory; 4) studies that question the appropriateness of either PTCA or CABG; 5) frequently the paucity of exercise testing to determine functional ischemia among patients with stable symptoms who are immediately subjected to catheterization and "same sitting" PTCA; and finally, 6) the profound economic incentives and high hospital reimbursements that are the life blood for many of our colleagues and institutions.

References

1. Data from the National Center for Health Statistics and the Commission of Professional Hospital Activities: Washington DC, 1992–1993.
2. American College of Cardiology—ACCEL Recording, October 1993.

3. CASS Principal Investigators and their Associates. Coronary artery surgery study (CASS): randomized trial of coronary bypass graft surgery: survival data. *Circulation.* 1983;68:939–950.
4. Bonow RO, Kent KM, Rossing DP, et al. Exercise-induced ischemia in mildly symptomatic patients with coronary artery disease and preserved left ventricular function: identification of subgroups at risk of death during medical therapy. *N Engl J Med.* 1984;311:1339–1345.
5. Mark DC, Hlatky MA, Harrell FE, et al. Exercise treadmill score for predicting prognosis in coronary artery disease. *Ann Intern Med.* 1987;106:793–800.
6. Reeves TJ, Oberman A, Jones WB, Sheffield LT. National history of angina pectoris. *Am J Cardiol.* 1974;33:423–430.
7. Chang J, Atwood JE, Froelicher V. Prognostic impact of myocardial ischemia. *J Am Coll Cardiol.* 1994;23:225–228.
8. Ambrose JA, Tanenbaum M, Alexopoulous D, et al. Angiographic progression of coronary artery disease and the development of myocardial infarction. *J Am Coll Cardiol.* 1988;12:56–62.
9. Little WC, Constantinescu M, Applegate RJ, et al. Can coronary angiography predict the site of a subsequent myocardial infarction in patients with mild to moderate coronary artery disease. *Circulation.* 1988;78:1157–1166.
10. Topol EJ, Ellis SG, Bates ER, et al. Analysis of coronary angioplasty practice in the United States using a private insurance data base. *J Am Coll Cardiol.* 1992;19:138.
11. Hilborne LH, Leape LL, Bernstein SJ, et al. The appropriateness of use of percutaneous transluminal coronary angioplasty in New York State. *JAMA.* 1993;269:761 765.
12. Leape LL, Hilborne LH, Park RE, et al. The appropriateness of use of coronary bypass graft surgery in New York State. *JAMA.* 1993;269:753–760.
13. Topol EJ, Califf RM. Scorecard cardiovascular medicine—its impact in future directions. *Ann Intern Med.* 1974;120:65–70.
14. ACC/AHA Task Force Report Guidelines for Percutaneous Transluminal Coronary Angioplasty. A report of the American College of Cardiology/American Heart Association Task Force on Assessment of Diagnostic and Therapeutic Cardiovascular Procedures. *J Am Coll Cardiol.* 1988;12:529–545.
15. Ryan TJ, Klocke FJ, Reynolds WA. Clinical competence in percutaneous transluminal coronary angioplasty. The statement for physicians from the ASCP/ACC/AHA Task Force on Clinical Privileges in Cardiology. *Circulation.* 1990;81:2041–2046.
16. Nicod PH, Gilpin E, Dittrich HC. Recent trends on the use of coronary angiography in the subacute phase of myocardial infarction. *Circulation.* 1989;80:410.
17. Every NR, Larson EB, Litwin PE, et al. The association between on-site cardiac catheterization facilities and the use of coronary angiography after acute myocardial infarction. Myocardial Infarction Triage and Intervention Project Investigators. *N Engl J Med.* 1993;329:546–551.
18. Gorlin R. Perspectives on invasive cardiology. The 24th Lewis F. Bishop Lecture. *J Am Coll Cardiol.* 1994;23:525–532.
19. Graboys TB, Headley A, Lown B, et al. Results of a second opinion program for coronary bypass graft surgery. *JAMA.* 1987;258:1611–1614.
20. Graboys TB, Biegelsen B, Lampert S, Blatt CM, Lown B. Results of a second opinion trial among patients recommended for coronary angiography. *JAMA.* 1992;268:2537–2540.

Editors' Comment

The preceding chapter by Dr. Graboys offers a sobering, staunchly conservative extremist rebuttal to the enthusiastic invasive approach to cardiovascular management presented throughout the remainder of this text. There is little doubt that if polled, the other authors would rebut or vigorously contest many of Dr. Graboys' contentions. However, Dr. Graboys' comments force us all to seriously reflect, even if we disagree, on the appropriate role for invasive diagnostic and treatment strategies.

With the current emphasis on cost containment, the requirement to justify invasive strategies will continue. One of our challenges in the future will be to delineate what procedures, devices, etc., are critical to improve outcome for patients with cardiovascular disease. The availability of technology is not an indication for its use unless the application leads to an improved outcome not achievable by other, presumably less complex means. Conversely, optimal patient cardiovascular disease outcomes should not only include relief of symptoms, but also a better quality of life in terms of safe optimum exercise performance for vocational and recreational activities. Lastly, morbidity and mortality should be maximally reduced, including therapy related complications. While these are important goals, the ability to document relative effectiveness remains a challenge.

We have advanced substantially in our technical abilities over a short period of time. Some advances have undoubtedly produced significant improvements in patient outcomes, but just as penicillin is not the cure for every infection, we need to continue to define the appropriate role for invasive diagnostic and therapeutic methods. The benefits of invasive strategies are real and significant, but Dr. Graboys reminds us that we must still define appropriateness of use.

Index